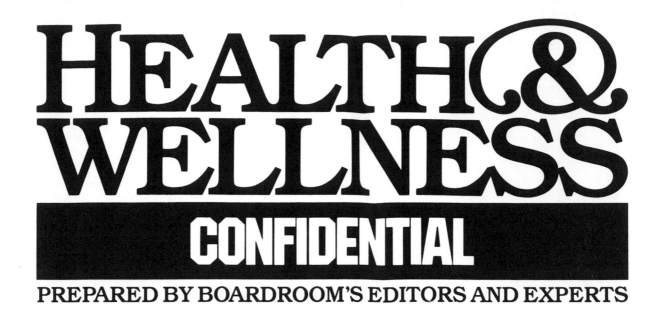

# HEALTH & WELLNESS

## CONFIDENTIAL

PREPARED BY BOARDROOM'S EDITORS AND EXPERTS

BOARDROOM CLASSICS

### Third Printing

Library of Congress Cataloging in Publication Data
Main entry under title

Health & Wellness : Confidential.

    Includes index.
    1. Health   I. Boardroom Reports, Inc.   II. Title:
Health and wellness.
RA776.H4355       1986      613      86-13678
ISBN 0-932648-71-1

Boardroom® Books, a division of Boardroom® Reports, Inc.
330 W. 42nd Street, New York, NY 10036

Printed in the United States of America

# HEALTH & WELLNESS CONFIDENTIAL
# Contents

**Your Child's Health and Safety**

**Parenting**

## 13   WHAT YOU SHOULD KNOW ABOUT TECHNOLOGY AND DRUGS . . . . . . . . 331

## 14 THE MIND: PROBLEMS AND SOLUTIONS

## 15 WHAT YOU SHOULD KNOW ABOUT DOCTORS AND HOSPITALS

# 1. Coping with Medical Emergencies

# Coping with Medical Emergencies

## DEALING WITH A MEDICAL EMERGENCY

In a medical emergency, emotions can run high. Knowing how to get someone to the hospital quickly and efficiently can not only calm the patient, it may even save his life.

### Whom to Call

It is best to call your local municipal emergency number for a public ambulance. The response time is usually quicker, because a central dispatcher sends an ambulance from the nearest hospital. A private ambulance must come from a single headquarters, which may be farther away.

### What to Say

When you call an emergency number, the dispatcher may ask you questions about the condition of the victim. The answers determine the priority of your call. A broken leg, for example, may not get assistance as quickly as a heart attack.

Tell the dispatcher exactly what condition the patient is in, as clearly and calmly as possible. Simply saying "I think he is having a heart attack" is not enough. Try to be specific about all the symptoms you have observed. Also helpful:

• Don't hang up until the dispatcher does. Let him decide when he has enough information.

• Give the dispatcher your phone number even if he doesn't ask for it. If something happens to delay the ambulance, he may need to reach you.

• Give careful directions that include your street address, prominent landmarks and any other information that will help the ambulance crew find your location quickly.

Very helpful: Tell the dispatcher that you will have someone wait outside, put the porch light on, or hang a bed sheet out the window so the driver can see where you are right away.

### While Waiting for the Ambulance

Stay with the victim (keep him in sight). Gather all relevant information, such as insurance numbers, medical history, medications currently being taken (the actual bottle of pills is even better) and anything else that concerns the patient's condition. Recommended: Keep all medical information about your family in a packet so you can grab it quickly in an emergency.

### The Ambulance Ride

You can usually ride with the patient. Exception: If the patient is in critical condition and needs emergency procedures in the ambulance. In that case, get the name and address of the hospital and the care unit where the patient will be admitted, and go there on your own. Don't speed after the ambulance or run lights in your anxiety to reach the hospital. Another accident won't help.

### At the Hospital

Find out who is caring for the patient, and let the floor nurse know that you are there. Offer to expedite the admitting-office paperwork.

**Source:** Interview with Brian Maguire, director of training, BRAVO (Bay Ridge Ambulance Volunteer Organization), Brooklyn, NY.

## IF YOU'RE ALL ALONE AND CHOKING

A choking person can save himself by falling so that a table or chair hits his diaphragm, thrusting it up against the lungs. It is the forced expulsion of air from the lungs that blows out the obstruction.

**Source:** Henry J. Heimlich, M.D., originator of the "Heimlich maneuver" (whereby a second person saves the choker).

## TIP FOR GAGGERS

If you gag when the doctor applies a tongue depressor, it helps to sing "Ah" in falsetto. You may feel silly, but you'll avoid the scary gagging reflex.

## BEST SKIN ANTISEPTICS

Isopropyl (rubbing) alcohol and ethyl alcohol are the skin antiseptics you should choose. None of the other commonly used antiseptics, including old standbys such as iodine and mercurochrome, were judged both safe and effective by the Food and Drug Administration.

## NEW ADHESIVE STRIPS

New bandages seal a wound, keep it moist and speed healing by 40%. And these super bandages won't stick to your cut as gauze bandages do. Brand names: Duo-DERM, Tegaderm, OpSite and Vigilon.

## BLISTER CARE

Clean the area of the blister with soap and water. Pierce the blister with a sterile needle (hold the needle over a flame for 60 seconds) and drain it. You may have to repeat this as many as three times in the next 24 hours. Keep the blister covered with a bandage until it heals.

## TO STOP HICCUPS

• To cure hiccups, swallow a teaspoonful of granulated sugar or eat crackers. The slight irritation in the back of the throat interrupts the hiccup cycle. Alternatives: Suck on a lemon wedge soaked in Angostura bitters. Or induce sneezing by sniffing pepper. Or

take a sniff of something with a strong aroma, such as vinegar.

**Source:** *Harvard Medical School Health Letter, Cambridge, MA.*

• Rub a cotton-tipped swab gently across the roof of your mouth at the middle of your soft palate (the part that vibrates with speech). A minute of light rubbing should squelch virtually all cases.

**Source:** Steven Goldsmith, M.D., Baystate Medical Center, Springfield, MA, quoted in *McCall's.*

## TREATMENT FOR A STIFF NECK

Stiff necks are usually caused by muscle strain. They generally go away when the strain is relieved. Heat packs are helpful. When to see a doctor: The stiffness is accompanied by other symptoms, such as pain in the arm...or the problem persists for more than a few days.

**Source:** Timothy Johnson, M.D., medical columnist, writing in *The Washington Post.*

## TWO THINGS THAT WON'T HELP A HURT ANKLE

Soaking a swollen ankle in hot water does it no good. Nor does wrapping a sprained ankle in an elastic bandage.

## BIG HELP IN LITTLE EMERGENCIES

• To remove a sticky bandage without pain, first soak a cotton ball in baby oil and douse the bandage with it. The oil significantly reduces the bandage's adhesion.

**Source:** *Parents,* New York.

• A quick, handy ice pack in an emergency is a bag of frozen vegetables (like peas or corn niblets). The bag is clean, water-tight and pliable enough to fit almost any part of the body. (It is, of course, only a stop-gap substitution.)

**Source:** *Harvard Medical School Health Letter,* Cambridge.

• To remove a ring from a swollen finger, use a few feet of string. Slip a few inches under and through the ring toward the wrist. Then wind the long end of the string tightly down the finger toward the tip, with the loops touching one another. (In most cases this will not be painful.) Finally, take the short end of the string and pull on it toward the fingertip. As the coil unwinds, the ring is pulled along until it falls off.

**Source:** *Emergency Medicine*, New York.

• Muscle trick to relieve cramps and spasms: Contract the muscles in the muscle group opposite the one that is cramped. This confuses the troubled muscle, making it relax. (Example: If your calf cramps, tighten the muscles in the front of your lower leg to relieve the discomfort.)

**Source:** *American Health.*

• Treating burns with butter or greasy ointments is dangerous. Neither is sterile and either can make subsequent treatment by a doctor more difficult. Better: Flush a burn with cold water or immerse it in cold water for up to 30 minutes. Alternative: Apply cold compresses. Cover with clean bandages. Never puncture a blister. For serious burns, seek a doctor at once.

**Source:** Gustavo Colon, M.D., associate professor of plastic surgery, Tulane University Medical School, quoted in *Vogue*, New York.

## ABOUT HIVES

The cause of hives—those red, itchy, raised skin blotches—is unknown for nine out of ten patients. Best treatment in such cases: Reassurance that the condition is not serious. . .and antihistamines. The side effects of stronger drugs such as cortico-steroids may prove to be more harmful than the hives.

**Source:** Barton Inkeles, M.D., New York Hospital—Cornell Medical Center, writing in *Drug Therapy.*

## LEG-CRAMP RELIEF

Leg cramps can usually be alleviated by firmly pinching your upper lip for 20–30 seconds.

**Source:** Donald Cooper, M.D., former US Olympics team doctor, in *Sportswise.*

## FIRST AID FOR CHEMICAL BURNS

Chemical burns to the eye usually don't cause permanent damage if rinsing starts within 15 seconds. After that, chances of recovery decline rapidly. Any innocuous watery fluid can be used. Continue flushing for at least 20 minutes.

**Source:** John Paul Wohlen, Bradley Corp., Menomonee Falls, WI, writing in *Plant Engineering.*

## WHAT TO DO IF SOMEONE FAINTS

Old-time fainting remedies are dangerous. Placing a fainter's head between his legs could cause brain damage. Most smelling salts contain ammonium hydroxide, which can cause chemical burns of the nose and lungs. Better: Lay the fainter on his back. Then raise his legs. Gently massage the calves to return blood to central circulation. Wait about 20 minutes and then raise the person in stages.

**Source:** *RN.*

## TAKING A SPILL

Relax and give in to your fall. Try to slide as you touch the ground. Drop any packages right away. If you tumble forward, put open hands out to break the impact and protect your face. When falling backward, try to sit as you go down, to protect your spine. If you catch a foot in a hole, drop to the side that's caught.

After the fall: Breathe deeply and get up very slowly—so you won't get dizzy and fall again.

**Source:** *Woman's Day,* New York.

## PERSONAL MEDICAL INFORMATION AT A GLANCE

There is a wallet-sized card that records all your vital medical information on a microfilm strip. On an opposite corner there's a tiny magnifying glass. In an emergency, a doctor can bend the card until the lens is over the microfilm. Details covered: Major ailments, allergies, blood type, names of physician and others to contact, insurance numbers, baseline electrocardiogram reading. Cost: $11.20.

**For an application:** Send a self-addressed, stamped envelope to National Health and Safety Awareness Center, 333 N. Michigan Ave., Chicago 60601.

## TOLL-FREE HELP LINES

Cocaine abuse: (800) COCAINE. Drug abuse: (800) 241-9746. Incest/child abuse: (800) 421-0353. Runaways: (800) 231-6946. Venereal Disease: (800) 227-8922.

• National referral hotline directs callers to help in fighting addictions, sexual dysfunctions and compulsive behavior (from gambling to overeating). Policy: Callers are never asked to identify themselves. The Dulcinea Foundation's data bank lists more than 7,000 self-help groups, treatment centers and other referrals. Phone: (800) 622-8466.

## FREE MEDICAL AID

National Health Information Clearinghouse will answer your questions on general health and medical topics. They'll also tell you whom to call for additional information on specific medical problems. Phone: (800) 336-4797

## EMERGENCY SERVICE FOR LIVE-ALONES

Help for the sick or elderly who live alone can be provided by an electronic panic-button service that brings assistance within minutes. Called Lifeline, the system connects to each household through the telephone, but the actual alarm button can be clipped to a belt or kept in a pocket.

How it works: The subscriber falls, for example, and can't reach the telephone. He pushes the alarm button, which activates a call light at the local response center. A trained coordinator phones to ask what's wrong. If there is no answer, the coordinator alerts a nearby responder who is on call. The responder rushes to the home to check out the situation and phones the coordinator to arrange appropriate medical help.

Backup: A phone timer can be set to trigger the call light every 12 or 24 hours. If the subscriber is unconscious, help is summoned automatically. Endorsed by the US Department of Health and Human Services, the service allows single people to be discharged from hospitals sooner and to stay out of nursing homes. There are currently 700 such systems in 47 states. A bill is pending in Congress to fund their use through Medicaid.

**More information:** Lifeline Systems, Inc., 400 Main St., Waltham, MA 02254.

# 2. Traveling Healthy

# Traveling Healthy

## SPEED KILLS

Although France installed a mandatory seat-belt law in 1973, the auto death rate continued to rise until the speed limit was slowed from no limit to 70 MPH. A year later, the death rate had dropped 57%.

**Source:** *Forbes* magazine, New York.

## 55 MPH UPDATE

The 55 MPH speed limit has saved close to 4,000 lives a year, prevented a slightly greater number of severe injuries, and staved off as many as 62,000 lesser injuries. About half of the highway safety improvement in the US since 1974 can be attributed to this nationwide speed limitation.

**Source:** National Research Council, Washington, DC.

## SEAT-BELT TRUTHS

Seat-belt myth: Passengers are better off being thrown clear of their car in a serious accident. Reality: You are 25 times more likely to be killed if thrown from the car.

**Source:** National Traffic Safety Institute, Alexandria, VA.

• Seat belts are vital to auto safety even when you're traveling slowly. Four out of five fatal serious car accidents involve cars going less than 40 miles per hour.

**Source:** Jane Brody in *The New York Times.*

## CAR SAFETY

The safest car travel: In a heavy car whose occupants are wearing seat belts. A new study found that belts reduce the risk of injury by two thirds. Also: The injury risk drops another 25% with every additional thousand pounds of car weight.

**Source:** Insurance Institute for Highway Safety, Washington, DC.

## WHY SMALLER MAY BE BETTER

Smaller cars have fewer crashes than larger ones. A study conducted by the General Motors Transportation Research Labs verifies this. Other findings: Drivers tend to be more cautious in smaller autos because they perceive they're at greater risk. They take fewer risks, drive more slowly and use their seat belts more.

**Source:** *NAFA Bulletin,* New York.

## NEW LOOK AT DEFENSIVE DRIVING COURSES

Defensive driving courses designed to reduce the likelihood of being in a crash don't seem to do much good. Finding: Five scientifically rigorous tests have shown that taking such courses does not make drivers less prone to involvement in auto crashes. Course graduates do have slightly fewer moving violations, though. And the courses can still pay off in some states, where graduates are eligible for lower insurance rates.

**Source:** Study by the Institute for Highway Safety, reported in *Journal of American Insurance,* Schaumberg, Il.

## WORST NIGHT TO BE ON THE ROAD

Saturday night is a bad time to be on the road. One out of every 10 drivers that night is likely to be drunk. Drunk drivers kill more than 25,000 people a year now. . .and injure one-half million.

**Source:** Runzheimer and Co., consultants on travel and living expenses, Rochester, WI.

## TRAVELING MEDICINE CHEST MUSTS

Travel health kits should include several prescription drugs purchased *before* the trip abroad. Reason: The foreign equivalents of these drugs may contain impure or toxic ingredients. For constipation: Alophen. Diarhea: Lomotil. Motion sickness: Antivert. Heartburn and indigestion: Glycical. Also useful: Aspirin, a sore throat remedy, a sunscreen and an insect repellent.

**Source:** International Health Care Service, New York Hospital–Cornell Medical Center, New York City.

## LEGAL WAY TO TRAVEL WITH NARCOTICS

To avoid severe penalities from US Customs on medication containing narcotics, get a written statement from your doctor that the medicine is essential for your health. Good practice: When traveling, carry the drugs in their original containers, and don't arouse suspicion by bringing more than necessary.

**Source:** US Customs brochure *Know Before You Go,* Washington, D.C.

## QUICKEST WAY TO FIND AN ALL-NIGHT DRUGSTORE

Call the police. They know which pharmacies are open late. Many people waste precious time calling every drugstore in the *Yellow Pages* or running all over town in a frantic search.

## HOW TO FIND AN ENGLISH-SPEAKING MD

Before going overseas, write to the International Association for Medical Assistance to Travelers and ask for its free directory listing well-trained, English-speaking doctors

around the world. Important: Write six to eight weeks before your trip.

IAMAT, 736 Center Street, Lewiston, NY 14092.

## IF YOU GET SICK IN GREAT BRITAIN

US travelers to the British Isles should be aware that Americans who need medical attention in the United Kingdom must pay to use the National Health Service. The British public health facilities offer free care only to citizens of countries that offer reciprocal privileges to the British. Americans, of course, still have the option to use (and pay for) private doctors and hospitals when in Great Britain.

## AFRAID OF TROPICAL DISEASES?

Have your physician call the International Travel Clinic at Yale–New Haven Hospital (203–785–4179) for up-to-date information on vaccinations appropriate to specific countries and regions within countries.

## ONE VACCINATION YOU MAY WANT TO AVOID

Avoid a cholera vaccination unless the country you're going to requires it. Reasons: The chance of contracting cholera is low if you avoid risky food and water. More to the point, the vaccines don't prevent the infection—and are only about 50% effective in reducing symptoms.

**Source:** *Travel & Leisure*, N.Y.

## PREVENTING MONTEZUMA'S REVENGE

University of Texas Medical School researchers have discovered that the primary ingredient in Pepto-Bismol (bismuth subsalicylate) can help to prevent the most common traveler's ailment. A group of new students in Mexico received four tablespoons of the medication four times a day (for 21 days). Others were given a placebo. Diarrhea developed in 14 of 62 students on medication versus 40 of 66 students on the placebo.

## FOREIGN PHRASES FOR THE DIETING TRAVELER

*The Special Diet Foreign Phrase Book* by Helen Jacobson assists dieters with the language and gives other information for Mexico, Spain, Germany, France and Italy. Includes guidelines for low-salt, diabetic, low-fat, low-cholesterol and custom diets, as well as sources of medical aid.

**Source:** Rodale Press, Emmaus, PA.

## SPECIAL LOW-CALORIE HOTEL MENUS

Weight-conscious travelers can try special menus now being offered by major hotel-chains. Although the names differ (Hilton's *Fitness-First Fiesta*, Hyatt's *Perfect Balance*, and Sheraton's *Eat, Drink and Be Healthy*), the goal is the same: To make low-calorie meals both interesting and tasty.

**Source:** *Nation's Restaurant News,* New York.

## SPECIAL AIRLINE MENUS

Airline meal options now range from the diet-oriented (low-calorie, low-cholesterol, diabetic, salt-free) to the ethnic (kosher, Mormon, Hindu, Moslem) to vegetarian and seafood choices. To get what you want, call the airline at least 48 hours before take-off time.

**Source:** *U.S. News & World Report,* New York.

## WHO SHOULDN'T FLY

Don't-fly basics: Those who have had a heart attack within four weeks of takeoff...a stroke within two weeks...surgery within two weeks...or a deep-diving session within 24 hours should wait to fly. Don't fly at all if you have severe lung problems...un-controlled hypertension...epilepsy not well controlled...severe anemia...a pregnancy beyond 240 days or threatened by miscarriage.

**Source:** *Pocket Flight Guide/Frequent Flyer Package,* Oak Brook, Il.

• Flying can be hazardous for victims of chronic obstructive pulmonary disease, Reason: Sudden changes in atmospheric pressure can deplete oxygen levels in the bloodstream. Possible consequences: Shortness of breath, dizziness, collapse and even heart arrhythmias. Pulmonary disease sufferers should have blood oxygen levels checked several days before a scheduled flight.

**Source:** *Medical World News,* New York.

## IF YOU HAVE A HEART OR LUNG PROBLEM

Air travel is much safer than once believed for those with heart and lung problems. Reason: Even though you get 80% as much oxygen in a cabin at 35,000 feet as at sea level, your body stays at rest, thereby cutting its workload. There remain, however, several wise precautions: Don't exhaust yourself before the trip with last-minute activities or packing. Arrive at the airport early, and don't carry your own luggage. Get a seat as far away from the smoking section as possible. Drink plenty of fluids while in the air. Minimize the use of antihistamines, tranquilizers and other medications. Walk up and down the aisle once an hour, or do exercises in your seat. Fly the Concorde when possible—you'll suffer less jet lag and fewer problems from ozone.

**Source:** *Travel & Leisure,* New York.

## EASY WAY TO UNBLOCK YOUR EARS

Swallowing and yawning are the easiest ways to unblock your ears during descent in an airplane. Both serve to open your Eustachian tubes, which, in turn, equalizes pressure on both sides of your eardrums.

Last resort: Pinch your nostrils shut and take a mouthful of air. Then use cheek and throat muscles (*not* the chest or abdomen) to force air into the back of your nose. When you hear a loud pop, you've succeeded. Also effective: A decongestant pill or nasal spray taken an hour before descent. This shrinks the membranes and makes the ears pop more easily. Recommended: Allergy sufferers should use the same treatment before takeoff, as well as before descent.

**Source:** American Academy of Otolaryngology, Washington, DC.

# HOW TO AVOID JET LAG

• Don't change your watch or habits for brief stops.

• Stay at an airport hotel with 24-hour food service and a quiet room.

• Schedule meetings soon after you arrive if you get there before the end of your normal working day. Example: An executive regularly flew from California at 8 A.M. to the East Coast, arriving at 5 P.M. New York time. He knew from experience that he'd have problems "getting started" the next morning, so he scheduled his meeting at 6 P.M. just after he arrived, since it was only 3 o'clock for him.

• For longer stays, be fully rested before departure. Don't rush to the airport. Plan arrivals as close as possible to your normal time for going to sleep. Don't take pills or alcoholic beverages. They hinder the deep sleep vital to recharging mentally.

• Don't plan important hard work for the first or second day of a long trip.

• When traveling, wear comfortable, loose clothing and shoes. Exercise during the flight, isometrics, etc. Don't overeat or drink heavily.

• Important tip: If crucial work must be done immediately after arrival, precondition your mind and body to the destination's time zone for several days before the trip.

# WORST TIMES OF THE YEAR FOR MOTION SICKNESS SUFFERERS

Motion sickness affects people most severely during the spring and fall—the same seasons when people tend to have the greatest mood swings. Theory: We may be more dependent than we realize on changes in the sunlight cycle.

**Source:** *Brain/Mind Bulletin*, Los Angeles, CA.

# MOTION SICKNESS UPDATE

A tiny adhesive patch is being used to combat motion sickness. Available by prescription only, *Transderm Scop* is placed on the skin behind the ear—much like an ordinary adhesive bandage. The patch contains an effective anti-motion-sickness drug (scopolamine), which is absorbed through the skin and passes into the blood system over a 72-hour period. Warning: Not for the elderly or children

# MOTION SICKNESS REMEDY

Ginger, available in health food stores. It has proven more effective than Dramamine and other anti–motion drugs and does not induce drowsiness. Recommended: Two or three gelatin capsules, each containing 500 milligrams of powdered ginger root, half an hour before the expected motion.

**Source:** Daniel B. Mowrey, M.D., Brigham Young University, Provo, UT.

# TRAVELING WITH TODDLERS

Sitting in the front seat helps children avoid car sickness. Reason: Motion sickness can be avoided by keeping your view about 45 degrees above the bouncing horizon. That's practically impossible for small children in a car unless they sit in a safety seat high enough to let them see out a window, which seldom works out in the back seat.

## HEALTH HINTS FOR HIGH PLACES

One out of three travelers to altitudes of 7,000 feet above sea level (Vail, CO, for example) experiences some symptoms of altitude sickness. By 10,000 feet (Breckenridge, CO), everyone is affected. Common complaints: Headaches, nausea, weakness, lack of coordination and insomnia.

Cause: Barometric pressure lessens as you climb higher, making the percentage of oxygen in the air lower. You must take in more air to get the same amount of oxygen that you are accustomed to. Your system will adjust itself within a few days if you give it a chance. (Full acclimatization takes three weeks.

To minimize the effects:

• Take it easy the first two or three days. Get plenty of rest and don't schedule vigorous activities.

• Eat a little less than usual. Avoid hard-to-digest foods such as red meat and fats. Carbohydrates are good.

• Drink more liquids than usual. (Breathing harder in dry air drains your system.)

• Avoid alcohol, smoking and tranquilizers. Their effects are compounded at high altitudes.

## MOUNTAIN-SICKNESS Rx

Many people traveling to high altitudes for vacations experience acute mountain sickness. Symptoms: Severe headaches, sometimes accompanied by nausea and vomiting. Four milligrams of dexamethasone, a prescription drug, taken four times a day for several days is effective in preventing the symptoms of acute mountain sick-

ness and in reducing the swelling of the brain thought to be responsible. Side effects are minimal.

**Source:** *The New England Journal of Medicine*, Boston, MA.

## FOR NON-SMOKERS ONLY

Smoke-free travel is almost possible. More public facilities are catering to the non-smoker. Some 20% of US restaurants offer non-smoking sections. Hotels offer rooms that have "never been smoked in," and travel agencies are offering nonsmoking vacations.

More information: Action on Smoking and Health, 2013 H St. NW, Washington, DC 20006.

• Rented cars now offer a no-smoking option. *Thrifty Rent-A-Car* is now allocating part of its fleet (at selected locations) for the non-smoker who wants to avoid smelling leftover cigarette or cigar odors.

• Hotels for non-smokers offer no-smoking rooms. Drapes, bed-spreads, carpets and walls have been thoroughly cleaned, and no ashtrays are provided. Among such hotels are Best Western, Four Seasons, Hilton, Hyatt, and Westin.

**Source:** *Airfare Discount Bulletin*, Riverside, CT.

## BATHROOM DANGER

Dirty hotel bathtubs can transmit athlete's foot, skin rashes and other infections. Make sure your tub is dry, smooth and free of cracks. When in doubt, clean it with Comet or a similar product.

**Source:** Yehudi M. Felman, M.D., clinical professor of dermatology, Downstate Medical School, Brooklyn, NY.

# 3. Deducting Medical Expenses

# Deducting Medical Expenses

## HOW TO BEAT THE DEDUCTION LIMIT

Everyone has medical expenses and everyone faces a limit on deducting them—you can only deduct those expenses in excess of the percent of your adjusted gross income allowed by law. But there are ways to beat the limit. . .

• Double up. Maximize your medical deductions by bunching payments in alternate years. If you're not going to meet the threshold percent this year, defer paying medical bills until next year, when your combined expenses may put you over the limit.

On the other hand, if you're clearly going to meet the limit this year, stock up on medicine and drugs, pay outstanding medical and dental bills before year-end, and consider having planned dental work and voluntary surgery done (and paid for) this year, rather than next.

• Hold off. If you plan not to itemize your deductions this year, but know that you're going to itemize next year, hold off paying medical bills until January. You'll get no deduction for them this year, while next year you might.

• Charge it. Medical and dental expenses paid by credit card are deductible in the year you sign for the charge, rather than in the year you pay the credit card company. You can boost your deductions this year by putting year-end medical expenses on your credit card.

• Drugs. Only prescription drugs and insulin can be deducted as medical expenses. Tip: Many over-the-counter drugs can also be bought on prescription. Ask your doctor for prescriptions for patent drugs you use. Trap: The price, as a prescription, may be higher.

• Dependents. You are entitled to include in your deductions medical expenses you pay on behalf of a dependent. Bonus: You can deduct medical expenses for a family member who meets all the requirements for being claimed as your dependent except that he or she has too much income (over $1,000). Suggestion: Make your support dollars do double duty by paying the medical bills of a person you're helping support. Those payments could get you both a dependency deduction and a medical expense deduction.

• Life care. The medical expense portion of a lump-sum life care fee paid to a retirement home for a parent is fully deductible as a medical expense in the year the fee is paid. You may be better off taking a deduction now for future medical care rather than making annual payments.

• Separate returns. It is sometimes advantageous for a married couple to file separate returns when one spouse, but not the other, has heavy medical expenses. On a joint return, medical expenses must exceed the legal percent limit of a couple's combined adjusted gross income. But if separate returns are filed, only the income of the spouse with the big medical bills is considered for the deduction limit. (The only way to tell for sure whether it's better to file jointly or separately is to work out the figures both ways).

### Doctor's Orders

Obvious medical expenses include prescription drugs, doctor, dentist and psychiatrist bills, hospital costs and laboratory fees. Less obvious expenses include:

• Transportation costs back and forth to the doctor's office or the dentist's, by cab, train or bus. If you drive, you can deduct as a medical expense either your actual car expenses or the IRS mileage allowance (plus tolls and parking, whichever method you use.)

• Lodging. Thanks to the new tax law, a patient and an individual accompanying him can each deduct up to $50 per night of lodging expenses—but not meals—on a trip to an out-of-town hospital facility to get necessary medical care.

• Marriage counseling is deductible if performed by a licensed psychologist or psychiatrist. So is sex therapy.

• Home improvements that are medically required are deductible to the extent they do not increase the value of your property. (If a pool for an arthritis sufferer costs $10,000 to install, and increases the value of the house by $6,000, the deduction is limited to $4,000.)

• Travel simply for a change of scenery is not deductible. But trips recommended by a doctor to treat a specific ailment are deductible. Example: A trip to Arizona by an asthma victim or by a person whose postoperative throat condition is aggravated by cold weather.

• Weight-loss programs prescribed by a doctor as treatment for a specific medical condition such as hypertension are deductible. Not deductible: Weight loss to improve general health and well-being. Get a letter from your doctor recommending a specific program as treatment for a specific disorder.

Also deductible if prescribed by a doctor as treatment for a specific medical condition are:

• Stop-smoking programs.
• Speech therapy.
• Health-club visits.
• Special filters for air conditioners. Ionizers to purify the air. Filters to purify drinking water.

Other deductible medical expenses include:

• Hair transplants, nose jobs, face lifts and other cosmetic surgery.
• Birth-control pills, abortions that are legal under local laws, vasectomies.

• Acupuncture, hearing aids, eyeglasses, contact lenses, dentures and braces.
• Orthopedic shoes, medically required shoe lifts, support hose and surgical belts.

**Source:** *Tax Hotline* interview with Edward Mendlowitz, partner, Siegel, Mendlowitz & Rich, CPAs, New York.

# TAX DEDUCTIONS CONFIDENTIAL

Keep a diary of your medical expenses. Include doctor and dentist bills and prescription drugs. The diary can be used both as proof for the IRS in case you are audited and as a reminder to yourself when filing your return.

Some not-so-obvious medical expenses that have been allowed by the courts and the IRS:

• A health club membership when prescribed as treatment for a specific medical condition. Strategy: Ask your doctor to put this in writing as he would any other prescription. This way, if you are audited a few years later, you'll have the prescription and be safe from the risk that you or your doctor may not remember the exact circumstances of the health club membership.

• A trip taken for the relief of a specific medical condition.

• Transportation to and from your doctor's office.

• Clarinet lessons taken on a doctor's advice to correct a dental defect.

• A dust-free room for an allergy sufferer.

• Legal fees for committing a mentally ill spouse.

• A wig bought to alleviate stress caused by hair loss—when prescribed by a doctor.

• Maintenance costs of a home swimming pool. (Has been approved when recommended by a doctor for people suffering from medical problems such as emphysema, heart problems, back problems. . .)

• Trained cat to alert its hearing-impaired owner to unusual sounds.

• New house siding for a person allergic to mold.

• Reclining chair bought on a doctor's orders to alleviate a heart condition.

## FOR CORPORATIONS ONLY

One of the healthiest tax benefits you can provide for yourself or your key employees is a corporate medical reimbursement plan under Section 105 (b).

You get full reimbursement of medical expenses without reduction for the percent of adjusted gross income limitation on medical expenses.

Medical expenses that are reimbursed to you or are paid directly for your benefit are fully deductible by the corporation as compensation.

The amounts reimbursed to you or paid for your benefit are not included in your gross income.

Simply put, all medical expenses for you and all your dependents can be paid by your corporation without your having to pay one penny of income tax on the benefits.

Uninsured (self-insured) medical expense reimbursement (pay) plans have to meet the breadth-of-coverage requirements applicable to qualified pension plans. In order for medical expense reimbursements to be excluded from the employee's income, the plan must not discriminate in favor of key employees (highly compensated individuals and certain stockholders).

**Source:** *The Book of Tax Knowledge,* by Irving L. Blackman, Boardroom Books, New York.

## MEDICAL INSURANCE TIP

Medical expenses are deductible to the extent they exceed the current allowed percent of your income... and weren't reimbursed by insurance. Included: The cost of medical insurance.

## INSURANCE TRAP

Insured medical expenses are not deductible, whether or not a claim is filed with your insurance company. In one case, a person didn't file a claim because of the paperwork involved. IRS ruling: The taxpayer could have recovered his costs through insurance, so he was entitled to no deduction.

**Source:** *Letter Ruling* 8102010.

## DOUBLE TAX BENEFIT

The IRS denied medical-expense deductions taken by a quadriplegic taxpayer who won a $4 million lump-sum damage award in a malpractice suit. IRS: The tax-free award covered future medical expenses. If he also deducted his medical expenses, he would get a double tax benefit—the right to exclude the award from income and tax deductions. Court of Appeals: For the taxpayer. Tax law permits the double tax benefit.

**Source:** *Kelly B. Niles,* CA-9, No. 82-4278.

## ABOUT DEPENDENTS

You can deduct medical bills paid for a dependent, even if you can't take a dependency exemption for that person, as long as you paid more than half that person's support in either the year the bills were run up or the year they were paid. Similarly, you can deduct bills paid now for a former spouse, as long as you were married when the bills were incurred.

## NURSING HOME DEDUCTIBLES

Nursing home residents pay a "resident fee" and a "monthly service fee." A portion of both fees is used for medical care. IRS ruling: The part that is used for medical care is deductible as a medical expense.

**Source:** *Letter Ruling* 8502009.

## MOTHERAID

A son paid his mother's medical expenses with money he withdrew from her bank account under a power of attorney. The IRS disallowed the son's deduction for these expenses, saying the money was really the mother's. But the Court of Appeals allowed the deduction. The money was legally his—a gift from his mother to him.

**Source:** *John M. Ruch, CA-5, 82-4463.*

## LIFETIME CARE

A one-time medical payment for a lifetime of medical care was fully deductible in the year paid. It didn't matter that treatment might take place in later years.

**Source:** *Acquiescence in Estate of Smith, 79 TC 313.*

## PREPAID INSTITUTION FEES

• A taxpayer prepaid a fee for the lifetime institutional care of his mentally retarded dependent son. The IRS ruled that the entire fee was deductible in the year it was paid, even though the taxpayer will receive a refund if his son dies within five years. The refund, of course, will have to be declared as income.

**Source:** *Letter Ruling 8310057.*

• The parents of an autistic child planned to make a lump-sum payment to an institution for lifetime care of the child. The payment would be partially refunded if the child died within 10 years. IRS ruling: The full prepayment is deductible as a medical expense despite a possible refund.
**Source:** *Letter Ruling 8309011.*

## A CHANGE OF SCENE FOR A DEPRESSED CHILD

A teenage girl suffered from depression. After conventional therapy failed, her parents decided to take her on trips that would provide her with new experiences. The girl's condition improved, but the Tax Court said that the travel costs were not a deductible medical expense. Reason: The trips were not prescribed by a doctor and did not amount to standard medical care.

**Source:** *Joseph R. Levene, TC Memo 1982-5.*

## WHEN A TRIP IS DEDUCTIBLE AND WHEN IT'S NOT

A doctor suggested that a change in environment could improve a taxpayer's parents' condition. So, the taxpayer sent them on an all-expenses-paid trip to Houston, Texas. Can he deduct the cost?

The IRS will usually allow a medical trip to be deducted if it is made on the advice of a doctor to treat a specific condition, when a change in locale is medically recognized as treatment for that condition. Example: A trip to Florida by a person recovering from throat surgery in a northern city, when cold air could aggravate his condition. Limit: Only travel costs (including meals and lodging en route) are deductible. Living costs at the destination are not.

Trips to promote general health are not deductible. So a doctor's recommendation that a "change of scenery" might help one's general condition won't get a deduction.

Finally, to get a medical deduction for your parents' expenses, you must have provided more than half of their financial support for the entire year.

## MEDICAL TRIPS

Parents who drove their disabled son to an out-of-state clinic for treatment could deduct travel costs plus expenses for lodging on the trip.
**Source:** *William L. Pfersching, TC Memo 1983-341.*

• A taxpayer's dependent adult son had an operation in an out-of-state clinic. The parent flew to the clinic each day during the post-operative period. IRS ruling: The parent's airplane fare was a deductible medical expense. So was the cost of renting a car to drive to the clinic and hospital. Key: The clinic required someone to attend patients during their post-operative period.
**Source:** *Letter Ruling 8321042.*

## LONG-DISTANCE TELEPHONING

Telephone counseling was deductible as a medical expense when a person's psychologist was located 350 miles away. The long-distance telephone bills were a necessary part of a post-drug addiction recovery program.

**Source:** *Letter Ruling 8034087.*

## THREE SPECIAL SCHOOLS THAT WERE DEDUCTIBLE AND ONE THAT WASN'T

• Taxpayers were advised by psychiatrists to put their emotionally disturbed child in a psychiatrically oriented boarding school with a strong guidance program. IRS ruling: Since the school fit the tax law's definition of a "special school," the tuition was deductible as a medical expense.
**Source:** *Letter Ruling 8447014.*

• The cost of a special school for a child with a specific learning disability was deductible. Key: The school has a specialized curriculum, and it required neurological and psychological testing before admission.
**Source:** *Letter Ruling 8445032.*

• The IRS ruled that parents could deduct the cost of sending their child, who suffered from dyslexia, to a special school for children with learning disabilities. Key: The school had a specialized professional staff providing services that weren't available in regular schools. Also deductible: The cost of transporting the child to and from school.
**Source:** *Letter Ruling 8401024.*

• Two children suffering from language learning disabilities were sent to a special school. Costs were $1,800 above regular tuition. The parents deducted that amount as a medical expense. But the IRS disallowed the deduction because the school had no trained psychiatrists or psychologists on staff and because the special schooling had not been recommended by a doctor. Tax Court: For the parents. The childrens' disorders were severe enough to make normal education impossible. And, while the school's staff members did not qualify as medical personnel, they had been

trained in special-education techniques.
**Source:** *Lawrence F. Fay,* 76 TC 408.

## HOME IMPROVEMENTS ARE DEDUCTIBLE...BUT

Medically required home improvements, such as elevators, air conditioners and swimming pools, qualify in part as deductible medical expenses. But, in order to get the deduction, the taxpayer making the improvements must have a property interest in the home. Recent ruling: A polio victim who had a specially designed swimming pool installed at his parents' home could not deduct part of the cost. Although he lived in the house, he had no ownership interest in it.

**Source:** *Letter Ruling 8249025.*

## CHILD SAFETY

The cost of removing lead-based paint from areas within a child's reach was ruled to be deductible as a medical expense when the purpose was to prevent the lead poisoning of a child who had been exposed to the paint. Not deductible: The cost of removing the paint from areas not within the child's reach, and the cost of repainting.

**Source:** *Revenue Ruling 79-66.*

## WHEN SWIMMING IS ALLOWED

• A patient with emphysema and bronchitis was advised by his doctor to exercise by swimming. Because local pool hours didn't coincide with his work schedule, he built his own indoor pool. He deducted the cost of fuel, electricity, insurance and other maintenance expenses. IRS position: The existence of a diving board and the lack of medical equipment showed that the pool was for nondeductible personal use. Tax Court: Expenses were deductible. The patient's need to exercise his lungs didn't require any medical equipment except the pool. Recreational use by his family was incidental.
**Source:** *Herbert Cherry,* TC Memo 1983-470.

• A special "lap" swimming pool for a sufferer of osteoarthritis was a deductible medical expense to the extent that the cost of the pool exceeded the resulting increase in the value of the property.

**Source:** *Revenue Ruling 83-33.*

• Swimming pool fees are a deductible medical expense when the pool is used following a doctor's recommendation. A couple could deduct the $100 a year they paid for their son to have access to a local pool, when a doctor had prescribed swimming as therapy for the son's arthritis.

**Source:** *Letter Ruling 8326095.*

## WHEN YOUR DOCTOR PUTS IT IN WRITING AND WHEN HE DOESN'T

• A taxpayer with high blood pressure was urged by his doctor to take a 13-day diet and exercise program at a health institute. IRS ruling: The cost of the program was a deductible medical expense. Key: The course was prescribed as treatment for a specific physical illness. The doctor put his recommendation in writing.

**Source:** *Letter Ruling 8251045.*

• Spa fees didn't reduce taxes. A woman claimed she was told by her doctor to join a health club. But she couldn't prove it because he died. Tax Court: Disallowed a medical deduction. Reason: Lack of doctor's proof that the payments were directly related to her medical care. Expenditures made for general health benefits aren't deductible.

**Source:** *May Gayle Strickland,* TC Memo 1984-301.

• Roy Disney, Walt's brother, claimed a medical expense deduction for a mechanical exercise horse. Disney's doctor had suggested more exercise and had recommended various kinds of gym equipment. But the doctor had not specifically prescribed use of a mechanical horse. Result: Deduction denied. Lesson: Have your doctor put his recommendations in writing and make sure they are specific.

**Source:** *Roy O. Disney,* DC-Calif., 413 F. 2d 783.

## HOW TO STOP SMOKING, LOSE WEIGHT AND GET A DEDUCTION

No-smoking and weight-reduction programs to improve your general health are not deductible, even when recommended by a doctor. But a weight-reduction program prescribed as treatment of hypertension, obesity, and hearing loss was ruled deductible. Key: The program was prescribed to treat specific ailments. The IRS would probably rule the same way on a no-smoking program prescribed by a doctor for a specific ailment, such as emphysema.

**Source:** *IRS Revenue Ruling 79-162; IRS Letter Ruling 8004111.*

## WHEN A SPECIAL CAR ISN'T DEDUCTIBLE

A back injury made it difficult for Donald Robb to drive a normal car, so a doctor recommended the purchase of a specially equipped van which made driving easier. Tax Court: The cost was not a deductible medical expense because the van had no therapeutic value.

**Source:** *Donald G. Robb,* TC Memo 1982-687.

## IF VITAMINS ARE PRESCRIBED

The cost of vitamins was deductible when they were prescribed as treatment for a specific medical condition . . . in this case, arteriosclerosis and related heart ailments.

**Source:** *Garnett Neil,* TC Memo 1982-562.

## UNUSUAL MEDICAL DEDUCTIONS

• Whiskey prescribed for heart disease.
• The cost of electrolysis qualifies as a deductible medical expense.
**Source:** *Letter Ruling 8442018.*

• A clarinet and clarinet lessons were deductible medical expenses when prescribed as treatment for a child's dental defects.

**Source:** *Revenue Ruling 62-210.*

• A doctor prescribed a wig to relieve the mental distress of a person whose hair fell out. The cost of the wig was a deductible medical expense.

**Source:** *Revenue Ruling 62-189.*

• Sex therapy treatments are deductible as a medical expense.

**Source:** *Revenue Ruling 75-187.*

• Legal costs related to the commitment of a taxpayer's mentally ill spouse to a hospital were held to be deductible as a medical expense.

**Source:** *Carl A. Gestacker,* 414 F2d 448.

# 4. Medical Insurance

# Medical Insurance

## GOOD NEWS ABOUT LONG-TERM HEALTH COSTS

Individual hospital and doctor bills will rise at only the general inflation rate over the next 25 years. Contrast: In the 1970s, they sometimes outpaced inflation by a two to one margin.

**Source:** US Dept. of Health and Human Services, National Center for Health Statistics, Washington.

## CREDIT CARD UPDATE

A medical charge card will soon enable you to pay immediately for dental work, vision care and other items not covered by your insurance package. Marketed by the Medical Bankcard Corp., it will be available in more than a dozen eastern states. The annual fee: $18. Average credit line: $1,000–$2,500.

**Source:** *Sylvia Porter's Personal Finance*, New York.

## ABOUT HMOs

By 1990, 15% of all individuals with health coverage will belong to health maintenance organizations. National firms, including Blue Cross/Blue Shield, are joining the trend and have set up HMOs in different areas that are under a single national management umbrella.

**Source:** *Innovation & Performance Report*, New York.

• Health maintenance organizations actually reduce the cost of medical care. Prepaid group practice typically costs 25% less than services of private doctors. Reason: The greatly lowered hospitalization rate among people participating in HMOs. The economic factor is a strong influence on keeping patients out of hospitals because the costs of hospitalization have to be paid out of the HMOs' own revenues.

**Source:** A study by the Rand Corp., Santa Monica, CA, reported in *Resource*, Alexandria, VA.

## COST OF HEALTH INSURANCE AROUND THE WORLD

The average US health insurance premium (per capita) runs in excess of $900. Only Switzerland has a higher average (near $1,000), with Canada a distant (under $650) third.

**Source:** Insurance Information Institute, New York.

## SINGLE PREMIUM PAYMENT STRATEGY

Insurance discounts for annual single-premium payments are often no bargain. Reason: Many large companies offer only a 3%–6% reduction. You may do better by paying monthly and keeping the balance of your premium in an interest-bearing account. Calculate it out.

**Source:** *Good Housekeeping*, New York.

## LIFE INSURANCE DISCOUNT

Call your insurance agent after joining a health club. Your membership may be accepted as evidence that you're leading a healthful lifestyle—and get you a discount on life insurance and health insurance premiums.

**Source:** *Medical World News*, Houston, TX.

# ORGAN TRANSPLANT UPDATE

Organ transplants—from corneas to hearts—are now covered by most employee health insurance policies. Reason: Use of the drug cyclosporine, which suppresses the body's rejection of an organ, has significantly increased the success rate of these operations.

**Source:** Dr. Thomas Culley, Aetna Life and Casualty Co., quoted in *USA Today.*

# GENERIC DRUG BARGAIN

Mail-order prescription services that sell generic drugs at a discount can reduce a company's insurance premiums and provide a welcome benefit to employees. How it works: Rather than taking a prescription to the pharmacist and then submitting a claim for reimbursement, employees mail the prescription directly to the dispensing service, which mails the drugs to employees. Discounts via generics can run as high as 46%. Hidden savings: Employees can't obtain prescription drugs for ineligible dependents or friends. Added bonus: No start-up costs to the company, only a $3 fee per prescription.

**Source:** *Venture,* New York.

# MEDICARE: WHAT IT DOESN'T COVER

Don't fool yourself that all your old-age medical needs will be taken care by Medicare. This program is riddled with coverage gaps. Be aware of what not to expect from Medicare.

### What Is Medicare?

Medicare must be distinguished from Medicaid, which is the federal program providing medical coverage for the indigent of all ages. Most elderly people wind up on Medicaid when their assets are exhausted paying for what Medicare doesn't cover. This can be a tragedy for people who

had hoped to leave something to their children.

Medicare is an insurance program for people over 65. It is subsidized by the federal government through the Social Security Administration. Each month, elderly people pay premiums to private insurance companies (Blue Cross/Blue Shield or companies like them), which act as fiscal intermediaries for Medicare. The program is overseen by a watchdog agency, Professional Standards Review Organization (PSRO), which makes sure hospitals are not used improperly. Drawbacks: Private insurance companies, acting in their own best interests, tend to deny benefits whenever possible. PSROs interpret Medicare regulations restrictively, since they must save government money.

### Major Problems with Medicare

• Congress passed much of the Medicare legislation with the intention of helping the elderly by keeping them out of institutions. However, the local agencies administer Medicare restrictively in a misguided attempt to save money. Actually, money is being wasted by forcing the elderly into nursing homes unnecessarily. Result: Benefits we thought would go to the elderly simply don't materialize.

• Medicare does not deal with the problem of custodial care. It is geared toward rehabilitation, which is hardly realistic for the population it serves.

• Medicare is part of an overall supply-and-demand problem. There are simply more and more old people every year, as modern medicine enables us to live longer. While the over-65 population expands, nursing homes are filled to capacity and have long waiting lists, and Social Security benefits and services to the elderly are being cut back. Fear for the future: Some see the frightening possibilty that euthanasia may be discussed.

### Hospital Cutoffs

Hospitals cutoffs are the biggest problem with Medicare today. Example: An elderly woman goes into the hospital with a broken hip. After surgery, she cannot go home because she can't take care of herself. She needs nursing home rehabilitation or an around-the-clock companion at home. Because of the shortage of these long-term-care alternatives, she has to remain in the hospital, though everyone agrees she is ready to leave. But Medicare cuts off hospitalization benefits, claiming that she no longer needs hospitalization. The family gets a threatening letter from the hospital—if she isn't out in 24 hours, the family will have to pay privately. At approximately $300 per day for a hospital bed, the family's assets will be wiped out very quickly.

### The Appeal Process

The only way to deal with such unfair (and inhumane) bureaucratic decisions is to appeal them aggressively. Appeal is a long and costly process, but a $300 per day hospital bill is even more costly. Also, as good citizens, we must make our government accountable for benefits promised but not delivered.

Chances on appeal: Very good. At the highest level, Federal Court, the reversal rate on Medicare cases is extremely high.

There are four levels of appeal:

• Reconsideration is a paper review by a bureaucrat. You can request this when Medicare is first denied. Some 95% of reconsiderations confirm the original denial of benefits.

• An administrative law judge will review the case after the reconsideration is denied. You present evidence at this hearing, and a lawyer is recommended. Some of these judges are competent and sympathetic. However, many judges fail to understand the issue.

• The Appeals Council in Washington is the next step. They will usually rubber-stamp the decision of the administrative law judge.

• Federal Court is your final crack. You do stand a good chance of winning here because judges at the federal level are not employees of the Social Security Administration. They tend to be less sympathetic to the agency's viewpoint.

At this level, a lawyer is necessary. Important: No new evidence can be presented in Federal Court, so be sure all your facts are presented to the administrative law judge.

### Medicare and Nursing Homes

Under the law, up to 100 days of skilled nursing care in a nursing home are to be paid for by Medicare. In fact, Medicare pays for an average of only five days, claiming that nursing homes do not provide skilled care. This is another patently unfair decision that must be appealed on an individual basis.

Beyond 100 days, you're on your own as far as nursing-home care is concerned. Medicaid will take over only after your assets are totally exhausted. At an average cost of $30,000 per year, few families can afford long-term nursing-home care. Important: Plan ahead for this possibility well before a nursing home becomes necessary. Transfer your assets to your children or set up a trust fund that the government can't invade. Be aware: You may be liable for payment if your assets have been transferred within less than an average of two years before entering a home, depending on the state.

Recommended: Consultation with a specialist in geriatric law. Ask your lawyer or a social worker in a local hospital or nursing home to recommend one.

### Home Care

The home care situation under Medicare is also dismal. Medicare will pay for a skilled person to come into the home occasionally on a doctor's orders to perform tasks such as giving injections or physical therapy. There is virtually no coverage for the kind of help most elderly people need—a housekeeper/companion to help with personal and household tasks. Many senior citizens groups are currently lobbying for this type of home custodial care to be provided by Medicare.

Assignment rate:

As far as general health care is concerned, Medicare supposedly pays 80% of the "reasonable rate" for medical care as determined by a board of doctors in the community. In reality, the "reasonable rate" is usually set so low that most doctors will not accept it. So, instead of paying 20% of their doctor bills, the elderly frequently wind up paying 50% or even more.

Suggestions:

• Don't drop your major medical insurance when you retire. If you keep it up, it will cover the gaps in your Medicare insurance. It is extremely difficult to buy such coverage after you reach 65.

• Be wary of insurance-company policies that supplement Medicare. You must be extremely careful when you buy one. Be sure it complements rather than duplicates Medicare coverage.

• Get together with other senior citizens to create consumer leverage. If a group of 50 seniors goes to a doctor and all promise to patronize him providing he accepts the Medicare assigned rate, it might be worth his while.

**Source:** Charles Robert, an attorney specializing in geriatric law, Hempstead, NY.

# TO FILL THE MEDICARE INSURANCE GAP

People generally assume that after retirement they'll no longer have to worry about medical insurance—that Medicare will foot the bills. Nothing could be farther from the truth.

Retired people covered by Medicare today are, on the average, reimbursed for only about 50% of their medical expenses. Medicare has many limitations and restrictions. Savvy older people are buying insurance to cover Medicare's gaps (often called "medigap" insurance). Unfortunately, many of these policies are overpriced rip-offs. In order to protect yourself, you have to understand both how Medicare works and what to look for in a Medicare supplement policy.

### How Medicare Works

Medicare comes in two parts: Part A covers hospital expenses and Part B covers doctor bills and other medical costs. Part A is free, while Part B, which is optional, re-

quires a premium of $14.60 per month. The coverage offered by Part A is fairly decent. Part B coverage, however, is inadequate in most areas.

What Part A covers: When you enter the hospital, you pay a deductible of $356. Then Medicare pays the full costs of only the first 60 days. For the rest of your stay:

• From the 61st day to the 90th you pay $89 per day.

• From the 91st day to the 150th you pay $178 per day.

• After 150 days you pay all hospital expenses.

Part A also covers private-duty nursing for the first 20 days and partially thereafter.

What Part B covers: After a $75 deductible, Medicare covers 80% of what it deems "reasonable charges" for doctor visits and other skilled medical services on an outpatient basis. Included are such services as medical tests, speech therapy and physical therapy. Prescription drugs are not covered.

### What to Look For

Most medigap policies pick up the $356 deductible on Part A, plus the extra $89 per day from the 61st day to the 90th day and the $178 per day after the 91st day. Some pay up to one year beyond the 150th day.

Find out which costs are covered. Is there a maximum per day the policy pays, or does it pay the hospital's semiprivate rate? Does it give you a new benefit period, or does it follow Medicare guidelines? That's important because, according to Medicare, you're not eligible for full coverage unless you've been out of the hospital for 60 days. If, for example, you spend 45 days in the hospital, go home for a week, and have to be readmitted, Medicare will stop full coverage 15 days later. Does your policy pick up at that point?

Most policies also pick up the 20% that Medicare doesn't pay on Part B. However, they don't solve the real problem of Part B, which is that Medicare pays 80% of the "reasonable" costs of covered services. "Reasonable" means what Medicare has decided is the usual doctor's bill in your area. Unfortunately, its estimation of "reasonable" may be well below what you actually paid.

Example: You have a heart operation for which the doctor charges $3,000. Medicare decides the "reasonable" bill for open heart surgery in your area is $2,000, so it gives you 80% of that, or $1,600. You are out of pocket $1,400.

Will the policy pick up the difference between Medicare's "reasonable" costs and the amount you actually paid?

Look at the policy's definition of "reasonable." Does it use its own scale or Medicare's? This kind of policy can be hard to come by and costs about $300 more than the standard medigap policy. But if you want the best-quality medical care, the price is probably worth it. If you can't find such a policy in your state, contact the American Association of Retired Persons(AARP).*

Costs: Medigap policies cost $250–$600 annually. Some have sliding scales, depending on age. These scales of course mean lower prices for younger buyers, so those over 75 should look for a policy that has a standard price regardless of age.

### What Else You Should Know

• Do not buy medigap insurance without doing some serious research and comparative pricing. Every state has an insurance department that authorizes the sale of policies in that state. Many of those departments issue booklets comparing the benefits of policies offered in the state. Write to your state's department of insurance. If your state doesn't issue such a booklet, you might write for the free one issued by New York State to get a basis for comparison.** Usually, any policy sold in New York or California can be sold anywhere else because these states have most stringent regulations.

• Medicare is designed to pay only for hospital expenses and skilled medical services. It specifically excludes anything deemed custodial care or nonskilled care, either in the home or in a nursing home. There is absolutely no provision for long-term care for the chronically ill, which many elderly people, if not most, will need eventually. No insurance sold covers such care. What to do: Plan in advance, so your family's assets aren't totally drained by a chronic illness. See a trusts and estates lawyer who is familiar with financial planning for the elderly.

• Don't allow your existing health coverage to lapse when you retire without careful consideration. The better policies are obtainable only when you're under 65. Play it smart: Find out if you can keep your current policy when you retire and use it to supplement Medicare. If you can't, consider buying another major medical policy a couple of years before retirement, even though you don't plan to use it until after retirement. Opt for the highest deductible to keep the price low—you can increase your premium and lower the deductible after retirement. Such a move may give you better protection than any medigap policy.

• Don't forget your spouse's coverage. One big problem: The husband retires at 65 and drops his company policy, assuming he'll be covered by Medicare. He forgets about his wife, who at 60, is not old enough to be covered by Medicare. She then has no coverage.

*Request the AARP Medicare Supplement Portfolio and Group Hospital Plans from AARP, Group Health Insurance Program, Box 13999, Philadelphia, PA 19187.

**Write for the *Medicare Supplement Insurance* pamphlet, New York State Insurance Dept., 160 W. Broadway, New York 10003.

**Source:** Interview with Peter J. Strauss, attorney, Strauss and Wolf, New York.

# SOCIAL SECURITY SECRETS FOR THOSE *UNDER* 65

It's your right as a working person to apply for disability insurance from the Social Security Administration if at any point you're unable to work because of a mental or physical disabilty. Before applying, you should know how the system works, who is eligible and what kind of medical criteria a decision is based on. When dealing with any government agency, the more you know before you walk in, the better your chances are of walking out with what you want.

### Who Can Collect—And How Much

There are two disability programs under

Social Security. One is the needs-based program, Supplemental Security Income Program. SSI is basically a nationalization of welfare benefits for the unemployable. The other, which applies to working people, is the basic insurance program that you pay into as the FICA tax: Old Age and Survivors Disability Insurance (OASDI).

Although the disability criteria for acceptance are the same under both programs, you don't have to prove financial need for OASDI. You're eligible if you've worked and paid into the system for 20 quarters out of the last 40 (five years out of the last 10) and have the necessary years of work credit, depending upon your age. If your last day in the system was 10 years ago or more, you're not eligible for disability benefits now, though you may be eligible eventually for retirement benefits.

Benefits are based on what you've paid into the system. The maximum benefit for an individual is currently $709 per month. For a family, benefits can go over $1,000 per month, since dependents are taken into account. The average benefit for a disabled male wage earner with a wife and children is $835 per month.

### How the System Works

• The first step: File an application with your local Social Security office. You'll be interviewed by a claims representative, who will ask you basic questions about your disability: What is the nature of it? When did you stop working? How does it interfere with your daily activities and ability to work? Which doctors and hospitals have treated you? You'll be asked to sign medical releases so Social Security can obtain information from your medical sources. The interviewer will also note any evidence of your disability that he observed.

• This material is sent to a trained disability examiner at a state agency, who will contact your medical sources.

• If the medical information you have submitted isn't sufficient, the agency will send you to a consulting specialist, at the government's expense, and this information will become part of your file.

• If you've met the medical disability re-quirements (which are extremely stringent), you'll be granted benefits. But you can still be found disabled even if you don't meet the medical requirements. Age, past work experience and education are also taken into account. Example: Anyone over 50 is put in a special category because his vocational outlook is less favorable. A 55-year-old construction worker with minimal education who suffers from mild heart disease might be eligible—he can't do his past work and probably wouldn't be able to find another job. Another construction worker of the same age and disability, but with more education and skill, might be expected to find light or sedentary work. The approach is individualized throughout the process.

• The final eligibility decision is made and signed by the disability examiner, together with a physician who works for the state (not the consulting physician).

• If benefits are denied, you can appeal the decision or reapply.

### Proving Your Disability

Social Security's definition of medical disability: The inability to do any substantial, gainful activity by reason of any medically determinable physical or mental impairment which can be expected to result in death, or which has lasted, or can be expected to last, for a continuous period of not less than 12 months. To meet the definition you must have a severe impairment that makes you unable to do your previous work or any other gainful work that exists in the national economy. How to prove it:

• It's crucial that your doctor submit very precise medical information, including all test results—the same kind of information a doctor would use in coming up with a diagnosis and treatment plan. Social Security won't accept your doctor's conclusions. It wants the medical evidence that led to the conclusion.

• Social Security has a long list of impairments under which your disability should fall. The listing, broken down into 13 body systems, covers about 99% of the disabilities that people apply for. This listing outlines exactly what tests must be met for eligibility. Examples: An amputee is eligible only if he has lost both feet, both hands, or one hand and one foot. Angina pectoris victims must show certain results on a treadmill test and/or a number of other listed tests. Recommended: You and your doctor should take a look at the listings before you apply. If your doctor answers in enough detail, you might avoid a visit to the agency's consulting physician.

### Filing an Appeal

When benefits are denied, a notice is sent. A brief paragraph explains the reason in general terms. At that point, you can go back to the Social Security office and file for a reconsideration, which is simply a review of your case.

If the reconsideration is denied, you can take your case to an administrative law judge within Social Security's Office of Hearings and Appeals. You don't need a lawyer for this hearing, but many people do have one. At the hearing, you present your case, review the evidence in your file, add other relevant evidence and personally impress the judge. The reversal rate ot this level is fairly high (40%–60%).

If denied at this hearing, you can go to the Appeals Council and then up through the courts. The chances of reversal improve at each level. Most people just go up to the administrative law judge level. If they're turned down there, they file a new claim and start all over. Often, delay works in a claimant's favor, since disabilities may worsen over time.

### What Else You Should Know

• Look into state disability programs. If your disability is temporary, you might be covered by your state. State programs bridge the gap for people who are disabled for less than a year. Be aware: Many state disability programs and private insurance companies require that you apply for Social Security first, before you can collect from them.

• File soon. Don't wait until you've been disabled for a year. There's some retroactivity (up to 12 months), but the sooner you file, the better.

• Call the Social Security office before going in. You can save yourself a lot of trouble. Find out first what you should bring with you and which are the best days and times to come in.

• Ask at your local Social Security office for the Listing of Impairments, or look them up in the library. Request the Code of Federal Regulations—see 20CFR404 and 20CFR416.

**Source:** Interview with Dan Wilcox, disability program specialist, Social Security Administration, Disability Programs Branch, New York.

# ALL ABOUT DISABILITY INSURANCE

When disability strikes, you have to replace your income with something or face losing your house, your life-style, savings and investments. Ironically, most people routinely buy life insurance to protect their families in case they die, but they neglect to buy disability insurance. Fact: Chances of being disabled during your working years are four to five times greater than chances of dying during the same period.

### How Much Is Enough?

First assess what resources you already have that would enable you and your family to manage. Compare these resources with your expenditures. Then, make up any gap with disability insurance. Key questions:

• Would you get partial pay from your employer? How much? For how long?

• Do you have a benevolent family member you could count on to keep you going or at least help?

• What assets do you have that could be converted quickly?

• Are you already covered by disability insurance policies?(Don't forget to check what's provided by credit cards and association memberships.)

• What could you expect from Social Security?

### Comparing Policies

*Concern #1:* How the policy defines disability. You want the broadest definition you can find and/or afford. Some policies, for example, define disability as inability to perform any of the duties required by your occupation. Caution: Under many definitions, including that of Social Security, disability is the inability to perform any occupation. Under that definition, you get no payment as long as you can work at something, even if the job you can perform after being disabled is low paying.

A split definition of disability that's often used: Strict for a specific period of time and broad for the duration of the benefit period.

*Concern #2:* The length of the benefit period. Will the policy continue to pay you after age 65? Many policies stop paying then and you may still need funds. Unless another retirement fund kicks in, you'd have an income gap.

Also check the waiting period, the time between the start of the disability and the actual beginning of payment of benefits. If you can wait 90 days before you need income, the premiums will be significantly lower than if you wait only 30 days.

Example: A person who is 45 years old wants a disability policy that will protect his income of $55,000 a year. Yearly premiums with a 30-day waiting period will cost $1,900...with a 60-day wait, $1,700...and for a 90-day waiting period, $1,550.

Reassess your disability coverage when:

• Income changes. Almost everyone increases life-style and financial needs when income increases.

• Financial responsibilities increase. Examples: You have a new child, a new mortgage, build a new house.

Investigate both individual and group coverage offered through your company, professional or other organization. Get quotes from several different companies. Also check to see what occupations they primarily insure. Some companies specialize in insurance for white-collar executives, while others insure blue-collar workers or high-risk occupations and charge much higher premiums.

### Choosing an Insurer

When you talk with insurance salespeople, avoid their jargon. Insist on concrete examples by using "what if" stories to obtain the real facts from them.

Example: What if I were hit by a car and after six months could go back to work only part-time? How much would I be paid? Only policies with a residual benefit would pay in such a case.

Be wary of some group policies advertised on TV or sold by mail. Their definitions and coverage are usually so restrictive that you may never be paid.

There's a Social Security trap to watch out for in planning your insurance needs. To get disability payments from Social Security, you must have paid into the system for 40 quarters. But there are errors in the Social Security records, and you may find out too late that records are wrong and you're not covered.

Safeguard: Write to the Social Security Administration (6401 Security Blvd., Baltimore, MD 21235) every three years for a copy of your account. If there's a mistake, correct it immediately (you have a three-year time limit to make changes).

**Source:** Interview with Karen P. Schaeffer, certified financial planner and branch manager, American Financial Consultants, Inc., Silver Spring, MD.

# FIGHTING BACK WHEN AN INSURANCE CLAIM IS DENIED

Even though the bureaucracy of a giant insurance company may seem intimidating, it's often worthwhile to challenge the company when reimbursement for a medical bill is denied or inadequate. An employee-benefits consulting firm recently found that health claims submitted were erroneously processed over 60% of the time.

Dealing with health insurers has become so complicated (particularly for people covered by two or more policies) that a new type of service industry has sprung up. Within the last five years, several companies have been formed to help people cope with the huge amount of paperwork that accompanies large medical and hospital bills.* Their services are targeted at elderly people covered by Medicare, who also have supplemental private insurance (often called

Medigap policies), and at successful executives, who are too busy to be bothered filling out stacks of forms.

Usual charge: $45 to $50 an hour. A consultation over billing problems connected with a lengthy hospital stay might be $75. While that might seem steep at first, the service can get you significantly more benefits.

It is also possible to challenge a health insurance company on your own. Most carriers have a fairly straightforward appeals process.

Blue Cross and Blue Shield of Greater New York is typical, although policies among companies do vary. At Blue Cross, a complaint is first reviewed by someone at a level higher than the examiner who made the initial determination. If the consumer is still dissatisfied, the complaint is reexamined by an examiner with a technical background (such as a nurse or lab technician). Next, the complaint is sent to the company's medical advisory staff of physicians. Top level of review: The physician who serves as the company's medical director. Only 1% to 2% of challenges ever get this far.

Under the Employee Retirement Income Security Act (ERISA), subscribers can file appeals within 60 days after the complaint.

Officials in charge of claims handling at insurance companies suggest putting a complaint in writing. That usually gets a more searching review than a gripe made over the telephone. (Many claims-handling departments, though, will accept collect calls from dissatisfied customers, or will call back at company expense.)

When challenging a company's reimbursement decision: Include as much pertinent information as you can. Specifically: Past bills and doctors' treatment records, if you have them. Sometimes, a dispute is resolved in a consumer's favor when a doctor provides additional details.

Example: Blue Cross, under one of its common contracts, will pay only $425 for gall bladder surgery. But it paid an extra $280 when the doctor repaired the patient's ulcer at the same time.

Some battles concern new or experimen-

tal medical procedures. Example: The use of elaborate new home equipment that tests the blood-sugar levels of people with diabetes. A company might challenge the use of the equipment, which costs $500, compared with 20 cents for the standard paperstrip tests. But, if the physician argues that the machine is necessary because the patient needs a very accurate reading, the decision might be reversed.

If you are still unhappy after exhausting the internal appeals process within a company, you can take your dispute to the peer review committee of the local medical society. The committee has no formal legal power to overturn either the insurance company's finding, or the doctor's fee, that both you and the company feel is higher than customary. But its findings are frequently followed up.

Another complaint route: Appeal to your state insurance department. While some experts say these agencies are not set up to handle consumer complaints, others find that they can be very powerful allies. One company's experience: 13% of the complaints about medical reimbursements filed with state insurance departments were found to be justified, and the company's decision reversed.

Final step: Take the company to small claims court. While tedious and time-consuming for the consumer, it is even more inconvenient for the insurance company. Result: The insurer doesn't put up much of a fight, and the subscriber emerges victorious.

*The companies include: MediClaim, Inc., with offices in Oakland and Santa Cruz, CA; Mediform in Cleveland; and the Health Claims Assistance Company in New York City.

## PERSONAL INJURY PAYMENTS

A 14-year-old injured in an accident needed constant care for over six months. The child's mother left her job and stayed home to care for her daughter. A court ruled that she was not entitled to personal injury payments under their accident insurance policy. The policy called only for payments to the injured person or to substitutes performing services ordinarily performed by the injured person. There was no provision for services by third parties.

**Source:** *Yeasky v. Reliance Insurance Co.,* S. Ct., N.J., 463 A2d 966.

# PREGNANCY BENEFITS

Pregnancy benefits don't have to be continued if the employee fringe gets to be too expensive. A 1978 law says that employers who offer long-term disability benefits of any kind have to include pregnancy among the conditions covered. But a recent court decision says a company has to comply for only one year. Thereafter, it can drop its long-term disability program entirely.

**Source:** *EEOC v. Wooster Brush,* USCA Sixth, 2/8.

# 5. Healthier Environment at Home and at Work

# Healthier Environment at Home and at Work

## TO REMOVE STALE CIGARETTE SMOKE

Ion-generator air cleaners can be effective in removing cigarette smoke from a closed room. The ions collide with and charge the particles, which are then drawn to walls, floors and other surfaces. Best model: The Bionaire 1000. Less effective: Fan/filter air cleaners. Most economical: A simple fan, provided the room has an open door or window.

**Source:** *New Shelter.*

## MOST COMMON INDOOR POLLUTANTS

Indoor pollution may be as much as 10 times worse than outdoor pollution. Most common pollutants: Asbestos. . .carbon monoxide. . .sulfur dioxide. . .formaldehyde (especially in new homes built of plywood and other cheap materials). . .aerosol sprays. . .cleaning products. . .dry-cleaning chemicals. . .and cosmetics. Highest risk: Well-insulated homes that trap pollutants inside.

**Source:** Report by the Consumer Product Safety Commission, in *Moneysworth.*

## SAFER WOOD BURNING

A new liquid catalyst spray called Anti-Creo-Soot (made by Rolfite in Stamford, CT) can be sprayed on wood before burning. It reduces unburned hydrocarbon emissions, keeps stoves and chimneys clean and prevents fires caused by creosote buildup. (The use of wood stoves, which boomed during the energy crisis, has been declining because of pollution problems.)

**Source:** *Chemical Week.*

## SAFE ASBESTOS SUBSTITUTES

Insulation alternatives to asbestos. When asbestos is removed from buildings, replace it with:

• Fibrous insulations (fiberglass, mineral wool): Easiest to install but lack durability for industrial use.

• Calcium silicate: More durable, but must be cut with a saw, increasing installation costs.

• Cellular glass: Lightweight and moisture-proof, best used underground where temperature is consistently low or in areas where chemicals are used. Difficult to cut and may shatter.

• Foam plastics (urethane and polystyrene): Lightweight and very efficient but tend to shrink under high heat and ignite more easily than other materials.

**Source:** *Energy User News.*

## HOT TUB HAZARD

Communal hot-tub bathing sometimes causes severe infections. Several cases of major ear infections were traced to a tub where the redwood itself was harboring the infectious organisms. Other users developed skin infections requiring intravenous antibiotics. Recommendations: Adequate chlorination, disposable liners for redwood tubs, frequent cleaning of the filtration system and maintenance of the pH at 7.5

**Source:** *Internal Medicine News*, New York.

## GERMIEST SPOTS IN THE HOUSE

Disease-causing bacteria are very much at home the same places you are. They're most populous in kitchens and bathrooms. Germiest spots: Sinks and bathtubs, U tubes, dishcloths, cleaning cloths, facecloths and bathmats. Surprisingly, researchers found toilets to be relatively germ-free. It may be that flushing is an effective disinfectant.

**Source:** *New Scientist.*

## HOW HAIR DRIERS CAN BECOME LETHAL

Bathtub electrocutions are often caused by appliances that aren't turned on at the time. If an appliance is plugged in and falls into the tub, the water will complete the circuit. Most frequent cause of electrocution deaths: Hair driers.

## NON-STICK PAN ALERT

Non-stick pans (such as Teflon® or Silver-Stone®) can be dangerous if allowed to boil dry. At 400°F, the pans may release toxic fumes after 20 minutes—enough to make a person sick. Especially susceptible: Birds and other pets.

**Source:** *Glamour*, New York.

## CHRISTMAS TREE SAFETY

Keep a natural tree's base in water until ready to set it up. (Cut the butt end diagonally one or two inches above its original cut, fill the holder with water to cover the cut line, and refill as necessary.) Keep both natural and plastic trees away from heat sources. Get rid of the tree when the needles begin to fall off in great quantities.

**Source:** *Mothers Today.*

## PRETTY PLANTS THAT CAN BE DANGEROUS

Many common plants are poisonous and can be fatal. Included are daffodils, buttercups, lily of the valley, sweet pea, oleander, azalea, rhododendron and yew. Warn children not to eat anything you're not absolutely sure is safe. If poisoning occurs: Call the nearest poison control center and your physician. If possible, collect a sample of the plant for identification, and estimate the amount consumed.

## HOW TO FIGHT NOISE POLLUTION IN YOUR HOME

To squelch noise pollution within your house: Line a wall with bookshelves filled with books. . .keep closets filled with clothing. . .plug all openings around pipe fittings and electrical outlets with fiberglass. To insulate from outside noise: Use weatherstripping and caulking to close all openings in outside walls. . .keep storm windows closed whenever possible.

## WHAT COLOR TO PAINT WHAT ROOM

Warm colors (yellow, rose, earth tones) create a cozy sense of well-being in the home. But soft green, off-white and cool blue can make you feel melancholy if they're overused. Where cool colors work best: In rooms that are intended for study or meditation.

**Source:** Jacqulyn Yde, a Miami designer and color consultant, in *USA Today.*

## INTERIOR LIGHTING: KEY TO A PEACEFUL HOME

Innovations in fixtures and even in the types of bulbs available make the lighting of rooms as important as the furniture or color scheme in achieving the effect you want.

Proper lighting can make the rooms of a house work efficiently and feel comfortable. Bad lighting in a room imposes psychological stresses on the people who spend time there, leaving them with a vague feeling of tension and strain.

### Living Room

Because it is used for so many purposes, this focal area of the house needs several lighting systems. Best: To keep lighting flexible, use dimmer switches on the main lamps and fixtures.

For entertaining, general brightness is important. That can be achieved with indirect lighting fixtures such as torchere lamps. Dark-colored walls and furniture require more wattage.

Track lighting is good for spotlighting paintings and plants. Halogen or quartz bulbs give the clearest, most natural light for art works. (However, they are more expensive and burn hotter than incandescent bulbs.)

Plants can be made dramatic at night with underlights. Use small floor or table fixtures that hold reflector bulbs. Experiment with using these lights to throw interesting patterns on the walls and ceiling

New low-voltage spotlights or floodlights throw soft light on prized objects such as sculpture or an antique table, or they can illuminate an heirloom rug. Low-voltage lights use a transformer to produce 5½-volt or 12-volt beams made up of cool rays that will not harm fabrics or wood.

For reading, writing or playing board games in the living room, individual lamps need to be strategically placed to give good, strong light on the work areas. When the television is on, the indirect lights can be turned low to prevent eye strain. Sharp contrasts between dark and light areas are the most fatiguing.

### Kitchen

Bright, even lighting is most beneficial to the cook. Fluorescent bulbs—the longer the better—are a practical, economical choice. If the room is L-shaped, use two fixtures. For natural color, use cool white bulbs in blue or green kitchens and warm white bulbs in red or yellow ones. Warm white deluxe bulbs have extra yellow for a sunny effect. Although under-cabinet lights shouldn't be necessary in a properly lighted kitchen, they give a cozy glow for midnight raids of the refrigerator when the overhead lights seem too much.

### Bedroom

Convenience dictates. Bedside lamps should be controlled by easy-to-reach switches and directed so that one person can sleep while another is still awake and reading. "Task lighting" (a separate fixture for each need) is best.

### Dining Room

This is the one room where a chandelier makes sense (unless the entryway is considered a room and has the necessary height). A shimmering glass fixture will catch light and play with reflections from your table silver and crystal. For a softer mood, use low-voltage indirect lights on dimmers.

### Bathroom

For women who apply makeup at the bathroom mirror, fluorescent lights are a poor choice because they distort colors. To get even, wide-spectrum light, use strips of 25-watt incandescent bulbs. Most bathrooms can be well lighted with a total of 200 watts spread the length of the room. Strips made up to specified lengths have recently become available.

**Source:** Interview with Miri Small-Kesten, vice president of Lighting Associates, a designer-lighting showroom in New York.

# DO-IT-YOURSELF ROACH KILLER

Powdered roach killers work better and last longer than liquids or foams—and without a noxious odor. Do-it-yourself formula: Mix boric acid with a little sugar and a little non-dairy coffee creamer. You might also add a silicate gel (for greater adhering power) and pyrethrum (a natural insecticide from African chrysanthemums). For best results: Put the powder in a plastic squeeze bottle and apply a thin line against baseboards and around cabinets, refrigerator and stove.

**Source:** Al (Bugs) Burger, president of Bugs Burger Bug Killers, Washington, DC.

## BEST INSECT REPELLENTS

Insect repellents vary in the amounts of active ingredients they contain and their effectiveness. Active ingredients: N, N-diethyl-metatoluamide (deet) and ethyl hexanediol. Most effective: Deet. Spray with highest deet level: Repel (52%). Liquid with highest deet level: Muskol (95%).

## BUGPROOF CLOTHING

Best bugproof clothing for mosquito, black-fly and no-see-um country is lightweight, waterproof rain gear of Gore-Tex, Klimate or coated nylon. These breathable fabrics are so tightly woven that bugs bounce off as easily as raindrops. The garments have tight closings at wrists, neck and ankles and can be adapted to different temperatures by changing the number of layers worn beneath. Extra protection: Take a head net and light cotton work gloves for badly infested areas.

**Source:** *Sports Afield.*

## LIGHTNING AND YOUR HEALTH

The odds of being struck by lightning are low. But they could be made a lot lower by taking a few simple precautions during a thunderstorm: (1) Move indoors quickly or get into your car. (2) Get off and away from golf carts, bicycles and motorcycles. Put down your golf clubs. Keep away from tractors or metal farm equipment. (3) Stay away from wire fences, clotheslines, metal pipes and rails. (4) If caught in an open area and your hair stands on end, drop to your knees and bend forward with hands on knees. Do not lie flat on the ground. (5) Never seek shelter under a tree.

**Source:** National Oceanic and Atmospheric Administration, reported in *Modern Maturity.*

## DANGEROUS DOG PLAY

Games of tug-of-war or fetch in which the owner tries to pull something from the pet's mouth may be dangerous. By learning to clamp hard onto passing objects, even good-natured dogs become potential biters.

**Source:** *The Weekend Dog* by Myrna M. Milani, Rawson Associates, New York.

## DISEASES YOU CAN CATCH FROM YOUR DOG

The family dog may pass on contagious diseases, particularly streptococcal sore throats. About 100 diseases can be transmitted from animals to humans. Point: If the family is bothered with persistent infections, especially sore throats, take the dog to the vet for testing. When the dog is cured, the family problem with diseases may also disappear.

**Source:** *Ladies' Home Journal.*

## PET FOOD TIPS

Dogs can be poisoned by chocolate. The villain in the chocolate is theobromine, a caffeine-related stimulant that can lead to urinary incontinence, seizures and death. Advice: Avoid giving your dog chocolate treats.

• Pet-food labels tell the story. A can labeled "beef" must be 95% pure, but "beef dinner" or "beef stew" may contain as little as 25% beef.

**More Information:** For a free booklet titled *Food Fit for a Fido,* send a postcard to the Food and Drug Administration, Office of Consumer Affairs, 5600 Fishers Lane, Rockville, MD 20857.

## SMALL PET—BIG DANGER

Pet turtles can be hazardous to their owner's health. They're often reservoirs of salmonella bacteria. Even though selling turtles under four inches long is illegal, they're still available in many pet stores.

**Source:** *The Harvard Medical School Health Letter.*

## PESTICIDE DANGER

Many unlabeled, so-called "inert" ingredients in pesticides, such as mercury, cadmium, lead, benzene, trichlorethylene, arsenic and asbestos are actually extremely dangerous substances. A recent investigation by the Environmental Protection Agency revealed that 50 of the inert ingredients used in pesticides are known or suspected carcinogens or are highly toxic; 30 are active ingredients in other pesticides. Presently, the law requires that only active ingredients be labeled on pesticides, even if inert—and toxic—ingredients make up most of the product.

## CHEMICAL CONFIDENTIAL

Of the 53,000 chemicals in wide commercial use, only one in seven has been even partially assessed for potential health hazards. Among drugs and drug ingredients, such data is available on only 36%...on pesticides, 34%...on food additives, 19%...on cosmetic ingredients, 16%...on chemicals in general use, 10%.

**Source:** The National Research Council.

## LEAD UPDATE

The level of lead in the blood of the average American dropped 37%, to .09 parts per million, in a four-year period. Reason: The decreasing use of lead in gasoline, which still accounts for about 90% of the lead in the air.

**Source:** Study by the National Council for Health Statistics and the Centers for Disease Control, quoted in *Science*.

## MOTOR OIL WARNINGS

Do-it-yourself mechanics should avoid prolonged skin contact with used motor oil. It may be carcinogenic. Suggested precautions: Wear gloves—or at least wash the oil off as soon as possible. Discard oil-soaked clothing. Don't tuck oily rags in pockets or under your belt. Discard the used oil at a designated disposal location.

**Source:** Environmental Protection Agency.

## SAFER VIDEO SCREENS

99% of all radiation from VDTs (video display terminals) and TV screens can be eliminated. (Doctors have voiced concern over scatter radiation's potentially harmful effects on VDT viewers—particularly pregnant women and children.) Solution: Transparent plate containing lead—fits easily. Bonus: Also enhances picture contrast and reduces glare. Cost: $100 to $150.

**Source:** Biflyx/Design West, Irvine, CA.

## VDT UPDATE

• VDT users do not suffer from more musculo-skeletal or visuo-ocular stress than other office employees. They *do* report feeling less staff support, job autonomy and physical comfort, and they complain about greater work pressure and supervisory control. However, they don't complain about lighting any more than non-VDT users.

**Source:** *Office Systems Ergonomics Report*

• Radiation from VDTs (video display terminals) has been ruled out as a cause of office-related lethargy, eyestrain and headaches...according to the latest studies. True causes: The boredom and monotony felt by isolated VDT users. Poor posture. Bad lighting. Glare on the screen.

**Source:** Study by the National Institute for Occupational Safety and Health, Washington, D.C.

• Video display terminals are not likely to contribute to the development of cataracts. However, they can cause tired and strained eyes, headaches and blurred vision. Prevention: Avoid strong overhead lights, uncomfortable furniture, long work periods and poorly designed screens.

**Source:** National Academy of Sciences, Washington, DC.

## BETTER CHAIRING

A good desk chair can add as much as 40 minutes to your workday. Reason: You don't develop fatigue-induced problems. . .back strain, leg cramps, etc.

What to look for in a chair:

• Seat: Made of porous material to let body heat dissipate.

• Front of seat: Rounded or padded so it doesn't cut off circulation in your legs.

• Backrest: Extends the width of the chair, conforms to your spine, and supports the lower and middle back.

• Height: Your feet should rest flat on the floor. Otherwise, circulation to your feet is slowed. This also takes some of your body weight off your lower back.

• Swivelability: This enables you to face your work at all times. You'll avoid eyestrain from moving your eyes back and forth.

Important: Don't sit for longer than 60 minutes at a time or you will tire your body.

**Source:** *Do It at Your Desk: An Office Worker's Guide to Fitness and Health,* Tilden Press, Washington, DC.

## HOW TO SIT CORRECTLY

Even if you have the perfect office chair, you can develop physical problems from prolonged sitting unless you align your body properly. Suggestions:

• Keep your neck and back in a straight line with your spine. Bend forward from the hips. Do not arch your lower back.

• Use a footrest to relieve swayback. Your knees should be higher than your hips.

• Move your feet up and down frequently to ensure constant circulation.

• Move your neck and shrug your shoulders to relieve the tension that results from prolonged sitting.

**Source:** *Office Hazards: How Your Job Can Make You Sick* by Joel Makower, Tilden Press, Washington, DC.

## GOOD AND BAD NEWS ABOUT THE NEW BACKLESS CHAIRS

The new backless chairs (the kind with knee rests) are creating some unforeseen problems. Among them: Chronic knee or leg problems are aggravated by pressure from the knee rest. . .There's danger of sliding down the chair seat when wearing slippery fabrics. . .Users are unable to strech backwards effectively. Major advantage: Users with chronic back pain say the chairs improve posture and relieve back strain.

**Source:** *The Office.*

## PERSONALIZED WORK-STATIONS ARE BEST

Adjustable work-stations make sense because experts don't agree on the ideal sitting posture or work-station design. Moreover, these systems make it possible for workers to adjust the stations to their own bodies, and the fact that they're comfortable minimizes their complaints.

**Source:** *Office Systems Ergonomics Report.*

## OFFICE POLLUTION PRESCRIPTION

To avoid office pollution: Keep carbonless copy paper stored away in closed cupboards (the chemical can be irritating). Never tear paper (it generates troublesome chemical dust). Keep copying machines outside the room you work in. Make sure your office is well ventilated and no warmer than 68°F.

**Source:** *Ultrahealth* by Leslie Kenton, Delilah Communications, Ltd., New York.

## CAN COMPANIES INSTITUTE RULES AGAINST EMPLOYEE SMOKING?

Yes. . .and there are several good reasons why they might want to:

• Employee surveys clearly show that an overwhelming majority (as high as 80% in some surveys) of workers favor a ban against smoking.

• Research strongly suggests that smoke from other person's cigarettes is harmful to nonsmokers.

• Smoking workers have an absentee rate 50% greater than non-smokers and cost employers an average of over $4,000 more than non-smokers.

The company can legally discriminate against smokers. Instituting a smoking ban may actually head off trouble in the form of lawsuits brought by nonsmokers who demand a healthful, smokefree work environment.

Effective antismoking rules:

• Total ban. Institute a policy like that of the Boyd Coffee Co. of Portland, Oregon. Employees may smoke only in the company parking lot, and then only during work breaks and on lunch hours. This rule was upheld by an arbitrator after the filing of a union grievance. And it applies to everyone, including top management, visitors and customers.

• Workstation ban. Smoking is prohibited in working areas but allowed during work breaks in specified areas.

Softer policies such as dividing the work area between smokers and nonsmokers rarely work.

When instituting a no-smoking program, these steps are obvious:

• Notify employees when the no-smoking rules will go into effect.

• Offer smokers the opportunity to join a stop-smoking program held on the company's premises.

• Circulate a memo specifying the designated areas in which smoking is permitted (if any) and reminding employees that smoking outside those areas is a punishable offense.

Most importantly, enforce the rules against all offenders.

**Source:** Dr. William L. Weis, Albers School of Business, Seattle University, Seattle, writing in *Personal Journal.*

# 6. Good Nutrition and Dieting

# Good Nutrition and Dieting

## WHAT AMERICANS ARE EATING

Americans are eating more sugar (up to 11.6%) but less beef (down 8.1%) than in 1970. Also down: Eggs (15.4%), dairy products (9.8%), pork (1.6%). More popular foods: Poultry (up 28.6%), vegetable oils (14.6%), cereals and baked goods (5.6%), fruits (1.9%), vegetables (1.4%).

**Source:** US Department of Agriculture, Washington, D.C.

## JUNK FOOD FACTS

The food industry—and some scientists—mislead the public with lines like *there's no such thing as junk food . . . just a junk diet.* They are trying to convince us that, within the "proper diet," there's plenty of room for junk food.

The reasoning is harmful. Few people have enough information to decide how to include junk food in the balance. Potato chips, for instance, are not totally bad, but they should be eaten sparingly.

While potato chips do contain some vitamin C and complex carbohydrates, and less salt than most people think—less than in one serving of canned soup—they're still a harmful food. Reason: Their salty taste encourages people to want more salty food and to add more salt to their diet . . . contributing to high blood pressure. Worse: Extremely high fat content in potato chips.

We classify foods as junk foods when they're *high* in fat, especially saturated fats, and cholesterol, sodium and sugar . . . and *low* in vitamins, minerals, protein, complex carbohydrates and fiber. Note: Our standards are higher than the ones used by the government.

### Ratings

The Center for Science in the Public Interest has developed its own rating scale to help people make more informed choices about the foods they eat. It's an open-ended scale that is based on a comparison of the beneficial components of a food to its harmful components. The higher the rating, the more nutritious the food.

In the snack food category, carrots have the highest nutritional rating, 48, because their high vitamin A and fiber content far outweigh, any detrimental components. Following are green peppers, 44 (vitamin C and fiber); apples, 23 (fiber, iron, pectin); unbuttered, unsalted popcorn, 19 (fiber, eating satisfaction); celery, 17 (fiber, trace minerals); and potato chips, 15.

On the low end of the snack food scale are Twinkies, –34 (fat, sugar); jelly-beans, –38 (sugar, no nutrients); and Hershey's milk chocolate without nuts, –42 (sugar, cocoa, caffeine).

Desserts: Canteloupe, 60, is rated highest, followed by strawberries, 34. Vanilla ice milk, 7, is rated higher than vanilla low-fat frozen yogurt, 3, which ranks much higher than vanilla ice cream, –22. And, then there's: Sara Lee chocolate cake, –26 and chocolate eclairs, –30.

"Nouveau junk food" eaters cringe at the thought of a Twinkie or a slice of Velveeta cheese, but they go for foods like Dannon Fruit Yogurt—each cup of which contains the equivalent of six teaspoons of sugar. The newly trendy croissants are extremely high in fat, each containing about 4½ pats of butter. A Roy Rogers croissant with ham has the equivalent of 11 pats of butter. In Pepperidge Farm and Sara Lee's all-butter croissants, 59% of the 200 calories come from fat, in contrast to the 5%–10% fat in breads, muffins and bagels.

Quiche is another of the nouveau junk foods. More than half the calories in the crust come from fat. The basic filling of cheese, eggs, cream and bacon contains 25–27 grams of fat per serving...the equivalent of 7 teaspoons of lard.

The new vegetables-in-pastry products also fall into this category. Pepperidge Farm's Asparagus Mornay, Dijon Mushrooms and Zucchini Provencal each contain as much fat as a slice of Sara Lee cheese-cake—13–18 grams of fat per serving.

Gourmet TV dinners are junkier than others. All of them are too high in salt. The difference lies in their fat content. Lean Cuisine and Weight Watchers dinners have a lower percentage of fat than the others, but Le Menu and Armour Dinner Classics contain as much fat as the old-line Banquet or Morton dinners.

Snacks: Granola bars, which used to be more nutritious than chocolate bars, are getting more and more junky as the manufacturers begin adding more candy ingredients. Per ounce, Nature Valley Granola clusters contain 3.3 teaspoons of added sugar, the same amount that's in a Snicker's bar, and more than in Nestle's Crunch, Hershey's milk chocolate with almonds or Mr. Goodbar, which contain only 2.7 teaspoons added sugar. Quaker Honey & Oats Granola Bar is the best of the lot, with only 1.5 teaspoons of added sugar...less than half the sugar of a Nature Valley bar.

Low-calorie crackers: More deceptive and junkier, too, than consumers are led to believe. Wheatsworth Wheat thins make you think they're full of whole-wheat flour...but they contain 10 times more white flour than wheat, and 42% of their calories come from fat. Similarly, Keebler's Harvest Wheat Crackers are labeled "a blend of hearty wheat," but that's not the same as whole wheat. White flour and fat provide 51% of the calories in these crackers. The more truthful label we would have preferred: "A blend of white flour, fat, sugar, salt and small amount of whole wheat added."

Best in class: Crackers whose first listed ingredient is whole wheat and which contain little, if any, sugar, fat and salt. Example: Scandinavian and Scandinavian-style crackers like Wasa Fiber Plus, which contains 26% dietary fiber. Ingredients: Rye whole-grain flour, wheat bran, vegetable shortening, yeast, salt, lecithin. Per cracker: 35 calories, 4 grams carbohydrate, 1 gram protein, 1 gram fat.

**Source:** Interview with Bonnie Liebman, a nutritionist allied with Ralph Nader as director of nutrition at the Center for Science in the Public Interest, Washington, DC.

## HEALTHY WAY TO ORDER FAST FOOD

Fast food may not provide the most balanced of meals, but you can cut its fat and salt content 10%–40% through judicious ordering. Hold the sauce, mayonnaise, ketchup, pickles or cheese on your Whopper or Big Mac. With pizza, avoid pepperoni, sausage and extra cheese. Try McDonald's English muffin without butter. Get Kentucky Fried Chicken's original recipe, not the extra crispy. Eat salad without dressing.

**Source:** *Nutrition Action*, Washington, DC.

## THE DIET/BEHAVIOR CONNECTION

Diet probably does affect behavior, but not always in the expected way. Example: Refined sugar and carbohydrates supposedly make children hyperactive and incite criminals to act aggressively. Fact: People who eat a high-carbohydrate meal are sleepier two hours later than those who have eaten a high-protein meal.

**Source:** MIT research reported in *Science*.

## TIP-OFFS TO WHAT YOUR BODY NEEDS

Food cravings often signal an inadequate diet or special nutritional needs. Cola and chocolate craving: A need for "instant energy," better met by whole-grain cereals and other B-vitamin foods. Cheese: A calcium and phosphorus deficiency, better relieved by fresh vegetables. Salty foods: An adrenal insufficiency, which results from stress. Relieve the stress, and cut down on salt.

## TROUBLE FOR THE WORKING WOMAN

Working women tend to have poor diets. A recent study found that the more hours she worked (and the more money she earned), the more fat a woman consumed. Reason: People who rely on fast foods and processed foods eat more fat (and calories) and fewer fruits, vegetables and whole grains.

**Source:** Research at Cornell University.

## BEST WAYS TO FUEL MUSCLES

• Steak and eggs may be the classic football-team breakfast, but they provide insufficient energy for physical performance. Muscles store little fat and no protein. Best muscle fuel: Complex carbohydrates such as brown rice, pasta and vegetables.

**Source:** *Eat to Win* by Robert Haas, M.D., Rawson Associates, New York.

• A candy bar on an empty stomach won't pump up your tennis game—or any other physical activity. After quickly boosting the glucose in your blood, the sugar is stored in your liver or in fat deposits. To fuel muscles during prolonged exercise, you would have to eat sugar every half hour.

**Source:** *The New York Times Guide to Personal Health* by Jane Brody, Avon Books, New York.

• Sweet snacks for athletes are not a good idea. Although they do give quick energy right before a sporting event, they also can cause a quick letdown soon afterward. For even, sustained energy: Snack on foods with a variety of nutrients, not just carbohydrates.

**Source:** Clinical Research Center, University of Rochester Medical Center, Rochester, NY.

## THE WRONG PLACE TO GO FOR ADVICE

Health-food stores are an unreliable source of medical advice. One investigator visited 24 stores, saying his mother had an eye problem. He then described the symptoms of acute glaucoma, which can cause blindness if not treated, but he didn't name the illness. Twelve health-store employees offered erroneous diagnoses. Several others prescribed vitamins and minerals, some of them in risky doses. Only six employees advised (correctly) that the woman see a doctor immediately.

**Source:** Study by American Council on Science and Health, reported in *Science Digest*, New York.

## WHAT YOU DON'T KNOW ABOUT FOOD LABELS CAN HURT YOU

Labels on food packages are nothing more than another form of advertising designed to sell the product. They're not there to help you make informed choices about the foods you eat. They're not a promise that what you're buying is nutritious. And unless a food claims in its advertising or on the label that it has a particular nutritive benefit, there's no law mandating that nutrients be listed on the label.

Federal law specifies only that label information be truthful . . . and truthful can sometimes mean misleading.

### What Labels Mean

• Natural. Nothing more than "anything occurring in nature." That includes artificial additives, fats and sugars. (Even strychnine is natural.) Natural doesn't necessarily mean healthy.

• Servings per container. The determination of serving size is completely at the discretion of the manufacturer. Because it's an arbitrary measure, comparing different brands for calories per serving is a meaningless exercise. As a rule, serving sizes are slightly smaller than an average person's appetite. This makes calorie and fat counts appear lighter than they really are.

• Sodium. Currently, there is no law requiring the listing of sodium content. Only foods low in sodium advertise it as such and list it in the nutrient list.

• Sugar-free. This only means the product is free of sucrose, not free of honey or corn syrup sweeteners. Once natural sweeteners are broken down by your body, they're all the same: Empty calories.

• Low-calorie. The FDA defines as low-calorie any food with fewer than 40 calories per serving. It doesn't matter whether the calories come from healthful fruit and grains, or from pure sugar and saturated fats.

• Lean...or low fat. Defined as 25% less fat than the manufacturer's standard form of the same food, which very well could be loaded with fat.

• No artificial flavors...but flavors aren't the problem. More dangerous are the artificial preservatives that have been found to be carcinogens and to which some people are severely allergic.

• No cholesterol. This means that cholesterol hasn't been added as an ingredient, but saturated, cholesterol-raising fats might have been. And they'll raise your cholesterol levels.

• May contain one or more of the following, followed by a list of five different kinds of shortening or oil. Decoded: The manufacturer used whichever oil was cheapest at the time of production. You could be getting unhealthy saturated fats from palm or coconut oils.

• Ingredient lists. They are required by law, and ingredients are listed in descending order by weight. Note: The law permits additives to be listed by code number (red dye #2), making it impossible for consumers to identify them. Some potentially dangerous additives (sulfites or sodium) aren't re-

quired to be listed at all. A typical label might read "...and other artificial additives."

• Vitamins. Don't rely on the label for useful information. There are about 70 essential vitamins and minerals, and only 20 or so are regularly listed on food labels. Food companies are required to list only the product's name, the manufacturer's name and address, and a list of ingredients. It's impossible to make informed judgments on nutrition and are relying on the label as the source of nutritional information.

# FOOD TRICKS: WHAT YOU SEE & WHAT YOU GET

Unfortunately, consumers are unable to find out much from reading food labels because of the many omissions and deceptions those labels contain. A typical "weasel word" is *natural,* for which the Federal Drug Administration actually has no definition. Technically, any company can call its products "natural." But clearly, consumers have a different idea of what natural means. They're misled because they think it means pure and unadulterated. A hypothetical example of this deceptive labeling is Mrs. Smith's Natural Juice Pies. The implication is that the entire pie is natural. Actually, however, only the juice is pure. The other ingredients in the pie include artificial flavors and colors and preservatives.

### Cereal Sugar Gangsters

Cereal manufacturers are among the greatest offenders. Cereals take up an entire aisle in most supermarkets. Because there is really not much difference among the cereals themselves, marketing is all-important. It creates perceived differences. Recognizing that consumers are concerned about sugar, Kellogg has dropped "Sugar" from Sugar Frosted Flakes' name, but not from its ingredients. Now it's Kellogg's Frosted Flakes. Kellogg's Sugar Smacks is now Kellogg's Honey Smacks, because honey is perceived to be more healthful. In fact, Honey Smacks contains 50% sugar and corn syrup, while honey contributes only 7%.

Post also sells sugar in the guise of cereal. The company has changed the name of Post's Super Sugar Crisp to Post's Super Golden Crisp and advertises its "golden goodness, golden wheat," emphasizing that it contains no artificial flavors or colors. But it is still over 50% sugar.

The New Cabbage Patch cereal boasts that it contains no artificial flavors. That may be true, but when you discover that it contains artificial colors and BHA preservative, you may feel tricked. (Artificial flavors are fairly harmless. Artificial colors and preservatives are considered much more dangerous to health.)

General Mills' Lucky Charms cereal advertises its "whole-grain goodness," but the marshmallow-filled cereal contains 39% sugar.

Adult cereals contain deceptive labeling too. Nabisco's 100% Bran cereal is "naturally sweetened with fruit juice." However, the amount of juice is minuscule. . .only one-tenth of a teaspoonful of fig juice and prune juice per serving. The cereal is 18% sugar, and it also contains even more salt than fruit juice.

### Cholesterol Enemies

Concern about cholesterol has uncovered another area of deceptive food labeling. Many products are labeled "no cholesterol" or "made with 100% vegetable shortening." But saturated fats raise blood cholesterol and are just as dangerous an ingredient as cholesterol itself.

A label that states a product is "made with 100% vegetable shortening" is no guarantee of healthfulness because two vegetable oils—palm oil and coconut oil—are highly saturated cholesterol-raising fats. The label for Crisco "pure vegetable shortening" says no cholesterol, but one of its main ingredients is palm oil. Remember: "Contains no cholesterol" does not mean it won't raise yours.

### Baked Fat

Baked goods may be even more difficult to interpret. Typically, labels say "may con-tain any or all of the following" and list five types of shortening. From such labeling, consumers can't determine whether the cakes and cookies they buy are made with lard, beef fat, or cottonseed, soy, corn, palm or coconut oils.

### Meat Enemies

Fresh-meat packagers, too, are guilty of deceptive labeling when they put "nutri-tion" labeling on fresh meats, a new marketing ploy co-sponsored by the American Meat Institute, the National Live Stock and Meat Board, and Food Marketing Institute. The new labeling is designed to reassure American consumers, whose largest dietary source of fat is red meat, that meat has been made much leaner and is perfectly all right to eat in quantity. However, the truth is that beef is only 10% leaner than it used to be. . .90% of the fat is still there. In pork, only the external fat, used to make lard, has been bred out. The fat content of the meat is still as high as ever.

Worse, consumers are deluded by the low calorie count on the meat labels. To achieve those deceptive low numbers, the marketers use figures based on meat that has been trimmed with a scalpel; no consumer does that. Then the marketers quote calories for a three-ounce portion of meat. It's low, but totally unrealistic—the average adult portion is five ounces, making the calorie count 67% higher than that displayed on the label.

**Source:** Interview with Bonnie Liebman, director of nutrition, Center for Science in the Public Interest, Washington, DC.

# HOW TO FIND LOW-CALORIE FOODS

"Light foods" have no legal definition. By federal law, "low-calorie" means a food has 40 fewer calories per serving than the regular version of the product. Reduced-calorie foods legally must be one-third lower in calories than the standard. Some so-called light foods are simply marketed as low-calorie as a sales pitch. Example: A soup once sold as a hearty meal, now touted as light, has always had 90 calories per serving. Good news: Some light products such as beer and wine do cut down on calories by one-third. (They also reduce the alcohol content.) Bottom line: To find the lowest-calorie products, read the calorie content on the label, not in the headline.

# HOW BAD OR GOOD IS YOUR DRINKING WATER?

The quality of drinking water in the US is persistently questioned by media reports, environmentalists and concerned citizens. To get an idea of the state of the water that flows from taps in various regions of the country, we commissioned independent laboratories to test samples of drinking water taken at random from systems that get their supply from both above ground sources (reservoirs and rivers) and underground sources (wells).

Samples of water were taken from public systems in Berkeley Heights, NJ; Baltimore, MD; Marietta, GA; Streamwood, IL; Austin, TX; and Los Angeles, CA.

Independent laboratories were then asked to test the water for specific contaminants: Arsenic, cadmium, chromium, lead, mercury, iron, manganese, nitrate, dissolved solids and trihalomethanes (choloroform, bromodichlorimethane, dibromocholoromethane and bromoform).

The results of each water analysis were then compared with the national drinking-water standard.

We next reviewed the findings with water expert Dr. Fred Gollob, director of his own independent analytical service.

### Good News
The drinking water from every region tested is safe. When the levels of contaminants are matched against maximum allowable standards set by the government, only two entries are beyond normal water specifications.

One is the nitrate reading for drinking water in Los Angeles (12 milligrams per liter vs. an allowable standard of 10). This is not a health hazard, but it may affect the taste of the water slightly. You couldn't brew perfect coffee with it.

The other abnormal reading is for the total dissolved solids in the Streamwood, IL, water—622 milligrams vs. a standard of 500. Increased levels of dissolved solids are not particularly harmful to the human body in this slight excess. Streamwood has an underground water source. These solids are picked up as water drips through areas of the ground that contain chemicals such as calcium carbonate. Some of the chemical dissolves in the water. In larger amounts, the total dissolved solids could be distressful to humans, but this level makes the water hard. Hard water often deposits a sediment in the pots it is boiled in or leaves a residue that closes up water pipes. It is difficult to get soap to lather in hard water, too, but these are inconveniences, not major health problems.

The contaminants in drinking water fall into two categories: Chemicals found in nature that are relatively dangerous to drink over long periods of time, and industrial chemicals that often seep into the water table.

### Danger of Trihalomethanes
The most publicly discussed—and feared—contaminants are a class of chemicals called the trihalomethanes. These are compounds that contain chlorine and bromine, chemicals that do not occur in water naturally. They are the results of a reaction between chlorine, which is added to drinking water to purify it, and other harmless organic matter that is present in the water.

No one knows the long-term effects of ingesting trihalomethanes on a daily basis in humans, but we know they are harmful to animals in a lab. To be cautious, the government has set a limit of only 100 parts per billion in drinking water.

As might be expected, the highest trihalomethane counts are in areas where the water is heavily chlorinated to purify it. This is true of Marietta, GA, where the count is 76, and also of northern New Jersey (43). (If you live in such an area, you can rid your water of trihalomethanes by boiling it or aerating it before you drink it or use it in cooking.)

The alternative to chlorine to purify water is ozone. A number of European countries have successfully switched to ozone. Problem: It has no residual purifying effect. Once the water is treated, it could pick up pollutants en route to users in water pipes.

### Groundwater Problems

Because industrial wastes and sewage often spread through the ground to reach the water levels below, most problems with water contamination come from groundwater supplies.

There are different levels of ground water. Dig down 30 feet and you will hit the first level of water. However, if you drill farther, through the underlying stratum of impervious rock, you reach much purer water that has been filtered through the ground, a natural purification system. Problem: In some areas, there is a natural limit on how deep you can go for water. On New York's Long Island, for example, going too far down can mean striking salt water.

### Caution

Water tests, such as the ones made for this story, provide only a general idea of the water quality of those places at the time the tests were made. And these tests did not analyze every component of the water. Water quality is subject to change, particularly when the source is from the ground. Well water in one location may be pure, while only a short distance away the water table could be tainted.

**Source:** Interview with Fred Gollob, Ph.D., Gollob Analytical Service, Berkeley Heights, NJ. Water tests were made by Dr. Gollob; Stan S. Zaworski, vice president of lab operations, Aqua Lab, Streamwood, IL; Francis Ptak, Gascoyne Laboratories, Baltimore, MD; IT Analytical Services, Cerritos, CA; Law Engineering, Atlanta.

# TESTING YOUR WATER

If your water is supplied by a municipal company, you have no need to test it. (The water company must make periodic checks

of its own.) However, if you have your own water from a well or other source, you should check its purity. The old-fashioned tests for biological impurities are not enough. Unfortunately, tests for more complex pollutants can be very expensive.

Use common sense in ordering tests. The basic tests for natural contaminants and for trihalomethanes are a first priority. The latter will also pick up common industrial pollutants such as benzine. If you have a shallow well in a heavily agricultural area, consider tests for pesticides. If you buy a new house that was recently treated for termites and it has a well, you should test the water for traces of chlorodane. If untreated sewage is a problem in your area, order tests for biological pollutants. If you are near an industrial complex, you might want to check out chemical waste products in your water.

The cost can be as high as $500 for a sophisticated battery of tests. If the first analysis shows nothing to be alarmed about, wait a year and test again. If the results are the same, you can rest easy for another 10 years unless, of course, the environment of the house changes radically.

### Filters

A good charcoal filter system absorbs most impurities from water. However, these impurities gradually build up in the filter. If it is not changed frequently, you run the risk of doing more harm than good. An overloaded filter discharges its chemicals into the water that goes through it and makes the filtered water more dangerous than the water from the original source.

**Source:** Interview with Fred Gollob, Ph.D., Gollob Analytical Service, Berkeley Heights, NJ.

# TAP VS. BOTTLED WATER

Myth: Bottled water is safer and more healthful than tap water.

Fact: Safety standards for bottled water are no stricter than those for water from your kitchen faucet. In one government study of 110 brands of bottled water, club soda, and seltzer, more than 40% were found to contain traces of organics, metals and sulfates. Ten percent actually failed to meet local drinking water standards.

Best bet: Support high standards for local water-supply sources.

**Source:** The Suffolk County (NY) Department of Health Services, quoted in *Vogue*, New York.

## TREATING YOUR TAP WATER

Home water distiller produces up to four gallons a day. End product is free of bacteria, viruses, salt, rust and chlorine. Includes boiler and four storage bottles.

**Source:** Hammacher Schlemmer, New York.

## BEST WAY TO RECONSTITUTE JUICE

Orange juice concentrate mixed with water from copper pipes may lose its vitamin C. Reason: Heavily mineralized water (such as water left sitting overnight in copper pipes) destroys the vitamin C. Best: Mix frozen juices with pure bottled water instead of tap water, or run the tap for two to three minutes before using the water.

**Source:** *The Consumer's Medical Journal*, Philadelphia, PA.

## KITCHEN ALERT

Antibiotic-fed livestock can produce meat that contains drug-resistant bacteria. When eaten, these bacteria can lead to serious illnesses such as salmonella—especially in people who recently took antibiotics themselves. Prevention: Before cooking raw beef and poultry, rinse them under cold running water. If you chop the pieces, wash the utensils and cutting board with hot, soapy water before they touch other food. Also: Avoid eating rare meat, especially hamburger. (Heat kills bacteria.)

**Source:** *Tufts University Diet & Nutrition Letter*, New York.

## REMOVING PESTICIDES FROM PRODUCE

Pesticides cling to fruits and vegetables even after a water washing. Best: Scrub the produce with a vegetable brush under running water. To be extra sure, use a mild detergent. Soak apples and pears in water containing one-fourth cup of vinegar before scrubbing.

**Source:** *The Practical Gourmet*, Middle Island, NY.

## BEWARE THE SPROUTED POTATO

It may contain elevated levels of natural nerve toxins called glycoalkaloids. If ingested, the substances can cause drowsiness, headache, diarrhea and even high blood sugar. Recommended: Store potatoes in a cool, dark place. If they sprout, peel at least one-eighth inch into the flesh before cooking. (The same goes for green, dried-up or bruised potatoes.) Always completely remove eyes and sprouts. Also: Baked potatoes contain safer levels of glycoalkaloids than fried potatoes.

**Source:** Research at Cornell University, in *American Health*, New York.

## BEST WAY TO COOK POTATOES

Frying potatoes does more than add cholesterol. Recent experiments showed that baking drives minerals into the potato's interior. Frying, however, reduces all minerals significantly.

**Source:** *Journal of Food Science*.

## LICORICE WARNING

• Large amounts of licorice may be hazardous. The chemical in licorice resembles steroid hormones and can have the same ill effects if you eat too much. How much is too much? You'd have to eat over two pounds a day for licorice to be harmful.

**Source:** Norman Farnsworth, Ph.D., University of Illinois, Urbana.

• Eating licorice or licorice-flavored products can be bad for your health. Hypertension and fatigue are just two of many conditions associated with glycyrrhizic acid, from which the familiar licorice flavor comes. Note: Ex-smokers and alcoholics are particularly susceptible to licorice's harmful effects..

**Source:** *Science Digest, New York.*

## SECRETS FOR CHOOSING THE FRESHEST SEAFOOD

Look for bright, metallic-looking skin...bright eyes, with translucent corneas and full, black pupils...red gills, free of slime...firm flesh that is elastic to the touch. A mild ocean or seaweed scent is good...but not the smell of ammonia.

**Source:** National Fisheries Institutes, Chicago.

• Clams, oysters, mussels: Pick tightly closed shells. (If the shell is slightly open, it should shut when you tap it gently.) Crabs, lobsters, crayfish: Check for moving legs. A live lobster curls its tail under the body when it's picked up. Scallops, shrimp: Aroma should be mild and fairly sweet. An iodine or ammonia-like odor in shrimp is a sign of spoilage. Frozen shrimp, crab, lobster tail: Be sure any exposed meat is well glazed and white, with no yellowing.

**Source:** *Sunset,* Menlo Park, CA.

## GOOD WAY TO COOK PORK

Safe-to-eat pork will emerge from a microwave oven if the meat is cooked inside a sealed plastic bag. By holding in moisture, the bag prevents surface evaporation and cooling, so all parts of the meat become hot enough to kill the trichina parasite.

**Source:** American Council on Science and Health, New York.

## KEEPING FOOD FROM BECOMING TAINTED

When in doubt, throw it out. This is the general rule concerning frozen food that has thawed too long or dishes that haven't been properly handled. Example: Cheesecake left on a counter to cool overnight could easily go bad.

Food should be kept at temperatures below 45°F or above 160°F. The longer food remains at temperatures suitable for the growth of bacteria, the greater the chances of its becoming tainted. Time limit: Food left away from heat or cold for two to three hours is probably unsuitable for eating. This is particularly true of foods that are moist, high in protein and low in acid.

Ways to prevent spoilage:

• Refrigerate leftovers as soon as possible. Don't let them sit at room temperature for more than two hours.

• Reheat food in wide, shallow pans rather than deep, narrow ones. Place foods in a preheated oven, not one that's warming up.

• When refrigerating large quantities of dishes such as stews, spaghetti sauce or chili, pour them into large, shallow containers. Point: To expose the greatest mass to the preserving effects of the cold refrigerator.

• The best way to thaw frozen foods is to place them in the refrigerator. If thawing must be done quickly, immerse the food in cold water or use a microwave oven.

## HOW LONG SHOULD YOU KEEP FOOD IN YOUR FREEZER?

Storage times for frozen meats vary significantly. Recommended holding time in months: *Beef roast or steak, 12. Ground beef, 6. Lamb, 12. Pork roasts and chops, 8–12. Bacon and ham, 1–2. Veal cutlets and chops, 6. Veal roasts, 8–10. Chicken and turkey, 12. Duck and goose, 6. Shellfish, not over 6. Cooked meat and poultry, 1.

*Based on a freezer kept at zero degrees or lower.

## SAFER HOME CANNING

If you do your own food canning, preserve only enough food to eat within one year. After that time, its quality deteriorates.

The USDA has more than doubled its recommended boiling times for most home-canned fruits and vegetables.

## WHEAT-GERM CONFIDENTIAL

Beware of stores that sell wheat germ that's not vacuum-packed, frozen or in an airtight container that has been flushed with nitrogen. Reason: Wheat germ rapidly loses its nutritional value when it's exposed to the air. Look for high turnover of stock, and don't buy much in advance. Keep wheat germ stored in the freezer. Note: Avoid defatted wheat germ . . . most of the nutritional value is lost when the oils are removed from the wheat germ.

## MILK TIP

Supermarket milk retains its nutrition better in fiberboard cartons than in clear plastic containers. Reason: When exposed to fluorescent lights, low-fat or skim milk loses 90% of its vitamin A in 24 hours.

**Source:** Research at Cornell University, Ithaca, NY.

## SPOILAGE MONITOR FOR FOOD

Innovative bandage-like label attaches to packaging to monitor potential spoilage of foodstuffs continuously, cheaply and with complete accuracy. Eliminates uncertainty over freshness for retailers and consumers alike—and can save food producers millions by promoting proper handling of their products.

Background: Some products (milk, for example) have expiration dates stamped on their packages. But these are guesses at best—they don't take into account the way the package has been handled, whether or not it has been stored at the proper temperature, etc. Breakthrough: New spoilage monitor exploits sophisticated enzyme chemistry for far more accurate monitoring. . . .Changes color to show whether any perishable food is safe for consumption, as well as how much time is left before it spoils.

How it works: Each strip contains two compartments, one containing a fatty substance, the other a fat enzyme. Affixing the strip to a package mixes the two substances, initiating a chemical reaction that moves along at different rates depending upon the type of food being monitored, temperature changes, agitation and so on. Result: Color changes—green means "fresh," yellow means "caution" and red means "spoiled." Cost: about 20¢ apiece now—ecomonical for use on large cartons—but refinements could bring that cost to 1¢ or less. That should be economical enough for retailers to use on individual packages. Soon: Spoilage monitors that work on a broader range of products.

**Source:** I-Point Technologies, Ltd., Washington, DC.

## ALTERNATIVES TO ALCOHOL

New fruit juices for adults come in wine-type bottles, are alcohol- and caffeine-free, and cost $2–$3 a quart. Essentially sophisticated ciders and grape juices, these grown-up drinks come in sparkling and plain versions that range in taste from crisp to sweet. They are available at supermarkets and delicatessens.

Sparkling juices:
- Grand Cru Cider.
- Martinelli's Gold Medal Sparkling Cider.
- Challand French Sparkling Apple Juice.
- Ecusson Sparkling White Cider.
- Ecusson Sparkling Red Grape Juice.
- Meiers Sparkling Catawba.
- Meiers Pink Sparkling Catawba.
- Meiers Cold Duck.

Still juices:
- Grapillon French Grape Juice (white or red).
- Meiers Pink Catawba Grape Juice.
- Meiers Catawba Grape Juice.
- Lehr's Black Currant Beverage.
- Lehr's Pure White Grape Juice.
- Lehr's Pure Red Grape Juice.

## IN PRAISE OF TEA

Tea mimics the antidepressant drugs. Its caffeine helps the brain synthesize chemical stimulants. Then, its polyphenols help to keep those chemicals around longer.

Unlike coffee, tea doesn't raise blood cholesterol levels. It actually strengthens blood-vessel walls and may even cut cholesterol absorption.

Rich in fluoride, tea inhibits growth of decay-causing bacteria in dental plaque.

It's a good source of zinc, manganese and potassium, and its tannins help preserve vitamin C in the body.

Hot tea fights colds by doubling mucus flow, which help to wash out germs.

## HERBAL TEA CONFIDENTIAL

Herbal teas can be dangerous. They sometimes counter the effects of prescription drugs or cause serious side effects. Severe diarrhea: Senna (leaves, flowers and bark), buckthorn bark, dock roots and aloe leaves. Allergic reactions: Camomile, goldenrod, marigold and yarrow. Cancer: Sassafras. Toxic (possibly fatal) reactions: Shave grass, Indian tobacco and mistletoe leaves. Hallucinations: Catnip, juniper, hydrangea, jimsonweed, lobelia, nutmeg, wormwood.

## NEW FACTS ABOUT COFFEE ADDICTION

Coffee junkies may now have a chemical explanation for their addiction. Coffee contains a substance that binds itself to the brain's opiate receptors to behave like morphine. Substance X is found in fresh and instant coffee, including the decaffeinated kind, but is absent from tea or cocoa. Uncertain: If the coffee plants themselves manufacture Substance X or if it is formed in the roasting process.

**Source:** *New Scientist*, London.

## HOW MUCH COFFEE IS TOO MUCH?

- Coffee in excess (more than six cups per day) is associated with approximately a 10% rise in serum cholesterol and with heart irritation. But moderate coffee intake doesn't seem to elevate cholesterol levels.

**Source:** *New England Journal of Medicine*, Cambridge, MA.

- Two to three cups of coffee can raise blood pressure significantly, especially in those over 50.

**Source:** *American Journal of Cardiology*, New York.

## COFFEE HAZARDS

Too much caffeine can cause a loss of calcium and magnesium from the body. This presents a particular threat to women—who need extra calcium to prevent osteoporosis (a thinning of the bones) in later life.

**Source:** *Nutrition Research*, Elmsford, N.Y.

- Coffee can interfere with some drugs' effects. Example: Since caffeine reduces the body's iron absorption, it's inadvisable to drink coffee within two hours of taking an iron pill.

**Source:** *The Medical Letter*, New Rochelle, N.Y.

- A study of college students showed that Type A people (impatient and aggressive) ingest 50% more caffeine than do Type Bs.

**Source:** *Medical Aspects of Human Sexuality*, New York.

## NEW LOOK AT COFFEE DRINKING HABITS

Avid coffee drinkers may think they can tell the difference between regular and decaffeinated coffee, but a recent test reveals they rarely can. And many prefer the taste of decaffeinated coffee. Of 26 people who regularly drink brewed coffee, only 12 could tell the difference between regular and decaffeinated.

**Source:** *Prevention*, Emmaus, PA.

## DECAFFEINATION MAY NOT BE THE ANSWER

Decaffeinated coffee leads to significant stomach acid secretion, causing heartburn and indigestion in many persons. Caffeine was assumed to be the culprit. A new study shows that decaffeinated coffee is even worse. The effect is seen in doses as small as a half cup of decaffeinated coffee. People experienceing ulcer symptoms, heartburn and dyspepsia should avoid decaffeinated as well as regular coffee.

**Source:** *Journal of the American Medical Association*, Chicago, IL.

## HOW TO KICK THE COFFEE HABIT

Select a Friday to start kicking the coffee habit so you can have the weekend to start withdrawal. Gradually reduce your intake before cutting out completely. Avoid rituals such as coffee breaks. Substitute caffeine-free drinks for coffee. Accept your body's rhythms—you may naturally feel tired at points during the day. Expect occasional cravings, especially in times of stress. Don't drink decaffeinated coffee—it tastes too much like the real thing and will start cravings again.

## SWEET ALTERNATIVES

A host of health problems, from diabetes to tooth decay, are linked to excessive sugar intake. Yet the average American consumes about 150 pounds of sugar a year (which works out to 500 calories a day per person).

Whatever their source—table sugar, corn syrup, molasses or honey—sugars are transformed into glucose in the body. Normally glucose levels in the bloodstream are kept in balance by the insulin that the body generates. Our bodies need glucose to function, but complex carbohydrates provide that glucose more nutritiously and economically than sugar does.

The problem with table sugar (sucrose) is that it provides empty calories. There is no other nutritional benefit. It is a myth that brown sugar and raw sugar (unrefined sugar) are more healthful than white (refined) sugar. Nor is turbinado, a partially refined sugar, any more nutritious than the others. How the alternatives to table sugar stack up:

• The corn sweeteners—dextrose, corn syrup and high-fructose corn sweetener (HFCS)—are all refined from corn starch and are as nutritiously bankrupt as the cane and beet sugars.

• Maple sap straight from the tree is only 3% sucrose (and quite delicious), but the syrup made from boiling down the sap is 65% sucrose. Imitation maple syrup is 97% sucrose. Although pure maple syrup contains some calcium and potassium, it is not a prime source of either.

• Blackstrap molasses (made from sugar cane) and sorghum (made from the sorghum plant) have varying amounts of iron, calcium, potassium and B vitamins. The darker the color, the better the nutrition.

• Honey has small amounts of minerals and vitamins.

### Better Choices

Vegetables such as parsnips, carrots, winter squash and beets have 4%–9% sucrose plus fiber, vitamins and minerals. Fresh fruits have 10%–25% fructose and glucose, plus fiber, vitamins and minerals. Dried fruits are much sweeter, but they do contain iron. Date sugar (dried and crushed date particles) can be substituted for other sugars in baking. Use half as much date sugar as the recipe calls for in regular sugar. Grind it in a coffee mill or food processor to get a smooth consistency. You can buy date sugar at natural-food stores.

Bottom line: The sweeteners added to many of the foods we love are high sources of calories and not much else, and they can become almost addictive. The best line of defense: Stick to fresh fruits and vegetables and whole grain products. . .with an occasional molasses or date-sugar cookie if you must have a sweet.

**Source:** Leslie Cerier is a personal-fitness specialist, Charlemont, MA.

## HEALTHFUL SWEETENER

Rice syrup, in which enzymes have naturally converted rice starch to sugar. Unlike refined sugar or honey, rice syrup contains B vitamins, minerals and protein, rather than empty calories. Best of all: Brown-rice syrup, which is made from the whole grain.

**Source:** *Vegetarian Times*, New York.

## SUGAR ALERT

Common table sugar may pose a bigger health risk than many artificial sweeteners. Besides being packed with calories and causing tooth decay, sugar also appears to contribute to heart disease and diabetes.

**Source:** Sheldon Reiser, Ph.D., carbohydrate nutrition laboratory, US Department of Agriculture, quoted in *Technology Review*, Cambridge, MA.

## VIEWS ON ARTIFICIAL SWEETENERS

The controversy over the safety of artificial sweeteners still rages. Scientific opinion varies both about their advisability in general and about which ones are safe and which aren't. At this point, you simply have to choose for yourself. To help you decide, here's a roundup of experts to tell you the latest on saccharin, aspartame and the possible return to the market of cyclamates.

• *Jane Brody, health science columnist for* The New York Times *and author of* Jane Brody's Nutrition Book *and* Jane Brody's The New York Times Guide to Personal Health.

An important but often overlooked aspect of using artificial sweeteners is that it simply perpetuates your sweet tooth and doesn't teach you to like less sweet foods. There are too many tempting foods that will never be made with an artificial sweetener, such as pecan pie, imported chocolate or even most ice creams. If you don't reduce your sugar cravings across the board, you'll always be vulnerable to the temptation of calorie-laden sweets. And no artificial sweetener has ever been proved to help people really lose weight or to help diabetics control their disease.

As for the effects of aspartame, laboratory tests have shown that it changes the level of neurotransmitters in the brain (crucial chemicals that carry nerve messages from one cell to another). Its effect on behavior and intelligence isn't really known. Phenylalanine, one of its breakdown chemicals, is known to cause mental retardation when used in large quantities, and perhaps it is dangerous to those who are sensitive to it. There have been hundreds of reports to the FDA from people who claim that aspartame has caused all kinds of neurological symptoms, including dizziness, depression and headaches. Although the FDA has dismissed these reports as inconsequential, the Centers for Disease Control have analyzed them and suggested that they require more careful clinical analysis. Aspartame poses the additional hazard of breaking down into dangerous substances when heated. Although instructions say to use it only in cold foods, people are bound to try it in hot foods such as coffee.

As far as saccharin is concerned, repeated studies since 1952 have indicated that it may promote the growth of cancers. Since our environment is beset with all kinds of potential cancer-causing substances that we can't avoid, I don't see any point in putting an essentially useless substance into our systems. The main benefit of artificial sweeteners is psychological. They make you feel you're getting something for nothing. But a main side effect is to increase appetite, which may cancel out the something-for-nothing benefit.

As far as the return of cyclamates is concerned, there has never been a case where a substance taken off the market by the federal government because it was declared a potential carcinogen has ever been reinstated. Although a large segment of the scientific community would like to see the cyclamates returned, the issue has been kicked around for years without getting past first base. So I doubt that cyclamates will be brought back—even though the evidence seems to indicate that the move against them was misguided and that probably saccharin was the bad actor in the story to begin with. Animal studies indicate that cyclamates aren't dangerous, and they're still being sold in Canada. It's ironic that saccharin remains on the market and we lost cyclamates, which tasted much better.

• *Dr. Michael F. Jacobson, microbiologist and executive director, Center for Science in the Public Interest, Washington, DC. Dr. Jacobson, an expert on food additives, is the author of* Eater's Digest.

Saccharin, a weak promoter of cancer, should not be used. Even the FDA agrees that it's a carcinogen. It took a special act of Congress to permit its continued use.

Aspartame should have been better tested, even though it may be safe. There were serious questions about the laboratory procedures used in testing it, which, according to FDA scientists, were abominable. And the handling of the complaints about aspartame has been terrible. The FDA should invite the complainers to be tested in a controlled study, ending the controversy once and for all. But with typical bureaucratic self-protectiveness, the FDA simply insists the complaints are baseless. If you want to use aspartame, I suggest you limit your consumption to one or two servings per day. You should probably avoid it altogether if you experience any adverse effects.

From the evidence I've seen, cyclamates cannot be exonerated as potential carcinogens, but the FDA is bending over backward to readmit them. I predict a big battle with consumer groups on this issue. I have a hunch the FDA's position won't hold up under a fair analysis.

There is no real evidence that artificial sweeteners help people to lose weight. When a truly safe product is eventually found, it will be a boon to the food industry, since people will eat more. But the health value of any artificial sweetener will always be questionable.

• *Dr. Bruce Yaffe, a gastroenterologist in private practice in New York City.*

Aspartame seems to be an excellent sugar substitute. It has a very good safety record and has been thoroughly investigated by the Federal Drug Administration. A few people claim that it can occasionally cause headaches, nausea, fatigue and menstrual irregularities, but usually only in those people who use aspartame heavily. Although there's no proven connection between aspartame and these symptoms, people who experience them should consider the possibility that aspartame is responsible.

As far as saccharin is concerned, there's still a question of its causing cancer in laboratory animals. But it has passed all the FDA tests and has been used for years. There's little chance of a significant cancer risk. Since being overweight is a medical hazard, it's important to use artificial sweeteners to reduce the medical complications of obesity.

Cyclamates may be brought out again. The risk of cancer with this sweetener is so low as to be negligible. Also, many new substances are being investigated. I've been personally informed about a forthcoming product that's sweeter than aspartame and usable in foods. Hopefully that product and others will come on market in the next few years.

## MORE ABOUT ASPARTAME

The sweetener aspartame (trade name NutraSweet), the new low-calorie sugar substitute used in soft drinks, may lead to mood changes and sleep problems. According to preliminary research, it may also trick the brain into wanting more carbohydrates—hardly desirable in a diet drink.

Source: Research by Richard Wurtman, neuroendocrinlolgist, reported in *Science 83*, Washington, DC.

## SORBITOL WARNING

Sorbitol, an artificial sweetener, can cause unpleasant bowel symptoms. As little as 10 grams produce gas and bloating, and 20 grams may cause cause cramps and diarrhea.

Source: *Harvard Medical School Health Letter*, Cambridge, MA.

## SUGAR SUBSTITUTES JUST OVER THE HORIZON

Sugar substitutes now under study will play a significant role in the low-calorie food market: *Thaumatin,* a mixture of proteins from a West African fruit, is about 2,500 times sweeter than sugar and has a licorice-like aftertaste. Already in use in Britain and Japan is *Miraculin,* derived from the so-called miracle fruit native to West Africa but now found in other places, too.

Source: Study by Dr. Robert Aries, president, Bioteknomics, researchers, New York, quoted in *Beverage World*, Great Neck, NY.

## THE INBORN NEED FOR SALT

The craving for salt seems to be a deep-seated biological drive as fundamental as thirst, sex and maternal behavior.

When many animals, including humans, lack sodium, the brain reacts with a message to obtain salt. This response appears to be inborn, since it occurs spontaneously among animals at the first experience of sodium deficiency—not after learning by trial and error.

The cravings of pregnant women for special foods may be tied to this response. (Many of the desired items are salty.)

Trap: The drive to eat salt, if indeed it is inborn, makes it difficult for people to give

it up for diets aimed at decreasing sodium consumption.

Source: *The Hunger For Salt* by Derek Denton, M.D., Springer-Verlag, New York.

## SALT WATCH

You should consume no more than 1,100-3,300 milligrams of sodium per day. (One teaspoonful of salt = 2,000 mg.) Here's how to calculate the amount of sodium per serving, based on food-labeling regulations.

• Sodium free: 5 mg. sodium or less.

• Very low sodium: 35 mg. or less.

• Low sodium: 140 mg. or less.

• Reduced sodium: Usual level reduced by 75%.

• Unsalted: Processed without salt when salt is ordinarily used.

Source: The National Research Council, Washington, DC.

## JUST WHEN YOU THOUGHT IT WAS SAFE TO EAT SALT...

Only a few months ago some medical studies indicated that salt might not be as harmful as people once thought. Now better evidence is in, and the message is clear. Sodium contained in salt can cause or aggravate hypertension (high blood pressure), which leads to heart disease, stroke and failure of vital organs.

Problem: The vast majority of foods sold in stores are laden with salt. Moreover, since we've all eaten these foods for most of our lives, we're conditioned to expect the taste of heavily salted foods.

To cut down on salt intake, you must recondition your taste. That's not easy, and it takes a psychological approach to accomplish it. How to do it:

• Reduce salt gradually. When people are abruptly placed on a very-low-sodium diet, they develop cravings for salt that cause them to revert to their former eating habits. But a gradual reduction of salt will change your taste for salt...so much that food salted to its previous level will taste unpleasant. Time: Allow up to three months to adjust to a salt-free diet.

• Keep daily records of the amount of sodium you eat. This is now relatively easy because federal law requires most grocery store foods to be labeled for sodium content. A pocket calculator is sometimes useful as you shop, but don't think you'll have to keep count for the rest of your life. After a couple of months, separating high- from low-sodium foods will be almost automatic.

As you cut down on salt, a big change will take place: You'll become more aware of what you're eating and what it really tastes like. You'll get to appreciate the taste of foods with other flavor enhancers, especially herbs and spices.

Opportunity: If you have children, start now to condition their taste by not feeding them salty foods. For the first time, low-sodium baby food is now on the market.

**Source:** Interview with Cleaves M. Bennett, M.D., clinical professor, University of California at Los Angeles and author of *Control Your High Blood Preasure* Doubleday, New York.

## SODIUM INTAKE CHART

Latest medical research indicates people stay healthier and are less prone to hypertension when they limit sodium intake to 1,000–5,000 milligrams a day. Sodium content of typical foods:

| | |
|---|---:|
| Thousand Island dressing (1 tablespoon) | 200–350 |
| Apple pie (1 piece) | 450 |
| Cheese spread (1 ounce) | 460 |
| Green beans, canned (4 ounces) | 470 |
| Broccoli, frozen with sauce (3 ounces) | 500 |
| Milk (1 quart) | 500 |
| Cornflakes (2 ounces) | 640 |
| Chicken pot pie (8 ounces) | 950 |
| Baked beans, canned (1 cup) | 1,000 |
| Kosher dill pickle | 600–1,000 |
| Pizza, small (one-half) | 1,500 |
| Big Mac | 1,510 |
| Fried chicken, frozen (12 ounces) | 1,540 |
| Corned beef (4 ounces) | 2,000 |

**Source:** Cleaves M. Bennett, M.D., author of *Control Your High Blood Pressure Without Drugs*, Doubleday, New York.

## TAP-WATER ALERT

People on low-sodium diets should check out tap water as a source of salt intake. Some local water systems have eight times the amount of sodium (20 milligrams per quart) that people with heart problems or hypertension should use.

**Source:** *The Sodium Content of Your Food*, Consumer Information Center, Pueblo, CO.

## DRINKS TO WATCH OUT FOR

If you are trying to limit your sodium intake, you should avoid drinks that include powdered milk (fast-food shakes and prepackaged cocoa, for example). Reconstituted instant milk has at least 300 milligrams of sodium per cup. Also watch: Carbonated drinks. Most bottled mineral waters have 42 mg. per cup, and club soda has 39. Happy surprise: Colas, ginger ale and root beer have 24 or less. But fruit-flavored carbonated drinks tend to be slightly higher. Beer has less than 20 mg. of sodium per eight-ounce cup. Dry wine is also low in sodium. Some other good bets: Coffee, tea and fresh fruit juices.

**Source:** *Shake the Salt Habit* by Dr. Kermit R. Tantum, Ballantine Books, New York.

## BEST SALT SUBSTITUTES

Most commercial products billed as alternatives to salt are based on potassium chloride. Problem: Although potassium chloride does enhance flavor, it leaves a slightly bitter or metallic taste. And excessive potassium may be as bad for your mouth as too much salt. Alternatives to the alternatives...Mrs. Dash, a commercial blend of 14 herbs and spices. Lite Salt, a half-sodium, half-potassium blend.

• In place of salt try savory herbs and spices such as basil, black pepper, coriander, dill seed or cumin, curry powder, marjoram, oregano, onion or garlic, and tarragon. Fresh herbs are preferable to dried because they have a livelier flavor.

# BEST SOURCES OF FIBER

The foods that add fiber to your diet include far more than just bran and whole grains. Researchers are finding that perhaps even more valuable sources of fiber are beans, other vegetables and fruit. Best alternatives in vegetables: Peas, parsnips, potatoes, okra, broccoli, zucchini and summer squash. In beans: Kidney, white, black and pinto. In fruits: Apples, blackberries, pears and strawberries. Other high-fiber foods: Popcorn, sesame seeds.

# HOW YOU COOK HAS A LOT TO DO WITH FIBER CONTENT

How much fiber a food gives you depends considerably on the method of preparation. Leaving the skins on vegetables and fruits enhances their fiber content. Browning bread increases its fiber (which is why crusts have more fiber than the interior of a loaf). Stir-frying or sauteeing vegetables adds fiber more than boiling because less soluble fiber is removed. Deep-frying increases fiber, too, but at great cost in fat and calories. On the other hand, pureeing food decreases fiber, and reducing foods to juice almost completely destroys fiber content.

# THE FIBER/CALCIUM CONNECTION

Dietary fiber can prevent the body from absorbing calcium. Recommended: Eat high-fiber and high-calcium foods at different times.

**Source:** *American Health*, New York.

# BRAN WARNING

Excessive amounts of bran can strip the body of iron. Bran often unites with iron. The iron is thus carried through the body without being absorbed.

**Source:** *The 100% Natural, Purely Organic, Cholesterol-Free, Megavitamin, Low-Carbohydrate Nutrition Hoax* by E. Whalen and F. Stare, Atheneum, New York.

# GOOD NEWS FOR BRAN EATERS

Eating wheat bran raises the levels of HDL cholesterol in the blood, which protects against heart attacks. But . . . large quantities of wheat fiber often cause abdominal discomfort. A new purification technique concentrates the fiber content by removing the phytates responsible for stomach gas and cramping, allowing more people to take advantage of this way to reduce the risk of heart disease.

**Source:** *Human Nutrition*, Westport, CT.

# BEST WHOLE-GRAIN BREAKFAST CEREALS

Whole-grain breakfast cereals are a rich source of protein, vitamins, minerals and fiber. Bonus: They have lower percentages of cholesterol, fat and calories. Added bonus: Often the cheapest cereals are the best nutritionally. What to look for: Cereals in which the first listed ingredient is a whole grain—whole-grain wheat, oats (rolled or flour), whole corn kernels or bran. Buy cereals with three or more grams of protein per serving. Avoid cereals with sugar or other sweeteners (honey, corn syrup, fructose) as a main ingredient. Guide: Four grams of sugar equals one teaspoonful. Also avoid: Cereals with dried fruits. They are concentrated sources of sugar. Best: Add your own fruits.

# ALTERNATIVES TO WHOLE-WHEAT BREAD

Whole wheat isn't necessarily the only nutritious bread. Also healthful: Other whole-grain breads, including pumpernickel, rye and oatmeal. Key: Check the ingredient label on the package. The closer whole-grain flour appears to the top of the list, the more nutrients the bread contains.

**Source:** *Backpacker*, New York.

## BEANS AND SOCIETY

Virtually fat-free and high in protein, vitamins, iron and fiber, beans are a healthful alternative to meat in any diet. People often avoid them, however, because of their reputation for gassy side effects. Culprits: Gas-forming sugars and starches that your body can't digest. Simple solution: Soak beans in water for four to five hours before cooking to leach out the sugars. Simmering the beans in fresh water or broth for one to three hours will break down the offending starches.

**Source:** Nutritionist Bonnie Liebman, Center for Science in the Public Interest, quoted in *Self,* New York.

## CHEAPEST SOURCE OF PROTEIN

The cheapest protein is found in beans. The recommended daily allowance (60 grams) costs only 33¢. Most expensive protein source: Veal cutlets, at $5.55 for 60 grams. Other sources per 60 grams: Peanut butter, 72¢; eggs, 78¢; milk, 84¢; chicken, 96¢; ground beef, $1.32; American processed cheese, $1.41; frankfurters, $1.77; rump roast of beef, $1.80; ocean perch, $1.83; bologna, $2.40; sirloin steak, $2.91.

**Source:** Survey by US Department of Agriculture in *US News & World Report,* New York.

## IDEAL SUBSTITUTE FOR MEAT

Soy products provide complete protein nutrition and can act as a healthful meat substitute. When eight healthy adults ate soy as their exclusive source of protein for 84 days, they suffered no ill effects or body cell-mass deterioration.

**Source:** Study at Massachusetts Institute of Technology, reported in *American Journal of Clinical Nutrition.*

## HEALTH FOOD OF THE FUTURE

Soy milk is nutritious, tastes like a milk-

shake, requires no refrigeration and can be stored indefinitely.

**Source:** *American Health.*

## WHY MEAT EATERS NEED "SEED FOODS"

Eating plant seeds may reduce the risk of breast and colon cancer among those who consume lots of meat. Many seeds contain protease inhibitors, substances that block digestion of the seed itself—and also of meat. Protease inhibitors are found in peas, corn, rice, whole-grain cereals and potatoes.

**Source:** Walter Troll, M.D., professor of environmental medicine, New York University, New York.

## YOU NEED FAT. . .BUT NOT TOO MUCH

• Eating some fat is good for you. Fat insulates the body and pads vital organs. It provides essential fatty acids and transports such fat-soluble vitamins as A, D, E and K from the digestive tract to body tissues. Fat also makes us feel comfortably full after eating.

**Source:** *The 100% Natural, Purely Organic, Cholesterol-Free, Megavitamin, Low-Carbohydrate Nutrition Hoax,* by E. Whalen and F. Stare, Atheneum, New York.

• High-fat diets are directly related to higher blood pressure, according to a recent Finnish study. Patients who stuck to a low-fat diet (and favored polyunsaturated fats * over saturated ones**) showed a steep drop in blood pressure—8.9 points systolic and 7.6 diastolic. When they returned to a typically fatty diet, their pressure climbed back up. Surprise: The study found no correlation between salt intake and blood pressure.

*Vegetable fats such as corn oil, peanut oil and safflower oil.
**Animal fats such as butter, cheese, bacon and lard.

**Source:** *The Lancet,* London, England.

# CHOLESTEROL IS EVEN WORSE THAN YOU THOUGHT

A National Institutes of Health panel recently evaluated the whole body of evidence on cholesterol as a heart attack risk. The task of the panel was to come to some conclusions about how harmful cholesterol really is and what can be done about it. Four key questions answered by the panel are crucial to the health of every American:

*Does high blood cholesterol really cause coronary heart disease?*

Yes—an unequivocal yes.

*Does reducing blood cholesterol actually help prevent heart disease?*

Yes, again. More than a dozen clinical tests have shown a clear trend toward a favorable result when blood cholesterol is lowered. In some tests, the results have been strikingly favorable. The most impressive involved a 7- to 10-year study of 3,800 men with high cholesterol levels who had never had a heart attack or coronary heart disease. Half got a diet and a drug that lowered their cholesterol levels by 20%, and the other half were treated with a diet that lowered their levels by 5%. Those who took the full dose of the drug, combined with the special diet, reduced their risk of heart attack by 50%.

Under what circumstances and at what levels of blood cholesterol should treatment be started?

This was the most important issue the panel studied. The average cholesterol level in the US is much too high. The medical field usually defines normal as being the same as average. But that won't work for cholesterol levels. American cholesterol levels are significantly higher than Japanese levels, for instance. And the heart attack rate in Japan is much lower than ours. This is not due to genes. It's diet that's responsible. Japanese who move to the US and eat an American diet show an increase in both blood cholesterol and heart attack rates. Average blood cholesterol in Japan is 170, while the average here is 210–220. The panel's recommendation: A level no higher than 200 should be the goal for everyone. For men age 40 and over, a cholesterol level of more than 240 should be treated. A level of more than 260 means high risk. Women are ultimately just as vulnerable to coronary heart disease as men—although it doesn't begin to hit them until after menopause.

*Is there a simple answer?*

Yes. Instead of consuming 40% of your calories in fat (the current average), we recommend that no more than 30% should come from fat. Saturated fat (animal fat, butter and coconut oil) should be reduced to no more than 10% of caloric intake. At the moment, it's more like 20% of average. Polyunsaturates, such as vegetable oils, can be increased, but to no more than 10% of the calories in your diet. Even though they're less harmful than saturated fats, it's dangerous to overdo it on corn oil or safflower oil. Cholesterol intake should be limited to 300 milligrams a day or less. (Four ounces of lean meat has about 80 milligrams of cholesterol.)

### How to Change Your Diet

The panel agrees with the standard methods currently recommended by the American Heart Association to lower cholesterol levels. Its principal recommendations:

• Cut down on red meat. Eat only lean cuts, and substitute fish and skinless chicken whenever possible. Avoid bacon and sausage meats.

• Switch from whole milk to low-fat milk and yogurt.

• Avoid hard cheeses, cream cheese and semisoft cheeses. Stick to cottage cheese, ricotta, mozzarella and Parmesan.

• Replace butter and animal fats as much as possible with margarine and polyunsaturated oils—but don't overdo those either.

• Eat no more than two to four egg yolks per week.

• Avoid processed foods made with a lot of saturated fats, especially coconut oil and palm oil.

• Limit fatty salad dressings, gravies and sauces.

It sounds as though it would be very difficult for the American palate to tolerate such a diet, but you don't have to make radical changes right away. Just substituting chicken and fish for steak or hamburger three or four times a week goes a long way toward meeting the dietary requirements. Yogurt can often be used in place of cream and mayonnaise.

We've recommended that manufacturers label the cholesterol content of foods to make cholesterol counting easier. If compliance isn't voluntary, the government should institute regulations that insist on appropriate labeling. It would be very helpful if people could find tasty low-fat foods, and cholesterol labeling would encourage manufacturers to develop such products.

Eventually we'll see a different approach to cuisine. If you've ever eaten in a good Japanese restaurant, you know that low-fat foods can be delicious. The cheese shop in my neighborhood has just started selling a French skim-milk cheese that tastes like real cheese. More low-cholesterol products like that should soon be coming out on the market.

### Other Issues

• Special attention must be given to the management of other known factors that cause heart attacks—high blood pressure, smoking, diabetes and obesity. It seems, however, that cholesterol is the major risk factor. In the study mentioned earlier, heart attack risk was lowered by 50% without modification of smoking habits or anything else. And the Japanese tend to be heavy smokers, with higher blood pressure than ours.

• There is evidence that stress plays a role in heart disease by increasing the cholesterol level. A study was made on the role of adrenalin in raising cholesterol levels. It found that medical students had higher cholesterol levels on the day of the final exam than they had in the middle of the semester.

• We recommend a moderate exercise program, mainly because it helps maintain, or reduce, body weight. However, exercise does not lower cholesterol levels.

**Source:** Interview with Daniel Steinberg, MD and Ph.D. in endocrinology and metabolism. He served as chairman of the Consensus Development Panel of Lowering Blood Cholesterol for the National Institutes of Health and is director of the Specialized Center of Research on Atherosclerosis for the University of California at San Diego.

## YOUR DOCTOR MAY BE WRONG

"Normal" cholesterol levels aren't healthful, according to a recent study of 12,000 middle-aged men. Findings: At a level of 250 (which most doctors consider acceptable), the coronary death rate was 3.6%. But for men with levels below 159, the death rate was less than 1%.

**Source:** Study at Northwestern University reported in *Prevention.*

## THE CHOLESTEROL WAR

Results of an exhaustive, 10-year National Heart, Lung and Blood Institute study have put to rest any doubts about the links between high blood cholesterol levels and heart disease.

For most Americans, careful diet can keep cholesterol in control, particularly the dangerous low-density-lipoprotein (LDL) cholesterol. The American Heart Association recommends that you cut cholesterol consumption to 300 milligrams or less per day. Keep the percentage of calories from fats to 30% or less of the daily intake. Substitute polyunsaturated fats for saturated fats in the diet.

No foods that come from plant sources contain cholesterol. The most concentrated sources of edible cholesterol are egg yolks (one yolk from a large egg has 252 mg) and organ meats (three ounces of calf's liver has 372 mg). Cholesterol counts (in milligrams) of some other common foods:

| | | | |
|---|---|---|---|
| Bacon (2 slices) | 15 | Cottage cheese | |
| Beef (3 oz. lean) | 77 | (½ cup, 4% fat) | 24 |
| Beef kidney (3 oz.) | 315 | Cottage cheese | |
| Butter (1 tbsp.) | 35 | (½ cup, 1% fat) | 12 |
| Cheese (1 oz. cheddar) | 30 | Cream (1 tbsp. heavy) | 21 |
| Chicken (3 oz. light | | Flounder (3 oz.) | 69 |
| meat, no skin) | 65 | Haddock (3 oz.) | 42 |

| | | | |
|---|---|---|---|
| Ice cream (½ cup) | 27 | Salmon (4 oz. canned) | 40 |
| Ice milk (½ cup) | 13 | Sardines (3 oz.) | 119 |
| Milk (1 cup skim) | 5 | Turkey (3 oz. light | |
| Milk (1 cup whole) | 34 | meat, no skin) | 65 |
| Pork (3 oz. lean) | 75 | Yogurt (1 cup lowfat) | 17 |

While many fats per se have no cholesterol content, certain types of fats actually raise the cholesterol levels in the blood even if the rest of the diet contains very little cholesterol. Types of fats:

• Saturated fats. You can recognize these by their tendency to harden at room temperature. They contribute most to a buildup of LDL cholesterol. They include meat fats, butter, chicken fat, coconut and palm oils, vegetable shortening and even some margarines (read the label).

• Monounsaturated fats. These play a more neutral role in cholesterol chemistry, although, like all fats, they should be eaten in moderation. These are the fats found in avocados, cashews, olives and olive oil, peanuts and peanut oil.

• Polyunsaturated fats. When kept to a limited part of the total diet, these actually lower the amount of LDL cholesterol in the blood. Good fats: Corn oil, cottonseed oil, safflower oil, soybean oil, sunflower oil, and fats from nuts such as almonds, pecans and walnuts.

If you are overweight, reducing will lower your cholesterol level. Certain fiber foods such as carrots, apples, oats and soybeans also help reduce cholesterol. Aerobic exercise also can cut down the percentage of LDL cholesterol in the blood.

## FOODS YOU SHOULD BE EATING

Cholesterol fighters: Fiber foods rich in gums (oatmeal and dried beans) and pectin (apples, citrus fruits, green beans, potatoes, cabbage, strawberries and carrots). These fibers bind to the bile acids that digest fats and remove them from the body. Bonus: By coating the stomach, gums and pectin also slow sugar absorption, a special boon to diabetics.

**Source:** *American Health.*

## SHELLFISH UPDATE

Shellfish has considerably less cholesterol than previously assumed, according to new data by the US Department of Agriculture. Example: A 3½-ounce portion of shrimp has only 90 milligrams of cholesterol, well within the American Heart Association's 300-milligram daily limit. Even lower: King crab, American lobster, clams, oysters, scallops and mussels.

## MORE GOOD THINGS TO EAT

Fresh fruits and vegetables help protect you from an early stroke as well as from cancer, a British study showed. Key factor: Vitamin C. Getting the vitamin from foods rather than pills has an added advantage: A diet high in fruits and vegetables is low in sodium. Result: Less hypertension, less chance of a stroke.

**Source:** Research at Cambridge University in *Vegetarian Times.*

## POULTRY CONFIDENTIAL

Poultry is a low-fat, low-calorie food if you eat it "skinless" (the skin adds up to 100 calories per serving)... stick to white meat (dark meat adds up to 50 calories)... cook by roasting, broiling or poaching (deep-frying can add 240 calories).

**Source:** Angelica T. Cantlon, a Connecticut-based nutrition consultant, in *Self* magazine, New York.

• Chicken is still one of the cheapest (and best) sources of protein. It is virtually the same price now as 10 years ago.

## DESSERT TIP

Fruit and cheese are a nutritious (as well as fashionable) dessert combination. Reason: A protein or complex carbohydrate smooths out the highs and lows induced in the body by fruit sugar.

**Source:** *Foods for Healthy Kids* by Dr. Lendon Smith, Berkley Books, New York.

## GOOD NEWS ABOUT ONION AND GARLIC

• Eating onions and garlic can help prevent heart disease. Both these pungent vegetables reduce the blood's tendency to clot. Added benefit: Garlic may be a natural antifungal agent.

**Source:** Joe Graedon, writing in *Medical Self-Care.*

• An onion a day may help prevent heart attack or stroke. Recent research shows that eating raw onions raises levels of high-density lipoprotein, the "good cholesterol" that clears arteries of clogging fats. Best varieties: Yellow or white onions. The mild red ones were not effective. Alternative: Capsules of concentrated onion juice. Cooking, alas, reduces the beneficial chemical activity.

**Source:** Study by Victor Gurewich, M.D., professor of medicine, Tufts University, in *American Health.*

• Garlic is a cholesterol fighter, as well as a first-rate seasoning. As little as a clove or two a day can lower levels of both cholesterol and triglyceride in the blood. What those same cloves can do to a salad dressing or pasta sauce is almost as impressive.

**Source:** Julian M. Whitaker, M.D., director, National Heart and Diabetes Institute, Huntington Beach, CA.

## CHOLESTEROL UPDATE

Early signs of an association between low levels of cholesterol in the blood and cancer seemed to indicate that good preventive medicine against heart disease might bring on cancer. Further research shows that it is the cancer that lowers cholesterol. Bottom line: Limiting fats in the diet (especially saturated animal fats) is still a first line of defense against both heart disease and cancer.

## MEAT MYTH

Fattier cuts of meat contain virtually no more cholesterol than less-marbled cuts,

based on a recent study. Reason: Most of the fat is burned off during cooking.

**Source:** Study at Texas A&M University, College Station.

## SURPRISING TRUTHS ABOUT BEER VS. JOGGING

Three beers a day may control cholesterol as effectively as jogging, according to recent research. Moderate beer imbibing seems to increase the body's high-density lipoprotein (HDL), the type of cholesterol linked with reduced heart disease risk. Moderate exercise also raises HDL levels. The benefits appear to be either/or: Joggers who take up beer drinking do not register higher HDL.

**Source:** Study at Baylor College of Medicine, Houston, reported in *Journal of the American Medical Association.*

## GOOD DIET SUBSTITUTES

Refined grain products: Switch to wholemeal alternatives in bread, pasta, crackers, noodles and rice. Ice cream and milkshakes: Fresh fruit sorbets, frappes and yogurt products. Candy bars: Fresh nuts and dried fruits.

**Source:** *Ultra Health* by Leslie Kenton, Delilah Books, New York.

## NONDAIRY CREAMER WARNING

Nondairy cream substitutes, often used by those on low-fat diets, usually contain coconut oil and have a higher fat content than the dairy product for which they're substituting.

## COCONUT AND PALM OIL TRAP

Avoid coconut and palm oil. They are more saturated than animal fats. Nonspecified vegetable oils frequently mean palm or coconut. When purchasing margarine, choose the brand with liquid vegetable oil as the primary ingredient. It contains less saturated fat.

## WHAT YOU SHOULD KNOW ABOUT OLIVE OIL

Olive oil bonus. Monounsaturated oils (olive and peanut) reduce levels of blood cholesterol even more than polyunsaturated oils (safflower, sunflower, corn and soybean). For a healthier heart: Stick to olive and peanut oils for cooking and salads.

• Olive oil is even better for the heart than once thought. Its monounsaturated fat works as well as polyunsaturated fats to reduce the level of harmful cholesterol—low-density lipoprotein (LDL)—which has been associated with increased risk of heart attacks.

**Source:** *American Health.*

• Olive oil is good for more than salad dressings. It could prevent a heart attack. High consumption of olive oil appears to alter fat composition and lower the rate of coronary disease. Bottom line: In Greece, only nine of 1,000 men between the ages of 40 and 59 develop the disease. In the US, it's 57 in 1,000.

**Source:** Study by the University of Miami School of Medicine and The Institute of Child Health, Athens, quoted in *Glamour* magazine, New York.

## HOW TO STORE VITAMINS

Don't refrigerate vitamins. The supplements will collect moisture, causing them to lose their potency. (And because it absorbs moisture, always remove the cotton that comes in the bottle.) Store vitamins and minerals in a dark, cool, dry place such as a cupboard away from the stove.

## FASTEST WAY TO GET VITAMINS INTO YOUR SYSTEM

Timed-release vitamin supplements are least well absorbed by the body, contrary to popular belief. Best absorbed: Vitamin solutions, followed by chewable tablets and conventional tablets.

**Source:** *Understanding Vitamins and Minerals* by Christine McPartland, Rodale Press, Emmaus, PA.

## EXERCISE MAY MAKE VITAMINS WORK BETTER

Vitamins may work best when supplemented by regular exercise. When two groups were given daily doses of vitamins C and E for two months, there was little change in the immune system of sedentary people. Joggers, however, experienced a significant increase in immunity.

**Source:** *Sports without Pain* by Ben E. Benjamin, Summit Books, New York.

## VITAMIN DEPLETERS

Smoking: Drains up to 40% of vitamin C supplies. Alcohol: $B_1$, $B_6$, $B_{12}$ and C. Steroids: Calcium. Antibiotics and oral contraceptives: B vitamins. Strict vegetarianism: $B_{12}$.

**Source:** *Understanding Vitamins and Minerals* by Christine McPartland and Patsy Vigderman, Rodale Press, Emmaus, PA.

## OVERDOSING ON VITAMINS

The old advice is still the best—there is no reason to take more than the recommended dietary allowance (RDA) of any vitamin, except for relatively rare individuals who cannot absorb or utilize vitamins adequately.

A megadose is 10 or more times the RDA. This is the level at which toxic effects begin to show up in adults. Even in cases of actual vitamin insufficiency, megadoses are not generally prescribed. Therapeutic doses are generally smaller than 10 times the RDA.

Vitamins are becoming more popular because of a combination of successful merchandising by manufacturers in so-called health magazines, faddism, misinformation, and questionable practices by some professionals.

Most persuasive to hard-nosed executives are enthusiastic testimonials from other executives who have been persuaded by the placebo effect of vitamins that megadoses really do make them feel better.

Some of the medical problems adults may experience as a result of prolonged, excessive intake are:

• Vitamin A. Dry, cracked skin. Severe headaches. Severe loss of appetite. Irritability. Bone and joint pains. Menstrual difficulties. Enlarged liver and spleen.

• Vitamin D. Loss of appetite. Excessive urination. Nausea and weakness. Weight loss. Hypertension. Anemia. Irreversible kidney failure that can lead to death.

• Vitamin E. Research on E's toxic effects is sketchy, but the findings suggest some problems: Headaches, nausea, fatigue and giddiness, blurred vision, chapped lips and mouth inflammation, low blood sugar, increased tendency to bleed, reduced sexual function. Ironically, one of the claims of Vitamin E proponents is that it heightens sexual potency.

• The B vitamins. Each B has its own charactersistics and problems. Too much $B_6$ can lead to liver damage. Too much $B_1$, can destroy $B_{12}$.

• Vitamin C. Kidney problems and diarrhea. Adverse effects on growing bones. Rebound scurvy (a condition that can occur when a person taking large doses suddenly stops). Symptoms are swollen, bleeding gums, loosening of teeth, roughening of skin, muscle pain.

Vitamin C is the vitamin most often used to excess. Some of the symptoms of toxic effect from Vitamin C megadoses:

• Menstrual bleeding in pregnant women and various problems for their newborn infants.

• Destruction of Vitamin $B_{12}$, to the point that $B_{12}$ deficiency may become a problem.

• False negative test for blood in stool, which can prevent diagnosis of colon cancer.

• False urine test for sugar, which can spell

trouble for diabetics.

• An increase in the uric acid level and the precipitation of gout in individuals predisposed to the ailment.

Better than vitamin pills are:

• Four portions a day of grains (either cereal, bread or pasta).

• Four portions of fruits and vegetables (including at least one fresh fruit or vegetable or fruit juice).

• Two or three glasses of milk, or portions of milk products.

• Two portions of meat, fish, poultry, eggs, dry beans, peas or nuts.

For people who don't eat properly or want nutritional insurance, take a regular multivitamin capsule containing only the RDA of vitamins.

**Source:** Victor Herbert, *Nutrition Cultism: Facts and Fictions,* George F. Stickley Co., Philadelphia.

## TOO MUCH VITAMIN A AND D

Unlike some vitamins (the Bs and C) that are passed out of the body through the kidneys when taken in excess, vitamins A and D are stored in fat and the liver, where they can do damage. Problems from overdoses: Cirrhosis of the liver. Dry, itchy skin. Fatigue. Painful muscles. Loss of body hair. Note: A deficiency of vitamin A is believed related to the onset of cancer. But there is no evidence that increased amounts help prevent this disease. Best: Eat a balanced diet. Limit supplementary intake to the recommended daily dietary allowances.

**Source:** *The Health Letter.*

## GOOD SUNLIGHT SUBSTITUTES

Artificial vitamin D is just as beneficial as the natural vitamin derived from sunlight. Good sunlight substitutes: Fortified dairy products, vitamin D tablets, multivitamins and cod liver oil. For people with dietary restrictions, only 20–30 minutes of daily sunlight exposure is needed to maintain strong bones.

**Source:** Michael Hollich, M.D., Harvard Medical School Vitamin Research Laboratory.

# VITAMIN E SECRET

Natural vitamins are generally no better for you than synthetic vitamins. Reason: They are used by the body in identical ways. Possible exception: Natural vitamin E. Telling the difference: In vitamin E, the principal active compound is listed on the label (usually right under the product name) as d-tocopherol for the natural vitamin—but as dl-tocopherol for the synthetic.

**Source:** *Understanding Vitamins and Minerals* by Christine McPartland and Patsy Vigderman, Rodale Press, Emmaus, PA.

# B₆ ALERT

Those one-gram $B_6$ tablets sold in health stores can be dangerous. The body needs only one or two milligrams of $B_6$ a day. Overdoses may lead to loss of sensory and motor control.

**Source:** *New England Journal of Medicine*, Boston, MA.

# TWO GOOD THINGS THAT DON'T GO TOGETHER

Vitamin C and aspirin should not be taken together. Studies at the University of Southern Illinois indicate that combined heavy doses produce excessive stomach irritations which could lead to ulcers (especially for those with a history of stomach problems).

# AGING STRATEGY

Vitamin C may help slow the aging process, doctors now believe. Mechanism: Vitamin C seems to combat oxidation (considered by many the basis of aging) at the cellular level. Note: Vitamin E also retards aging,

but, unlike Vitamin C, it can be harmful if taken in excess.

**Source:** *New Scientist.*

# BEWARE CHEWABLE VITAMIN C

Chewable vitamin C is taken by millions of Americans in the hope of preventing colds. Hidden danger: Chewing the vitamin creates an acid imbalance in the mouth that erodes tooth enamel, particularly in the rear of the mouth. Excessive vitamin C in some fruit juices can create the same situation. Better: Vitamin C that's swallowed without being chewed.

**Source:** *Medical Tribune.*

# GOOD SOURCE OF VITAMIN C

Kohlrabi, a vegetable with a bulblike stem and turniplike leaves, is a good source of vitamin C. Bonus: One cup cooked is only 40 calories. Taste: Somewhere between turnip and cabbage. What to look for: Unblemished bulbs two to three inches in diameter. If leaves (usually not eaten) are left on, they shouldn't be wilted. Preparation: Bulbs can be sliced and boiled, added to soups and stews or served raw.

# TRACE MINERAL SUPPLEMENTS

Sometimes these supplements can be dangerous. Reason: These elements are in delicate balance in your body. It's easy to overdose, and an excess of one can lead to a deficiency of another. Better: Eat foods rich in these nutrients. Examples: Meat, liver and eggs (zinc and selenium). Oysters, nuts and chocolate (copper). Brown rice, tea and coffee (manganese).

**Source:** *Glamour*, New York.

## TO ABSORB MORE IRON

The iron in food is absorbed better when you eat foods rich in vitamin C at the same meal. Iron blockers: Tea, antacids, dietary fiber supplements.

**Source:** *The Washington Post.*

## MAGNESIUM LOSS AND DIURETICS

Magnesium loss is a frequent problem for people on diuretics (drugs to prevent water retention). This leads to changes in blood fats, which in turn increase the risk of heart disease. Magnesium supplements may be indicated. Food sources of magnesium include leafy green vegetables, nuts, cereals and seafood.

**Source:** *South African Medical Journal.*

## IF YOU DON'T GET ENOUGH ZINC

Zinc deficiency can lead to loss of appetite, diminished smell and taste, and delayed healing. Best: Eat a balanced diet. Liver, red meat and shellfish are very high in zinc. Other sources: Dairy products, soybeans, peas, corn, carrots, peanuts and lima beans. Avoid zinc supplements not prescribed by a doctor. They can create hazardous body imbalances.

**Source:** *Self*, New York.

## IF YOU GET TOO MUCH ZINC

Too much zinc can cause undesirable and potentially dangerous lowering of HDL, the high-density lipoprotein that helps to protect against the dangers of cholesterol. Right dosage: No more than 50 milligrams of zinc sulfate daily. Note: This dosage applies only to zinc sulfate, not to other zinc salts such as zinc gluconate. Reasons for taking zinc: To improve immunity, strengthen bones and preserve taste, smell and hearing.

**Source:** *US Pharmacist*, New York.

## KELP ALERT

Kelp is believed by many to help the bones heal faster. But those who overindulge in kelp tablets risk arsenic poisoning. And kelp is so rich in iodine compounds that prolonged use can affect the thyroid, causing metabolic disorders.

**Source:** *The 100% Natural, Purely Organic, Cholesterol-Free, Megavitamin, Low-Carbohydrate Nutrition Hoax* by E. Whalen and F. Stare, Atheneum, New York.

## TRUTHS ABOUT CALCIUM SUPPLEMENTS

Calcium supplements won't work if taken under the wrong conditions. Example: Calcium carbonate (the most common supplement) is absorbed by an empty stomach only in the presence of stomach acid. But in many older people, gastric acids may diminish or even shut off entirely. Solution: Always take calcium carbonate with a meal.

**Source:** *New England Journal of Medicine*, Boston, MA.

• Calcium supplements of bone meal and dolomite have high lead levels that can be injurious to the very young and the elderly, according to the FDA. Most vulnerable: Children allergic to milk who are prescribed heavy doses (10 grams a day). Also susceptible: Pregnant women. The lead from the supplements passes through the placenta to affect the fetus. The elderly who take calcium supplements to offset bone loss are putting themselves in double jeopardy. Lead is already being released as the bones undergo a natural breakdown. Safe doses: Five grams a day taken by adults who are neither pregnant, nursing nor elderly.

**Source:** *American Health.*

## TWO OPINIONS ON THE BEST TIME TO TAKE CALCIUM

Calcium supplements are best absorbed in small amounts and should be spaced throughout the day. Save one–third of your daily dose for bedtime, since the body loses more calcium when you sleep. Otherwise, take the tablets between meals, ideally with milk or yogurt. Recommended variety: Calcium carbonate, which is the least expensive and is tolerated well by most people.

**Source:** *Medical Self-Care.*

• Calcium supplements do the most good when taken at bedtime. Reason: Skeletal calcium tends to be drawn on more at night, when no food is being eaten. For maximum absorption: Have a glass of milk or some yogurt before taking the supplement.

**Source:** Martin Notelovitz, M.D., professor of obstetrics and gynecology at the University of Florida, Gainesville, in *Prevention*, Emmaus, PA.

## HOW TO GET MORE CALCIUM INTO YOUR MEALS

• Add a small amount of vinegar when-preparing homemade soup from bones. This will dissolve calcium out of the bones, and the vinegar taste will be eliminated in cooking.
• Substitute grated or shredded cheese (Parmesan is particularly good) for butter on vegetables.
• Use dark-green lettuce leaves in salads.
• Pickle fruits and vegetables with calcium chloride rather than with salt.
• Add powdered nonfat dry milk to skim milk, cream soups, casseroles and baked items. You'll get added flavor and calcium without extra fat.

**Source:** *Medical Self-Care.*

## WHY YOU SHOULDN'T TRUST HAIR ANALYSIS

Hair analysis to detect nutritional deficiencies is unreliable. Reason: The results can be distorted by sweat, shampoo, dust and beauty treatments. Further, it's debatable whether the amount of a substance in the hair truly reflects the amount elsewhere in the body. (Hair analysis may have some value in detecting toxic metals.)

**Source:** *Harvard Medical Health Letter.*

## YOU ARE WHAT YOU EAT

Obesity is the greatest nutritional problem in the US today. Estimate: 30% of all Americans exceed their desirable weight. One child in three is overweight.

**Source:** *The 100% Natural, Purely Organic, Cholesterol-Free, Megavitamin, Low-Carbohydrate Nutrition Hoax* by E. Whalen and F. Stare, Atheneum, New York.

• Excessively thin people may have a much higher death rate than their normal-weight counterparts. When adjusted for other risk factors, a recent study shows that the death rate was 63% higher among a large group of thin women than of women with average weight. It's 45% higher for thin men. Other findings: Death from cancer is significantly greater in thin people. . .and the greater the weight loss from maximum adult weight (not associated with illness), the greater the increase in the death statistics.

**Source:** *Cardiovascular News*, New York.

## NUTRIENT DENSITY MATH

To calculate nutrient density (the ratio of nutrients to calories): (1) Add the total percentages of the US Recommended Daily Allowances per serving for the first eight nutrients listed on the label. (2) Divide this total by the number of calories per serving. (3) Multiply by 100 to obtain a percentage reading. The minimal score for good nutritional value is 32—but the higher the better.

**Source:** *Modern Maturity*, New York.

## HOW YOUR THYROID AFFECTS YOUR WEIGHT

Common misconception: That an underactive thyroid can cause obesity. This is virtually impossible. Reason: The thyroid regulates the interaction of body metabolism and appetite. If the thyroid is underactive, appetite will not be great enough to create obesity. About 99% of people with an underactive thyroid are not overweight. Dangerous: Thyroid hormone to treat obesity. An excessive amount can induce hyperthyroidsim, causing severe side effects such as an overworked heart, muscle breakdown and psychological changes.

**Source:** Norbert Freinkel, M.D., Kettering professor of medicine and director of the Center for Endocrinology, Metabolism and Nutrition at Northwestern University Medical School.

## WEIGHT LOSS OPERATION SOME MDs WANT TO HAVE STOPPED

Intestinal bypass surgery for weight loss should be stopped. Reason: Danger of complications. They include liver failure, bone disease and nervous-system disorders. Causes: Metabolic changes following the operation and possible toxin buildup in the bypassed intestine.

**Source:** *Journal of the American Medical Association*, Chicago, IL.

## DIET PILL WARNING

Diet pills can be dangerous to the health of those who use them. Scientists have linked phenylpropanolamine, the principal ingredient of over-the-counter diet pills, with high blood pressure, seizures, kidney problems, irregular heartbeats and cerebral hemorrhages. Focus: Although these findings affect the entire American public, older women are most at risk. They're the greatest users of diet products and are already among the most susceptible to these risks.

## DIET MYTH

Spirulina, a blue-green algae, contains amino acids that suppress the appetite. Fact:

The amino acids in question are found in all high-quality proteins. There is no medical evidence that they reduce hunger. Better appetite curb: A large glass of water before meals.

**Source:** Christina Stark, nutritionist, division of nutritional sciences, Cornell University, Ithaca, NY.

## FAT FIGHTER THAT DOESN'T HURT YOUR APPETITE

On its way—a history-making drug that slims down dangerously obese adults. Situation: 80 million Americans are overweight—and nearly half of those are so overweight that their health is threatened. Obese people are especially vulnerable to diabetes, arthritis, hernias, arteriosclerosis, hypertension, kidney disease and cirrhosis of the liver. Most medications that attack obesity aim to suppress the appetite, usually with little success.

Better way: New drug mimics the effects of exercise on the body's metabolism by burning up fat. Taking the drug for a week or two effects no visible changes. . . but on a continuing basis allows an overweight person to lose weight gradually until proper body weight is achieved. The drug then ceases to be effective, and the attending physician discontinues the treatment. Forecast: The drug—sold by prescription only—will capture a large share of over $500 million spent on weight-loss aids every year.

**Source:** Roche, a division of Hoffman LaRoche, Nutley, NJ.

## BEFORE TAKING YOUR DIET TOO SERIOUSLY

Consider writer Franny Shuker's advice:
• If no one sees you eat it, it has no calories.
• If you drink a diet soda with a candy bar, they cancel out each other.
• When eating with someone else, calories don't count if you both eat the same amount of food.
• Food used for medicinal purposes never counts: Hot chocolate, brandy, toast, Sara

Lee cheesecake.

• If you fatten up everybody around you, you'll look thinner.

• Movie-related foods don't count because they're simply part of the entertainment experience, not part of one's personal fuel (Milk Duds, popcorn, Junior Mints).

## BEST TIME OF DAY TO EAT

Diets work better when you eat more of your food early in the day. When six people consumed food worth 2,000 calories for breakfast and none for the rest of the day, they lost an average of 2.2 pounds in one week. But when they ate the same amount of food exclusively at dinnertime, four gained weight after a week and two lost relatively little. Theory: Calories consumed early in the day are more likely to be converted to energy than stored as fat.

**Source:** Study by Frank Halberg, Ph.D., University of Minnesota, cited in *The Health Letter.*

## WINTER DIETING

Complex carbohydrates and low-fat proteins will keep you warm and provide needed energy. Good meal: A vegetable soup and salad. Ideal food: Pasta, at only 200 calories per cup.

Eat less food, but more often; you'll generate more constant heat by snacking between meals. Ground rules: Limit each snack to 150 calories, and don't eat late at night. (That's when your body stores fat.)

Sleep in a cold bedroom. You'll burn up calories just by maintaining body heat all night.

**Source:** *Harper's Bazaar,* New York.

## WEIGHT LOSS AND YOUR HEART

Dieters should lose no more than two pounds a week, doctors say. To plan a weight-loss program: Calculate the number of calories required each day to maintain your present weight. (Multiply your weight by 15 for a rough estimate.) Then cut that count by 1,000.

**Source:** Association of Heart Patients.

## HOW TO DIET LESS AND LOSE MORE

The diet naturally just doesn't work when it comes to long-term weight loss. The straitjacket approach will probably backfire as soon as you go off the strict regimen. To be successful, you have to analyze your eating habits and change them gradually.

### Raise Your Food Consciousness

First, look at what's going on when you're eating. Awareness is all-important. Start keeping a daily food diary, and review it after a week:

• Where did you eat? Do you have food stashed in your car's glove compartment, in your nightstand and in your desk at work? Maybe you eat in too many places. Best: Keep food only in the kitchen.

• What position were you in while eating? Do you eat while standing up in the kitchen, lying in bed, sitting in front of the TV or at your office desk? Learn to eat only when sitting at the table.

• With whom did you eat? Food can be a crutch for social interactions such as business lunches or family dinners. If you pinpoint such times, you can learn to deal with them.

• What was your emotional state while eating? Where you feeling anger, stress, etc.? Did you feel the need for security, protection or comfort? Find out what food means to you.

• Were there any visual cues associated with eating? Some of us eat when the clock says noon, rather than waiting until we're hungry. If you eat at noon every day, put lunch off for half an hour and see what happens.

• What was your eating style? Paradoxically, many overeaters don't really savor their food. They gulp it down quickly, as if they wanted to get the process over with. Practice eating slowly. Taste each bite and savor each flavor. If you pace your eating, you'll consume less but enjoy it more.

• Did any practical factors influence your eating? Were you late for work, missed breakfast in the process? Did you eat an enormous lunch instead? Did you overeat when you came home from work because you were too busy for lunch? Rearrange your schedule to permit planned, unhurried meals.

### Making Realistic Changes

After you become aware of how, when and why you eat, start making some behavioral changes in ways that you find most comfortable:

• Don't avoid food—manage it. There are no "good" foods or "bad" foods. You can eat small amounts of those favorite foods of yours that are forbidden by traditional diets—but be in control.

• Pay attention to portion size. We tend to use restaurant-portion sizes as a gauge. But restaurants serve much larger portions, especially of entrees, than most people really need. Suggested portions: Three ounces of meat, fish or chicken, rather than the customary six to eight ounces.

• Pay attention to quality. You might be just as satisfied with one small piece of Swiss chocolate as with two cheap candy bars. Half a glass of really fine wine goes a long way. A tablespoonful of real Vermont maple syrup on French toast is a pleasant substitute for drowning it in an inexpensive syrup. Develop a discriminating palate. Bonus: Quality foods will make you feel you're treating, rather than depriving yourself.

• Keep in mind that spices don't have calories. Use garlic, pepper, vinegar, curry and other herbs and spices liberally and creatively to add sparkle to your meals.

• Be creative. Today's markets offer a multitude of products that are low in calories even though they're not in the diet-foot section. Suggestions: Exotic fruits and vegetables. Whole-grain bread products (they're tasty, and they have more fiber and fewer calories than white bread).

• Make imaginative substitutions. For example, vanilla yogurt flavored with cinnamon and nutmeg is as good as fruit yogurt and has 50 fewer calories. Half an English muffin with mozzarella cheese and tomato sauce toasted under the broiler is a delicious pizza substitute.

### What to Expect

A weight loss of one to two pounds a week is very good. But success isn't measured only by the absolute amount of weight lost. Your physical health can improve from eating better foods, and your emotional health can improve by dealing with the source of your overeating. Example: If you're overeating out of frustration, begin dealing with the source of frustration rather than simply placating yourself with food.

We don't all have to be (and really shouldn't be) bone thin. Being 10-15 pounds overweight isn't necessarily unhealthy. And the stress from constantly going on and off diets may be a lot worse for your body than the extra weight itself.

**Source:** Interview with Janet K. Grommet, a doctor of nutrition and administrator of the weight control unit at St. Luke's Hospital Center, New York.

# PERILS OF CRASH DIETS

Crash diets actually make people fatter in the long run. Reason: When dieters consume fewer than 1,200 calories a day, they lose muscle tissue as well as fat. If they go far enough below that level, their percentage of body fat will increase, even though their weight may go down.

**Source:** *Berkeley Wellness Letter*, Berkeley, CA.

• Repeated crash dieting can increase the chance of heart disease. The faster weight is lost from the body, the faster it tends to go back on. It is this rapid accumulation of weight that results in higher levels of blood cholesterol. Quick weight gain also accelerates the rate at which cholesterol is deposited in the blood vessels.

**Source:** *The 100% Natural, Purely Organic, Cholesterol Free, Megavitamin, Low-Carbohydrate Nutrition Hoax* by E. Whalen and F. Stare, Atheneum, New York.

• Crash diets impair the immune system response and make dieters more vulnerable to infection. Special danger: Surgery patients with poor nutrition have a much higher rate of postoperative infections.

**Source:** Peter Lindner, M.D., director of continuing medical education, American Society of Bariatric Physicians, in *Prevention*, Emmaus, PA.

## WHO NEEDS A VERY LOW CALORIE DIET?

Very low-calorie diets (under 500 calories a day) are still risky propositions—even if they include carbohydrates, mineral supplements and high-quality protein. Mortality rate of such diets: 0.3%. Bottom line: These diets should be tried only be people with serious obesity (more than 30% above ideal weight), and then only under medical supervision.

**Source:** *New England Journal of Medicine*, Boston, MA.

## LOW CARBOHYDRATE DIETS

Low carbohydrate diets do not curb appetite better than the more balanced reducing diets. In a recent experiment, subjects on a 1% carbohydrate diet were compared with a control group on a 29% carbohydrate regime. Both ate equal amounts of protein (35% of their daily intake), but the low-carbohydrate subjects received 64% of their calories in fat while the others had 36% fat. There was no difference in how full or satisfied either group felt.

**Source:** Study by J. C. Rosen and others in *American Journal of Clinical Nutrition*, New York.

• Fad diets such as the Scarsdale, Atkins or Stillman are based on few carbohydrates (breads, potatoes and other starches). The emphasis is on other proteins, which the body burns for energy. Weight loss in the first weeks of low carbohydrate diets is due to water flushed out of the body.

## ALL ABOUT FAD DIETS

The trouble with the sensible approach to dieting is that it just doesn't work for most people. That's why each new fad diet, no matter how bizarre, is enthusiastically taken up by desperate dieters. Some of the fad diets are basically harmless, but others can do a great deal of harm if followed for very long. If science knew the answer to weight control, we'd put the faddists out of business overnight. But, as long as there is no safe yet easy way to lose weight, Americans are bound to keep going on fad diets. To protect yourself, it pays to know what each of the fad diets is all about.

• The Cambridge Diet is an extremely low-calorie liquid diet. (The FDA has issued a warning about it.) Whether there's any difference between 300 calories a day and starvation is a matter of debate. The Cambridge resembles the previously popular liquid protein diet, which caused some unexplained deaths. There's no doubt you'll lose weight on the Cambridge, but the evidence so far suggests that it's not entirely safe. Also: It doesn't give you anything to rely on in the long term. Recommended: If you do go on the diet, follow it for no more than two weeks at a time.

• The University Diet is essentially the same as the Cambridge, except that it applies only to lunch. You eat a relatively low-calorie diet for the rest of the day. If this helps you diet, it's a reasonable approach.

• The Scarsdale Diet isn't so bad. It's a reasonably low-calorie diet—though quite expensive. It has more protein than you need, making it more palatable than a lot of other diets. If you stick to it, it will work, because it comes to about 1,000 calories a day. No deviations are permitted. The foods allowed are tasty. If you're not concerned about money, this is a fairly acceptable diet.

• The Atkins Diet is a very high-fat, high-protein, low-carbohydrate diet. The objective is to produce ketosis, a bodily state that may be dangerous to normal people and is dangerous to diabetics. Ketosis will probably inhibit your appetite and make you feel somewhat ill. If you follow the Atkins, you'll almost certainly lose weight. But the diet's high fat content will increase your susceptibility to atherosclerosis and other diseases. This diet is not recommended.

• The Stillman Diet, a little like the Atkins, is essentially a high-protein diet with limited fat and carbohydrates. Stillman argues that digesting a lot of protein will burn off calories without converting them into fat. This very bizarre diet is certainly not well balanced nutritionally. I think it's an unwise choice.

• The Beverly Hills Diet is utterly ridiculous—a sure formula for malnutrition if followed for very long. The diet consists solely of fruit, eaten according to precise instructions. The book is absolute nonsense, laced with factual errors.

• The Pritikin Diet is essentially a vegetarian diet, very low in fat, sugar and salt. Originally designed to treat heart patients, it's reasonably well balanced and would, I believe, decrease your risk of heart disease, cancer and hypertension. Problem: It's very extreme. You must develop a whole new way of life to stay on it. Although it makes sense, I don't think it provides much of a solution for the long run. Most people would rather take their chances on a heart attack than live on the Pritikin Diet.

• The Never-Say-Diet Diet by Richard Simmons is primarily an exercise book by an author who's more interested in exercise than in diet. He gives a low-calorie diet that's also low in fat, cholesterol and salt. While the dietary instructions are reasonable, the book is intended mainly as promotion for his TV program.

### Why Diets Don't Work

All diets work for a few weeks, but most are simply too hard to adapt to the way we want to live. Statistics indicate that only 2%–5% of the people who go on diets keep the weight off for more than a year. Practically no diet works in the long run for most people, including the sensible diets. When it comes to fad diets, the built-in boredom factor is a blessing because it keeps people from staying on the diet long enough to harm themselves.

### Suggestions

• Don't go on any nutritionally unbalanced fad diet for more than two weeks at a stretch.

• Develop a diet that fits into your personal lifestyle. If a diet doesn't suit you, you won't stay on it.

• Try to go on a balanced diet that substantially reduces fat. Reason: Fat, the richest source of calories, influences the incidence of heart disease, cancer and stroke.

• Be aware that the latest research suggests that moderate obesity and middle-age spread have been overemphasized as a health hazard. Real risk factors: High cholesterol and high blood pressure.

• Avoid the seesaw syndrome. The evidence suggests that constantly losing weight and then regaining it is unhealthier than staying somewhat overweight.

**Source:** Interview with D. M. Hegsted, Ph.D., professor emeritus of nutrition, Harvard School of Public Health.

## BLACKMAIL DIET

A new road to weight loss, recently refined by author/psychologist John Bear, is to create a situation where you dare not fail. Keys: Pick a reasonable goal, devise an appropriate penalty (painful enough really to motivate you), and select a reliable trustee who won't allow you to wriggle out at the last minute. In Bear's case, he put $5,000 into a trust fund, payable to the American Nazi Party, if he failed to lose 70 pounds in a year. Result: He lost the weight.

## ALL ABOUT CRAIG CLAIBORNE'S DIET

When my doctor put me on a no-salt, modified fat, cholesterol and sugar diet, with limited alcohol consumption, I feared I would feel in a gastronomic straitjacket. Although he did say it would be acceptable to indulge in forbidden foods occasionally, it was a drastic change for someone who was a salt addict and who loves eggs, sausages and other high-sodium, high-cholesterol food.

I have found, however, that not only have the benefits been enormous—no more edema, a reduction in blood pressure, considerable weight loss and a feeling of well-being—but that I have also increased my food intake without increasing my weight. Other revelations: My sense of taste is much sharper. Foods to which no salt has been added are just as satisfying, if well prepared, as the foods I used to enjoy.

### Basics of My Diet

Do's:

• Low-sodium cheeses.

• Seltzer.

• Trim meat well.

• Skim all fat from the surface of stews and pan drippings.

• Use fish, poultry without skin, veal and lamb.

Don'ts:

• No eggs, except those used in food preparation.

• No added sugar, no drinks made with sweet liqueurs, no soft drinks.

• No canned or packaged foods or sodas with high salt content.

• No rich and/or salty products—bacon, gravies, shellfish, organ meats, most desserts except fruit and fruit ices.

• No salt added to food cooked at home.

### Tricks to Fool the Taste

Substitutions: If you leave out salt or fat, you must add something to compensate. Not all substitutions work. For example: I never could make oysters, which are lower in cholesterol than clams, satisfactorily stand in for clams in a sauce for linguine.

Pitfalls: You cannot use large quantities of herbs, spices, lemon or vegetables with a strongly assertive flavor. An excess of any of these can become tedious or overpowering. Try for a compensation in flavors while retaining a natural balance. Winners:

• The sweet-and-sour principle. A touch (sometimes as little as half a teaspoonful) of sugar and a dash of vinegar can add the sweet-and-sour flavor needed to fool the palate.

• Garlic. Essential in salad dressings and tomato sauces. Use it with rosemary to transform broiled chicken, broiled fish or roast lamb.

• Fine or coarse black pepper. When broiling and roasting meats and chicken, use as much as a tablespoonful for a welcome flavor. Use a moderate amount in soups, stews and casseroles (the pungent nature of pepper will not diminish in these as it will with broiling and roasting).

• Crushed hot red pepper flakes. A good flavor distraction or flavor addition. Not for every palate.

• Curry powder. Use judiciously and without a large number of other spices. Combine it only with a bay leaf, green pepper, garlic or black pepper. Add smaller amounts for rice, more for poultry or meat.

• Chili powder. Similar to curry, but you might want to add more cumin, oregano or garlic. Also try paprika, ground coriander, ground hot chilis. They're good with almost any dish made with tomatoes.

• Homemade hot-mustard paste. Dry mustard and water does wonders for salad dressing and grilled foods.

• Freshly grated horseradish. Goes well with fish or plain yogurt.

• Bottled green peppercorns. A welcome touch for bland foods.

### Accompaniments

Plain boiled or steamed rice, cold yogurt relish, chutneys and other sweet relishes are a good foil for spicy dishes. Sweet or sweet-and-sour relish complements simple food.

### Cooking Techniques

• Charcoal broiling: The flavor of charcoal helps compensate for lack of salt.

• Steaming: Preferable for fish and better than boiling for vegetables.

• No-salt soups: They are difficult to make palatable. Solution: A stockpot going on the back of the stove, to which you add bones, cooking liquid, vegetables. The more concentrated the broth, the greater the depth of flavor. Use only the freshest, ripest vegetables.

### Cheating

I like a frozen ice to end a meal. I make it with a considerable amount of sugar, but a small spoonful is enough to satisfy me.

Good judgment will save you from anxiety. I would not eat a stalk of raw celery or a serving of braised celery. Celery is high in sodium. But I would add a cupful of chopped celery to a Creole dish because the added sodium per portion would be very low.

### My Typical Meals

*Breakfast:* Grapefruit or melon, shredded wheat with a sliced banana and skimmed milk, tea without milk or sugar.

*Lunch:* An apple with plain yogurt, a sandwich made of no-salt French bread, low-sodium mayonnaise with leftover lamb or chicken, and no-salt-added buttermilk or seltzer. Alternatives: A low-salt soup and salad, a grilled chop, steamed fish or a veal patty.

*Dinner alone:* Broiled chicken, lamb chops, paillarde of veal or steamed fish with a light sauce. Vegetables: Spinach, tomato or couchet (tomato and shredded vegetables) and a salad with a light dressing. Dessert: Fruit.

*Dinner with guests:* Menus are built around dishes prepared without salt and with reduced amounts of fat and sugar. I put a salt cellar on the table, but guests rarely add salt to the food I serve.

*Snacks:* Fruit, a glass of no-salt-buttermilk.

**Source:** Interview with Craig Claiborne, food writer for *The New York Times.*

## TIPS FOR THE BEGINNING OF A DIET

The first week of a diet often makes the dieter feel weak, tired, even slightly nauseated. This passes by the second week. To help you through the bad time: Be sure the diet has sufficient salt (lack of salt causes depres-

sion) and potassium. If your diet is salt-free to speed off the pounds, add a pinch. You may lose weight more slowly. But you have a better chance of staying on the diet.

**Source:** *How to Eat Like a Thin Person,* by L. Dusky and J.J. Leedy, M.D., Simon & Schuster, New York.

## 5 PROVEN DIETING TIPS

When you feel the urge for something sweet, take a bite of pickle or lemon. Neither has any calories to speak of, and the sour taste will curb your craving. Another ploy: Brush your teeth. Nothing tastes good after that.

**Source:** *Stop Killing Yourself* by Susan Seliger, G.P. Putnam's Sons, New York.

• Put your fork down between bites, and sip water frequently during the meal. Stop eating for a full minute halfway through the meal. Then decide whether you are still actually hungry. Eat two–thirds of your normal portion, treating the rest as optional seconds.

**Source:** *Breaking the Diet Habit* by Janet Polivy and C. Peter Herman, Basic Books, New York.

• Eat some raw vegetables or fruit 30–40 minutes before your next meal to take the edge off your hunger. Choose foods that take time to consume (such as a clear soup) and eat with small utensils.

• Dieters can break the habit of eating when they are bored by keeping a list of projects and errands on the refrigerator door. Substituting constructive activity for eating can cut calorie intake and produce a feeling of accomplishment.

• Background music can help a dieter eat less at dinner. Reason: Soft, mellow tones tend to slow the meal. Then the stomach will have enough time to signal the brain that it's full.

**Source:** Stanley Title, M.D., of the Clinic for Weight Control quoted in *New Woman*, New York.

## WHITE WINE VS. RED

White wines have about the same number of calories as red wines. The chief caloric component of wine is alcohol, which runs between 11% and 14%. A five-ounce serving of any table wine generally contains about 110 calories. A half bottle contains slightly less than 300.

**Source:** Alexic Bespaloff, author of *The New Signet Book of Wine,* New American Library, New York.

## BEER MAY BE BETTER FOR YOU THAN APPLE JUICE

A 12-ounce bottle of beer contains 150 calories. That's fewer than in 12 ounces of apple juice (174) or milk (240). And light beers have only 75–100 calories. Beer's carbonation helps make the stomach feel fuller, turning off hunger signals. And, by soothing the mind and senses, it reduces nervous eating.

**Source:** *The I-Like-My-Beer Diet* by Martin R. Lipp, M. Evans & Co., New York.

## HELP FROM THE LABORATORY

Miracle molecules are fat enough to keep you thin. Polymers are molecules too big to be absorbed through the walls of the intestines. Molecules that can't be absorbed by the body can't be stored as excess fat, either. Unwanted additives that are bonded to such molecules also pass right through the system. Example: Polydextrose is a polymer with the texture and weight of sugar but only one-fourth the calories. Approved by the Federal Drug Administration, it is combined with artificial sweeteners and used in low-calorie baked goods, puddings, frozen desserts and candies. In ice cream, it reduces the need for both sugar and fats, cutting calories two ways. Other polymers under study: Polyvinyl, a sugar substitute that replaces both the bulk and the sweetness, and a polymer that can replace much of the fat in salad dressings, mayonnaise, margarine and baked goods.

## SUBSTITUTES FOR CREAM AND MAYONNAISE

Fat is the enemy of both the heart and the waistline. But, cutting back on fat-laden sour cream, cream and mayonnaise isn't easy, either psychologically or practically. With a few tricks, though, it can be done, and the best substitute to start with is yogurt.

Besides adding flavor, butterfat thickens cream, and egg yolks emulsify mayonnaise. Therefore, yogurt, which is low in fat, must be thickened by other means for satisfactory results. Suggestions:

• Commercial yogurt is too thin to use right from the container. To prepare it for use as a replacement, line a sieve with a paper coffee filter and place it over a bowl. Pour in the yogurt and let it drain until it is the consistency you want...that of light, heavy or sour cream.

• Drained yogurt provides an excellent base for any dip that originally called for sour cream. (If the yogurt seems too thick for your purpose, beat a little of the drained whey back into it.)

• To use yogurt in cooking or baking, replace each cup of cream or sour cream with ¾ cup of drained yogurt mixed with 1 tablespoonful of cornstarch. The yogurt should be at room temperature.

• In dishes such as beef Stroganoff, where the yogurt-cornstarch mixture replaces sour cream, fold it gently into the beef at the last minute...and let it just heat through.

### Basic Recipes

• Light mayonnaise: Mix ⅓ cup thickened yogurt into ⅔ cup mayonnaise.

• Light salad dressing: Mix ⅔ cup slightly thickened yogurt into ⅓ cup mayonnaise.

• Mock sour cream dressing:* Mix 1 cup drained low-fat yogurt with 2 tablespoons full of wine vinegar. Add a dash of sugar (or substitute), a bit of garlic powder, and ¼ cup vegetable oil. Mix and chill.

### Other Good Substitutions

Splendid as it is as a dairy replacement, yogurt is not the only one. Buttermilk and skim milk combined with dry skim milk are also useful substitutes. Suggestions:

• Replace the cream in cream soups with buttermilk, which is satisfyingly rich, yet low in calories. To eliminate any hint of buttermilk's slightly acidic taste, add a liberal amount of mild curry powder.

• Mix 1 cup skim milk with ½ cup dry skim milk. Add to soup to thicken it. This works with all cream soups, including vichyssoise.

The replacement won't duplicate the cream and mayonnaise you are used to. However, the new taste will be very good in a different way—and much better for you.

*The Low-Cholesterol Food Processor Cookbook* by Suzanne S. Jones, Doubleday & Co., Garden City, NY.

# THE HEALTHY GOURMET

You can have your coquilles St. Jacques and eat them (safely) too by following these general substitutions:

• Cut fat in your favorite recipes by 25%–50%. Example: If the recipe suggests one cup of oil, try ¾ cup. If that works, try ⅔ cup the next time. In many casseroles and soups you can omit the butter or margarine completely.

• Instead of sauteing vegetables in oil or butter, add several tablespoonfuls of water or broth and steam them in a covered pot.

• Compensate for lost fat flavor by adding spices and herbs.

• Use skim or low-fat milk instead of whole milk..evaporated skim milk instead of cream.

• In sauces that call for cheese, stick to grated Parmesan or Romano (about 25 calories per tablespoonful).

• Rather than starting sauces with a fatty "roux," add cold milk or fruit juice to the flour or cornstarch.

• Substitute veal, skinless poultry, or flank or round steak for fat-marbled cuts of beef.

• For bulk without extra calories, slice meats thin and add more vegetables to the meal.

**Source:** *Tufts University Diet & Nutrition Letter*, New York.

# LEAN CUISINES

You can stay on your diet even while dining at your favorite restaurants. Here's how to order to avoid excess fat, sugar, cholesterol or salt:

• Italian: Pasta dishes with marinara (meatless) sauce. Baked or broiled chicken or veal. Pizza with mushrooms, bell peppers and tomatoes (but ask them to go light on cheese). Minestrone.

• French: Grilled swordfish. Chicken breast with wild mushrooms. Steamed vegetable plate. Salade nicoise (with dressing on the side). Poached salmon. Raspberries.

• Mexican: Chicken taco in a steamed corn tortilla. Tostados (light on the avocado, sour cream on the side). Red snapper Vera Cruz. Avoid fried rice or beans.

• Chinese: Broccoli, scallops and mushrooms sauteed with ginger and garlic. Stir-fried bean curd or chicken. Steamed fish and rice. Ask for preparation without MSG or soy sauce.

**Source:** Dr. Cleaves Bennett, author of *Control Your High Blood Pressure without Drugs,* and Chris Newport, a Paris-trained nutritionist and chef, cited in *Los Angeles.*

# VACATION DIET SECRETS

• Bring a tight-fitting outfit to try on each morning. (A zipper that won't zip easily is the first sign you may be eating too much.)

• At dinner, wear an outfit that needs a belt—or one with a non-elastic waistband.

• Bring a scale so you can to check your weight every day.

• Use a tape measure to check body changes the scale doesn't show.

• Ask the concierge or room clerk about local (and light) food specialties.

• Reserve your room without meals, if possible. You'll likely save money, as well as calories.

• Plan your treats. Have bread, wine or dessert—but just one with any meal.

• Drink eight glasses of water each day (bottled if necessary).

• Drink alcohol in moderation. Too many drinks can lead to overeating.

**Source:** *Passport to Sensible Eating on the Go,* The Caryl Ehrlich Program, New York.

## HOLIDAY SURVIVAL

Diets and cocktail parties don't have to be incompatible. To avoid a binge:

• Eat before you go, and arrive late (it's fashionable and less fattening).

• Avoid fattening hot hors d'oeuvres. Stick to cold meats, fresh fruit, crudites.

• Nibble off the top of an hors d'oeuvre. Stuff the rest into a napkin.

• Don't eat even a single peanut. Then you'll be sure not to eat a handful.

• Ditto for potato chips and pretzels.

**Source:** *New Woman*, New York.

# 7. Looking Good, Keeping Fit

# Looking Good, Keeping Fit

## PROBLEM PERSPIRATION REMEDY

Problem perspiration can be controlled by prescription devices that pass a harmless electric current through the sweat glands. The devices (by Drionic) are applied to feet, hands or underarms. After 10 daily treatments, they reduce perspiration significantly for about 95% of users. Maintenance: One treatment every four to six weeks. Cost: about $100 a pair.

**Source:** Mervyn Elgart, M.D., professor and chairman of dermatology at George Washington University Medical Center, in *Self*, New York.

## SWEAT STRATEGY

Too much sweat can soften the outer layer of the skin, presenting a food source for bacteria and fungi. Prevention: Stick to exercise clothes made with absorbent cotton, rather than nylon or acrylics. Use powders with bacteriostatic and fungistatic ingredients. Use a strong antiperspirant containing aluminum chlorohydrate. Try an over-the-counter acne product (containing 10% benzoyl peroxide) on sweaty feet.

**Source:** *Outside Magazine*, New York.

## DEODORANTS VS. ANTIPERSPIRANTS

Deodorants cut down on bacteria but do not halt perspiration. Antiperspirants reduce perspiration by shrinking the openings of the sweat glands. They also control odor by fighting bacteria. Neither deodorant nor antiperspirants are toxic. But people with sensitive skin may find antiperspirants an irritant. (Such people should use unscented deodorants which are less apt to cause allergic type reactions.) Best underarm protection: either roll-ons or creams. Because they are water-based, they are less irritating.

## BEST TIME TO APPLY AN ANTIPERSPIRANT

To stay dry all day, it helps to put on antiperspirant at bedtime. The main ingredient (aluminum chlorohydrate) works by plugging sweat glands, and it does that best when they're dry as long as possible. You're dry longest when you're asleep. To build up sweat protection, it's best to use antiperspirant every day. It takes up to eight days for an antiperspirant to reach maximum effectiveness.

**Source:** Kenneth Hiller, Ph.D., coordinator, Procter & Gamble Beauty Care Council.

## COSMETIC-LABEL SECRET

Cosmetics labeled "unscented" can still cause the itchy, swollen skin known as dermatitis because they contain masking perfumes. Best bet: Look for "fragrance free" labels on makeup and creams. Dab perfume only on clothes or hair.

**Source:** American Academy of Dermatology, cited in *Women's Health*, New York.

## WASHING TIPS

Scrubbing your skin too hard removes the outer layer (the stratum corneum). This layer plays an important part in protecting the body, by keeping in body heat and liquid while keeping out bacteria and other foreign substances. On its own, the body replaces the stratum corneum. So normal washing is enough.

**Source:** Michael Gass, M.D., dermatologist, Davis, CA, quoted in *American Health*, New York.

• Two washcloths are better than one for a good, neat cleaning. You can get a couple of fine lathers with one, wash them off with the other. Different colors help on a continuing basis.

## DEODORANT SOAP WARNING

The right soap is the mildest one that still leaves your skin feeling clean. Never use a deodorant bar on your face. It only dries and irritates that sensitive area.

**Source:** *Harper's Bazaar*, New York.

## MILDEST SOAPS

If your skin feels dry and taut, it may be due to the harshness of the soap you're using. A number of popular soaps were rated on a scale of zero to ten. Those below a rating of one are mildest, and those above five are harsh: Dove, .5; Dial, 2.4; Neutrogena, 2.8; Ivory, 2.8; Jergens, 3.3; Irish Spring, 4.0; Zest, 6.1; Camay, 6.4

**Source:** Albert Kligman, M.D., professor of dermatology, University of Pennsylvania.

## SKIN WORKOUT

Do your heavy exercise before you shave to save your skin (perspiration can irritate clean shaven skin). Use moisturizers and colognes after exercise, but always on clean skin. Wait a few minutes after showering to apply powder or a deodorant (so that your skin will have time to dry completely).

**Source:** *Playboy*, New York.

## TREATING WINTER-DRIED SKIN

Limit yourself to three baths or showers a week. (In between, you can sponge-bathe face, armpits, groin and feet.) Keep bath water tepid, not hot. Use a low-alkali soap (such as Dove), with no washcloth. Dry by patting gently with a towel, not rubbing. If you add bath oil: Wait until after you've soaked a while. Otherwise your skin will be coated with oil before it can absorb moisture.

**Source:** Jane E. Brody, writing in *The New York Times*.

## REAL CAUSE OF WINTER SKIN PROBLEMS

Chapped lips and dry skin are not caused primarily by cold outdoor temperatures and winds. The real villain: Overheated homes and offices. To prevent chapping: Use a protective ointment or lipstick. Install a humidifier in living or work areas. (Open containers of water near heating systems also help.) Drink at least six glasses of water a day.

**Source:** Norman Orentreich, M.D., a dermatologist at New York University Medical Center.

## BATH-OIL HAZARD

Bath oils are good for dry skin, but they can also make the tub dangerously slippery. Safer: Apply the oil directly to your skin after bathing.

**Source:** *Consultant.*

## TANNING SALON WARNING

Tanning salons are still dangerous, even though modern facilties screen out "burning rays" (ultraviolet B). Fact: Even the milder ultraviolet A rays increase the risk of skin damage (leading to a wrinkled, leathery look) and edema. They're also a suspected factor in skin cancer. If you're taking a medication, you may experience side effects, such as swelling. If you go to a salon anyway: Don't put on a deodorant or perfume. Wear protective goggles.

**Source:** Report by the Food and Drug Administration.

## SUN SCREENS

You can now determine which sun screen is best for you, thanks to sophisticated tests that have established the degree of protection given by various sun-screen brands. The measure of protection a sun screen affords is its SPF number. This number tells the length of time it takes the sun's rays to penetrate the screen and burn your skin. The higher the number, the longer you can stay in the sun without burning. Example: If you're going sailing for four hours, you'll want a screen with the highest available SPF—15. The lowest SPF number is 2, virtually no protection against the sun's rays.

In addition to giving protection against the sun, a sun screen should be durable. It should not "wash off" as soon as you begin to perspire. Other important properties: It should not be toxic to your skin, smell bad, feel offensive or stain.

To find the best screens: Look for the Skin Cancer Foundation seal of approval when choosing a screen. The Foundation conducted tests of the leading sun screens to determine their actual effectiveness outdoors and the degree to which they have all the other important properties (durability, lack of toxicity, etc.). Their seal of approval was assigned to the brands that met these standards. The seal appears on the container.

Brands that don't have the seal of approval aren't necessarily ineffective. They may simply not have been included in the tests.

So-called "alternate" sun screens of aloe or coconut compounds are worthless as protection.

Tan gradually. Don't sit in the sun until

you get red. Redness means it's too late—the sun's rays have already damaged your skin.

**Source:** Interview with Perry Robins, M.D., associate professor of dermatology and chief of chemosurgery, New York University Medical Center.

## AGE AND SUNBURN

Sunburn causes more damage as you grow older. Your body becomes less efficient in repairing the sun-damaged skin. Recommended: Use a stronger sun screen to protect your skin. Try to tan gradually.

**Source:** Marianne Nelson O'Donoghue, M.D., associate professor of dermatology, Rush University Medical College, Chicago.

## WINTER SUNBURN ALERT

Skiing in winter sun can be harder on skin than summer sports. Because they are reflected off the snow, the sun's rays increase in intensity. Added risk: Skiing at a high altitude, which boosts exposure to ultraviolet rays. Recommended safeguard: Use a moisturizing sunscreen with a sun protection factor of 15 for winter activities on sunny days. Then apply a final "sealing" layer of petroleum jelly or a liquid foundation.

**Source:** Stephen Kurtin, M.D., co-founder of the Institute for the Control of Facial Aging, New York.

## SUNBURN R$_x$

To soothe a sunburn, apply wet compresses of cool tap water for 20 minutes, three or four times a day. Coat the burned area with a lubricating lotion or cream (not a heavy ointment). Take aspirin or acetaminophen as needed. Drink lots of water. Avoid the sun until your skin has healed completely.

**Source:** Skin Cancer Foundation, New York.

## MEDICATIONS AND THE SUN DON'T MIX

Many common drugs can make your skin more susceptible to burning. Major ones: tetracyclines (antibiotics), sulfa drugs (anti-bacterials), phenothiazine derivatives (major tranquilizers), grisofulvins (anti-fungals), sulfonylureas (anti-diabetics) and thiazides (diuretics).

**Source:** Maureen Poh-Fitzpatrick, M.D., Columbia University College of Physicians and Surgeons, writing in *Self*, New York.

## TO AVOID SUN RASH

Sun rash or a quick burn can result when people with sensitive skin put cologne or perfume on areas of the body exposed to the sun. (Some soaps and deodorants may also produce this effect.) The ailment: Photodermatitis. Remedy: Apply colognes and perfume to clothing, not to skin. Certain drugs and medications also make the skin supersensitive. Examples: Diuretics, antibiotics and sulfa drugs. When taking them, be careful to limit time in the sun.

## COSMETICS AND DRUGS

Photo-toxins in drugs and cosmetics can react with sunlight to produce mild rashes or burns, severe headaches, or nausea and vomiting. These ingredients can cause problems even when a strong sunblocker is used. Examples: Oil of bergamot and musk ambrette (used as a base in some perfumes). The "scent" in underarm deodorants. Hexachlorophene. Various plant extracts (used in bath soaps and lotions). Antihistamines, antibiotics, tranquilizers, diuretics, antipsychotics. . .and drugs used to treat diabetes. Recommended: If you use any of these products, consult your doctor or pharmacist before spending time in the sun.

**Source:** The Skin Cancer Foundation, New York.

## CLOTHING TIPS

Summer clothing is not necessarily a protection from the burning rays of the sun. You can get dangerous exposure outdoors even when fully dressed if your summer togs are made of airy, light-colored fabrics. Test your clothes by holding them up to natural light. Apparel that casts a good shadow will probably protect you from harmful ultraviolet rays. Natural fabrics with a denser weave are better shields than loosely woven, thin materials. Dark colors screen better than light ones.

**Source:** Gerald Milton, M.D., director of the melanoma unit, Sydney Hospital, Sydney, Australia, quoted in *American Health*, New York.

## SUMMER SKIN RASH CHECKLIST

Hot weather and outdoor activities can bring on a variety of skin problems that are a nuisance but not really dangerous. However, you should see a doctor if a rash is accompanied by fever and/or swelling around the eyes or the genital area.

Common summer skin problems and how to cope with them:

• Prickly heat. A reaction to hot weather caused by clogged pores that keep you from sweating properly. The rash has tiny, itchy pimples and blisters. What to do: Stay out of the sun, take cool baths and wear loose clothing. A pharmacist can recommend something soothing if the rash really bothers you.

• Poison ivy, poison oak and poison sumac. Most people have an allergic reaction to these. That means reddening, swelling and blisters that are very itchy and uncomfortable. Keep the affected areas dry. If you have a severe case, see your doctor. Best: Learn to recognize and avoid the pest plants, and keep your legs covered when you hike in unfamiliar areas. If you think you've had skin contact, wash yourself immediately with a strong soap. . .and your clothes, too.

• Insect bites. Try not to scratch bites. Scratching may cause longer-lasting secondary infections. If an extreme reaction sets in right after a sting or bite, get to a doctor or hospital immediately. Some people are super-allergic to bites. . .even to mosquito bites. And some ticks cause a serious disease—Rocky Mountain spotted fever. For normal irritating, itchy bites (chiggers, gnats, no-see-ums, etc.), you can get a prescription from your doctor that will reduce the itching if it's really bothersome. Protection: Insect repellant applied to your skin.

• Athlete's foot. This fungal infection starts with cracks, reddening and scaling between the toes. The first line of defense is keeping your feet clean and dry and wearing open shoes, such as sandals, as much as possible. If it gets worse or seems persistent, see a doctor. Home remedies can create worse problems than the disease.

**Source:** Interview with Neal B. Schultz, M.D., a Manhattan dermatologist.

## POISON IVY, OAK AND SUMAC

If you realize you have touched any of these three, wash your skin *immediately* with soap and water. If your first awareness is the rash, you need a soothing agent to reduce the itching. Use crushed aloe vera, plantain or jewelweed leaves, vitamin E oil, or a paste of baking soda, Fels Naptha soap and water. Cover the rash with a clean cloth to keep from scratching it.

**Source:** *Spring*, New York.

## INSECT-BITE REMEDIES

Insect-bite remedy combines ammonia with mink oil (which helps to keep the skin from drying). *After Bite* comes in a pen-size cylinder with a pocket clip or as a package of throw-away wipes.

**Source:** Tender Corp., Littleton, NH.

• Mosquito-bite relief. Turn your hair dryer on the bite for a minute. The warm, dry air dulls the itch.

## JEWELRY SECRETS

Platinum jewelry is ideal for those with sensitive skin. Reasons: It does not rust, tarnish or corrode. And, unlike gold, it doesn't require the addition of base metals for strength, so it is almost pure.

• Nickel is the culprit that most commonly causes skin irritations from jewelry. Used to strengthen softer metals, nickel is alloyed with white gold, chrome and other metals for stone settings and watch backings. Sweat leaches the nickel out to start allergic reactions in pierced ears and under rings. Safest jewelry for sensitive skin: stainless steel, plastic, sterling silver, yellow gold, platinum, brass and pure aluminum.

**Source:** *Changing times* New York.

## MEN AND WRINKLES

Because a man's skin is naturally both thicker and oilier than a woman's, he will show his age at a slower rate. Natural lubrication, plus thicker protection from the sun's radiation give men up to a ten-year jump on women in eluding the aging process's most visible gauge, wrinkles.

**Source:** *Sexual Signatures: On Being a Man or a Woman,* John Money, Little Brown & Co., Boston.

## ACNE INDUCER

One of the few proven substances that can bring on flare-ups of acne is iodine. Excessive, long-term intake of iodine (a natural ingredient of many foods) can bring on acne in anyone, but for people who are already prone to the condition, iodine is especially damaging. Once iodine hits the bloodstream, any excess is excreted through the oil glands of the skin. This process irritates the pores and causes eruptions and inflammation. Major sources of iodine in the diet: Iodized table salt, kelp, beef liver, asparagus, turkey, and vitamin and mineral supplements. For chronic acne-sufferers, cutting down on these high-iodine foods and looking for vitamins without iodine may bring relief.

**Source:** *Dr. Fulton's Step-by-Step Program for Clearing Acne* by J.E. Fulton Jr., M.D., and E. Black, Harper and Row.

## PIMPLE PREVENTION

Acne-prone preteens (generally those whose parents had it) can be tested and treated before their skin erupts. An oil-sensitive tape monitors sebum level and bacterial count. If readings are high, antibiotic ointments are applied. If they don't work: Internal antibiotics are used. For stubborn pores: Vitamin A (retinoic acid).

**Source:** Research by James J. Leyden, M.D., dermatologist at the University of Pennsylvania, reported in *American Health*, New York.

## PSORIASIS TREATMENT

When waterproof tape was applied to scaly skin areas for one week, many lesions cleared completely. Some stayed clear for a month or more. Others partially cleared. In general, the results were better than those obtained with cortico-steroid ointments or creams.

**Source:** Ronald N. Shore, M.D., Johns Hopkins School of Medicine, writing in *The New England Journal of Medicine* Boston, MA.

## WARTS UPDATE

When removed, new warts often grow nearby. A new treatment—injections of bleomycin (Blenoxane), which is a cancer-chemotherapy agent—has proved 81% effective in removing warts permanently. Problem: The treatment is unpleasant and somewhat painful to patients. This procedure is not recommended for children. Antiviral substances such as interferon are also promising.

**Source:** *Journal of American Academy of Dermatology,* New York.

## HELP FOR BIRTHMARKS

Port-wine birthmarks, the harmless purple-red blotches often found on the face and neck, can now be treated with lasers. The birthmarks are cauterized under local anesthetic, creating a superficial burn. The resulting crust disappears within three weeks. Results: In 65% of cases, the stain disappears. In 20%–30% of cases, it's much less noticeable. Who can't be treated: Children under 10; patients whose stains cover eyelids or upper lips.

**Source:** Ross Levy, M.D., dermatologist, Albert Einstein College of Medicine and Montefiore Medical Center, New York.

## ABOUT AGE SPOTS

Age spots—the brown freckle-like blotches on skin—usually first appear in the thirties and are a natural part of maturing. But if an age spot is raised, inflamed or bleeding, see a dermatologist. To fade them: Simple prescription bleaching creams (stronger than the over-the-counter variety) work best. You should see results in six weeks.

**Source:** *American Health.*

## ROSY-CHEEKS MYTH

Rosy cheeks are not the sign of health that most people assume. Fact: The rosiness comes from weak, dilated capillaries in the skin. In severe cases the capillaries break, leaving tiny, spidery veins. A simple way to control capillary dilation: Hold your hands over your cheeks for five seconds after coming indoors from the cold.

**Source:** *Working Woman,* New York.

## HELP FOR SPIDER VEINS

Spider veins are minor varicose veins (typically red or blue, with no bulging) that occur just below the skin surface. Although they pose no health hazard, they can be treated effectively for cosmetic purposes. The treatment is almost painless, causes no scarring, and is 90% successful. Several veins can be handled by your doctor at each office visit. Cost: $80–$100 per visit.

**Source:** *McCall's*, New York.

## FACTS ABOUT HAIR LOSS

First the bad news: Dermatologists still don't know why some people lose their hair. The good news: We can slow the process or replace the hair from other parts of the scalp. And if a revolutionary substance now under testing pans out, we may soon be able to grow hair back in places where it hasn't been seen for years.

A number of conditions can lead to hair loss: Thyroid disease, nutritional problems or secondary syphilis. Some nervous people literally pull their hair out. More common is *alopecia areata:* People wake up to find a round spot of hair missing or, in extreme cases, lose all their head and body hair.

The most common condition, however, is known as male pattern baldness. A testosterone by-product triggered by a person's genetic code causes the hair follicles to fall out. It's a mystery why it attacks some people more than others, or why it never touches the "horseshoe rim" at the back of the head.

Some 15% of the male population shows significant thinning (50% hair loss) by the age of 25, and 70% shows it by the age of 65. (Since the hormone is produced by everyone's adrenal glands, women can be affected as well, though generally to a lesser extent.) If you haven't had much thinning by age 35 or 40, you probably won't be bald later on.

What you can do about getting bald:

• Accept it, and grow bald gracefully. It's not the worst thing in the world. After all, hair serves no real function. Baldness can be distinctive: Telly Savalas and Yul Brynner have done very well without hair.

• Buy a toupee. The best look fairly natural. However, a good one costs at least $2,000, and it must be replaced whenever your natural hair gets grayer.

• Women should avoid unnaturally tight hair styles. They permanently damage the roots of the hair.

• Progesterone injections four times a year can retard hair loss for some people. They're not useful for women, however, because they upset the hormonal balance.

• Hair transplants offer a permanent solution. Using local anesthesia, a doctor transfers several hundred plugs of hair from the back of the head to the bare area. The procedure requires four to eight sittings. Cost: $4,000–$6,000. We aim for a partial restoration, with a receding hairline appropriate to the patient's age. You'd look silly with the hair of a 20-year-old. Warning: Avoid cut-rate clinics, even medical ones, where the procedure may be performed by a doctor with only a few days' training. Seek out a plastic surgeon or a dermatologist associated with a medical school or with the American Society of Dermatologic Surgery.

• An alternative surgical method rotates flaps of hair-bearing scalp from the back of the head to the front. Some people prefer this because it gives them "instant" hair. However, it requires general anesthesia and a hospital stay. The body sometimes rejects the flaps—an unpleasant complication. Cost: $3,000–$5,000, plus hospital fees.

Two recent developments offer new hope. The first is a drug, *spironolactone.* Although used primarily to fight high blood pressure, it also blocks testosterone and slows hair loss, so one may go bald in another 10 years instead of five. There are no hormonal side effects. However, it is a diuretic, and it can cause dizziness and fatigue in people who have normal blood pressure.

More exciting is *minoxidil,* another antihypertensive agent. (It's still being tested. When taken in pill form, it led to the growth of thick, excess hair on patients' faces and bodies.)

The Upjohn Company recently developed a minoxidil lotion to be applied directly to the scalp. Preliminary studies show that about one third of the subjects achieved natural hair regrowth with no apparent side effects. I've had similar results working with 25 or 30 balding doctors.

**Source:** Interview with Steven Victor, M.D., a specialist in baldness, New York.

## HOW STRESS CAN DAMAGE YOUR HAIR

Stress and emotional tension take the life out of your hair. Reason: Tension restricts blood vessels in the scalp, reducing its supply of oxygen and nutrients. For good-looking hair, eat well, get plenty of exercise, shampoo daily. . .and relax.

**Source:** Philip Kingsley, author of *The Complete Hair Book,* Grosset & Dunlap, New York.

## WORST TIME OF YEAR FOR DANDRUFF

Don't blame the cold if your dandruff gets worse during the winter. The real villain: Overheated rooms with forced-hot-air systems. The scalp dries out the same way skin does. Solution: Turn down the heat.

**Source:** *Cosmopolitan,* New York.

## DANDRUFF SHAMPOOS THAT DON'T WORK

Antidandruff shampoos can actually cause the condition, a new study shows. Reason: The harsh solutions irritate the scalp. Simply switching to a milder shampoo may control the problem. It's also a good idea to discontinue the use of hair oils. Suggestion: Visit a dermatologist, who can prescribe a topical antibacterial agent.

**Source:** *International Journal of Dermatology.*

## DON'T OVERUSE YOUR ANTIDANDRUFF SHAMPOO

Antidandruff shampoos can lose their effectiveness if used every day. To stay flake-free: Try alternating your dandruff shampoo with a regular shampoo (for normal hair) every other day or week.

**Source:** Vera H. Price, M.D., clinical professor of dermatology, the University of California at San Francisco, in *Glamour,* New York.

## HAIR-CARE TIP

Your hair will look better if you have regular trims. Trimming makes hair look healthier and fuller, especially if it's on the long side. Reason: Old hair is more prone to splitting. Trimming stops the split from traveling up the hair shaft. When trimming matters most: During warm weather, when hair grows fastest.

**Source:** Vera H. Price, M.D., clinical professor of dermatology, University of California, San Francisco, in *Glamour,* New York.

## HOW TO CHOOSE THE RIGHT HAIRBRUSH

The best hairbrush bristles come from boars. Their uneven surface cleans better than smooth nylon. Stiffest: Black bristles from the back of the boar's neck. Good for thick, heavy hair, these are the rarest and most expensive bristles. White bristles are better for fine and/or thinning hair.

**Source:** Jan Hansum, Kent of London, quoted in *The Best Report,* New York.

## HAIR-CREAM WARNING

Prolonged use of hair creams and lotions containing estrogen has caused breast enlargement in men and young children. Also: One hair product led to vaginal bleeding in women as old as 82. Problem: Because cosmetics are not regulated, no one knows which products contain estrogen.

**Source:** *The Harvard Medical School Health Letter,* Cambridge, MA.

## HELP FOR NAIL BITING

Nail biting can be cured if the biter becomes acutely aware of the habit. How to do it: Make a mark on an envelope every time a nail is bitten. Add up the number of bites every day, and enter the totals on a chart. Put every chewed-off piece of nail in the envelope. This gives you an idea of the amount of nail-biting. Also, keep nails clean and well filed. After a no-biting week, give yourself a reward. Extreme measure: Coat the nails with a bitter substance.

**Source:** *Stop It!* by S. Morris and N. Charney, Doubleday, New York.

## FOR HEALTHY FINGERNAILS

Clip nails when wet (dry nails are brittle). Use an emery board to smooth nail surfaces, especially near the edges. Replace old nail clippers as they get dull. Fix breaks and cracks with nail glue (cyanoacrylate). Never open a bottle seal or pull out a staple with your nails.

**Source:** Howard Baden, M.D., dermatologist, Harvard University, in *American Health*, New York.

## WHAT YOUR FINGERNAILS SAY ABOUT YOUR HEALTH

• Parallel, transverse white bands: You may have a protein deficiency.

• Brittle nails separating from the nail bed: possible sign of a thyroid disorder.

• Abnormally white color: You may have a liver problem.

• Thin, linear hemorrhages under the nail: could indicate a blood disorder or endocarditis (inflammation of the heart lining).

• Spoon-shaped nails: often a sign of iron-deficiency anemia.

• Thinning nails with longitudinal ridging and discolored nail bed: symptoms of a chronic skin disease (lichen planus).

• Thickened nail tips: Either a genetic trait or a sign of lung or heart diseases.

**Source:** *Harrison's Principles of Internal Medicine,* eighth edition, and *Symptoms and Signs in Clinical Medicine,* Chamberlain and Ogilvie, ninth edition.

## WHAT YOU SHOULD KNOW ABOUT YOUR FEET

Feet occupy a very strange position in our minds. I have yet to find an individual who likes his or her feet. Most people think they have ugly, smelly feet. Feet are phallic symbols that we hide and avoid discussing. Because people are embarrassed about their feet, they prefer to remedy foot pain with a store-bought product instead of seeing a doctor. This leads to chronic problems.

But times are changing. The recent running fad has brought feet out into the open. In the past five years there's been an explosion of knowledge about the foot. No matter how you feel about your feet, it's to your benefit to know how they function, how to take good care of them and when to seek medical help.

### If the Shoe Fits...

We must remember that the foot is a dynamic structure, constantly changing as we walk. Because our feet have developed on soft, grassy surfaces over the course of millions of years, our shoes should reflect the things our feet are best adapted for.

Specifics:

• Shoes should provide a lot of cushioning to match the type of surface the bare foot needs. Poor: A rigid, so-called supportive shoe. Shoes should be loose and giving. Good: The running shoe, the most physiologic shoe made. Soft and malleable, it provides cushioning and a little bit of support.

(Leather ones breathe best if your feet sweat.) Women: If you wear a high-heeled, thin-soled shoe, have a thin rubber sole cemented onto the bottom to cushion the ball of the foot.

• Too-small shoes are the most common shoe-fitting mistake. As we grow, our shoe size tends to lag behind actual foot size. I see people with hammertoes, red spots and corns who have no idea that their shoes are too small. To most people, a fairly tight shoe gives a feeling of normalcy. Fit shoes with your hands, not with your feet. There should be an index finger's breadth between the tip of the toes and the front of the shoe. Tell the salesperson to start with a half-size larger than you usually wear and work down. The shoe shouldn't be pushed out of shape when you stand. The leather should not be drawn taut.

• Women with a wide forefoot commonly have problems with loose-heeled shoes. Remedy: Pad the heel on the sides, not the back. Aim: to hold the heel, not push the foot forward.

• An ideal heel height for a woman is 1½–2 inches. This is not a magic number, simply the most comfortable. If a man wore a 1½-inch heel, he'd be more comfortable than in the traditional ¾-inch heel.

### Muscle Balance

Beyond properly fitting shoes, one of the biggest foot concerns is muscle balance. The body's muscles are interconnected. The calf muscle comes down to form the Achilles tendon, which attaches to the back of the heel. It then wraps under the heel, coming forward in the arch as a structure called the *plantar fascia* attached to the base of the toes. A tight calf muscle puts stress on the whole system.

Typical problems caused by calf-muscle tightness:

• Night cramps in the calf muscles. These are not due to calcium loss or vitamin E deficiency.

• Metatarsalgia (pain under the ball of the foot) and thick callus formation. The tight calf muscle drives the front of the pain and calluses. Also: Hammertoes, from cocking up the toes in an effort to relieve the pain in the ball of the foot.

• Burning in the arch from an overpull of the plantar fascia.

• Hell-spur syndrome. If the plantar fascia becomes overstretched, it becomes very thin at the heel, causing severe pain. The bone spur that shows up in an X-ray is a result of this syndrome.

• Achilles tendinitis is the same sort of problem, caused by excessive pull on the Achilles tendon.

Virtues of stretching: This is not a miracle cure, but it's extremely important. How to do it: Stand facing a wall at arm's length, and place your palms against the wall. Feet have to be kept together and flat on the floor. Bend your arms until your elbows touch the wall. Hold for 20 seconds. Do four repetitions three times daily. Move your feet one or two inches back from the wall every day until you get as far as you can go (about 30 inches).

### Other Foot Problems

• Flat feet are not bad feet. A flat, flexible foot is very functional. Most great athletes have them. Problem: The shoe industry doesn't make shoes to fit flat feet. Look for low-heeled shoes that feel balanced. They should not throw your weight forward on the balls of your feet or gape at the arches. If your feet hurt: Do toe raises and calf-stretching exercises. Toe raises help build the muscles that support the arch. Do five in the morning and five at night, increasing by three or four repetitions a week until you're up to 100.

• People who stand a lot need arch supports. Suggested: wooden clogs. They have built-in supports and heel elevation. Many surgeons wear them.

• Weekend athletes most commonly suffer from improper training and lack of warm-up. Runners get Achilles tendinitis and shin splints from shock overload. Remedy: Don't run on your toes. This negates the effect of the foot and ankle as a shock absorber. Tennis players get tennis toe, where the nail hits the shoe. Remedy: A long enough shoe. Important: Never run or play when overtired or not warmed up. Stop when tired or in pain. This is when most injuries occur.

• Ankle pain is often caused by an old sprain. While the torn ligament is recovering, the other leg is favored. Although the ligament has healed, the muscles haven't. Unless the ankle is rehabilitated, it can be an ongoing problem for years. I've seen people who still have ankle pain seven or eight years after a sprain. When they're put on the right exercise program, the pain goes away.

**Source:** Interview with orthopedist John F. Waller, Jr., M.D., chief of the foot and ankle section, Lenox Hill Hospital, New York.

# ORTHOPEDIST VS. PODIATRIST

An orthopedist is an M.D. who specializes in bone disease. Some orthopedists specialize in problems of the foot and leg. A podiatrist's training is similar to that of a dentist. His professional degree, a D.P.M. (Doctor of Podiatric Medicine), indicates that he has studied at a four-year podiatric college. He can take additional post-doctoral training. There are many differences of opinions between orthopedists and podiatrists on how to treat various foot problems. If surgery is recommended, it is wise to seek a second opinion.

# FOOTCARE: THE SIMPLE SECRETS

• Cut your toenails long (beyond the ends of the toes) and straight across. Rounded, too-short toenails can become ingrown.

• Soak your feet once or twice a week in warm water and Epsom salts. This will relax them. Your feet need the same tender, loving care you'd give your complexion.

• Make sure not only your shoes, but also your socks or stockings, are roomy enough. Your toes should be able to move freely.

• For corns or calluses, use pumice stone and a good skin lubricant. Recommended: Ureacin or Carmol cream or lotion. Don't

be a bathroom surgeon. If your corns and calluses are chronic and painful, see a doctor—either a podiatrist or an orthopedist who specializes in foot care.

• The protective padding sold commercially is helpful in alleviating shoe pressure or friction. Recommended: Moleskin for corns or calluses; lambswool in between toes.

• Don't use chemical preparations for corns. It's too easy to destroy surrounding tissue. People don't read the fine print, which says to surround the affected area with a bland ointment. That other skin could become ulcerated. Also: Don't use moleskin or padding impregnated with chemicals. A deep corn must be removed professionally. No corn remedy will get rid of it.

• Bunions, a hereditary condition, can be aggravated by improper foot care, weight or occupation or by short shoes or socks. The only real cure is surgery. Today's sophisticated podiatric bunion surgery can often be done in the office under local anesthesia. To help yourself: Buy bunion-last shoes. These shoes have a special pocket that accommodates the bunion.

• Don't walk barefoot in the house. Your feet will spread, and after several hours they won't want to go back into shoes. Recommended: Wear comfortable shoes at home. Dr. Scholl's sandals are good.

• For athlete's foot, use powder or spray twice a day. Good product: Tinactin. Look for tolnaftate, the active ingredient.

**Source:** Interview with podiatrists Nicholas Azzarello, D.P.M., and Stanley E. Dauber, D.P.M., New York.

# BUNION RELIEF

New bunion surgery reduces the full recovery time from one year to six months. Formerly a piece of the bone of the big toe was cut out. Now the joint is realigned and locked into proper position with two stainless-steel screws.

**Source:** Charles Gudas, D.P.M., director of the bunion clinic, University of Chicago Medical School.

# WHY WE'RE HAVING SUCH FOOT PROBLEMS

Foot supports are an answer to the ills of civilization, at least where aching arches are concerned. Our feet were designed to walk across the yielding surface of fields—without shoes. Instead, we walk on hard pavement, often in stylish footwear that doesn't fit correctly. With age, we lose muscle tone, and the problem becomes worse.

In time, the foot's ligaments and 26 bones go out of alignment. Nerves are pinched. Blood vessels are squeezed. Legs, pelvis and spine are thrown out of whack. It's an insidious process. Our body adjusts, and we don't notice the problem until our forties or fifties. Then we're distressed to find that we can barely walk without pain.

This is where custom-formed flexible foot supports come in. They return the foot to its natural position and function, or at least close to it. Slipped into any ordinary shoes, supports ease the shock of each step while at the same time maintaining the foot's normal flexing action. By easing unnatural friction, these devices can eliminate corns, bunions, callouses and hammertoes. In some cases, they even improve posture and balance.

**Source:** Interview with Harvey Rothschild, president of Featherspring International Corp., Seattle, WA.

# HOT FOOT

The temperature inside your shoes can reach 125° in summer. This slows down your circulation and causes fluid buildup. Best prevention: Take a walk. Muscles pump fluid back up the leg as you move. If your feet do swell: Prop your feet above the level of your heart for about 10 minutes. Massage toes, then instep, ankle and calf, moving the water up into the legs. Keep your feet moving. . .curling and straightening toes, rotating ankles, flexing knees.

**Source:** *Woman's Day*, New York.

# THERMAL-BOOT ALERT

Thermal boots keep your feet warm, but they can also build up perspiration. Result: Tender, water-logged feet that are painful to walk on. Prevention: Don't wear the boots for more than a few hours at a time, particularly indoors. Or get a model where the plastic liners are removable, thus allowing the feet to breathe. Best: The Moonboot, whose liner is designed to diffuse moisture away from the foot.

**Source:** Colin E. Blogg, M.D., consultant anesthetist at the Radcliffe Infirmary, Oxford, England.

# TIPS FOR TIRED FEET

To revive tired feet: (1) Run hot water over them for one minute, and then switch to cold. (2) Sit straight, point each foot and flex it 10 times. Then rotate each ankle 10 times in each direction. (3) Massage each sole with your thumb in circular motions. Then move to the top of the foot. (4) Grasp each toe, and tug and twist it gently.

**Source:** *Mademoiselle*, New York.

# CURE FOR FOOT ODOR

Foot odor is caused by perspiration and bacteria. Antidote: Keep your feet clean and dry. Use talcum powder or cornstarch between your toes, and wear cotton or wool socks. Wear shoes made of leather or another material that "breathes." Let shoes air out for at least 24 hours between wearings. For persistent or very strong odor, apply an underarm antiperspirant to your soles.

# STYLE VS. COMFORT

Aching feet plague almost 75% of Americans over 18 years old—and 62% think it's normal for feet to hurt. Most common problems: Blisters, calluses and corns. Women reported more pain than men, and 45% of the women said they wore uncomfortable shoes because they look good. But when asked if they'd give up style for comfort, 22% of the women said no.

**Source:** Recent Gallup Poll.

## BEST MEN'S SHOES

Comfortable men's shoes feel slightly roomy but not loose on the feet. Toe box: High and rounded at the base. The space between your longest toe and the shoe tip should be the width of your index finger. Heel: Snug but flexible at the back, three-quarters of an inch to one inch in height. Soles: Crepe or rubber (better shock absorbers than leather). Buy shoes later in the afternoon, since feet tend to swell during the course of the day.

**Source:** *Gentlemen's Quarterly*, New York.

## WHAT YOUR PLASTIC SURGEON *SHOULDN'T* TELL YOU

After elective, aesthetic surgery, you'll be living with the results. Since elective aesthetic surgery is not necessary for medical reasons and is purely a personal choice, it's best to know the pitfalls before making your decision. Here are warning signals that you *shouldn't* be getting as you query your physician:

• A new life. If a surgeon, a clinic, or its advertising leads you to believe that relationships, careers, etc., will improve with your new looks, don't be deluded. It may be what you *want* to hear, but the same old problems will still be there after you emerge with a new nose.

• Big promises. If you're not Marilyn Monroe, the most skilled surgeon in the world cannot make you look like her. Nor should any surgeon promise to. For this reason, before and after patient pictures or computer systems that produce a graphic image of *your* face with Cheryl Tiegs' nose can be misleading. Gimmicks such as these are not necessarily indicative of a good surgeon. Better: A surgeon who sends you to a medical photographer and then discusses your facial structure and potential changes using the photos.

• Numerical credentials. Your surgeon should be certified by a speciality board* and experienced in the procedure that you want done. But let your choice weigh equally on technique. One surgeon could have done three times as many chin augmentations as another, but if the patients don't look natural afterward, you aren't benefitting. Some surgeons are technically proficient; others have a fine skill. Find someone who has demonstrated both.

• Too-good-to-be-true bargains. If a surgeon in a "plastic surgery clinic" offers you a facelift at one-third the going rate, you can be sure he's planning to spend one-third the normal time and effort on the operation. The most important thing you need from a plastic surgeon is his time and attention. You must feel comfortable asking him questions about either the physical or the mental side effects, complications, etc. In turn, he must take into account your personality, age, skin elasticity, and general health before designing the proper surgery for you. If you opt for an assemblyline job, that's what you're going to get.

• "Free" consultation. These same clinics offer a free "consultation" which is really a meeting with a nurse who gives you a sales pitch. A thorough consultation with a qualified plastic surgeon should cost between $50 and $100.

• Bargain flat rates for surgery only. This implies that follow-up visits are charged separately. Make sure your surgeon charges a fee for surgery that includes all care for complications and follow-up visits.

Besides these safeguards, there are other *don'ts* that can apply to your decision:

• Don't bargain hunt through the Yellow Pages or advertising. For referrals: Ask your family doctor. . .Check with friends or relatives who have had plastic surgery done. . . Call or write the American Society of Plastic and Reconstructive Surgeons (233 North Michigan Ave., Suite 1900, Chicago, IL 60601) for a list of board specialists certified in your area.

• Don't be wary of a plastic surgeon who uses ambulatory facilities for operating.

*For a list, check the *Directory of Medical Specialists,* Marquis Who's Who, Inc., Chicago, IL.

Unless your health is unstable, they are a good money-saving alternative to hospital care.

• Don't ask for a look that may be trendy. An out-of-style face may be worse than one with uncorrected features.

• Don't be afraid to ask, "What if I don't like it?" If your doctor doesn't have a serious alternative to that question, then he is taking neither you nor your plastic surgery needs seriously.

**Source:** Interviewed with Robert G. Schwager, M.D., clinical assistant professor of plastic surgery at Cornell University Medical College in New York.

## COSMETIC SURGERY WARNING

Cosmetic surgery carries risks like any other medical procedure. Examples: Blepharoplasty, an operation to correct droopy eyelids, carries a .04% risk of damaging vision. Collagen injections, used to fill out wrinkles and scars, cause allergic reactions in some patients with arthritis. (In one case, a collagen injection resulted in sudden blindness.) People considering cosmetic surgery should be aware that complications can affect their health as well as their appearance.

**Source:** Dr. Henry Clayman, ophthalmologist, Miami Beach, quoted in *The Miami Herald.*

## NOT FOR WOMEN ONLY

Plastic surgery for men is catching on. In 1982 about 500,000 males had elective procedures—four times as many as 10 years before. Most common procedures: Nose jobs for men in their teens and twenties; eyelid surgery for men in their forties; face-lifts for those in their fifties.

**Source:** *Psychology Today,* New York.

## BLOODLESS SURGERY

A new skin-peel technique uses a computer-controlled laser beam to erase wrinkles,
acne scars, sun damage, etc. Advantages over "wire wheel" dermabrasion: A perfectly uniform peel. Bloodless surgery (the doctor always has a clear view). Less risk of infection, postoperative pain and swelling.

**Source:** Alan Schiftman, Laser Research and Treatment Center, Albert Einstein College of Medicine, New York, quoted in *Self,* New York.

## NEW FAT REMOVAL TECHNIQUE

Suction lipectomy, in which fat deposits are vacuumed away, can reshape a body without scarring. Popular in France, the procedure was recently endorsed by the American Society of Plastic and Reconstructive Surgeons. Who can benefit: This is not for the obese. The ideal patient is generally trim except for localized bulges in thighs, buttocks or abdomen. Best candidates are under 40, when skin retains elasticity. Potential dangers: Shock from fluid loss if too much fat is removed; loss of skin tissue; complications from poor postoperative care. The procedure calls for general anesthesia and often a brief hospital stay. Full recovery takes two months.

## THE INSIDE STORY OF A FACE-LIFT

Most people who undergo cosmetic surgery discover that they didn't know nearly as much as they thought about what was going to happen. No matter how well busy surgeons and their nurses try to prepare patients, there is a lot they generally leave out—details of consequence to those who actually undergo such surgery. Here's a first-hand account of what to expect during and after a face-lift and/or eyelid surgery, as related by a source who has had both (with, we add, stunning results).*

A full face-lift is an extensive surgical

* Advice and counsel were provided by Gerald Imber, M.D., a cosmetic surgeon in New York.

procedure, as you'll discover if you're awake throughout. This will be possible only if you've chosen a doctor who operates with the use of local anesthesia (much preferred) rather than full anesthesia. Injections of local anesthesia and strong narcotics are fed to you intravenously. Though wide awake, you will feel nothing (though you may notice a pull when work starts on your neck muscles). While chatting away with your surgeon, you will, in fact, hear the tearing of those muscles. This, it will surprise you to know, is not at all disconcerting. Consider: The noise of your own flesh being ripped sounds loudly in your ears—and you don't care. This cavalier unconcern for the sound of your tearing flesh is, you will later learn, nothing more than the effect of the powerful narcotic being pumped into your body.

You'll be on the table a long time. It takes two hours for a face-lift alone and from two and one-half to three hours if you're also getting your eyelids done. You may become a bit fidgety toward the end of the procedure, simply from lying on the table. When the surgery is over, a small circle of nurses will ask you to sit up while a helmet of bandages is wrapped fairly tightly around your head. This helmet consists first of an underlayer of white gauze, which you will fortunately be unable to see in its soon-to-be-blood-soaked condition. (A little blood on white gauze looks like a lot.) This gauze will then be covered by darker-colored gauze. The overall effect is of a turban covering your forehead, the sides of your face (including ears) and the area under your chin.

If you have had general anesthesia you will, of course, be aware of none of the foregoing. You will simply wake up bandaged. If you've had surgery with local anesthesia, you will be led to your bed. Now you begin to appreciate the advantage of surgery with local anesthesia. You will be experiencing none of the stupor, physiological depression and nausea that afflict patients waking up from full anesthesia. On the contrary, you will likely be in a state of mild euphoria—a combination of the residual impact of the drugs and your exhilaration that the deed has been done. Feeling no

pain, you will doubtless devour with zest the danish and coffee the nurse brings you. Roughly two hours later you will start to feel pain (for which you have been equipped with pain-killers.) It is neither unbearable pain nor mild pain, but a middle-size, "not-to-be-sneezed-at" pain, easily subdued with acetaminophen. (You will, of course, have been forbidden anything in the form of aspirin, which causes bleeding.)

You will by now understand that you are best off in bed, lying propped up on two pillows to help elevate your head and thus minimize swelling. Don't expect to be able to talk on the phone with your friends. Not only won't you be able to hear well through the bandages, but the slightest touch of the phone receiver will hurt your ear where, after all, the incisions are located.

You'll be sleeping a lot the first day and, if your eyelids haven't been done, watching television. If your eyelids have been done, you are strictly forbidden to look at television, but you will discover that during prime time you can follow perfectly well almost everything going on without looking at the screen.

Your face, this first day, will still seem to have most of its normal proportions. This will also be true the second day, though less so. The bandage around your head, you'll note, is becoming tighter and more burdensome. You may also not have had a first-rate night's sleep, what with swallowing acetaminophen every four hours or so and being allowed to sleep only on your back.

The third day, the nurse will remove the bandages. You will be told that you can go under a warm shower and wash gently with medicated shampoo to get all the encrusted blood out of your hair and from behind your ears. This is easier said than done. There are staples behind your ears, and stitches in front of your ears, along the sides of your head and in your hair. Your head behind the ears feels like a tangle of blood and barbed wire. You don't know what you're touching or just where the incisions are, and you don't want to know. You'll find yourself washing very gingerly behind your ears, the most heavily swollen area—afraid all the time that you'll rip something. You won't. It takes great strength to remove those staples, as you'll discover when the nurse tries to do it. The job will be a lot easier if you've washed away as much encrustation as possible, gently but firmly.

On the morning of the third day, you'll be in for a surprise—namely, seeing that your face is swollen beyond recognition. It's a surprise because your surgeon's nurses told you you'd have "moderate" swelling. This swelling is doubtless moderate compared with others the medical professionals have seen. But to you, it is a terrifying spectacle. Impossible as it may seem, this swelling will increase during the course of the day. By now, you will begin to understand the importance of having made careful plans to stay safely secluded for roughly 10 days. The extreme swelling will have largely disappeared by then, but your face will also be exhibiting patches of purple and yellow bruises around the chin, throat and eyes (where traces will linger longer).

The stitches and staples will be removed in stages on the fifth and tenth days after the surgery. At the end of the second week, you'll be able to walk around outdoors without betraying (to the causal eye, at least) that you've undergone surgery. But your face will still be puffy, especially around the jaw. If you've had your eyelids done as well, you'll still need dark glasses to cover lingering bruises around the eyes. By the end of week three, you can go anywhere, free of all disguises, and look quite good. Your face will still be rounder than it should be, however, due to a residual but subtle swelling that will diminish gradually within the next two weeks. But long before that (as early, in fact, as the first week of the surgery), you'll be delighted with the effects of the surgery. As soon as the bandages are off, you can see a dramatically restored neck, even through the swelling. It's hard to appreciate the aged looks that a subtly sagging neck can confer on all the rest of you until you've seen the effects of this magical transformation. It will take longer to appreciate the transformation your face has undergone fully. By the end of six weeks you should look quite good to yourself. After eight to ten weeks you should be absolutely ecstatic.

## MORE ABOUT FACE-LIFTS

• Choose a surgeon who gives local anesthesia rather than full. Most surgeons agree that full anesthesia is harder on your system and doesn't help the healing process (particularly since it can cause vomiting and coughing in some patients).

• Avoid having your face-lift done in conjunction with eye-lift surgery. Most surgeons believe you should save yourself time and healing problems by having both operations done at once. They, however, are not patients. Get your eyelids done first, perhaps nine months to a year before the face-lift. The postsurgery period after an eye-lift can be more uncomfortable than the one following a face-lift. Another reason: Having already had your lids done will make you something of a veteran, so that you walk into your face-lift surgery with much less apprehension.

• Don't listen to people who ask you why you think you need to have a face-lift or who tell you you don't need one. The only people to listen to are yourself and, most importantly, plastic surgeons. If two or three highly reputable surgeons concur that you could profit from a face-lift, that's all the reassurance you need. Of course you still look good—but you could look a lot better. The best time for a face-lift is while you still look fairly good. If you wait till you're obviously wrinkled and sagging, the transformation will come as something of a shock to the world. You'll also have wasted years looking just all right instead of splendid.

## HOW SMOKING DELAYS HEALING

A recent study shows that smokers tend to shed dead skin after the procedure thereby delaying healing and causing scars. Theory: Nicotine constricts blood vessels, cutting off the blood supply to vulnerable facial skin.

**Source:** Study by Thomas D. Rees, M.D., a plastic surgeon affiliated with the Manhattan Eye, Ear and Throat Hospital, New York.

## WHAT EXERCISE DOES FOR YOU

Regular exercise toughens the mind as well as the body. After working out three times a week for six months, one group was found to be 20% fitter. Bonus: They also scored 70% better in a test of complex decision making.

**Source:** Study by industrial engineer Gavriel Salvendi of Purdue University, in *American Health*.

## EXERCISE/AGING CONNECTION

Regular physical exercise, extolled for its healthful effects on the heart and circulatory system, is now believed to help delay the aging process. Once thought to add wear and tear to the body, vigorous physical activity has been shown to improve body tissues and functions that normally decline after age 25 in healthy people who do not exercise regularly. Some benefits of aerobics that slow down aging: More energy, less depression and anxiety, better digestion, stronger bones, reduced risk of cardiovascular disease. Problem: If regular exercise is stopped, the body loses its conditioning very quickly, even in a matter of weeks. Good news: Conditioning can be regained just as quickly, and even people who have been sedentary all their lives can improve their physical condition dramatically in as little as a month.

**Source:** *Total Fitness* by Lawrence Morehouse and Leonard Gross, Simon & Schuster, New York.

## IS EXERCISE AN APHRODISIAC?

Researchers and common sense have long held that exercise enhances health and makes people feel better about themselves and their bodies. This, in turn, makes them more sexually attractive and responsive. Now studies are suggesting that exercise is a potent stimulus to hormone production in both men and women. It may, in fact, chemically increase basic libido by stepping up the levels of such hormones as testosterone.

**Source:** *Whole Body Healing* by Carl Lowe, Rodale Press, Emmaus, PA.

## ACTUARIAL STRATEGY

Regular physical workouts do indeed help you live longer, according to USLIFE. It now gives 17% discounts to exercisers who don't smoke. Smaller discounts go to fitness buffs who do, however, smoke.

**Source:** *Prevention*, Emmaus, PA.

## ABOUT PEOPLE WHO EXERCISE

Of people between the ages of 18 and 34 who earn more than $25,000 a year, 54% exercise regularly. Only 32% of those over 50 exercise. And just 34% of people with incomes of less than $15,000 ever work out. Irony: Of those surveyed, 88% agreed that exercise is good for them, but 55% said they never get any.

## BEST FATIGUE-FIGHTER

Exercise is a better way to fight late-afternoon fatigue than the traditional cup of coffee, soft drink or cigarette break. These can leave you feeling just as groggy an hour later. A brief walk or 25 jumping jacks does a better job of waking up the body. Eating the right food earlier in the day also helps—protein for breakfast and a light lunch.

**Source:** *Body Bulletin*.

## 5 WAYS TO AVOID FATIGUE

Fatigue rarely comes from overexertion. Underexertion is a more likely cause. Ways to avoid fatigue: (1) Eat well-balanced meals. Don't skimp on breakfast or you'll get tired at work. (2) Exercise more. Exercise increases energy. Evening exercise will also help you sleep better. (3) Sleep more. If you often become drowsy during the day, get an extra hour of sleep at night. (4) Work at your peak. Schedule tough jobs for the time of day you usually feel most energetic. (5) Take breaks. Even if you love your job, it helps to stop, stretch, walk or just relax.

# FITNESS VS. HEALTH

Considering the promotion of exercise over the last decade as the panacea for practically everything from heart disease to depression, it boggles the mind to look at the actual medical facts. Almost everything you've heard about the benefits of exercise in terms of health is untrue. Exercise is not only not good for your health, but it can be positively dangerous and even fatal. The only thing exercise will do for you is make you physically fit—fitness being defined as the capacity to do physical activity comfortably. But, contrary to popular misconception, fitness and health are two separate things.

If you want to be an athlete, or even just physically fit, you must exercise. However, you should know the risks and should recognize that you won't be improving your health but you will be putting yourself in danger. Don't fool yourself into thinking that exercise is an all-benefit, no-risk proposition.

### Heart Health Myths

There are three main myths about exercise and coronary health:

• Myth: Exercise makes your heart healthier. Many people, including physicians, have mistaken mechanical efficiency of the heart for health of the heart. Exercise does make your heart mechanically more efficient—it makes it possible to do more physical activity more comfortably. But your heart isn't healthier just because it's beating more slowly. This would be true only if each of us were allotted a certain number of heartbeats per lifetime. There is no such allotment. I have patients in their nineties who have had fast heartbeats all their lives.

• Myth: Exercise improves your coronary circulation. Everyone now agrees that this is untrue, even avid exercisers. Jim Fixx was the most dramatic example. His coronary arteries were badly clogged. The original idea that exercise improved coronary circulation was based on an early-1950s study done with dogs under highly artificial conditions. The tests had nothing to do with anything resembling human life. Also: Exercise does not stimulate your body to grow collateral blood vessels around the heart. The only thing that does this is the clogging of your original arteries.

• Myth: Exercise reduces your coronary-risk factors. High blood pressure and cholesterol are the risk factors exercise is supposed to reduce. But . . . most hypertension specialists would agree that the likelihood of reducing blood pressure to a significant degree via an exercise program is very small. A California study of trained distance runners found that they had the same range of blood pressure as nonrunners. Common misconception: That lower heart rate means lower blood pressure. One has nothing to do with the other. It's been claimed that there are several types of cholesterol: HDL (high density lipoprotein), the "good" cholesterol . . . and the "bad" ones, LDL (low density lipoprotein) and triglycerides. Exercise supposedly raises the level of the good ones and lowers the bad. Problem: There's no proof that the "good" kind is really so good. The latest evidence suggests that even when your HDL goes up after exercise, it may be the wrong kind of HDL. Some studies show that HDL doesn't go up with exercise and that triglycerides and LDL don't go down. There's even an important study that shows the opposite actually occurs. So far, a low-fat, low-cholesterol diet is the only reliable way to lower cholesterol levels.

### Other Health Myths

• Myth: Exercise makes you live longer. No one really knows why some people live longer than others. Innumerable factors contribute to it, including genes, marital status, number of social contacts, resistance to stress and educational level. There's never been an unflawed study showing that exercise prolongs life. Just as many studies "prove" it as "disprove" it. The ones that make extravagant claims for exercise have gotten all the publicity. An interesting book called *Living to Be 100* analyzed 1,200 centenarians. Avoidance of stress was a common denominator.

• Myth: Exercise makes you feel better. A lot of people do feel better when they exercise. But many other people would feel much better curling up with a good book. Although many claims have been made that exercise alleviates depression and anxiety, the data are contradictory. Some studies claim benefits, others don't. Some studies comparing the benefits of exercise with those of meditation and relaxation have found no difference.

### The Dangers of Exercise

There is extreme danger to the heart during exercise. Eighty percent of sudden cardiac deaths occur during moderate or vigorous exercise. Jim Fixx was an example of this syndrome—underlying coronary disease (usually blocked coronary arteries)—despite years of running. The sudden-death rate during running and among runners is seven to nine times greater than among sedentary people.

The most common danger of certain types of exercise, especially running, is orthopedic injuries. Podiatrists and orthopedists are doing a brisk business. Every year, two—thirds of all runners injure themselves sufficiently to have to give up running for a while. Worse: Today's runners may be tomorrow's arthritics.

There are other medical dangers to exercise. Intestinal bleeding is a common phenomenon among runners even after only a few miles. No one knows what causes this, but it's suspected to be something like gangrene—insufficient blood flow caused by diverting blood from the stomach to the muscles. You can bleed from the kidneys while running. Some runners develop asthma or other allergies, even if they've never had allergies before, and others develop intense constriction of the bronchial tubes. Young women are vulnerable to osteoporosis (brittle bones)—which usually affects only postmenopausal women. The loss of body fat is sufficient to alter their hormone systems.

### What Should You Do?

Don't engage in strenuous exercise. Among the risk factors for coronary disease, physical inactivity ranks near the bottom. You can counter this small risk by getting a little exercise. I recommend walking—the safest, easiest, least expensive exercise going. If you walk a mile twice a day at a pace of 20 minutes or less per mile, you'll surely get enough exercise to undo the risks of inactivity. Even a mile once a day is probably enough. That's all it takes to get the health benefits of exercise.

**Source:** Interview with Henry A. Solomon, M.D., a cardiologist who practices in New York City, where he is on the faculty of Cornell University Medical College.

# POGO-STICK THERAPY

Exercising an injured knee conventionally can be quite painful. However, recovering athletes have a new therapy, too—the pogo stick. Orthopedic specialists say that the child's jumping stick allows people with knee problems to strengthen their quadriceps and hamstring muscles without moving the injured joint unduly. Result: No pain while you're in the process of increasing knee stability.

**Source:** *The Physician and Sportsmedicine.*

• High-tech pogo stick tones abdominal, arm and leg muscles and improves heart rate and respiration. The Jetstar comes in red or blue, with three models for adults of different weights: 100, 150 or 200 pounds.

**Source:** Trileen, Inc., Costa Mesa, CA.

# EXERCISER'S WOE

Swollen fingers or toes during or after exercise are not necessarily cause for alarm. Hikers experience the phenomenon, as well as those who work out indoors. Reason: Since vigorous activity often leads to muscle trauma (muscles must be broken down in order to be built up), some minor swelling may occur in the extremities due to this trauma. Consult a doctor if the swelling persists or is accompanied by discoloration or pain.

**Source:** Bruce Yaffe, M.D., a gastroenterologist in private practice in New York.

## HELP FOR SPRAINS AND STRAINS

Ice packs can stave off joint problems as well as treat sprains and strains. Applying ice to joints after a strenuous workout can prevent inflammation, swelling and soreness.

**Source:** Orthopedic surgeon Paul Bauer, quoted in *Medical World News.*

## WORST THING TO DO IF YOU WANT A MORE DEMANDING WORKOUT

Wrist and ankle weights often do more harm than good to runners and aerobic exercisers. Reason: Every added pound requires 3.5% more effort, but most people fail to compensate by reducing their workouts. Also, weights often strain ligaments and tendons in the joints. Recommended alternative: For a more demanding workout, increase your mileage or exercise time.

**Source:** *Rodale Report,* Emmaus, PA.

## HOW TO KNOW WHEN YOU'RE DOING TOO MUCH

Overdoing on exercise can make your body more susceptible to injury and infection. Testing your limits: After exercising, rest for exactly five minutes. If your pulse still registers more than 120 beats per minute, you're pushing yourself too hard. (Limits

for people over 55 are lower.) Good rule: Never exercise so hard that you're gasping for breath.

**Source:** *Personal Lifeplan for Health and Fitness* by Dennis and David Singsank, American Health and Nutrition, Madison, WI.

## WORKOUT WARNING

Regular, moderate exercise is more healthful than more intensive but sporadic workouts, a comprehensive analysis confirms. Data from 66 studies show that a person lowers "bad" cholesterol and raises "good" cholesterol in proportion to the time spent in physical activity. But high intensity of exercise, by itself, has no effect. Bottom line: A brisk walk or slow jog for 30 minutes a day is better than a heavy weekend workout.

**Source:** Research at the University of Colorado, cited in *The Harvard Medical School Health Letter.*

## COOLING OFF

Keep your postworkout shower lukewarm. Hot water makes you start sweating again and drains energy. Best: Finish off with a 30-second cold shower. Cold water benefits both circulation and muscle tone.

**Source:** *Ultrahealth* by Leslie kenton, Deliah Communications, Ltd., New York.

## HOW TO AVOID A POSTEXERCISE HEART ATTACK

Postexercise heart attacks do not exclude any age group. Even for young, healthy people, stopping strenuous exercise abruptly is dangerous. Blood pressure falls drastically (in one recent study, the average drop was from 189/78 to 137/70) and increases the risk of a heart attack. Mandatory: A cooldown period. Conclude the strenuous exercise gradually and lie down afterwards for a few minutes.

**Source:** *Journal of the American Medical Association.*

## DRUG WARNING

Drugs and exercise can be a hazardous combination. Aspirin can mask the pain that should tell you to stop. Antihistamines can cause drowsiness and strain the heart and muscles. Decongestants raise overall blood pressure. Diuretics can lead to dehydration and cramping. Tranquilizers, besides robbing you of your competitive edge, dull your perception of pain. Best: Take a new drug at least twice and gauge your reaction before adding to the stress of vigorous exercise. And never combine different drugs with exercise without consulting your doctor.

**Source:** Richard H. Dominguez, M.D., co-medical director, Sports Performance and Rehabilitation Institute, Carol Stream, IL.

## IMPORTANCE OF STICKING TO IT

The average exercise or diet regimen lasts only four days. Before you start one, see if you can imagine doing it regularly and for the long haul.

**Source:** *Stress Management* by Edward A. Charlesworth, Atheneum, New York.

• Exercise layoffs quickly erode gains made in heart and lung capacity. Steepest drop: During the first 12 days of inactivity. After that, the fitness decline continues at a slower rate. Advice: After suspending exercise because of illness, resume your workout at a lower level to give your body time to work back up.

**Source:** Research at Washington University Medical School, St. Louis, MO.

## INVERSION—A SENSELESS NEW FAD

Hanging upside down is a new fad, a particularly senseless one. It does absolutely no good to anyone, and can dangerously raise blood pressure, especially if a person tries to exercise or lift weights in this position.

**Source:** *Harvard Medical School Health Letter.*

## SOME EXERCISES TO AVOID

Harmful exercises: (1) Bouncing (tears connective tissue between muscles). (2) Locking knees and elbows (puts excessive stress on tendons and ligaments). (3) Back bends and full waist circles (can injure discs). (4) Jumping jacks with swinging arms (tear muscle fiber). (5) Deep-knee bends, squat thrusts, deep pushups, (strain ligaments and tear cartilage). (6) Any exercise if it is done too fast.

**Source:** *Vogue.*

## EXERCISE BY COMPUTER

New software allows the home-computer owner to choose among 18 different routines that vary in length of workout, level of difficulty and part of the body to be exercised. Aerobics–video display features a woman exercising accompanied by synthesized music.

**Source:** Spinnaker Software, Cambridge, MA.

## RATING THE EXERCISE VIDEOTAPES

Video workout tapes seem to offer the best of both worlds—a challenging fitness routine with the convenience of doing it at home. But they share one major flaw: They don't teach you how to exercise properly. Even the programs with narrative voiceovers don't compare correct techniques with the wrong ones. They may tell you not to hyperextend your leg, but they never show you what they mean and often they fail to practice what they preach. (As Jane Fonda urges you not to "bounce," she herself is bouncing a good deal of the time.)

Without individual monitoring and supervision, beginning exercisers can do themselves serious damage. Advice: Before buying an exercise tape, take a class with a qualified teacher. There you'll learn body awareness and the right alignments. Then you can safely follow a tape as either a supplemental or primary form of exercise. With that caveat, I would rate some of the more popular videotapes as follows:

• *Every Day with Richard Simmons' Family Fitness*, $59.95. This is probably the best one for beginners. It's a good overall workout, varied and well paced, with nothing really harmful. And unlike many exercise videotapes, it offers superior production values. Simmons knows how to motivate people. The program holds your interest. But like most workout tapes, Simmons's falls short on aerobics. He offers five minutes of running in place—far short of what you need for real cardiovascular benefits. Suggestion: Stop the tape at this point and continue on your own for another 15 minutes. Protect your feet with sneakers (not worn on the tape).

• *Jane Fonda's Workout*, $59.95. It has value, but only if you discard several dangerous stretches and exercises. Examples: The drop-over, where you stand and stretch your head down to your knees. (If you round your back—and if you're less flexible than Fonda, you will round it—you could pop a disk.) Stretches with locked knees. (You could hyperextend and rip the knee joint.) The "plow." (Could pinch the upper spine and interfere with blood circulation of the brain.) The "V" sit-up. (Unless you have extremely strong abdominals, you'll arch your back and possibly strain the lower back.) The abdominal drills demand too many repetitions for the beginner. You should stop your workout halfway through if you're feeling too much "burn." This tape is really geared to the intermediate exerciser.

• *Jane Fonda's Workout Challenge*, $59.95. This does not include some of the more dangerous routines. Still, this workout is suitable only for dancers and extremely advanced exercisers. The stretches include too much bouncing, which can tear muscles. Better: A gentle pulsing, as you try to hold a stretch and push lightly on each beat of the music.

• *Jacki Sorensen's Aerobic Dancing "Encore,"* $39.95. You get 30 minutes of true aerobic conditioning in a program paced for beginners. Drawback: Although the dance steps

are fairly simple, they may be too intricate for many men. And there's little material here that provides strength or flexibility training.

• *Jayne Kennedy's Love Your Body*, $59.95. The warm-ups are fine. But the music is too sluggish for adequate aerobics. The tape includes several dangerous exercises (the plow, the hurdler's stretch, straight-leg lowering for the abdominals). Another problem: Kennedy shifts from beginning moves to advanced moves without warning or development.

### Tapes to Avoid

• *Let's Jazzercise*, $39.95. This is a cutesy-pie mishmash with no logical progression. It may have some toning value for those who are very out of shape.

• *Texersize*, $39.95. Leader Irlene Mandrell is a prebeginner herself. This tape has no redeeming features.

• *Aerobicise: The Ultimate Workout*, $29.95. Too many of the exercises are done by scantily clad women with arched backs and tilted pelvises—a dangerous example to follow.

### Bottom Line

Since no hour-long videotape can satisfy all exercise goals, for experienced exercisers I would recommend the Sorensen tape for aerobics and the Simmons and Fonda tapes (with caution) to develop strength and flexibility. Alternating the tapes (each three days a week, with a Sunday rest), gives you an optimal workout.

**Source:** Interview with Jackie Rogers, president of Aerobics 'n' Rhythm, a national exercise program based in Westfield, NJ.

# R$_x$ FOR STRESS

Regular aerobic exercise seems to improve the way we handle stress. Results of a study: When students without aerobic conditioning were told they'd done poorly on a test, they showed increased blood pressure, muscle tension and anxiety. But the aerobic-conditioned group reacted with less tension and anxiety and no rise in blood pressure—a key measure of stress reaction.

**Source:** *Berkeley Wellness Letter,* Berkeley CA.

## HOW FAST SHOULD YOU GO?

Aerobic exercise is safest when you keep it at a "conversational" pace. Even at highest intensity, you should be able to talk—in a slightly halting (but not gasping) manner. By observing this precaution you'll help to avoid stress on the heart.

**Source:** Dr. Franklin Payne Jr., Medical College of Georgia, Augusta, GA.

## NOT FOR ADULTS ONLY

Aerobic exercise benefits children as much as adults. A new study has found that children between five and 13 showed improved heart function after participating in 20-minute sessions several times a week. Theory: These children will have reduced risk of heart attack later in life.

**Source:** Study by William Stone, department of health and physical education, Arizona State University, Tempe.

## WHEN YOU'RE READY TO STOP

Keep moving for at least five minutes after an aerobic workout until your heart rate drops below 120 (below 100, if you're over 50). The most dangerous period is just after a workout. A cool-down is necessary because the heart is starved for blood when blood pressure and heart rate both drop.

**Source:** *Employee Health & Fitness.*

## AEROBIC-DANCING ALERT

Aerobic dancing may not be so good for your health. Injuries plague 50%–70% of the estimated 18.7 million participants in this energetic exercise. More than half the injuries involve the lower leg: Shins, calves and feet.

**Source:** *Medical World News,* Houston, TX.

## TRY JUMPING ROPE

Jumping rope can be an ideal fitness supplement for endurance, muscle strength and agility. The rope should be heavy enough that you can develop a steady rhythm (the leather ones with ball-bearing handles are very good) and long enough so the ends reach your armpits when you stand on the center. Caution: Jumping rope can raise the heart rate too high for those not already in shape.

**Source:** *Berkeley Wellness Letter.*

## IDEAL AEROBIC EXERCISE

"Rebounding" on a mini-trampoline. Like swimming or running, rebounding strengthens the heart and lungs and firms muscles. And the continuous changes in gravity stimulate cellular metabolism and elimination. Result: A gradual detoxification of your whole system. Added advantage: Because the activity is easy and enjoyable, people tend to stick with it longer.

**Source:** *Ultrahealth* by Leslie Kenton, Deliah Communications, Ltd., New York.

## SPACE-AGE GYMS

The sophisticated machinery that has turned old-fashioned gyms into today's health clubs and fitness centers is indeed revolutionary. Designed to improve the training of serious athletes, equipment, such as the Nautilus system, offers great benefits to more ordinary mortals as well.

To understand how these machines can fit into a normal person's health regimen, we interviewed a physical therapist who directs the program of a fitness center in

New York City.

What is revolutionary about machines such as the Nautilus?

The equipment is designed to offer continuous resistance during each of the movement exercises you use it for. This is a much faster, more efficient way to build muscle strength than using weights, for example. Reasons: These new machines demand consistent effort throughout. Also, they are carefully programmed to work on all the major muscle groups in the body. This requires different sets of exercises for different machines, but the option of dealing with any specific problem is there.

So, if I did all the exercises for all the muscle groups on a regular basis, would I be perfectly fit?

No. This equipment builds muscle strength. But strength and fitness are not equivalent. Although muscle strength is a component of fitness, you also need flexibility and heart-lung capacity. Stretching exercises make you flexible, and aerobic exercises such as running and bike riding build up your heart muscle and your lung capacity.

Why is building muscle strength important if it isn't helping my heart or making me more limber?

If you are active in any kind of sport, building up muscle strength improves your performance. Even more important, strong muscles prevent injuries that result from poor muscle tone. . . particularly lower back pain, the number-one orthopedic problem in the US. You are much less likely to suffer from sports injuries if you follow a good muscle-strengthening regimen.

Can working out on these machines help me lose weight?

There is a common myth that strengthening exercises turn fat into muscle. It doesn't work that way. People who are overweight need to follow a calorie-restricted diet and do aerobic exercises, which trigger the body to use up fat. Working out on machines only builds up muscle under the fat layer. However, combining a weight-loss program with strengthening exercises can improve body tone as the weight comes off.

Are these machines dangerous?

Not if you follow proper instructions. Ideally, a trainer should be supervising you and giving you feedback the whole time you are on each machine. (To cover the entire body, you must work out on 12–15 different ones, each designed for a different group of muscles.) You need to learn the proper technique for using each machine, including proper breathing, before you are allowed on the equipment alone. On the Nautilus, for example, all the straps must be secured before you start. If one is broken or missing, don't use the machine. Poor form on the machines can lead to serious injuries. So can using the wrong weight settings.

How can I tell if I am using the right settings?

As your muscles get stronger, you will want to work against harder and harder resistance. This is how you make progress. However, working against too much weight can cause muscle strain. Good rule of thumb: Use a weight setting that lets you do 8–12 repetitions comfortably. If you must struggle to get beyond five, the setting is too heavy. If you complete 10 without feeling any fatigue at all, it is too light. You will have to experiment with each machine to get the right setting. Then, from time to time, you can adjust the weights upward. But be cautious. Pushing yourself too hard not only invites injury, it also discourages you from sticking to the program on a regular basis.

**Source:** Interview with James S. Cardone, program director and director of physical therapy, Bio-Fitness Institute, New York.

## MACHINES VS. WEIGHTS

Working out with a machine, such as Nautilus or Universal, is easier to learn and safer than working with free weights (barbells and dumbells), since there's nothing to fall on you. Machines are also more effective in building the lower body. However, free weights do a better job for the chest, shoulders, forearms and back.

**Source:** *USA Today.*

## ABOUT WEIGHT-LIFTING

Moderate weight-lifting is good for the heart, according to a recent study of 14 nonexercisers who worked out regularly with weights for 16 weeks. All showed an increase in HDL ("good") cholesterol and a decrease in LDL (harmful) cholesterol. In another study, eight body-builders also showed a healthy HDL-to-LDL ratio.

**Source:** *Journal of the American Medical Association, Washington, DC.*

## INDOOR EXERCISE MACHINES

• Multipurpose gyms: To develop major muscle groups, not cardiorespiratory fitness. Check for: Smoothly tracking weights. A sturdy, level bench. Padded levers. Steel pulleys. Coated cables. Cost: $400 and up.

• Stationary cycles: For cardiovascular fitness, injury rehabilitation and lower-body strength. Check for: A rigid frame. A heavy flywheel. A seat post that can be locked into position. Cost: $100–$400.

• Treadmills: For cardiovascular fitness through running or walking. Check for: Comfortable, secure footing. Cost: $700 and up.

• Rowing machines: For cardiovascular fitness, all major muscle groups and injury rehabilitation. Check for: A smoothly sliding seat. A track that allows full leg extension. Oars with equal resistance. A covered flywheel. Cost: $150–$600.

• Skiing machines: For cardiovascular fitness, major-muscle development. Cost: Around $500.

**Source:** *Changing Times,* Washington, DC.

## BEST EXERCISE MACHINE

The stationary bicycle is safe, aerobic and noncompetitive. You can ride it rain or shine, and because you work out continuously without pauses, you can work off more calories per minute than in a stop-and-start sport.

**Source:** *Spring.*

## STATIONARY BICYCLES: HOW TO PICK AND USE THEM

A good in-home stationary bicycle should be made from sturdy steel (not lightweight aluminum). It should have a comfortable, adjustable-height seat, smoothly rotating pedals, and a selector for several degrees of pedal speed and resistance (simulated "uphill" pedaling that makes your heart work harder). A heavyweight flywheel creates a smoother and more durable drive system. Sophisticated electronic gadgets such as "calories burned" or "work-load" meters are frills.

Our picks of stationary cycles:

• The Fitron ($1,000). The Fitron is really designed for the heavy use and different needs of health clubs, not for just one home cyclist. But we would rate it the best among stationary bicycles.

• The Body Guard 955 Home Ergometer (around $450). This bike has the smoothest flywheel rotation of any we've found.

• The Home Tenturi Ergometer (around $425).

• The Monarch 865 Ergometer (around $425).

To choose the right cycle: Visit a large sporting goods store and try a variety of models. The one that works you hard and still feels comfortable is right for you.

To ride without pain or injury:

• First, check with your doctor, especially if you have any heart, knee or leg problems.

• Raise the seat on your cycle high enough so that in the downward position your foot just reaches the pedal with your knee slightly bent. This is the proper mechanical position for cycling.

• Always warm up and cool down with your bicycle set on a low resistance level. After a three- to five-minute warmup, set a constant pedal speed and increase the resistance to the level of difficulty at which you want to work. Cool down with a lower resistance setting, again for three to five minutes.

• When you begin a stationary bicycle program, work at 60% of your predicted maximum heart rate. To calculate the rate: Subtract your age from 220. Sixty percent of that figure is the number of times your heart should beat per minute during your workout. If your heart is beating faster, then you are overdoing it. As you become more fit, you can work at up to 80% of your predicted maximum heart rate. But remember to keep the increase slow and gradual.

• Start cycling in 10-minute sessions. Then increase to 15, then 20, and then 25 or more minutes per session. Gradual increases over a period of weeks help prevent injury to muscles and joints. Once you build up your physical strength, you can pedal for as long as you feel comfortable.

**Source:** Interview with Anthony Saraniti, director, and Alan Kroll, program director, Eastside Sportsmedicine Center, New York.

## ALTERNATIVES TO FORMAL EXERCISES

Vigorous exercise isn't the only way to stay healthy. An easier way to help circulation and relax your nervous system: Lie on your back on the floor. Raise your lower legs and rest them on a chair, with knees relaxed and slightly bent. Keep them there five to 10 minutes. Do this once or twice a day.

**Source:** *Sports without Pain* by Ben E. Benjamin, Summit Books, New York.

• If you hate formal exercise, you can still stay fit through natural activity. Walk for 20 minutes a day in loose-fitting clothes and soft shoes. Try the "M&M" policy: Move more. Take stairs instead of elevators. Walk for the paper. Stow your golf cart, and carry your own bags.

**Source:** Norbert M. Sander, Jr. M.D., founder of the Preventive and Sports Medical Center, New York City.

## CHINESE SECRETS OF INNER STRENGTH

If you've ever seen a TV documentary on China, it probably included a shot of people performing *tai chi chuan*. It's for the Chinese what jogging is for us—something like a national exercise. However, tai chi is a total body-and-mind exercise.

### How It Works

The ancient art of tai chi (pronounced *tie-jee*) uses a series of very slow, fluid movements, which are imitations of natural animal movements. Each movement is supposed to benefit a different part of the body. Some movements are meant to strengthen internal organs, others to promote muscle strength.

The objective is to release tension, relax the body and calm the nerves. Relaxation is important, because it is seen as the natural state, while tension is unnatural.

The short form of tai chi consists of 37 movements that take about seven minutes to complete. The traditional long form has 108 movements and takes about a half hour. The long-form movements are more expansive, rounder and more graceful.

While doing tai chi, one must concentrate on breathing correctly and visualizing bodily energy flowing in certain directions. This concentration gives tai chi a meditative quality, which is probably why it works so well for stress reduction.

### Who Can Benefit?

Although Oriental martial arts such as kung fu and karate share a common origin in tai chi, nowadays tai chi is done mostly to improve health. Physical therapists in China prescribe it for heart problems, arthritis and respiratory ailments. The least aggressive and most graceful of the martial arts, tai chi is actually non-strenuous and is appropriate for many heart patients, the elderly and those in fair or even poor physical condition.

Physical benefits: Tai chi helps posture and lower-back problems because it aligns the spine and strengthens the lower back.

Many movements are done with the leg bent, and these movements strengthen the leg muscles.

It has also helped to lower high blood pressure, improve breathing, alleviate respiratory illnesses such as asthma and bronchitis and strengthen organs such as the bladder and kidneys as well as the joints in the knees and ankles.

### Self-Discipline

Psychological benefits: Tai chi reputedly improves sensitivity to others. The slow, gentle movements increase awareness, facilitating more attentive listening and quicker adjustment to changing situations. The almost hypnotic quality of the movements slows the mental pace, reducing nervousness and promoting a sense of inner peace. Some practitioners claim the calm and self-discipline that tai chi promotes help overcome such habits as smoking and drinking.

You don't need a gym or complicated equipment to practice tai chi. It takes about 24 classes over three or four months to learn the movements, after which you can practice it yourself every day to keep fit. Fifteen minutes a day is enough to maintain health and strength. Many people do it outdoors as the Chinese do.

To find a school, visit the facility and watch a class and the instructor. The classroom should be spacious and the instructor should project calm and relaxation himself. Important: A school that emphasizes health, not self-defense. Recommended: A school that's been in business for several years.

**Source:** Interview with tai chi master Don Ahn, who in 1970 founded the Ahn Tai Chi Studio in New York.

# TO LOSE WEIGHT SUCCESSFULLY

More and more research is pointing to exercise, rather than reduced calorie intake, as the key to shedding excess pounds. Among the new insights:

• Aerobic exercise—the sustained kind of workout that conditions heart and lungs— raises your metabolism and helps you burn off calories at a higher rate. Jogging, pedaling, swimming or jumping rope not only use up calories in the doing, they also speed up the calorie-burning of your other activities. Regular exercise can boost a slow metabolism 20%–30%. A single aerobic workout can keep your metabolism up for as long as 15 hours.

• Drastic dieting triggers a loss of water and protein from your body in the first few weeks. This drain causes you to feel tired, which in turn makes you less active. You will need even fewer calories to maintain your weight. It takes several weeks for your body to start burning fat. If you are still on the diet, it will have to be even more restricted to be effective.

• Cutting calories slows down your metabolism, making your body conserve calories as a defense against starvation. If you go off a diet regimen that doesn't include exercise, you will gain weight even more quickly than before the diet.

• Vigorous exercise draws on fat for energy. Fat does not burn off as quickly as muscle protein, but the pounds are more likely to stay off.

• Aerobic exercise suppresses appetite and relieves stress. (Stress causes many people to overeat in the first place.)

• Regular aerobic exercise turns fat into muscle, a double benefit. Muscle takes up less space, so you look trimmer. Muscle also needs more calories to sustain itself, so you can eat more without risking a weight gain.

**Source:** *The 200 Calorie Solution* by Martin Katahn, Ph.D., Berkley Publishing, New York; *The Dieter's Dilemma* by William Bennet, M.D., and Joel Gurin, Basic Books, New York; and *California Diet and Exercise Program* by Peter Wood, M.D., Anderson World Books, Mountain View, CA.

# TO GET RID OF FAT

To burn away stored fat, you must exercise at least three times a week for 30–60 minutes each time. Shorter periods of exercise, even with high intensity, burn only stored carbohydrates.

**Source:** *Ultrahealth* by Leslie Kenton, Deliah Communications, Ltd., New York.

## EXERCISE AFTER EATING

Working off a big meal is easier than you think. Exercising soon after eating is an efficient way to burn off excess calories. Reason: Since both eating a good meal and exercising raise your body's metabolic rate, you use up more calories exercising after a meal than before one. (Conversely, cutting back on calories lowers your metabolism and makes you work harder to burn off what you do eat.) Minimum requirement for working off a meal: A 20-minute walk within 45 minutes of eating.

**Source:** David Levitsky and Eva Obarzanek, Division of Nutritional Sciences, Cornell University.

## A LITTLE EXERCISE GOES A LONG WAY

Modest physical activity for 30 minutes per day will knock as much as 15 pounds off your weight within six months—assuming, of course, that calorie intake is not increased.

• Fit people burn more calories after eating than do less trim individuals. An average person's metabolic rate jumps about 30% during the two hours after a meal (that's why you feel warm after a heavy lunch). But for dedicated joggers and the like, the jump is even higher and lasts longer. The difference: An extra 40 calories burned a day.

**Source:** Study by Dr. Jim Davis, a psychologist at the University of New Hampshire, in *American Health.*

## TRUTH ABOUT CELLULITE

Cellulite is not a special fat that resists diet and exercise. It is simply the dimpled fat found on the hips and thighs of many women. Since it is ordinary fat, it can be reduced as part of any respectable weight-loss program.

**Source:** *Vitamins and "Health" Foods: The Great American Hustle,* by Victor Herbert, M.D., and Stephen Barret, M.D., Stickley Publishing.

## EXERCISES TO DO IN THE CAR

(1) Double chin: Lift chin slightly and open and close mouth as though chewing. (2) Flabby neck: Move head toward right shoulder while looking straight ahead at the road. Return head to center, then toward left shoulder. (3) Pot belly: Sit straight with spine against back seat. Pull stomach in and hold breath for count of 5. Relax, then repeat. The exercise also relieves tension and helps fight sleepiness.

## STOMACH FLATTENER

Sit or stand upright and suck in your stomach. Hold for about 20 seconds, breathing normally. Repeat about once every waking hour. You should see results within four weeks.

**Source:** Dr. David Bachman, former assistant professor of orthopedic surgery, Northwestern University Medical School, Chicago.

## CALORIES AND GOLF

A 180-pound man playing 18 holes of golf will use 850 calories if he carries his clubs and 760 if he pulls them. Hazard: Each 12-ounce glass of beer at the clubhouse puts back about 150 of those calories.

**Source:** *Modern Maturity.*

## STEAM BATH AND SAUNA MYTH

Sweat therapy won't deflate the "spare tire" around your waist—or even help you lose weight. Reason: Saunas, steam baths and body wraps cause dehydration. But since body fat contains only a trace of water, it is unaffected.

**Source:** Dan Riley, conditioning coach for the Washington Redskins, quoted in *The Washington Post.*

## 15-MINUTE SAUNA CAN EQUAL A 2-MILE JOG

Sauna bathing for only 15 minutes uses as many calories as a mile or two of jogging. Even after you replace the water you've lost, a regular sauna program helps you lose weight. Reason: Working up a sweat acts to speed the body's metabolism.

## FITNESS SECRETS

Between the ages of 30 and 50, the average sedentary person declines by 15% in cardiovascular and muscular fitness. But our studies have shown that this decline is neither inevitable nor irreversible At least half of it stems from simple atrophy through disuse. That portion can be regained with proper fitness training. (In fact, some middle-aged people end up in better shape than they were in at 30.)

The key here is to follow a good exercise program conscientiously. (I recommend Kenneth Cooper's *Aerobics* and *Aerobics for Women.*) But some people try to do too much too soon. They think they're immortal. They retain the same competitive mindset they had as college students. After 20 or 30 years of relative nonactivity, they try to get back to where they were by participating at their old level. But their muscles aren't toned to hold their joints in place. Result: Severe injuries to the ankles, knees and hips.

Before launching a fitness program, anyone over 40 should have a complete physical examination, including an electrocardiogram. If there are any abnormalities, a stress test should be performed to check the heart's capacity.

We advise against jumping into a racquet sport or a basketball league. Instead, prepare your body with a six-month program of walking and stretching. Light jogging and weight training are also helpful. (This is especially important for middle-aged women, whose muscles are generally less developed starting out.)

When you're ready to take on a rigorous sport, the same philosophy carries over. Break each workout into five parts. First walk or jog in place for two or three minutes (critical for people who frequently pull muscles). Then warm up with 10 minutes of stretching. When you move into your sport, take the first five minutes at a slow pace (a relaxed volley in tennis, for example) until you break into a light sweat. After that you can pour on some more coal. Recommended peak activity: For the first few months, aim for 40%–60% of your maximum heart rate.* After six months you can go to 70%. After nine months (and to keep improving fitness), vigorous exercisers can shoot for 85%. Finally take 10 minutes to cool down with slow jogging and more stretching.

"Going for the burn" may be fine for a young athlete, but it's all wrong for the middle-aged. You'll know you've gone too far if it aches to take a step the next day.

There is no ideal sport for everyone. Swimming is easy on the joints but it lacks the healthful stress needed to build bone strength. (A recent study found that tennis players had 20% more calcium and phosphorous in their spines than swimmers.) Running and racquet sports provide good aerobic workouts but can be hard on the knees and ankles. Cycling is a fine alternative, but it does little for upper-body strength. Rowing works most major muscle groups, but many people find it boring.

Solution: Choose a complementary activity to go along with your primary sport. A swimmer might walk or jog two days a week. A runner could work with weights. In any case, the longevity of the program is the key. It doesn't help to train every muscle intensively for a week and then do nothing for two months. It's also dangerous. Weekend warriors are prime heart attack victims. Minimum frequency for increasing fitness: Three sessions a week, at least 30 minutes per session.

Bottom line: Find a sport you enjoy, and then stick with it.

To calculate these goals, subtract your resting heart rate from your maximum rate—220 minus your age—and multiply by the desired percentage. Then add your resting rate to get your goal. Example: A 45-year-old man has a maximum heart rate of 175 and a resting rate of 60. To perform at 70% of maximum, he should reach a rate of 140.

**Source:** Interview with Everett L. Smith, director of the Biogerontology Laboratory, Department of Preventive Medicine, University of Wisconsin, Madison.

## DANGEROUS SPORTS

Football is not the most dangerous college sport. Lacrosse is the riskiest, followed by gymnastics and ice hockey. The rates of death and permanent injury per 100,000 participants: Lacrosse, 20.25; gymnastics, 14.27; ice hockey, 12.73; football, 9.33; tennis 6.83; basketball, 6.63; swimming, 3.55.

**Source:** Study by The University of North Carolina, Chapel Hill.

## AEROBIC RATINGS OF SPORTS

Best for cardiovascular fitness: Stationary bicycling, uphill hiking, ice hockey, rope jumping, rowing, running and cross-country skiing.

Moderately effective: Basketball, outdoor bicycling, calisthenics, handball, field hockey, racquetball, downhill skiing, soccer, squash, swimming, singles tennis and walking.

Nonaerobic: Baseball, bowling, football, golf, softball, volleyball.

**Source:** Franklin Payne Jr., M.D., Medical College of Georgia, Augusta, GA.

## BUYING ATHLETIC SHOES

When buying athletic shoes, shop in the late afternoon. Your feet will be most swollen at that time—and closest to the size they reach during sports activities.

• Of 50 million Americans who own running shoes, only 20 million actually run. And only 12 million hit the road more than a few times a year. How many run 40 miles per week? 700,000.

**Source:** Report by American Sports Data, White Plains, NY.

## BEST PRE-WORKOUT SNACK

A banana is an ideal preworkout snack. It's easily digested and converts rapidly into energy. It compensates for body losses of potassium. And, a single banana provides

20% of the RDA of vitamin $B_6$ (essential for building muscle tissue).

**Source:** Robert Keith, Ph.D., a nutritionist at Auburn University, in *The Runner.*

## TRUTH ABOUT HIGH-SUGAR SNACKS

Is athletic performance improved if you eat a high-sugar snack just before competing? Surprisingly, the answer is no. In tests, the exercise time to exhaustion was 25% longer when runners drank a sugar-free drink than when they drank one with sugar. After the sugar-containing drinks, sugar levels rose rapidly but then sank quickly. . . a drop-off that seems to be responsible for more rapid exhaustion. This goes against the conventional wisdom of eating a candy bar before a big race.

**Source:** *Physician Sports Medicine.*

## DRINK OF CHAMPIONS

For top athletic performance, make sure your body gets enough water. Guideline: Drink two cups of water 15 minutes before exercise or competition. . .one cup every 15–30 minutes during the activity. . .and at least two cups beyond thirst requirements when the activity is over. Less effective: "Sports" drinks. These contain sugar and salt and take longer to reach the bloodstream than pure water.

**Source:** *Eat to Win* by Robert Haas, Rawson Associates, New York.

## FITNESS MYTH

Stretching is the best way to warm up before exercise or a sports activity. Reality: Stretching doesn't generate enough heat to warm up muscles. Better: Start the activity at a slower rate. Take a fast walk before you run. . .toss a ball easily before throwing it hard. (Stretching, however, has its own value in keeping muscles flexible.)

**Source:** Mona Shangold, M.D., director of The Sports Gynecology Center at New York Hospital-Cornell Medical Center.

## BEST WARM-UP TECHNIQUE

Stay flexible. If you don't, the tendons that attach muscles to bones will shorten . . . and movement will become painful and restricted. Proper routine: First, warm up gradually by running in place or walking a block or so. Then slowly begin to stretch arms, legs and torso. Don't bounce. Stretch smoothly, and stop before it starts to hurt. Warm up and stretch before participating in any vigorous activity. Equally important: Stretch and cool down afterwards.

**Source:** *The Health Letter,*

## SPORTS STRATEGY

Taking regular breaks from your favorite sport improves your power and reduces the chance of injury. Good rule: Rest two to four minutes after every 30 minutes of vigorous activity. This gives your muscles a chance to recoup their oxygen supply. Alternative: Use the opposite set of muscles every so often. Examples: Alternate swimming on your stomach and your back . . . Volley with your left hand in between tennis matches.

**Source:** *Sports without Pain* by Ben E. Benjamin, Summit Books, New York.

## WHAT TO DO IF YOU GET HURT

Sports injuries that damage tissues or joints immediately develop swelling, pain and inflammation. To reduce the possibility of long-term damage while also alleviating pain, take an anti-inflammatory drug such as high-dose aspirin (Naprosyn or Motrin). Tylenol will reduce the pain but not the inflammation.

**Source:** *Pharmatherapeutica.*

## HOW TO BUY THE RIGHT BIKE

Commuters have special biking require-ments. If you're in the suit-and-tie crowd, you'll want fenders to keep yourself clean. You may want a rack on the back for a newspaper or side racks for your briefcase. They're making bicycle sacks (panniers) of heavier nylon now, with stiffeners to retain their briefcase shape. Although rubber pedals are less durable than steel, they'll help preserve your leather soles. Finally, every city rider needs a topnotch lock. The U-bolt models by Kryptonite and Citadel are among the best ones.

What kind to buy:

Touring bikes are right for most people. They have a longer wheel base for a "Cadillac" ride. Racing bikes offer a "Fiat" ride. With their shorter wheelbase, you feel the road more, but you get better handling and efficiency.

The Japanese have learned how to make bikes better and more cheaply. A European bike of equivalent quality will cost at least 20% more. Although there are 30 different Japanese makes, they're all produced by one of two corporate families, so they're about the same.

The best American bikes offer better frames, with superior materials and handcraftsmanship. But you sacrifice quality on components.

Choosing parts:

A good frame design for women is the mixte (pronounced mix-tay). Two parts run from the head tube to the rear axle for added stability. With longer skirts, many women can use a man's 10-speed, and they do. The men's models are lighter and stronger.

For those who find bicycles uncomfortable to sit on, a new anatomically designed saddle may be the answer. These seats, made of leather with foam padding, feature two ridges to support the pelvic bones, with a valley in between to avoid pinching the sciatic nerve.

Mixte handlebars, which project almost perpendicularly to the frame, are good for all-around cycling, as are racing (or drop) bars. The traditional curved bars are not recommended for city riding. They keep you sitting erect, so your spine is jolted by each bump. And foam grips will absorb more road shock than standard cloth tape grips.

In buying a helmet, look for a low-impact plastic shell. In a typical biking accident, this will protect the head better than a high-impact motorcycle helmet.

Padded bike gloves make good shock absorbers. Sheepskin bike shorts provide added comfort. Bike jerseys with rear pockets will keep your keys from digging into your leg with each push of the pedal.

**Source:** Charles McCorkell, owner, Bicycle Habitat, New York.

## CYCLING BY SEX

Female bike riders should point the seat slightly downwards to avoid irritating the genital area. Men should point the seat upward, to avoid problems such as irritation of the urinary tract and injury to the testes.

**Source:** *Physicians Sports Medicine.*

## MORE ABOUT BIKE SEATS

A bicycle seat can be uncomfortable or even dangerous if it's not at the right height and angle for your body. To gauge the optimal saddle height for your 10-speed: Measure 109% of your inseam size from the inner spindle in the pedal to the top of the seat, with the crankarms for the pedals parallel to the seat tube. The forward end of the seat should be a forearm (elbow to fingertip) away from the handle bar stem. When you are seated, the handlebars should obscure your view of the axle at the center of the front wheel.

**Source:** *Sportswise*, New York.

## ABOUT TENNIS ELBOW

The principal physical difference between serious tennis players and their week-end-only counterparts is the strength of their racket-holding wrist and finger extensions. (All players have a stronger racket-holding arm.) Doing exercises to build up that extension will not only prevent tennis elbow—it might also improve your game. Sample exercise: Hold your arms and hands out in front of you, palms down, at shoulder height. Without moving your arms, tilt your fingers toward the ceiling. You will feel the wrist and finger extension muscles. Relax and repeat. Variation: Try the exercise while holding small bar bells.

**Source:** *The American Journal of Sports Medicine,*

Tennis elbow is usually caused by insufficient arm strength or a hitch in your swing. Symptoms: Sharp pain on the court and a lingering ache thereafter. Remedies: Heat treatments, ice packs or, in extreme cases, cortisone shots. Stretching, wrist curls, and weights, to build up muscles strength. Then, lessons to correct your stroke.

## PREVENTING TENNIS ELBOW

Most important factor in preventing tennis elbow is your swing. While pros usually develop the pain on the inside of the elbow (from their service), recreational players get the condition on the outside of the arm (from the backhand).

• Solution: Switch to a two-handed stroke. Also: Be especially careful not to turn the wrist upward as you come through the backhand stroke. And keep the elbow firm at the time of impact.

Other preventives:

• Racquet: Metal rather than wood; flexible rather than rigid; light head rather than heavy; as large a handle as is comfortable, perhaps a 4⅝-inch grip if you have a big enough hand. Don't string with nylon. Choose 16-gauge gut, and avoid tight stringing—52 or 54 pounds will be the right tension for most amateur players.

• Balls: Avoid pressureless balls. Beware of heavier balls, particularly the Italian imports. Be careful, if you are vacationing in the mountains, about using balls bought for sea-level play: they will bounce faster, forcing you to stroke before you've gotten your body ready.

• Courts: A problem only if you switch to a faster court from a slow clay surface that you are used to. Makes you prone to taking the strokes late.

**Source:** *Physicians and Sportsmedicine,*

## BEST TENNIS RACKET FOR OLDER PLAYERS

The flexible wood racket probably jars the arm less than a metal racket. Older players will likely be more comfortable with lighter-weight rackets, and they may improve their game by using a racket that has been loosely strung.

**Source:** *Tennis Begins at Forty,* Pancho Gonzales, Dial Press, New York.

## HOW TO CHOOSE ICE SKATES

Most important: A stiff boot with a snug fit. Toes should reach the tip of the boot but lie flat. Lace the boot tightly through the toe area, very tightly through the instep, comfortably at the top. To check the fit. Walk. If your ankles wiggle even though the lacing is correct, ask for smaller or stiffer skates.

## CROSS-COUNTRY SKIING

Cross-country skiing is the most time-efficient aerobic exercise. It's more intense than running because it involves the arms and shoulders as well as the legs.

**Source:** Franklin Payne, Jr., M.D., Department of Family Practice, Medical College of Georgia, Augusta.

## FIGHTING FROST BITE ON SKI SLOPES

For warm hands and feet, a good hat helps. Reason: If your head and torso (the body's first priorities) are kept warm, blood circulates freely to the extremities. Most versatile hat: Wool with an acrylic liner gives you warmth without itchiness.

**Source:** *Skiing Magazine, New York.*

## WHAT YOU DON'T KNOW ABOUT SKI INJURIES

Skiers' thumbs are injured more than any other part of their bodies, according to a recent study. The classic ankle and shin injuries are at least 60% less common than in 1972. Reason: Better boots and safer ski bindings. Overall, the injury rate has declined from 7.6 injuries per 1,000 skier visits in 1960 to 2.2 per 1,000 visits in 1980.

**Source:** Study by Jasper Shealy, Ph.D., industrial engineering professor, Rochester Institute of Technology.

## BUYING SKI BOOTS

A snug, proper fit immobilizes the heel, instep and ball of your foot but leaves toes free to wiggle. The boot should flex forward comfortably, with no pressure on the shin or upper ankle. Note: A boot that feels a bit soft in the warm ski shop will stiffen slightly in the cold. Trying boots on: Begin with one model on the left foot and another model on the right. Walk around for 10 minutes. Then replace the less comfortable boot with a third model. Continue until you find the best for you.

**Source:** *Ski Magazine, New York.*

## BEST SKI PANTS

Stretch ski pants look great, but not all models are warm enough—especially for the novice or intermediate, who burns fewer calories and generates less heat. What to look for: High wool content (preferably with the wool floated to the inside, nearest your body). Terry lining (traps insulating dead air). For those who get cold easily: Newly marketed insulated stretch pants, with a three-layer sandwich construction.

**Source:** *Ski* Magazine, New York.

## GETTING THE MOST FROM THE BEST EXERCISE OF ALL

Swimming helps the entire musculature of

the body, particularly the upper torso. It tones muscles, but does not build them. Greatest benefit: To the cardiovascular system.

For weight loss: Running is better than swimming. Reason: In running, the heat generated is sweated away, burning off more calories. Water, however, cools the swimmer. The heat is dissipated into the water, and fewer calories are consumed.

Best strokes for a workout: Crawl, butterfly and back strokes. They are the most strenuous.

Less taxing: The side, breast and elementary breast strokes. These strokes are usually used for long distances to remain in the water for extended periods without tiring yourself.

Applications: The elementary back stroke is best for survival. The face is clear of the water for easy breathing, and the limited muscle use saves energy. The side stroke is traditional for lifesaving. It can be performed with one arm, which leaves the other free to tow someone. It is very relaxing—and effective.

In swimming, the legs do not receive as much exercise as the arms and shoulders. To build up the legs: Hold a kickboard while swimming. This forces propulsion by the legs alone. Or swim with the flippers favored by divers. Their surface increases the resistance to the water, making the legs work harder.

**Source:** Interview with James Steen, swimming coach at Kenyon College, Gambier, OH.

## TIPS IF YOU DO YOUR SWIMMING IN A POOL

When swimming in a pool, wear goggles to protect your eyes from chlorine. After swimming, place a drop of alcohol in each ear to help ward off infections. Have your indoor pool cleaned regularly to kill algae.

**Source:** Kenneth Cooper, M.D., in *USA Today.*

## SWIMMER'S HEADACHES

Some types of underwater goggles apply pressure in the wrong places. Best: Buy the kind with soft rubber rims around the eyes.

## SNORKELING SUCCESS

Snorkeling is an expensive way to get cardiovascular exercise. Since many of the most spectacular sights are at shallow depths, you don't need to be an especially strong swimmer. And, because your body is buoyed by water, snorkeling is an ideal activity for people with lower back pain, arthritis or trick knees. Advice: Stick to the leeward (away from the wind) sides of islands, where the water is calmer and clearer. Look but don't touch—some species of coral can cut and burn your skin.

**Source:** *Prevention,* Emmaus, PA.

## WHY YOU SHOULD CONSIDER ROWING

The ideal exercise may be rowing. It offers more benefits than jogging, swimming, bicycling or calisthenics. Rowing burns calories, eliminates body fat, improves endurance and boosts muscle strength and flexibility. And, it can be done indoors at any time. It's even suitable for arthritics and individuals who have orthopedic or joint injuries.

**Source:** *Gallagher Medical Report.*

## WHY PEOPLE RUN

Recreational runners do it to promote fitness, prolong life and feel better. Running is also associated with a desire to lose weight and stop smoking. Result: It provides positive feedback to 75% of those surveyed. Problem: More than one—third of the runners suffered injuries during a recent year. Irony: The more miles run, the greater the weight loss—but also the more chance of musculoskeletal injury. Who runs: Most are college-educated professionals, both men and women.

**Source:** A survey of runners in the annual 10-kilometer Peachtree Road Race in Atlanta by a team, headed by Jeffrey P. Koplan, M.D., as reported in *The Journal of the American Medical Association, Chicago, IL.*

## JOGGING PITFALLS

Running on the balls of the feet causes an estimated 60% of all injuries suffered by distance runners. When the front of the foot rather than the heel absorbs the shock of each stride, the calf muscles tighten. This, in turn, leads to a variety of ailments such as runner's sciatica, hamstring pulls, pains in the Achilles' tendon, shin splints and assorted ankle and foot strains. Treatment: Run so that the *heels* make contact first. But don't force this stride if it does not come naturally—the results of forcing can be as bad as running on the balls of your feet. Always stretch the muscles in the backs of the legs before running. Also, try running shoes with higher heels, or use heel inserts.

**Source:** Richard Schuster, M.D., New York City, writing in *The Runner*.

## CAN RUNNING IMPROVE YOUR SEX LIFE?

Running can improve a man's sex life if he doesn't take it too seriously, according to recent surveys of runners. Those who clocked less than 35 miles a week reported increased sexual desire, a more frequent sexual activity and greater sexual satisfaction. However, more than half the runners training for marathons and covering more than 35 miles a week admitted to sometimes feeling too tired for sex.

**Source:** *The Runner, New York.*

• Marathon men leave much of their passion on the road, according to a recent study. Men who run 40 or more miles per week were found to have 30% less testosterone and prolactin—the hormones required for male sexual drive. Theory: The lower hormone levels may explain why some runners have less sexual desire during intensive training.

**Source:** *Journal of the American Medical Association, Chicago, Il.*

## MUSIC AND JOGGING

Jogging seems easier for those who listen to rock music with stereo headphones while they work out. Joggers who listened to music had lower lovels of endorphin (a natural painkiller) after finishing their exercise. Conclusion: The music lowered the runners' need for endorphin because they felt less pain.

**Source:** Eric Miller, researcher at Ohio State University, in *USA Today*.

## TO PREVENT RUNNING INJURIES

Avoid sudden increases in training, workouts or distances covered. Use proper running shoes in good repair. Stretch and warm up before you run . . . and cool down when you are finished. Don't always run on hard surfaces.

**Source:** David Drez, Jr., M.D., chairman, American Academy of Orthopedic Surgeons' Committee on Sports Medicine, Las Vegas.

## WHO NEEDS TO RUN BUT SHOULDN'T?

Overweight runners are more prone to injury than their slimmer colleagues. Extra pounds aggravate the stress on joints and bones. The irony, of course, is that jogging is an ideal exercise for using up extra calories and helping dieters lose weight. Better: Start a serious weight-reduction program with walking or working out on an exercycle or rowing machine. When you reach your ideal weight, take up running for maintenance.

**Source:** *Medical World News, Houston, TX.*

## JOGGER'S ALERT

• Over-zealous runners threaten their mental stability. Those who take jogging so seriously that it is a compulsion often become irritable and restless, have trouble sleeping, and grow preoccupied with guilty thoughts.

**Source:** Psychiatrist Michael Sacks, addressing the American Psychiatric Association in New York.

• About 70% of those who run more than

40 miles a week will suffer injuries, compared with only 30% of those who run less than 10 miles a week.

**Source:** Study by Carl Caspersen, M.D., and Kenneth Powell, M.D., Centers for Disease Control, Atlanta.

• Running can be harmful during the summer. Air pollution is at its peak during hot, muggy days, which adds to the intake of pollutants (such as carbon monoxide) to into your body. Running increases that intake even further because you breathe more air. Suggestion: Work out indoors instead.

## FATIGUE WARNING

Sports anemia is a common problem among long-distance runners. Cause: The loss of small but significant amounts of blood through the stomach and intestines. In advance cases, the runners feel abnormal fatigue. Treatment: Iron supplements.

**Source:** David Ahlquist, M.D., a consultant to the Department of Gastroenterology at the Mayo Clinic, cited in *Outside.*

## HOW YOU BREATHE MAY HURT YOUR KNEE

"Runner's knee" sometimes can be eliminated by a shift in breathing patterns. Most of us are "footed," meaning we lead off consistently with the same foot. We also exhale consistently either on the right foot or the left one. Left-footed breathers occasionally experience pain in the right leg, and vice versa. Why? Exhalation helps absorb shocks better than inhalation. If you have a painful leg: Try exhaling on the other foot.

**Source:** Study by Dennis Bramble and David Carter, zoologists, University of Utah.

## NEW WAY TO DETECT STRESS FRACTURES

Runners' stress fractures can be detected early (before they become full breaks) with a new tool that measures sound waves traveling through bone. Modified acoustic emission is more sensitive than X—rays and more accurate than bone scans. If you test

positive: Give up all activity for at least four to six weeks. To get back in shape: First work out with weights (strengthens bones and ligaments). Cut back your old running program by at least half and then increase it by 10% doses.

**Source:** Lyle Micheli, M.D., director of sports medicine, Children's Hospital, Boston.

## IF YOU GET SIDE CRAMPS

Don't try to run "through" those stitch pains. Better: Slow to a walk or easy jog. If the spasm persists for five minutes, call it quits. Pushing too hard could result in a serious strain on the diaphragm. Prevention: Warm up thoroughly before you run.

**Source:** *Sports without Pain* by Ben E. Benjamin, Summit Books, New York.

## PICKING THE RIGHT RUNNING SHOES

The choices seem endless. Where do your feet fit in the race for the perfect pair?

There are five things to look for in running shoes:

• A heel counter still enough to hold your heel in place and keep it from rolling in and out.

• Flexibility in the forefoot area so the shoe bends easily with your foot. (If the shoe is stiff, your leg and foot muscles will have to work too hard.)

• An arch support to keep the foot stable and minimize rolling inside.

• A fairly wide base for stability and balance. The bottom of the heel, for example, should be as wide as the top of the shoe.

• Cushioning that compresses easily. (Several different materials are used now.) The midsole area absorbs the most shock and should have the greatest amount of padding. However, the heel (which, particularly for women, should be three-quarters of an inch higher than the sole) needs padding, too. Too much causes fatigue, and too little causes bruising.

Running shoes do not need to be broken

in. They should feel good the moment you try them on.

Fitting:

• Start with manufacturers' least costly shoes and keep trying until you find the one that feels best.

• Try on running shoes with the same kind of thick socks you will be wearing with them.

• Light people need less cushioning than heavier people.

• If you have a low arch or tend to flat feet, pick a more stable shoe with more rear foot control, called a "cement" lasted or boarded shoe. ("Last" is the foot shape that the shoe is built around.)

• For a high arch, try a softer, more curved last (called a "slip" last).

• Be sure you have adequate toe room (at least one-half inch of clearance). Running shoes, particularly in women's sizes, run small, and women often need a half-size or whole-size larger running shoe than street shoe.

**Source:** Gary Muhrcke, proprietor of the Super Runners Shop, New York.

## BEST SHOES FOR BIG RUNNERS

Heavy runners need sturdier shoes than the norm, preferably leather uppers with only moderate spring. They also need to replace their shoes more often, since their soles tend to compress and "bottom out." Most suitable models: Nike Odyssey and Epic, New Balance 670 and 565, Tiger Striker, Avia 680, and Brooks Chariot.

**Source:** *The Runner,* New York.

## SHOES THAT AREN'T FOR RUNNERS

Jogging in tennis shoes is unwise. They are designed to facilitate the quick directional changes that tennis players must make and don't provide sufficient heel and toe support for runners.

**Source:** Richard Lampman, Ph.D., exercise physiologist, University of Michigan School of Medicine, Ann Arbor.

## BEST SOCKS TO BUY

No-blister running socks have two thin layers to keep the sock from sliding against the skin or moving about in the shoe. Runique socks are absorbent rayon wrapped in nylon. They also feature flat toe seams, no-slip construction and a 1,000-mile guarantee.

**Source:** Runique Socks, Carversville, PA.

## WINTER RUNNING WEAR

For areas with wet and relatively mild weather, your best bet may be a waterproof shell garment over light polypropylene underwear. (Unlike cotton, polypropylene wicks sweat away from the skin and insulates even when wet.) For cold, dry winters: A skintight Lycra suit or polypropylene long johns under running shorts. In areas with freezing rain and/or chilling winds: A Gore-Tex or coated nylon suit.

**Source:** *Outside,* New York.

## TWO GOOD SUBSTITUTES FOR RUNNING

Racewalking provides excellent conditioning, exercises the entire body and promotes weight loss around the midsection. It also involves only a fraction of the foot stress caused by running, and injuries are rare.

Brisk walking is a good substitute for jogging. It not only helps maintain vigor and stamina but can also sharpen the mind. Progressive walking—starting at a slow pace and increasing speed over time—can improve short-term memory and reasoning power, especially for those 55 or older.

**Source:** Health Insurance Association of America, New York.

## DUBIOUS NEW SPORT

"The National Survival Game," also known as "Skirmish" and "The War Game." The sport is based on capture-the-flag, but with a twist . . . rival armies try to kill each other off by shooting gelatin pellets filled with colored dyes. A harmless outlet for agression? Some psychologists disagree, noting that hostile behavior is often a rehearsal for future action. Added drawback: Reports of eye injuries from "head shots."

**Source:** Georgia Lanoil, a psychologist on the board of the *Journal of Preventive Psychiatry, New York.*

# A DANGEROUS KIND OF FUN

Recreational water slides can be dangerous.

Several fatalities, as well as almost 3,000 fractures, concussions and other serious injuries, occurred last year, mostly to inexperienced slide users. Additional hazard: People with allergies can get grasses and pollens imbedded in their skin during the ride, triggering life-threatening allergic reactions. With more than 600 such slides in operation around the country, parents should be aware of the potential dangers.

**Source:** *Morbidity and Mortality Weekly Report, Centers for Disease Control, Atlanta, GA.*

# 8. Courtship and Marriage

# Courtship and Marriage

## THE SINGLE LIFE

(1) Of the 50 million Americans between the ages of 20 and 55 who are single, only one-third of the men and one-fifth of the women are alone by choice. (2) Women divorced twice or more suffer five times as much physical abuse from men met at bars as women divorced only once. (3) Fifty percent of single women sleep with a man on the first to third date.

**Source:** *The New Americans* by Jacqueline Simenauer and David Carroll, Simon and Schuster, New York.

• Unattached heterosexual women over 50 years old outnumber men in the same category by more than five to one.

**Source:** *Love, Sex, and Aging* by the editors of Consumer Reports Books, Consumers Union, Mount Vernon, NY.

## ABOUT FRIENDSHIP

• Most men—whether married or single—believe a real friendship with a woman is impossible without sex. But women generally seek close platonic relationships with both sexes.

**Source:** Study by Gerald Phillips, Ph.D., professor of speech communication, Penn State University.

• Sex without love is unenjoyable and unacceptable in the opinion of 29% of the men and 44% of the women in a recent survey. (In 1969, only 17% of the men and 29% of the women felt that way.) The ingredients of love: Friendship, devotion and intellectual compatibility.

**Source:** A poll of 12,000 people aged 13–86 by *Psychology Today*, New York.

• Man-woman friendships are far more common now than they were 20 years ago. Reasons: Since people are marrying later, they turn to friends of the opposite sex for the companionship they are missing. And with more occupations open to both sexes, men and women have more shared interests.

**Source:** Marilyn Ruman, Ph.D., a psychologist in Encino, CA.

## TRUTH ABOUT ABUSIVE DATING

Almost half of college students surveyed say they've been abused, abusive or both in dating relationships. Most likely offender: A traditional male who was abused as a child or saw frequent abuse between his parents.

**Source:** J.L. Bernard, professor of psychology, Memphis State University, writing in *Medical Aspects of Human Sexuality*, New York.

## GREAT PLACE TO MEET AN ATTRACTIVE WOMAN

Date idea for young men with honorable intentions but modest budgets: A good place to meet attractive women is at the cosmetics counter of a large general department store. Such stores often put their most charming saleswomen in this department. (And the customers aren't bad, either.) Reasonable approach: Say that you are shopping for a gift for your sister or your mother, and let the conversation take its course from there.

**Source:** *The Cheap Date Handbook* by Bruce Brown, New Lifestyle Publishing, Los Angeles.

## SECRETS OF SUCCESSFUL BLIND DATES

Blind dates work on the same principles as a direct-mail campaign...a 2% return is phenomenal. Suggestions: Never build up your hopes. Restrict blind dates to weekdays, which have less psychological importance. Avoid blind dates for dinner. (If it doesn't work out, the meal will seem interminable.) Better: A meeting for drinks, which can always be extended. As a courtesy, report back to your Cupid at once with at least one nice thing to say about your date.

**Source:** *Honorable Intentions* by Cheryl Merser, Holt, Rhinehart and Winston, New York.

# ONE WOMAN'S VIEW OF PERSONAL ADS

The personal classified ads in *The New York Review of Books, New York* magazine and *The Village Voice* are becoming an increasingly useful social medium. Here's advice from a very talented, beautiful woman in her early forties, recently divorced, who wanted to develop a group of interesting male friends. She answered several ads. . .and placed others. . .and feels good about the experience. Her suggestions:

• Don't lie. Even white lies do damage. One man who said he was a college professor actually taught occasional courses in night school at several local colleges. Though this is merely stretching the truth, it's as bad as lying because it sets up unrealistic expectations, and your "date" is certain to be disappointed. Important omissions also count—like the man who didn't mention that he walked with two canes or the one who never said he weighed 300 pounds. Anyone who answers an ad that includes such information already knows what to expect, and that will prevent a great deal of awkwardness for both parties.

• Look in the mirror. Don't say you're handsome, beautiful or very attractive if you're not. My favorite ad, placed by a man I still date, said "Gruff, beat-up face". . .Another said "OK guy. Average looking." And still another merely said "Presentable." You have a better chance being honest because different people want different things.

• Don't ask for photos. When it comes to wallet-size portraits, they lie at worst. At best, they say nothing. When you like someone,

that person becomes better-looking to you. And when you don't like someone, it doesn't matter how good-looking he is. Besides, some very attractive people photograph badly. . .and vice versa. You'll get the best sense of a person from the letter, not from the picture. Gender bias: Using *New York* magazine for a survey, I found that 90% of the men ask for photos, but only 30% of the women do. I never send one.

• Try humor. It always gets a reponse. I placed a funny ad in *The New York Review* and received a 50% better response than is the average for that publication. It went like this:

"Tall, blonde, excruciatingly bright DWF, 41. Great teeth. Wishes she were a ballerina. Looking for a nice man. Well-spoken. Hair—no dandruff. Should be able to read."

Responses were witty and open. One man wrote that he wished he were old enough for me. Another man is now a very close friend. We laugh a lot together.

• Avoid attractiveness requirements. Just on general principles I don't answer any ad by a man who asks for a "very beautiful " woman or a woman with a "fabulous figure." If he's preoccupied with looks, he's too superficial for me. Even ads that go on to say ". . .but of course personality is most important" are from men to whom looks are ultra-important. They just feel obliged to say something about personality.

• Don't limit yourself with age requirements. Why do men in their fifties consistently ask for women in their twenties and thirties? That really implies terrible things about 50-year-old men. By eliminating the forties and fifties, a man misses a large group of what could be the most interesting, exciting women. Unless you want children, don't limit your possibilities.

• Don't brag. This unpleasant trait breeds skepticism and distaste in the reader.

• Be sincere. Nothing catches a woman's attention more surely than a sincere, straightforward, informative letter. When you answer an ad that looks inviting, let the person know why. Respond to the particulars in the ad in a warm and personal way. Talk honestly about yourself, your likes and dislikes, favorite vacations, funny anecdotes, etc. And never, never, never send a photocopy response. I don't respond to them. They make me think the man answered every woman's ad in the Personals section.

• Try again. I really liked one man's ad. When he didn't answer my response, I wrote again. He called, we had a nice evening, and he commented favorably about my persistence.

• Don't be discouraged. Chances are you won't be attracted to 99% of the people you meet this way. But that will also be true of singles you meet other ways. This is more efficient, however, since the people are already preselected. They're singles who want to meet someone—just like you. And most of them are very nice, decent people. I never feel that I've wasted my time.

## TIPS FOR WRITING ADS THAT PAY OFF

With more and more people seeking romance via the classified personal ads, a special vocabulary has evolved. Words to watch out for: Rubenesque (it usually means fat). Unpretentious (it probably means dull). Words that work: Men respond to women who describe themselves as affectionate, sensual, and good cooks. Women like men who say they are compassionate, sharing and successful.

**Source:** Personal Touch, a New York agency that specializes in writing personal ads, quoted in *The New York Times*.

## EIGHT KINDS OF PERSONAL ADS

Classified ads—the personal kind—are attracting attention. A recent sampling from several publications turned up ads that were. . .

### Sincere

"Balance, harmony, full of awareness and joy of existence is what I strive for in my life. Often easy, sometimes not, but definitely achievable. Have natural need to share with woman of similar inclinations. Respond only if your life is already richly textured. SWM, 42, passed and successfully resolved mid-life crisis."

"I'm tired of swimming upstream & fighting currents & want man, not salmon, snorkeling easily in the same direction as I: Exclusive committed relationship. I'm just 40, tall, attractive, well-employed, creative, love to dance &, at the moment, take myself too seriously. YOU: 35-50, non-smoker, tender, playful, humorous, reasonably cultured, attrac, not 'slick,' successful, formerly married, & READY!"

### Sexy

"Brilliant attr. imaginative modest creatively kinky SWM Md-Ph.d 38 sks clever imaginative liberated lady of 18-38 to explore our wildest fantasies."

"Winsome wench SWF, 29 attractive, fun-loving, sybaritic, seeks older, successful, sophisticated man 55 + ."

### Funny

"Lois Lane—Where Are You? Lusty, loving Superman, 48, tired of leaping over tall buildings. I need a caring lady to share earth's joys and vices. Have phone booth, will travel. It sure is cold flying around in my damn tights. Come warm me up."

"Prince Charming I'm not looking for, because Snow White I'm not. What I am is average, 50yo W/S/F with good sense of humor and intelligence. Looking for average, 45plus W/M who likes good music, drama, dancing, and cares about others."

### Poetic

"Lover, be my cover. In the long cold nights ahead. I'm warm, witty & wonderful, pretty and playful. Come on. Make me smile."

"Dear Man, do not go into the nite gently, there's life, joy & experiences a-plenty. I'm tall blonde & nifty. I'd welcome meeting a charmer above 50."

### Self-Assured

"I'm terrific: the question is, are you SWF seeking straight, single WM who's bright, witty & believes friendship & romance are equal elements in love. Send letter & photo and maybe you'll find out how terrific I really am."

"Unique & Rare. Middle East, feminine; modesty prevents me from flogging mundane advertisement adjectives, but the heading is true. Cultured, diplomatic backgrnd, 10 languages. UN posting & prerogative. Travelling the world in luxury. Meeting a vast int'l crowd at cocktails, concerts has not led me to Monsieur Ideal. Surely amidst NY's maddening crowd, a Gentleman 38–50 w/similar backgrnd, tall and tender, serious & secure, apprec my int'l cooking, music, sports, bridge, reading, dancing, painting, discussing foreign affairs! I am tall & redhead. My selective sensibilities exclude addicts, scroungers, uncouth, short & bald gentlemen."

### Extracurricular

"Moderately charming young (33) married man, handsome, stylish, urbane, amoral and athletic. I yearn for a soft attractive woman with good teeth, skin and breeding for an old fashioned guilt-ridden volcanic but most illicit love affair."

"A pretty, shapely, married WF 44 seeks handsome, bright, very successful MWM 43-55 for platonic lunches and frndshp first, then we'll see."

### Semicommercial Arrangements

"Struggling NYC beautiful slim blonde SWF coed, 25, seeks MWM of means for discreet encounters."

"Traveling Companion. Desired for handsome 34 year old president of international co. If you are an intelligent, petite, attractive woman who enjoys sailing, world travel, fine dining & clothes, send letter to. . ."

### Exotic Adventures

"Manhattan couple with private country retreat, frequent European travelers, seek slim aesthetic young intelligent man for varied pleasures."

"Is it possible for a classy etc etc happily married woman 33 and her super etc etc husband to meet through these columns a super etc etc bisexual lady without all of us being embarrassed out of our minds?"

| Abbreviation Key |
| --- |
| SWM or F: Single White Male or Female. |
| SBM or F: Single Black Male or Female. |
| NR: Nonreligious. |
| GWM: Gay White Male. |
| BWM: Bisexual White Male. |

**Source:** *Harvard Magazine*, Cambridge, MA.

# HOW TO FLIRT

Making an overture to an attractive stranger can cause the most courageous of us to quake with fear. Somehow that humiliating moment in sixth grade when no one asked you to dance, or everyone turned you down, keeps coming back to haunt you. Luckily, the art of flirting can be learned. Matchmaking is a thing of the past, so if you hope to find that special someone, you have to know how to go about it. With practice, an activity that once seemed totally alien will start to come naturally.

### Pickup Do's and Don'ts

When you spot a stranger whom you'd love to meet, approach him/her tactfully. Here's how:

• *Don't* come on with obvious lines or a standard act. You'll be seen as crude or a phony.

• *Don't* get too personal. Make your conversational opener about something neutral, or you may be seen as pushy.

• *Do* pick up on an innocuous topic and comment on it. Good: That's a lovely ring you're wearing. Is it Art Deco? Poor: You have the most beautiful hair.

• *Do* make eye contact—but not for too long. According to a psychological study, three seconds is optimal to indicate interest without seeming to stare.

• *Don't* touch the person right away. Women, especially, are very put off by men they consider "grabby." You might even move away to create allure.

• *Do* show vulnerability. People love it when you're not Mr. or Ms. Self-Confidence. If you're nervous, say so. Your candor will be appealing. Also: Your admission will allow the other person to admit that he or she is nervous, too. This breaks the ice, and then you both can relax.

• *Do* ask for help as a good conversation opener. Example: I don't know this area well. Could you recommend a good restaurant around here?

• *Don't* feel you have to be extraordinarily good-looking. If you have confidence in yourself as a person, the rest will follow. Whatever your type may be, it is certain to appeal to someone.

• *Do* be flexible. The same approach won't work with everyone. If you're sensitive and alert, you can pick up verbal and nonverbal cues and respond appropriately.

• *Don't* let your confidence be shattered by a rejection. It may not have anything to do with you. You may have approached someone who is married, neurotic, recovering from a devasting love affair, in a bad mood, or averse to your eye color. The best remedy: Try again as soon as possible.

### Now That I Have Your Attention

You may be a whiz at starting a conversation—but if you don't know how to keep it going, you won't get anywhere. A conversation depends totally on give and take. It should be like a tennis game: You hit the ball to the other person, who hits it back to you, and so on.

*Don't* oversell yourself or feel compelled to give all your credits. Make the other person feel like the most important person in the world to you at that moment. Being interested is just as important as being interesting (if not more so). Really listen. Don't just wait until the other person finishes a sentence so you can jump in with your own opinion.

**Source:** Interview with Wendy Leigh, author of *What Makes a Woman Good in Bed* and *What Makes a Man Good in Bed.*

## ARE YOU READY FOR LOVE?

At one time or another most single people want to fall in love. But usually they don't pay any more attention to what they think

would work for them in a loving relationship than they do to ordering dinner. At The Godmothers we have learned that you can profit from past successes and failures. We ask clients to write biographical sketches that reveal patterns that can help direct or redirect behavior so that it will be more productive.

### Love Resume

The love resume can help you think or rethink what it is you really want and what you respond to. Sometimes just the act of writing can change your thinking. Like a work resume, it may show a tendency toward instability. Or it may show a logical progression from one "job" to the next. You can discover your own patterns in relationships.

*A. Write a detailed report\* about your three (or more) most serious relationships, including:*

• A description of the person and what you did and didn't like.

• What worked and what didn't work.

• How it ended and how you got over it.

• What you think you would have done differently.

• What your partner would say worked or didn't work, and why it ended.

• Would you be attracted to such a person today?

*B. Write a description\* of the person you would like to meet now, including:*

• Is this person like the ones in past relationships? If not, why not?

• What sort of relationship you want (marriage, a companion for weekends, an escort, etc.).

• Characteristics you would avoid.

• Your three highest priorities.

\*Do this before you go on to read the scoring section that follows.

### Scoring

*Scale 1:* Use a red pencil to underline the times you have written *I* or *me.* Count them, and put the score in a box.

Use a blue pencil to underline the times you have written *he, she, we, us* or *both.* Count them. Put this score in another box.

Add the numbers in both boxes. Divide the total into the number of red underlines. If the percentage is anywhere up to 35%, you're *Available* for a relationship. From 36% to 50% means you are *Borderline* (okay on short-term dating but unable to sustain long-term relationships). Over 50% indicates a *Counterfeit* lover. Your concern for yourself and lack of empathy for others almost guarantee that nothing will work, no matter who the partner is.

We have discovered that when you are available for a relationship, you find one. When you're not, you don't.

*Scale 2:* Look at the phrases underlined in red. If a feeling is expressed ("I was hurt"), underline it a second time. Count the number of underlines and put the total in a red box.

Underline the other person's feelings a second time in blue. Divide the numbers as in Scale 1, and average your score to see whether you get an A, B or C rating.

We have found this scoring of the love resume 95% reliable in predicting whether a client will connect successfully with a partner.

### Content Analysis

Help for Borderlines: When you read over the love resume, patterns will emerge. People often function on old assumptions and scripts that don't meet their current needs. How does the person you think you want to meet fit in with your lifestyle? A man who asks for a gracious social hostess may not have the sort of life that demands an ongoing heavy-duty hostess. He'd manage nicely with someone who is able to cope with the logistics of small dinners.

How realistic are your demands? You say, "I want a woman who likes the work she's doing but who also has time for me." A woman with a full-fledged career isn't going to be available to you all the time.

The love resume can help you to see that some of the things you thought were important in a relationship really aren't. Example: You may think you want a man who isn't so dependent on you—but when you found one in the past, you didn't like that either because you didn't know where you fit in.

The resume may reveal that you are one of the people who set arbitrary time limits. Recommendation: Relax and let matters take their own course. One client finally changed her situation because she turned 44 and abandoned the idea of having a child that had given her the need to lock in a relationship.

Help for Counterfeits: Counterfeits reject everyone they date. If everything isn't perfect, they won't go out a second time. They say they don't have time to waste.

If you scored Counterfeit, you might want to examine the resume for clues to what is holding you back.

If you find a pattern of choosing inappropriate partners, ask yourself: Do I select them because I'm more comfortable with them or because I really don't want a relationship? People who want an out write their own ending: This isn't going to work and I really have a good reason—look at the person I've chosen.

If you can isolate the anger, lack of trust or whatever is holding you back, you're a step ahead. You can work on it. Some people need therapy. Others, once they identify a problem, can refocus it. You don't necessarily have to get over the problem—just be careful not to dump it on somebody else.

**Source:** Interview with Abby Hirsch, founder and director of The Godmothers, a dating service, New York, Washington (DC), and Philadelphia.

# OPPOSITES ATTRACT... OR DO THEY?

The opposites attract theory of mate selection is most successful when the characteristics of one partner complement those of the other. Examples: A dominant person is drawn toward one who is more submissive. Extroverts are attracted to introverts. Hitch: Research evidence indicates that partners who are similar have more attraction and compatibility than those who are complementary. Similarities that pull people together: Economic status, intelligence, educational level, physical attractiveness, race and even height. People often evaluate themselves through social comparison.

**Source:** Robert J. Pellegrini, Ph.D., and Robert A. Hicks, Ph.D., professors of psychology, San Jose University, San Jose, CA, writing in *Medical Aspects of Human Sexuality*, New York.

## WHAT MEN LOVE IN WOMEN

Brunettes come in first with 36% of the men, 29% go for blondes and 32% are indifferent to hair color. Favorite eye color: 44% select blue, 21% like brown and 20% prefer green.

By two to one, men choose curly hair over straight.

The trait men first associate with a beautiful woman: 42% say personality, 23% think of the smile, 13% say eyes and only 6% zero in on the body.

Their favorite look: Striking and sophisticated is first, with 32%. Least favored: The preppy look, preferred by only 3%.

Biggest turnoffs: Heavy makeup, 26%; excess weight, 15%; arrogance, 14%.

**Source:** A poll of 100 men age 18–40 conducted by *Glamour*, New York.

## WHAT MEN HAVE THAT WOMEN LIKE

The ideal man is tall, dark and handsome. Backup: In a recent poll, 57% of the women who responded liked men with black or brown hair and 54% for tall men. What defines handsome? Personality, 33% say; 18%, the smile; 14%, eyes; 14%, finely chiseled features; 12%, a good body; 9% say something else. Also:

• An older, well-coiffed man is a favorite. Fifty-two percent prefer going out with an older man, and 62% choose men with hair cut like the average businessman's.

• Physically, the greatest asset is the face, 37%. Surprising second: The buttocks, 24%. Chest wins 19%, shoulders and legs, 6% each.

• Favored body: A muscular build is chosen by 51%, and 44% like a hairy chest.

• Favorite look: Rugged is best, with 38%. Sophisticated is second, with 34%. Preppie

and poetic are way back at 10% and 4% each.

• Biggest turn-offs: An inflated ego, 27%. Others: Poor grooming, 17%. Bad teeth, 16%. Flabby body and no class, 11% each. Badly dressed, 10%. Pet peeves: Smoking, weird shoes.

• Turn-ons: A great smile, 24%. Personality, 15%. Sensitivity, 11%. Athletic look and good grooming, 8% each. Sense of humor and great eyes, 6% each. Back of the pack: Sexiness, 4%.

Bottom line: The male dreamboat is tall, handsome, dark-haired and muscular, with an air of confidence. He is well-groomed without flaunting it. His charming personality shows in his smile, his eyes and the way he moves.

**Source:** A survey of 100 women conducted by *Glamour*, New York.

## WHAT WOMEN *REALLY* LOOK FOR IN A MAN

What women say they look for in a man are personality, character and intelligence. Correlation studies of dating couples and psychological experiments suggest otherwise. A man's physical attractiveness overwhelmingly determines his appeal as a romantic partner to women.

**Source:** Alan Feingold, psychologist, Brooklyn College, City University of New York, writing in *Medical Aspects of Human Sexuality*, New York.

## HOW WOMEN FEEL ABOUT PREMARITAL SEX

Premarital sex is gaining more acceptance among women. In a recent survey, only 44% frowned on sex before marriage, as compared with 51% in a similar survey the year before. Key variable: Age group. Two thirds of women aged 18–24 thought premarital sex acceptable, but only 30% of women over 55 agreed. Still taboo: Extramarital sex. Four out of five women disapproved.

**Source:** *Glamour*, New York.

## THE "EXPERIENCED" WOMAN

When asked how many sexual partners the average mid-thirties female would have had, women estimated 18–30. But men said the typical woman would have had only three to nine partners. Theory: Men are uncomfortable with the notion of "double-digit" women—even when they've had that much experience themselves.

**Source:** Carol Cassell, president of the American Association for Sex Educators, Counselors and Therapists.

## MODERN LIVING

Unmarried couples living together have more than tripled in number (to 1.9 million) since 1970. Also on the rise: Young adults living with their parents. Women delaying their first marriage until their thirties.

**Source:** U.S. Census Bureau.

## LIVING TOGETHER VS. MARRIAGE

Living together is not a satisfying alternative to marriage. In fact, it is a caricature of marriage.

Practitioners are usually 18- to 30–year-olds who are separated from their families while going to college or working in a city. The major motivating factors: To assuage loneliness. To avoid the anxiety of finding dates. To escape the shallowness of fleeting liaisons.

Sexual relations are generally more satisfying to the men than to the women. Sexual dissatisfaction is the main reason for breakups between those who live together.

Problems: Living together is an uneasy alliance with pseudo-intimacy. The good times are shared, but the bad times and the bad self are hidden. Result: There is really no commitment to a shared life. True commitment seldom occurs until after a marriage ceremony.

Hard fact: Living together is not a replication of, nor a preparation for, marriage.

It may, in fact, actually postpone or complicate the mature intimacy needed for a satisfying marriage. Often major changes occur between people who have lived together once they have exchanged marriage vows. Reason: They have not thought out the serious, long-range side of their relationship.

**Source:** Observations based on many years of discussions with couples as compiled by E. Mansell Pattison, M.D., chairman, department of psychiatry, Medical College of Georgia, Augusta, for *Medical Aspects of Human Sexuality*, New York.

## LIVING TOGETHER CAN BE BAD FOR A MARRIAGE

Living together before marriage can be a trap. Marital satisfaction tends to decline in the first decade. Since co-habiters have already been together for awhile, they may feel the strains earlier. They have already established a residence, so marriage is just a new set of responsibilities with little excitement. People who marry without having lived together feel they are carving a mutual identity in the community.

**Source:** Roy E. L. Watson, Ph.D., University of Victoria, British Columbia, writing in *Medical Aspects of Human Sexuality*, New York.

## BREAKING UP

Women suffer more often than men after a romance ends. A new study found that 88% of women (compared with 74% of men) suffered physical effects—insomnia, overeating or loss of appetite, chest pains or headaches—if their partner initiated the breakup. Even when they were the "breakers," 50% of the women reported physical symptoms, compared with only 26% of the men.

**Source:** Research by Robin Akert, a psychologist at Wellesley College, MA.

## GOOD THING ABOUT LATE MARRIAGES

First marriages are occurring an average of 1.5 years later in life than they did 10 years ago, according to the US Census Bureau.

Men now marry at an average age of 24 years, 8 months and women at 22 years, 3 months. This is good news. Couples who marry before the age of 21 double their probability of divorce.

**Source:** *Medical Aspects of Human Sexuality.*

# MARRIAGE/DIVORCE—THE NEW STATISTICS

At one time, the nuclear family (husband, wife and one or more children) constituted a majority of households in the US. Now, only one in seven, or 14%, of US households can be considered a nuclear family.

There is growing evidence now that, despite the statistics, people want to return to the nuclear-family model. The collapse of the family has changed our lives in ways that many people consider negative.

### Economic Impact

The single-parent household simply doesn't have as much money as the traditional household of the past. About 90% of single-parent families are headed by women, who don't have the earning power of men. Their combined job and child-support income can't match what they had before.

If the trend continues:

• Housing. Families will be living in smaller, less expensive dwellings. The move toward suburbia will slow as single parents realize that urban life is less isolating and offers closer and easier access to work and child care. The demand for housing will increase as families split into two households, but the type of housing demanded will be different.

• Consumer goods. The single-parent family will have a major impact on the way goods are marketed. The trend toward smallness will continue, and markets will become better defined.

• Education. A single parent will not be able to assume the financial burden of sending children through college, especially as government grants and loans are cut back. This will mean that fewer and fewer youngsters will be able to attend college. Those who do will have to shoulder part of the burden themselves by working their way through. Advantage: Many youngsters who felt pressured to attend college because of parental expectations will be free to pursue other careers.

• Employment. The massive entrance of women into the lower-paying end of the labor market has created competition between women and minorities for the same jobs. As unemployment increases, so will tension between these two groups. Female heads of households will put increasing pressure on a sagging economy to create enough jobs to fill the demand.

### Social Changes

Despite, or perhaps because of, the social upheavals created by the decline of the nuclear family, the US is clearly drifting toward conservatism. The more rapidly things change, the more people seem to want to return to the value of the past. These include:

• Sex. The trend toward casual sex and lack of involvement seems to have peaked: Commitment is again in fashion.

• Marriage. The 1950s were a time of "staying together for the sake of the children" and "keeping up with the Joneses." Couples stayed together because of what the neighbors would think. Now people are interested in the nuclear family for its own sake, for the sense of stability, security and happiness it offers, rather than to keep up a front of normality.

• Morality. As part of the conservative trend, there is a growing force opposed to pornography. Too much personal freedom is seen as leading to exploitation.

• Goals. A home of one's own and a good marriage are still the dominant elements of "the good life" for a majority of people. Since 1975, material things such as a car, TV set and travel have risen in importance, while social goals, such as the desire for a job that contributes to society, have fallen off.

### What the Future Holds

I don't think the new conservatism means that people will stop trying to be true to the self or be willing to return to the hypocrisy that characterized much of family life in the past. There's a scintilla of evidence in our recent research that couples will be trying to explore personal growth within the family instead of leaving the family to find themselves. The tightened economy, which forces couples to choose between economic security and personal freedom, has been a strong influence.

There were more marriages last year than at any other time in US history. This statistic, plus people's changing attitudes, may be a harbinger of a return to the dominance of the nuclear family.

**Source:** Interview with Charles E. Wilson, executive vice president of Starch, INRA & Hooper Mamaroneck, NY, parent company of the Roper Organization.

# ALL ABOUT MARRYING AND REMARRYING

Today, with predictions that two out of every three marriages will end in divorce, couples who are marrying need all the help they can get. Here is some advice for a good start:

• Choose the right person for the right reasons. The most important thing the couple should do is to consider why they want to marry and whether they have selected the best person to meet those goals.

Too often, they have made the wrong choice—because they have needs they don't admit even to themselves. They know what they want, but even though the person they plan to marry doesn't fill the bill, they think he/she will change.

• Have realistic expectations about the marriage. Another person can do only so much for you. No one person can fill every need. It is important for both partners to develop their own lives and interests and not depend solely on each other.

• Learn to communicate. Get issues out on the table and talk about them. Try to reach conclusions regarding conflicts rather than letting them stay unresolved. My father was so right when he said, "Never go to sleep on an argument."

• Respect the other person's style of communication. People express affection in different ways. Women tend to be emotional and want flowers and wine as signs of love. Men tend to be more practical and to express their caring in their actions. Example:

A patient who had been out of work for some time finally got a job. When she called her husband to share the good news, he began to ask her questions about health insurance and other benefits. She thought he was indifferent to her feelings of relief and joy. However, he was treating her as he would have liked to be treated under the same circumstances—with concern that she got the best possible deal.

Instead of expecting a spouse to react as you do, try to be sensitive to what he or she is telling you in his/her own way.

• Respect the other person's feelings about space and distance. Many people have difficulty understanding someone else's needs for privacy and time alone. Some like a lot of separate space. Others want to constantly merge. Deciding what kind of distance to settle on is a major task. Important: Remember, conflicts about space needs can be resolved by trial and error—and patience.

• Create a new lifestyle. Each partner comes with different concepts about customs, handling money, vacations, etc. One may be used to making a big thing about celebrating holidays and birthdays, the other not. Combine the best elements to get a richer blend that is distinctly your own.

• Draw up an agenda of important issues. Many people are put off by legal contracts concerning property settlements, but consider a written list that makes you talk about how money, sex and vacations will be handled, whether or not you want children, how the household chores will be divided, etc. You don't have to agree on everything. You can agree to disagree on certain points or to explore a solution together. But at least you will have opened a dialogue on expectations, roles and beliefs, one that can be continued periodically.

**Source:** Interview with Barbara C. Freedman, CSW, director of the Divorce and Remarriage Counseling Center in New York.

## THE "AVERAGE" BRIDE

The average US bride spends $4,376 on the wedding. She is probably not a virgin (60% are not virgins), and she expects her husband to share equally in child-care duties (57%).

**Source:** *Bride's Magazine.*

## 5 REASONS GAY MEN MARRY WOMEN

Gay men who marry women may compose 20% of the total adult male homosexual population. Why they do it: For a home and family. Parental expectations. Professional protection. A desire to be "cured." Genuine love for their wives.

**Source:** *Woman's Day.*

## THE TWO STAGES OF A GOOD MARRIAGE

A successful marriage must go through two stages. Initially, people fall in love with ideals, not other people. They see what they want to see—usually an image of what they themselves would like to be—and they fall in love with that image. Then, disillusionment sets in when they discover the spouse isn't that ideal. When people can accept their disappointment and acquire a realistic image of the other person, the marriage has a chance to survive.

**Source:** Psychiatrist Howard Corwin, Tufts University School of Medicine.

## KEYS TO A GOOD MARRIAGE

• Intellectual differences are not a major factor in a successful marriage. Kindness, interest, forbearance and self-knowledge make up for any disparity in intelligence.

**Source:** Charles William Wahl, M.D., University of California, writing in *Medical Aspects of Human Sexuality.*

• A happy marriage doesn't depend on great sex, a new study shows. More important elements : Mutual respect and enjoyment. Avoiding trivial arguments. Knowing how to fight fairly. Keeping communication open.

**Source:** Study of 350 couples married 15 years or more by Robert and Jeanette Lauer, professors at the United States International University, San Diego.

## SEX AND THE SEXES

Physically, lovemaking is more important to men than to women as a key to a happy marriage. However, both husbands and wives agreed that "love and affection" is most important in married life. Men ranked sexual relations second. . .followed by respect, communication and time spent with spouse. The women rated time spent with spouse second. . .followed by respect, sexual relations and "open, honest expression of feeling." '

**Source:** Research at Michigan State University, reported in *Journal of Marriage and the Family.*

## SEX COMPLAINTS

Husbands (particularly young ones) gripe most about *infrequency* of sex within marriage. But wives are more critical of the *quality* of sex. Most common dissatisfaction: A lack of communication, sharing and togetherness. . . both during the sex act and in the marriage as a whole.

**Source:** Study by Dr. Michael McGill, professor of organization behavior, Southern Methodist University, Dallas.

## COMPROMISE TRAP

Compromise can actually harm a marriage if it's overdone. Some marital conflicts cannot be resolved. In a compromise, both sides lose something. Alternative: Give in on issues you care less about, and expect the same from your partner.

**Source:** Gayla Margolin, associate professor of psychology, University of Southern California, Los Angeles.

## WHAT IS THE STATE OF YOUR UNION?

Couples in a long-term committed relationship seldom take the time to evaluate their marriage. Conflicts are ignored, whether consciously or unconsciously, only to bubble up periodically in times of anger, stress and despair. Unknowingly, the partners may fall into a state of unhealthy resignation and frustration concerning the union.

### Unearthing Potential Trouble

Each of the partners marries for individual needs and purposes, and each usually imagines that the relationship is guided by a hypothetical contract. This is not a clearly defined legal tract but rather a collection of assumptions, convictions, ideals and beliefs that are more felt than delineated. Often, each partner is guided by a different set of assumptions, which, however, neither ever makes clear to the other. Result: The partners are susceptible to feeling hurt, angered or betrayed when they think the spouse has neglected to fulfill his/her part of the bargain.

Below is a test that will help you define the current state of your union. It may help uncover trouble areas, or it may reaffirm your strengths. If nothing else, it should stimulate your thinking about marriage.

Keep in mind that some differences are to be expected. Maxim: If there is no conflict, something is wrong with the marriage. But most of these conflicts are helped by defining them clearly and seeking solutions. Significant differences that defy resolution, however, should be taken up with a marriage counselor.

*Test procedure:* Each partner should write out responses to each item separately. Compare notes upon completion.

### Expectations of a Marriage

Here are some generally held expectations. Determine which ones apply to you and answer whether they are being met.

*I expected a mate who would:*

• Provide constant support against the rest of the world. Positive answer: My spouse always takes my side when I'm in trouble. Negative: When critical remarks are made against me, my partner never defends me.

• Be loyal, devoted, loving and exclusive, a person I would develop with and grow old with.

• Provide sanctioned and readily available sex.

• Insure against loneliness.

• Attain a respectable position and status in society.

### Psychological and Biological Needs

These areas often exist beyond our distinct awareness of them. They are often the hidden causes of problems in a marriage. Some of these sources:

• Who controls whom in the relationship? Do you abdicate power to your spouse? Do you leave decisions to your partner and then complain about them? Are you competitive with your mate? Would you prefer not to be?

• How much closeness and intimacy do you want with your mate? An oft-heard complaint is that a spouse claims to desire closeness but pushes the partner away when true intimacy develops.

• Do you feel good about yourself? This truism is still valid: If you don't love yourself, you can't love others.

• Does your mate turn you on? Are the physical and personality characteristics you desire evident?

• Do you love your partner? Is that love returned?

### Common Complaints

• Do you use openness and clarity in speaking to and listening to each other?

• Are your lifestyles, interests, work and recreational activities similiar? Do you need to agree to do things together?

• Are you in accord about child-rearing practices? (This is a persistent battleground between some spouses.)

• Are your children used in alliance against either parent? Is any child identified particularly as yours or your mate's?

• Are there differences over the control, spending, saving or making of money?

• Who initiates sex? How frequently? Are there alternative sex partners or practices? Is sex pleasurable and gratifying?

• Do you share friends, or does each partner have his or her own? Do you and your mate each have friends of the opposite sex? Does this cause problems?

• Do you share the same values? Include those related to sex and equality and to cultural, economic and social class.

• Does gender determine the roles and responsibilities of each partner at home and socially?

• How do you react when you feel let down or deceived?

Finally, write down any additional relevant thoughts that may have occurred to you during the completion of this survey.

When you review your responses with your spouse, you will have a pretty clear idea of the state of your marriage and the steps that are needed to forge an even stronger bond.

**Source:** Interview with Clifford J. Sager, M.D., clinical professor of psychiatry, New York Hospital—Cornell Medical Center.

## AGE CONFIDENTIAL

The woman is older in only 14% of marriages in the US. But studies suggest that the men in these marriages tend to be happier than their more traditional peers. Reason: Older women—less likely to be emotionally and finacially dependent on their spouses—are generally less demanding and more understanding.

**Source:** *Psychology Today.*

## 10 GAMES YOU CAN'T WIN

Games people play kill relationships. Even if you "win" by entrapping your partner, you both lose in the end. Particularly dangerous: Jealousy...The Silent Treatment ...Withholding Sex...Bargaining... Keeping Score...Getting Even...Complaining to Outsiders... Using Children ...One-Upmanship...Buying Love.

**Source:** *The Love Test* by Harold Bessell, William Morrow & Co., New York.

## IMPORTANCE OF SPENDING TIME TOGETHER

Marriage myth: The amount of time you spend with your spouse is less important than the quality. In a recent survey, more than 90% of the couples who considered their marriages strong and close also said they spend a great deal of time together. Conversely, divorced couples usually had spent little time together before the split.

**Source:** Study by Nick Stinnett, chairman, department of human development and the family, University of Nebraska.

## FOR MORE INTIMATE INTIMATE RELATIONSHIPS

When assertiveness training orginated back in the 1960s, it focused primarily on getting people to stand up for themselves with bosses, co-workers and the outside world in general. It zeroed in on issues like how to avoid being pushed around, how to deal with manipulative people, how to say no without feeling guilty and so on.

But a whole element was missing in early assertiveness training...how to deal with intimate people in your life. Today we're teaching people to take emotional risks, express deep feelings and help others to get their feelings out. Our results are very encouraging, especially with couples. Good communication is vital to a happy marriage, and assertiveness is crucial for good communication.

### Assertiveness and Couples

Definition of assertiveness: The honest, open and direct expression of feeling without maliciousness. With many couples, communication problems arise because one spouse (usually it's the husband) isn't adequately communicative about his feelings. He doesn't let his partner know what he's experiencing. His feelings of annoyance, appreciation and love all go unstated. Partners often express anger indirectly by being too tired for sex or hiding behind a newspaper.

Many people, men particularly, simply haven't learned to tune in on, identify and express feelings. Using various exercises, we help the couple learn the language of feeling.

### The Feeling List

We provide the couple with a list of a couple of hundred different feelings that human beings experience. . .warmth, ambition, joy, anger, annoyance, bitterness, jealousy, sadness, etc. The list includes positive and negative feelings. Throughout the day, whenever either partner is experiencing an emotion, he or she reviews the chart and tries to pinpoint the exact feeling—tuning in on the feeling and writing down the context in which it's occurring. For 20 minutes that evening, first the wife and then the husband merely state things they felt about the other during the day. Examples: Honey, I really felt loved when you made breakfast for me this morning. I felt annoyed and jealous when you told me about your lunch meeting with your boss.

Important: The other person should just listen without comment. Reason: People's greatest fear about expressing feelings is that they're going to be put down, censured or somehow invalidated for revealing themselves. Many people had this experience as children. Men especially fear ridicule when they express feelings, since they've been taught that being open means showing weakness.

If this exercise is done every night, the couple slowly learns to express feelings spontaneously throughout the day. Result: Anger and resentments can't build up. If feelings are expressed directly, hidden agendas are undercut, and couples stop acting out their anger in indirect ways.

### The Caring List

A number of studies have shown that the major difference between successful and unsuccessful couples is that the winners give goodies to each other. They know how to give what the spouse needs to feel cherished. Most couples don't know how. Typical complaints: He doesn't appreciate me. She's not my friend.

We tell couples to create caring lists consisting of 15 or 20 items that would make each of them feel cared about. Examples: I'd like him to give me a backrub every day. I'd like her to initiate sex once in a while. They post their lists, and each day the couple is assigned to communicate directly and assertively at least two or three items from the list. When one does, the other puts a checkmark on the list.

Result: Couples stop waiting for the other person to break the ice. Each acts independently, building trust, confidence and better communication. Attempts at mind-reading are also eliminated. The notion that *I know what she wants* or *She should know how much I love her even if I don't tell her* is nonsense. Most people don't know how much they're loved until it's clearly communicated.

**Source:** Interview with Barry S. Lubetkin, Ph.D., clinical director, Institute for Behavior Therapy in New York.

# HOW A GOOD FRIEND CAN HELP YOUR MARRIAGE

The happiest marriages are made by people who talk intimately with a close friend.

Theory: Problems in a marriage that aren't broached with the spouse can often be talked through with a friend.

**Source:** Study by the University of Colorado, Boulder.

## SECRETS OF HAPPY COUPLES

The happiest couples don't deny or avoid difference between them, but consider such differences enriching. Cornerstones for a successful marriage: A wife with a long-standing interest outside the home. A husband who is able to talk about his feelings.

**Source:** Donna Hulsizer, Ed. D., Harvard University, in *Vogue.*

## WHO NEEDS MACHO?

It was no surprise when recent research found that husbands were happiest when their wives were most "feminine" (warm, tender, loyal, sympathetic). But the same study showed that wives were happiest when their husbands exhibited these same traits. Couples were happiest when both spouses scored high. And what of masculine traits such as ambition, dominance and aggression? They bore no relationship to happiness.

**Source:** Research by John K. Antill, Ph.D., reported in *Vogue.*

## THE SUFFOCATING MARRIAGE

If you need more time to be by yourself, explain your feelings to your partner. (Be patient in waiting for changes.) Reserve a set time for solitude in your daily schedule. Develop outside interests. When the desire for "space" may mask a problem: You're uncomfortble when you spend time with your mate. You avoid discussing problems with each other. You're frightened by the feelings that go with intimacy.

**Source:** Dr. Stuart S. Asch, professor of clinical psychiatry, Cornell University Medical College, in *USA Today.*

## SECRETS OF A HAPPY VACATION

Although trips taken together may relax a couple, they can also result in disappointment and frustration. To make a joint vacation work, clarify expectations beforehand. Do you want to get into better physical shape or just lie on the beach? If you expect to indulge in lots of lovemaking, plan for privacy and minimal outside distractions. For some couples, bringing the children along alleviates the tensions of too much togetherness and provides an organizational focus for the trip—but get away from them for an evening or two. On any vacation, be mentally prepared for mishaps such as illness or bad weather.

## RULES FOR FAMILY FIGHTS

Conflict is an inevitable part of marriage—especially in the modern, two-income variety. The traditional marriage was a set piece, with each spouse's role well defined. In the modern marriage, roles tend to overlap and compete. Both partners are under multiple demands and heavy stress: Should I take the promotion if it means more travel?. . . Is the time right to have a baby?. . .etc., etc., etc.

Very often, there are basic disagreements. Result: A constant series of marital readjustments that must be talked through in order to be properly resolved.

It's important that both parties understand and accept the talking-through process. It does a marriage no good to avoid conflict. If a couple never fights, it's usually because one spouse is submissive and afraid to get out of line. Tensions are never ventilated. Under a surface of stability there is great unfairness—and a high potential for eventual explosion.

Of course, marital arguments can also be destructive. In the Albee play "Who's Afraid of Virginia Woolf?", George and Martha show just how not to fight. They sandbag and belittle each other, quarrel in front of guests, and drink heavily. Like many real-life couples, they stretch their relationship until the love bond is torn.

Essential: Fighting fair. Every couple must develop its own rules of combat, but we think the following are generally sound.

• Never go for the jugular. Everyone has at least one soft, defenseless spot. A fair spouse attacks elsewhere.

• Focus on a specific topic. Don't destroy your spouse with a scorched-earth campaign. Fair: "I'm angry because you don't make breakfast before I go to the office." Unfair: "I'm angry because you're useless, and my mother was right—you're not tall enough, either."

• Don't criticize things that probably can't be changed. A physical blemish or a spouse's limited earning power is not a fair target. On the other hand, it's dangerous to stew in silence if your partner drops dirty socks on the floor or chews with mouth agape. These may seem like minor irritations hardly worth mentioning, but they fester with time.

• Don't leave the house during a fight. According to popular myth, a "cooling-off" period will make you more reasonable. In fact, it will do just the opposite. You'll be talking to yourself—your own best supporter. Result: A self-serving reconstruction of what happened, rather than an objective view of the situation.

• Argue only when sober. Alcohol is fuel for the irrational, but disagreements are beneficial only if you use reason.

• Keep your fights strictly verbal. A fight that turns physical is both abusive and ineffectual. It intimidates rather than resolves.

• Don't discuss volatile subjects late at night. It's tempting to sum up your day at 11 o'clock. But everything seems worse when you are tired . . . and if you start arguing at 11, you'll be still more exhausted the next morning. Better: Make a date to go at it when both sides are fresh.

• Always sleep in the same room, no matter how bitter the fight. The bed is a symbol of the marital bond, and it's more difficult to stay angry with a spouse there. Maybe you haven't resolved the issue, but you can still come together as friends. We're not necessarily recommending sex under the circumstances. But a friendly hug never hurts . . . and it may ward off insomnia.

• If you are getting nowhere after a long stretch of quarreling, simply stop. Don't say a word. Your spouse will have great difficulty arguing solo. You can always resume the next day.

• Don't sulk after the real fighting is over. Pride has no place here. When we disagreed with more gusto than we do today, we had an unspoken rule: The winner of the fight was the one to initiate the reconciliation.

• Consider outside help. If you never seem to resolve an issue despite both parties' best efforts, use other resources . . . not necessarily a 10-week course or a formal session with a counselor. You might simply cultivate a couple whose marriage you admire and try to profit by their example.

• Don't give up too easily on either the fight or the relationship. A strong marriage demands risk-taking, including the risk of feeling and showing extreme anger. The intimacy of marriage is won through pain and friction as well as through pleasure. You have to push further and harder than in any other relationship.

Down the road, an old fight can be a source of great satisfaction. You can turn to each other and say, "Look, we made it through that argument. It didn't destroy our marriage."

**Source:** Interview with Kevin and Marilyn Ryan, co-authors of *Making a Marriage*, St. Martin's Press, New York.

# BETTER CONVERSATIONS AT HOME

If conversation is a lost art, nowhere is the loss more keenly felt than in the family. Up against the tyrannies of tight schedules, pervasive television watching and all the other stresses of modern life, some families only go through the motions of real communication.

That's a shame, because the potential is so great. The intimacy of marriage makes possible a special kind of language between husband and wife. It can be uniquely comfortable, candid and free. You don't have to rehearse before you speak to a spouse. You don't have to put on "company manners" (though marriage should not be a license for rudeness). You're free to be yourselves.

But conversation within marriage still demands a great deal of effort—if only because men and women use language with essentially different styles and purposes.

In our recent study, we found that men tend to be both direct and directive. Their talks with other men are filled with practical advice. Male talk thrives on humor, camaraderie and playfulness. It often involves competition and one-upmanship. It typically moves fast and deals mostly with surface subjects, such as sports.

But when women talk with other women, they're primarily seeking empathy and understanding. They're more supportive. They're better listeners. . .they don't feel the need to talk all the time. They move into intimate subjects more quickly and easily, even with people they don't know so well.

This works fine in same-sex conversations. But when a husband talks with a wife, their styles often clash. He'll tell her what to do, and she'll resent being told. He'll ask for advice and get impatient if she's indecisive.

To bridge the gap: Don't expect to change the other person's style. But you can learn from each other. Example: Instead of "solving" his wife's problem, a husband could encourage her to talk it out, letting her arrive at her own solution. Key: Consider the needs of the other person by reflecting on what he or she is saying.

Spouses can make an effort to share the content of their lives through talk—a special challenge in two-income families, where shared time is at a premium. If they pursue different hobbies or interests, that may nudge them farther apart. Better: Ask penetrating questions about the other's passion. At the very least, you'll grow closer. You might even discover and develop a shared enthusiasm.

Of course, you may already share an inexhaustible source of conversation—your children. Then your challenge is to bring them into the discussion. . .which needs a somewhat different approach. Suggestions:

• Avoid sarcasm when talking to children. A biting quip that might be funny among adult friends can frustrate a child, who lacks the ego and intellectual maturity to respond.

• Praise more and criticize less. Criticism makes adults uptight, and children react the same way. You'll do better by rewarding appropriate behavior. Example: "I'm really happy with the way you dealt with that school-bully problem."

• Keep in mind that arguments are inevitable. The key is handling them constructively. Instead of accusing, try to understand why your spouse or children feel the way they do.

• Seize the moment. If your child runs in with important news, sit down and talk about it. If you put if off because you're busy, you've lost it.

• Be patient, and don't interrupt. When you cut children off, it may confirm their notion that they can't or shouldn't express themselves. Finally they'll stop trying.

• Limit television time. People who are watching sitcoms can't pay attention to one another—even if they're talking.

• Cultivate the time-honored tradition of dinner-hour conversations. It may not be possible to coordinate everyone's schedule every night, but aim for at least a few nights a week. Keep the conversation light. Save heavier topics for family meetings after dinner.

**Source:** Interview with Mark Sherman, associate professor of psychology, and Adelaide Haas, associate professor of communications, State University of New York at New Paltz.

# INSIDE MARRIAGE

Wives who feel their marriages are very satisfying sexually and who characterize themselves as excellent lovers give these reasons for the success:

• They view sex as a pleasure and a priority, not a duty. More than half say they make it a point to go to bed when their husbands do, not lingering over a book or TV program.

• An overwhelming majority prepare for bedtime by wearing sexy lingerie, perfume and a little makeup.

• Almost all these wives report that their husbands like to have them initiate lovemaking occasionally.

• While making love, most whisper compliments, tell what pleases them and express pleasure. Key: Letting their husbands know that they love and admire them.

• During the sexual act, these wives think of nothing but sensory messages, closing out thoughts of personal and family problems. Result: More than three-quarters of them say they rarely have trouble climaxing.

• A clear majority make love whenever they or their husbands have the urge. Also, they sometimes have sex elsewhere than in the bedroom. Most popular places: The living room, the den, outdoors or in the car.

• Busy couples find that scheduling sex is a turn-on. They regard it as exciting, not calculating.

• Almost 90% say they enjoy the sexual experiments their husbands suggest.

• Just about every woman said she feels good about herself as a woman. Some of these feelings of self-esteem come from the workplace. More than two-thirds of the sexy wives have outside jobs.

Bottom line: The sexiest wives are usually the happiest wives and vice versa.

**Source:** A poll conducted by *The Ladies Home Journal.*

## BATTERED WIVES

Marital rape, defined simply as forced sex without the woman's consent, appears to be a common form of family violence. Recent studies show that battered wives are at highest risk. A survey of battered women in shelters in Minnesota revealed that 36% had been sexually abused by their mates. Other studies suggest that marital rape is twice as prevalent as rape by an outsider.

Only 11 states currently recognize this form of wife abuse as a prosecutable offense.

**Source:** Dr. Kersti Yllo, Wheaton College, and Dr. David Finkelhor, assistant director of the Family Violence Research Center, University of New Hampshire, writing in *Crime and Delinquency.*

## SEX IN LONG-TERM MARRIAGES

The importance of physical intimacy in long-term marriages depends on each couple. Sex is great and enjoyable, but in this country it's been overrated.

Many people like holding, cuddling and sleeping together but not intercourse. However, sex can be a matter of substantial importance if one partner (or both) doesn't find pleasure in sexual activity with a mate.

### Waning Sexual Interest

Some women want sex only to have children. And some men have sex with their wives only for children and go elsewhere for pleasure.

Many women used to feel that their sex lives were over after menopause. Today we know it doesn't have to be that way. And, an astounding number of men used to give up sex after 60. Men may need more stimulation and an increase in the refractory period (the period of time necessary before one can have another erection or ejaculation.) Both sexual pleasure for both men and women can go on and on.

### Desire for Change

It's not unusual for married couples in their late fifties or early sixties who haven't had sex together for several years to say, "We're happy, we enjoy each other and love each other, but maybe we're missing something."

If they come to me with a desire for more sexual expression, we first check physical causes for lack of sexual desire and then check psychological causes.

Many men and women are turned on by other lovers but not by a spouse. Familiarity is one cause. Outside partners always have an advantage because they don't have to deal with day-to-day problems. Sex is important to a person having affairs, but is it important in the marriage? If it is, then the big problem is how to redirect it to the marriage. It is not always possible. Example:

A patient of 73 with a wife of 65 couldn't get an erection with his wife, even though he wanted to. But with a woman friend two years older than his wife he had excellent sex a couple of times a week on a regular basis.

We worked on the problem for some time, without success. His abrasive, cold wife wanted sex only because she thought her husband was neglecting her. The other woman, who was warm and had a zest for life, really enjoyed sex.

### What to Do

I am seeing more people in long-term marriages who want to do something about the lack of sexual desire in their marriage. Those who've been married 20 years may not know how to cope with changes, and they may be drifting apart. But they don't want to run out on the relationship.

It is important to determine whether the cause or causes of reduced sexual interest are interactional (routinizing of sex, depression or other emotional problems) or organic in nature (arterial sclerosis of the arteries to the penis, postmenopausal problems in women, low levels of testosterone in men). A small number of partners are aware of the fact that over time their sexual desire has shifted from heterosexual to homosexual. Outside relationships may also preempt the interest of one or both partners.

We have a virtuous attitude toward extramarital affairs in this country, and until recently, it was a major cause of divorce. We can learn from other countries, where married people have a love relationship with somebody else but still maintain the family structure without bitterness, whether or not there is sex between husband and wife. Example:

A French patient and her husband both had lovers they talked about openly. The married couple had problems between themselves, and their seeing other people was part of their annoyance with each other. They wanted to improve their own relationship. They did get closer, but they had no intention of giving up the other partners.

Very often, people with sexual problems also have problems being open about other feelings. Increasing openness about sex helps. Suggestion: Talk about fantasies and try to incorporate them into your sex life.

Executives in high-powered jobs want to come home to a loving, relaxing place. They are impatient if their needs aren't understood...causing them to turn off sexually. So they sometimes look for sex outside (where they can find it quickly and easily on a short-term basis) rather than working out the problem at home.

**Source:** Interview with Clifford J. Sager, MD., director of family psychiatry, Jewish Board of Family and Children's Services, New York, and clinical professor of psychiatry, New York Hospital, Cornell Medical Center.

## ABOUT EXTRAMARITAL AFFAIRS

• Sixty percent of men and 45% of women in the US engage in extramarital sex at some time during their marriage.

**Source:** Survey of 262 marital therapists by Donald Granvold, social-work professor at the University of Texas at Arlington.

• Unlike men, women seek emotional intimacy more than physical pleasure. Most know their sexual partner as a friend first (only 2% are "swept away"). One woman in four feels guilt at the outset...but virtually none feel guilt as the relationship continues. An affair's average duration: One year.

**Source:** Study by Lyn Atwater, a sociologist at Seton Hall University, South Orange, NJ.

• Thanks to the women's movement and the sexual "revolution," extramarital sex has become commonplace. Fact: The American marriage remains highly traditional. In one study, more than 70% of marriage partners had never had an extramarital affair.

**Source:** Frederic Humphrey, marriage researcher at the University of Connecticut and past president of the American Asssociation of Marriage and Family Therapy.

# THE "NEW" WORLD OF EXTRAMARITAL SEX

The dramatic shift in economic and social conditions during the second half of the 20th century has led many successful people—both men and women—to have extramarital lovers.

The modern concept of such an arrangement stretches back to the European aristocrats, whose marriages were land and power contracts, not romantic liaisons. Any personal unions took place outside the marriage. Indeed, the romantic side of chivalry was concerned with extramarital affairs. Camelot was not unusual in this regard.

Attitudes changed with the rise of the mercantile middle class. A tremendous cultural and religious force was directed against anything that interfered with the marital bond. Reasons: The family was the primary economic unit. Marriages united families in a way that facilitated the orderly transfer of acquired wealth as an inheritance to offspring. In addition, the emerging middle class had not yet acquired the cynicism and decadence of the aristocrats. They felt morally bound by the strictures that reinforced the marriage vows as expounded by the churches of the major faiths.

After World War II, with the help of the movies from Hollywood, marriage came to be regarded as an institution inspired by romantic love that could be reevaluated periodically. People began to place more emphasis on individual satisfaction. If needs were not being met in the marital relationship, alternatives were seriously entertained. Key: Economic success no longer depended on class, land holding and family achievement. It was based on individual ability. One person became the economic unit. Each successful person had the time, finances, propinquity and opportunities to form relationships apart from the marriage.

This liberation spawned many new concepts. One was the open marriage, which tries to incorporate sexual relationships as an adjunct of marriage. But statistics show that marriages under these open contracts seldom survive for more than three years. Usually, the desire for an open contract is only an attempt to ameliorate serious troubles between spouses.

Others have followed the aristocratic patterns. Some are extramaritally promiscuous. Others are serially monogamous—true to each new love until a newer one appears. Some even have a monogamous relationship with a lover as well as a similar relationship with a spouse. Examples: A busy executive has a spouse at home and colleague/lover who is a constant companion on any business trip.

What is the attitude of friends and colleagues toward this extramarital lover? Tricky. Necessary ingredient for all parties: Tact and diplomacy.

Example: A friend, without clearing it with you in advance, shows up at your party with the lover rather than with the spouse. The guest is committing a gross indiscretion. Any lover is potentially an unwanted guest. Minimum courtesy: The guest should call the host to explain that the spouse is indisposed and ask permission to bring the friend. People who flaunt their indiscretions are both rude and foolish.

The financial etiquette of keeping a lover is set by negotiation. In the old days, the lover, usually a mistress, was economically dependent on her wealthy patron. Now, the person who is the wealthiest at the time picks up the larger expenses of maintaining the relationship. This includes items such as travel costs and the checks at fancy restaurants. It rarely includes support-system payments.

Insight about etiquette: The close friends of a woman support her affairs. A man's friends ignore his affairs or offer support from a distance. Prime reason: Women tend to talk about these relationships much more. Males are usually not as involved in sharing details of their personal lives. Exception: The locker-room braggarts. They are also the ones who bring a lover to a party without prior clearance with the host, especially if they are squiring younger consorts.

Bottom line: In general, marriages do not survive a series of extramarital relationships unless they are temporary transitional crises of adult life.

**Source:** Interview with Martin G. Groder, M.D., a psychiatrist and business consultant who practices in Durham, NC.

## PROS AND CONS OF LONG-DISTANCE MARRIAGES

Long-distance marriages (where spouses live more than 50 miles apart because of job demands) do not necessarily lead to extramarital affairs. Although 8% of the couples studied started having affairs after having moved apart, 11% stopped having them. In all, fewer than one-third of the spouses had affairs.

**Source:** Study by Naomi Gerstel, a sociologist at the University of Massachusetts, Amherst.

## WHAT TO DO IF A SPOUSE IS GOING BACK TO SCHOOL

A spouse's return to school tests a marriage. Reason: The student develops new friendships or starts to regard the partner as an intellectual inferior. To make the process easier: Before enrolling, enlist your mate's support. Agree in advance to share household chores. Don't let all conversations center around school. Develop new activities with your partner to establish a fresh common ground. To keep your sex life healthy, set aside unbreakable dates for time alone together.

## PARENTAL DRIVE

Wives in childless couples tend to be more competitive and career-oriented than their counterparts with children. But childless husbands are generally less competitive than fathers. Reason: Freed from breadwinning pressure, they seek career satisfaction over higher salaries.

**Source:** Jean Veever, Canadian psychologist, quoted in *Glamour.*

## WHEN BOTH PARTNERS WORK

• Dual-career marriages have become the norm. About 52% of American families (nearly 30 million) have two wage-earners. Does it work? Men with working wives are more likely to say they're happy than other husbands.

**Source:** Survey by the National Opinion Research Center, quoted in *U.S. News & World Report.*

• A wife's employment can unsettle a marriage if either wife or husband doesn't want her to work. In traditional marriages with nonworking wives, depression is more frequent among wives than husbands. But if the wife has to go to work for economic reasons, it's the husband who becomes more depressed. In households where both partners expect the wife to work, the level of depression is much less. But a working wife can become depressed if her husband doesn't help with the household chores.

**Source:** *American Demographics.*

• The younger the man, the more time he spends on housework and child care, a recent study shows. Most involved: Husbands of employed wives with preschool children (12 hours a week). Husbands with stay-at-home wives average five hours a week. Educated professional men are no more likely to do dishes or change diapers than blue-collar men.

**Source:** Study by Shelly Coverman, sociologist at Tulane University, in *USA Today.*

• Two-career couples are generally closer than more traditional couples. In dual-career marriages, 88% of the spouses said their partner was their best friend. Keys to their marital success: Equality, commitment and respect. Among the traditional couples, 77% said their best friend was someone outside the marriage.

**Source:** Study by Mary F. Maples, professor of counseling education at the University of Nevada, cited in *Self.*

## TIP FOR WORKING COUPLES

A second bathroom has helped to save many a two-career marriage, particularly at 7 A.M., when both people are trying to get ready for work. (On a smaller scale, the same can be said for handheld hairdryers.)

## MARITAL-THERAPY CONFIDENTIAL

Clinical psychologists spend about 40% of their professional time dispensing marital therapy. Embarrasing fact: Fewer than 1% of training courses for clinical psychologists offer even a single course on marital therapy.

**Source:** A survey by the American Psychological Association.

• Marital therapists bias their counseling based on their own gender and experience. When 72 therapists were shown a videotape of a couple in therapy, the females blamed the husband for incompatibility while the males blamed both spouses. The males were more doubtful about saving a marriage in which the husband had had an affair, whereas female therapists were most pessimistic when the wife had strayed.

**Source:** Research by Elena Aguiar-Stevens and Daniel R. Boroto, Florida State University, in *Vogue*.

## MOST DANGEROUS YEAR OF MARRIAGE

Divorces are most likely (over 10%) during the second year of marriage. They decline after that. Only 6% occur after the 25th year.

**Source:** *Medical Aspects of Human Sexuality.*

## RECOVERING FROM A DIVORCE

After a divorce, most people need from two to four years to regain their emotional bal- ance and recover from the stresses of the process.

**Source:** Dr. R. Vance Fitzgerald, clinical associate professor, department of psychiatry, Medical College of Ohio, Toledo.

## DIVORCE TRAP

The guilt feelings commonly associated with divorce often cause the individuals involved to fail to protect themselves financially. Partners may think they do not deserve any financial settlement. Recommended: Consult a psychiatrist during the divorce proceedings. The lawyer and psychiatrist can work together to protect the interests of both parties.

**Source:** G. Pirooz Sholevar, Jefferson Medical School, Philadelphia, addressing a psychiatric meeting in New York.

## DIVORCE AND THE HOLIDAYS

A divorced father had his three children over for a midafternoon Christmas dinner. He noticed they weren't their usual ravenous selves. "How come you're not hungry?" he asked. They confessed that they were going to their mother's house for dinner that night.

Where children of divorced parents should spend the holidays is a common problem. The parents have to map something out together. It only works to their own detriment if younger children try to do it themselves. Children shouldn't be put in that position. Even former spouses who aren't getting along well should be guided by what's best for the kids.

### Strategies

Possible solutions: Some families alternate Christmas and Thanksgiving. Others celebrate on different days—for example, Christmas Eve at one house, Christmas Day at the other. Occasionally both parents join in holiday festivities together. (This is rare, because after a while people get involved in other relationships. But when ex-spouses are on good terms, and it doesn't interfere with their current relationships, they sometimes continue to celebrate together even after the first few years.)

Variation: Occasionally, when there is still a warm feeling, the patriarch or matriarch of one family invites the divorced partner to a holiday party. This is fine, if the ex-spouse doesn't object.

Dividing children between parents: Unless there is an open rift and a child doesn't see one parent anyhow, it can be difficult and painful for a child to choose between parents.

Think ahead: If you don't have a regular arrangement, plan early. Otherwise, someone else will have issued an invitation—and you'll be stuck.

When one person gets left out: Don't let yourself be walked on. But be considerate and understanding when kids are in a bind, and don't insist.

Guard against being hostile to children if they choose not to come (unless there is really a breakdown in relations, in which case you'd better get help.)

Helpful: Arrange for other family and friends to be at your house for the holiday. That way, it won't be as much of a disappointment if children have a change of plans. And an ongoing party with other people, preferably ones the children know also, helps to create a normal setting and relieve any awkwardness.

### Problems

The former husband or wife may not want the kids to go to Daddy's or Mommy's house if a new love interest is there. This can be very worrisome for children and shouldn't become an issue.

Sometimes the person who doesn't have custody (usually the father) doesn't buy the right presents. He remembers only the capabilities and emotional level of the child when they last lived together. It is upsetting to the parent if the child doesn't like a present. It's better to ask than to try to guess.

Establishing patterns: At first, a mother might insist on having Christmas at her house. Later on, she should be able to reassess the situation. But by then a tradition might have been established. Going to the father's house is then difficult for the children because he does things differently. They feel strange. It's not Christmas.

Better: Establish sharing of holidays early. Some form of joint custody sets up a tradition of co-parenting. Otherwise, it is difficult for children suddenly to become part of a household just because it's a holiday.

One parent, usually the father, often has more money. He can take the kids away for the holidays on a ski vacation or to the Caribbean. It's not fair to leave the decision up to the children. The parents themselves should decide. If they can't, they should call in an arbitrator.

**Source:** Interview with Clifford J. Sager, M.D., director of family psychiatry, Jewish Board of Family and Children's Servies, New York and clinical professor of psychiatry, New York Hospital-Cornell Medical Center.

# 9. Health Problems and Solutions

# Health Problems and Solutions

## AIDS UPDATE: FACTS AND FICTIONS

Publicity about acquired immune deficiency syndrome (AIDS) has multiplied faster than the disease. And because the disease is frightening and its cause is still unidentified, public reaction has sometimes been excessively dramatic.

To find out how much of a threat to the general population AIDS has become—and what precautions citizens should be taking—we interviewed Dr. Carlos Urmacher, a pathologist at New York's Memorial Sloan-Kettering Cancer Center, who has been studying the disease for three years.

Is AIDS a threat to everyone? You are not likely to contract AIDS unless you belong to one of the well-defined risk groups—namely, promiscuous homosexual men and intravenous-drug addicts.

Are the high-risk groups equally vulnerable? No. Seventy-five percent of AIDS sufferers are male homosexuals. The other 25% is divided among intravenous-drug users (the majority), Haitians (who may actually fit into other categories and not be a risk group at all), and a small percentage of hemophiliacs.

How can you be sure of the definition of these high-risk groups? To date, 95% of AIDS cases have been reported among the high-risk groups. Also, since the epidemic started, no known case of AIDS has been reported among the laboratory technicians, nurses or medical workers who have worked closely with AIDS patients. There have been a few cases related to the receipt of blood transfusions among hemophiliacs, but not among the remaining population.

What do these risk groups have in common that makes them susceptible to AIDS? They all appear to already suffer from a deficiency in their immune systems. Hemophiliacs, for example, are known to

have impaired systems. Some infants have contracted AIDS through blood transfusions—but they needed transfusions because there were already problems with their immune systems. The same can be said of homosexuals who have a history of repeated infections that may affect their immunity.

What is known about AIDS so far? It seems that AIDS is an infectious disease, but we don't know what causes it. We think it is transmitted in a manner similar to hepatitis: through the use of needles and through sexual contact among promiscuous individuals.

What is the prognosis for AIDS patients? Grim. Most die within three years of contracting the disease. AIDS differs from most other diseases that we deal with in that we don't yet know a way to diagnose it early. We can't catch it or treat it in the pre-clinical stage.

What are the characteristic symptoms of AIDS? Inexplicable weight loss, enlarged lymph glands, difficulties in breathing combined with fever or coughing, protracted diarrhea, and, in some cases, the appearance of lesions that look like bruises throughout the skin.

What precautions would you advise for avoiding AIDS? You have virtually no chance of contracting AIDS unless you belong to one of the risk groups and you also have an impaired immune system. Precautions for the high-risk groups are difficult to establish as long as we don't know what causes the disease. It seems logical to assume that avoiding sexual promiscuity and the use of illicit intravenous drugs would control or diminish the incidence of the epidemic.

## ALL ABOUT SINUS TROUBLE

The sinuses are four pairs of spaces in the

human skull, each lined with mucous membranes. When these membranes swell, the drainage of mucus slows or stops, bringing painful discomfort. Causes: Primarily viral infections, such as a cold or flu. But sinus membranes also swell from pressure changes during air flights, from swimming or diving in chlorinated water, or from sudden changes of temperature, such as going from the hot sun to an air-conditioned room.

Over-the-counter drug tablets and capsules work only temporarily. When this medicine wears off, it leaves the patient with more pain, which requires more medication. The same is true for nosedrops and nasal spray.

Best: Apply hot-water compresses to the affected areas. Drink extra fluids. Use a humidifier or vaporizer in your room. If bacteria are the cause of the problem, try a week or 10 days of antibiotics prescribed by a physician.

# WHAT SINUSITIS IS AND HOW TO PREVENT IT

We've all suffered the discomfort of nasal congestion caused by a cold or flu. Unpleasant though it is, it usually goes away in a week or so. But a common cold can lead to sinusitis, a very troublesome condition that can be difficult to manage.

Sinusitis (which simply means inflammation of the sinuses) in its acute stage causes swelling of the membranes inside the sinus cavities, pressure, headache, low-grade fever and a general feeling of misery.

### What Are the Sinuses?

We all talk about our sinuses as though they were bodily organs. Actually they're not organs at all, but air-containing spaces located within the skull. If the skull didn't have sinuses, it would be solid bone, too heavy to hold on your shoulders.

There are four sets of sinuses. The maxillary sinuses, the largest ones, are lateral to the nose and underneath the eyes. The ethmoid sinuses are between the eyes. Behind the ethmoids, practically in the middle of the head, are the sphenoid sinuses. The frontal sinuses are in the middle of the forehead, between the eyes and above the nose.

Although medical science is well acquainted with all the things that can go wrong with the sinuses, nobody really knows exactly what they do. It's suspected that they're tied up with the body's immune system. The membrane within them secretes mucus, and, within these secretions, are substances that probably protect the body from infection.

Normally, secretions from the sinuses flow into the nose, then to the postnasal space, and finally into the pharynx, where they're swallowed or coughed out. Many people complain about that secretion, so-called post-nasal drip. But the mucus secreted is a normal mechanism for cleaning out the sinuses and nasal passages.

### How Trouble Begins

When the nasal passages are irritated—by smoke, pollution or allergies, for instance—these cells secrete a lot more mucus to clean out the pollutants. That's why you get watery eyes and nose and swelling as a reaction to the irritant.

Usually sinusitis develops when the patient has a cold or upper respiratory infection brought on by bacteria or a virus. This sets up an inflammatory condition of the nose and the sinus cavities that obstructs the flow of secretions. When the flow is obstructed, the secretions become polluted, just as a blocked stream of running water would. Infection follows, producing more swelling of the mucous membrane, which in turn produces more blockage—and a vicious cycle ensues. If something isn't done to break the cycle, it gets worse and worse.

Nasal polyps can also develop as a reaction to increased stimuli. The polyps themselves can cause obstruction, leading to more polyps. Eventually subacute or chronic sinusitis develops. Operative intervention must then be considered in order to break the cycle.

Most likely to get sinusitis:

• People with allergies.

• Those with anatomical deformities that block good nasal drainage. Example: a deviated septum (an irregular wall dividing the two sides of the nose).

• People who react abnormally to stress. Emotional problems can cause the nasal membranes to become terribly engorged, producing sinus obstruction and subsequent infection.

### What to Do About Sinusitis

Once you've got full-blown sinusitis, you'll probably need antibiotic treatment. One of the first things the doctor will do is put an instrument into the sinus and gently irrigate it with water or saline solution. Then he'll put a sample of the mucus under a microscope to see what type of bacteria is involved and which antibiotic is appropriate. An antibiotic, if you use the right one, will usually knock out the infection quickly. Most commonly used: Penicillin compounds.

If antibiotics alone don't clear up the problem, it may be necessary to open the sinuses with surgery (usually an office procedure). Just like a boil or an abscess, a sinus has to drain before it can heal.

In 10%–15% of cases an in-hospital operation is necessary. A deviated septum may have to be corrected. Or it might be necessary to make an opening between the nose and an obstructed sinus for maximum drainage.

### Avoiding Sinusitis

• Do take decongestants and use nasal sprays when you have a cold. They reduce the amount of swelling and inflammation, preventing the sinuses from becoming blocked and infected. But don't overdo them. They also dry up the secretions that fight infection. Nasal sprays shouldn't be used for more than 48 hours and should be administered under the care of a doctor. Decongestants should also be taken under a doctor's supervision.

• Use a humidifier or vaporizer when you have a cold, and don't sleep in a hot, dry room. Dry heat is the worst thing for the sinuses. Suggested: Leave your bedroom window open, even if you live in a cold climate. Your nasal membranes will respond to the cool, moist air by shrinking and maintaining the important flow of secretions.

• Avoid cigarettes and alcohol. Both are irritating to the nasal passages and sinuses. Smoking may cause a chronic cough that infects the lungs. The coughing can throw mucus and other contaminated secretions up the back of the nose into your sinuses.

• Hay-fever sufferers and other allergy victims should have their allergies treated.

• Eat a balanced diet and get plenty of exercise. Exercise is particularly important for promoting proper nasal and sinus function.

**Source:** Interview with Stanley M. Blaugrund, M.D., an ear, nose and throat specialist and director of the Department of Otolaryngology, Lenox Hill Hospital, New York.

## 4 WAYS TO AVOID SINUS PROBLEMS

Preventing sinus problems: Avoid abrupt changes in temperature. Stay clear of household aerosol sprays. Keep your oven clean (smoke can trigger congestion). Have regular dental checkups (tooth infections spread easily into the sinuses.) If congestion persists, consider allergy tests.

## NASAL SPRAY ALERT

Nasal sprays, even over-the-counter decongestants, can lead to hazardous side effects with chronic use. In one case, a heavy user was afflicted with severe eyelid spasms and facial grimaces. Suggestion: Avoid long-term use of sprays except under medical direction.

• Nasal sprays can backfire if used too frequently. Beyond losing effectiveness, the sprays can aggravate sinus distress by damaging delicate membranes. They may also lead to dependency, so that nasal secretions increase when the spray is stopped.

**Source:** Overlook Hospital Foundation, Summit, NJ.

## HOW TO BEAT ARTHRITIS

The statistics are staggering: More than 36 million Americans—one in seven people, one in every three families—have some form of arthritis. Each year, one million people will learn that they too suffer from the nation's most common chronic disease.

It is estimated that arthritis costs the US over $13 billion annually in medical care and lost wages. That's over and above disability payments and many of the costs to individual arthritis sufferers and their families. We spend almost $800 million a year on drugs to treat arthritis and almost $1 billion on unproved remedies. Yet many Americans know relatively little about the various forms of arthritis (there are over 100) and fail to take the disease seriously. Many people believe that arthritis is simply the minor aches and pains that are an inevitable—and untreatable—part of growing older.

Some little-known facts:

• Arthritis afflicts people of every age, including 250,000 children.

• Early treatment is the key to optimum management of this potentially crippling disease.

• People wait an average of four years after noticing the symptoms of arthritis before they seek medical help. Many needlessly suffer irreversible joint damage that could have been minimized had they not delayed proper treatment. Most of the money mentioned above is spent after joints have become disabled, not before.

Bottom line: Arthritis is serious—but highly treatable.

### The Warning Signs

• Swelling in one or more joints.

• Early-morning stiffness.

• Unexplained weight loss, fever or weakness combined with joint pain.

• Recurring pain or tenderness in any joint.

• Inability to move a joint normally.

• Obvious redness and warmth in a joint.

Naturally, if you twist an ankle it will swell. If you sleep in an awkward position, you may be stiff on awakening. But if the above symptoms continue for two weeks, or if they recur for no apparent reason, it's important to see your physician.

### Why Early Diagnosis Is So Important

Arthritis literally means "joint inflammation." In its most common forms, arthritis is chronic, progressive and degenerative. Simply put, this means that it doesn't go away, and, if untreated, it tends to get worse. Even in mild cases it is best to have a physician monitor the progression of the disease from its beginnings.

For every form of arthritis, proper early treatment offers the greatest success in slowing or even halting the progression of the disease. When arthritis is effectively controlled, pain and inflammation can be reduced, permanent joint damage can be minimized or even prevented, and the range of motion in joints is maintained or increased.

Treatment programs are tailored to the individual. They differ depending on the kind of arthritis diagnosed, its severity, the particular joints affected, the age and occupation of the patient, and other factors. Because the various types of arthritis can be difficult to distinguish at the beginning, it is important to obtain a correct diagnosis. This procedure may involve blood or urine tests, X rays and other tests, in addition to a standard physical examination.

It is normal for arthritis sufferers to have ups and downs—flare-ups and remissions. Many arthritis patients are content to self-treat their problems by dosing themselves with aspirin or other conventional arthritis remedies. During remission periods, they convince themselves that the disease is cured. Although this method may seem to work well for many patients, it is certainly not all that can be done to combat the long-term effects of the disease. There is more to controlling arthritis than merely taking aspirin.

A complete treatment program includes medication in prescribed dosages . . . some combination of rest and prescribed exercises designed to maintain a full range of movement in affected joints . . . and instruction in methods of joint protection to prevent undue stress on affected joints. In cases where overweight is creating problems in joints, a diet may also be prescribed. Treatment programs should be followed during remissions as well as during flare-ups.

Arthritis research is ongoing. Frequent advances are made in treatments and medications, so it is important to check in with your doctor periodically even after you begin a program of treatment.

### Can Arthritis Be Prevented?

Although arthritis has been around for ages—it has been found in Egyptian mummies and even in dinosaurs—its causes, and therefore its prevention, for the most part still remain unknown.

One type of arthritis, caused by viral infection, is quite curable. Some types may be related to genetic predisposition, and research in this area is lively. A lifetime of physical labor or injury to a joint may lead to a form of arthritis later on.

But arthritis is surrounded by myths. Chances are that cracking your knuckles in your youth will not cause arthritis, and wearing a copper bracelet will certainly not prevent or cure it.

### Where to Go for Help

Start with your family physician. He may refer you to a rheumatologist or other specialist if necessary. And take the time to become well-informed—the Arthritis Foundation publishes free pamphlets about all aspects of the disease. Visit your local chapter or contact national headquarters.

**Source:** Interview with Dorothy Goldstein, Director of Medical Affairs, New York Chapter, Arthritis Foundation.

# 6 TIPS FOR ARTHRITIS SUFFERERS

For arthritis relief: (1) Get at least 10-12 hours of rest each day, including naps. (2) Avoid fatigue by splitting up big jobs and resting in the intervals. (3) Never skip prescribed exercises—even when you have a painful flare-up. (4) Set your aspirin or other medicine on your night table, along with water and some crackers. Then take the pills an hour before you get out of bed. (5) Use "contrast baths" for aching hands and feet . . . place them in warm water for three minutes, then cold water for one minute. (6) Learn to respect pain. If a joint still hurts several hours after an activity, don't repeat the activity.

**Source:** *Rheumatoid Arthritis: What You Can Do for Yourself,* Arthritis Foundation, Atlanta.

# BED REST MAY NOT BE THE ANSWER

Rheumatoid arthritis sufferers don't necessarily need bed rest. According to a 10-year study, activity equaled or surpassed bed rest as a treatment. Moderate exercise keeps individuals functionally independent.

**Source:** *The Lancet.*

# BEST TIME OF DAY FOR ARTHRITICS TO HAVE SEX

Arthritic patients generally enjoy sex more in the afternoon or evening (after morning pain lessens) . . . by using pillows to prop various limbs . . . through open discussion and a willingness to experiment with positions to find the most comfortable.

**Source:** Susan M. Daniels, director, Rehabilitation Counseling Department, Louisiana State University Medical Center, New Orleans, in *Medical Aspects of Human Sexuality.*

# AID FOR DIABETICS

The new medicines Glipizide and Glyburide are up to 200 times stronger than other drugs on the market, enabling patients to use very small doses only once a day. They have fewer side effects and don't cause water retention, significant problems in patients with high blood pressure or other heart troubles. They're effective in 50% of patients who previously failed on other oral agents and may also aid those now taking low doses of insulin.

**Source:** *Medical Tribune.*

# HOW BREAST FEEDING MAY FIGHT ONE KIND OF DIABETES

Juvenile-onset diabetes declines as breast feeding regains popularity. And according to a recent study in Denmark, babies who are breast-fed for at least three months also have fewer viral infections than bottle-fed babies. Reason: Antibodies from mothers' milk help infants fight infection. Possibility: Juvenile diabetes may be caused by a virus.

**Source:** *New Scientist,* New York.

## THE STRESS AND INSULIN CONNECTION

Diabetics who control their sugar levels with insulin can expect to have higher sugar levels during periods of stress. Adrenalin, adrenal steroids and other hormones produced during stress tend to elevate the blood glucose. Solution: Control metabolism through drugs and exercise, and learn stress reduction techniques.

**Source:** *Psychosomatic Medicine.*

## GOOD SUGAR SUBSTITUTES FOR DIABETICS

• Aspartame has been found acceptable as a sugar substitute by the American Diabetes Association and approved for moderate use in diabetic meal planning. Since dietary needs vary with the individual, the Association recommends that diabetics consult their doctors about the use of aspartame in their daily meal plans.

**Source:** American Diabetes Association.

• Fructose, the sugar found in fruit, has more sweetness per calorie than ordinary table sugar and is useful for diabetics who require insulin. It may, however, increase the risk of heart disease. Reason: Fructose increases the cholesterol level, especially LDL-cholesterol, the type most involved in fatty-cholesterol deposits in the arteries.

**Source:** *American Journal of Clinical Nutrition.*

## FOR DIABETICS WHO WANT TO EAT SWEETS

Diabetics can eat at least some sweets

without adversely affecting their sugar or insulin levels, according to major new research. Three conditions: The sugar-containing food must be eaten as part of a well-balanced, high fiber meal. Daily caloric intake should remain steady. The patient needs to follow a regular physical fitness regimen. The findings apply to diabetics who take insulin as well as to those on pills.

**Source:** *New England Journal of Medicine.*

## CHROMIUM SUPPLEMENT TIP

Diabetics may benefit from a chromium supplement. Chromium is necessary for normal glucose metabolism. A group of diabetics not requiring insulin had significantly better control when taking a chromium supplement in the form of brewer's yeast.

## DIABETICS, BEWARE

Aspirin, cold remedies, decongestants and laxatives can all cause special problems in a diabetic. Many contain sugar, while some others contain alcohol.

**Source:** Ames Division, Miles Laboratories, Inc., Elkhart, IN.

## PAINLESS INJECTIONS

Painless insulin shots for diabetics are possible using a liquid needle injector. Cost: $925.

**Source:** Derata Corp., Minneapolis, MN.

## HEMORRHOIDS: WHAT THEY ARE AND HOW TO TREAT THEM

Just about everyone gets a hemorrhoid occasionally. But don't worry, with good medical and dietary management, you can almost always avoid surgery.

### What Are Hemorrhoids?
This seems like an easy question. However, there's been a big change recently in medical thinking on the subject. We no

longer believe that hemorrhoids are simply varicose veins around the anus. Studies show that what we call hemorrhoids—dilated blood vessels in the anal canal—are present not only in adults with hemorrhoid symptoms but also in children and even fetuses. So we can no longer consider them a disease as such. What we think of as hemorrhoids are actually vascular cushions. These blue swellings are entirely normal and are suspected to have something to do with maintaining continence (control of bladder and bowels). Abnormality (hemorrhoids) occurs when these vascular cushions protrude in some way and become enlarged, ulcerated, inflamed and bleeding.

### Causes

Although we like to relate every disease to our industrial society and fastlane lifestyle, hemorrhoids have been around since antiquity. (One of Hippocrates' essays is entitled *On Hemorrhoids.*) However, doctors do think they are related to both pressure and diet.

The pressure problem is seen most commonly in pregnant women. There's probably a relationship to constipation, too . . . or to straining during bowel movements, which is linked to diet. In the US, one bowel movement a day is considered normal. In the Third World, however, where a large part of the diet is fiber and grain (with very little animal protein), only one movement a day would be considered extremely unusual. Three or four essentially nonformed bowel movements a day would be the norm. Causes are relative, but straining seems to cause the vascular cushions to protrude outside the anus. Thus unprotected, they enlarge and often bleed.

### What to Do

The most common symptom of hemorrhoids is rectal bleeding. Most people are frightened by rectal bleeding, although in the overwhelming majority of cases the cause is benign. First get a medical checkup to rule out malignancy. Then the following measures are recommended:

• Increase your intake of dietary fiber. In a 24-hour period you should have close to 20 grams of fiber. Eat high-fiber cereals. (Look at the contents lists on the boxes and choose brands that have at least eight grams of fiber per serving.) To get your fiber from other foods you would have to eat two pounds of raw carrots or apples every day. In addition to the cereal, which you must eat religiously, also eat whole-grain bread, a daily salad, and fresh fruits and vegetables. Avoid refined foods. It's also wise to avoid irritants such as alcohol and spicy or constipating foods during an attack. With a change in diet there may be some initial discomfort, including cramping, an increase in gas, and more bulky, more frequent stools. This will improve as your intestine gets used to the increased fiber. Straining should decrease, though one might not be aware of the change since many people are so used to straining that they don't notice it. I don't recommend medical stool softeners unless the high-fiber diet turns out to be really intolerable to the patient.

• If you have pain and irritation, take sitz baths (warm baths), which are soothing to the area and keep it clean.

• Take mineral oil to lubricate bowel movement. Mineral oil is harmless in the short run—but don't use it for more than two weeks.

• Use any over-the-counter preparation that gives you relief. They're all about the same. But avoid steroid preparations, especially on a long-term basis. My patients have found that simply using petroleum jelly as a lubricant when wiping is usually adequate.

• Moderate exercise has a generally beneficial effect on colonic function. However, very strenuous exercise, such as weightlifting, can aggravate hemorrhoids, especially if it involves bearing down on the afflicted area. General rule: If the exercise is painful, don't do it.

### Medical Treatment

The most common complication of hemorrhoids is bleeding, which usually disappears with a change in diet. Another common complication is thrombosis, caused by a blood clot in the hemorrhoid. Thrombosis causes sudden acute pain, and the patient may notice a lump or mass that bleeds. A doctor can inject a little local anesthesia around the area of the lump and make a simple incision to remove the blood clot. The wound is left open. It usually heals without a problem while the patient is on a regimen of sitz baths and a high-fiber diet.

Prolapse (protrusion of the hemorrhoid) may also spontaneously reduce with dietary change and other simple measures, or the patient may be able to push the hemorrhoid back in himself. When a prolapsed hemorrhoid can't be reduced, the outpatient rubberband procedure is the most benign method of medical treatment, giving good symptomatic relief.

How it's done: A special type of rubber band is fitted onto an instrument that grasps the lining of the rectum and places the band just above the hemorrhoid. The tightening effect on the lining pulls the hemorrhoid back into the anal canal. The rubber band falls off by itself after 7 to 10 days. The area where it was applied will be somewhat scarred, keeping the hemorrhoid up in the anal canal. If the band is placed correctly, there will be very little discomfort. Most patients can go to work the next day.

Important: Find a doctor with extensive experience in the procedure. Improper placement of the band can cause pain, and the procedure won't be successful. Most experienced: General surgeons and proctologists.

Fewer than 5% of patients have very large, even gangrenous, hemorrhoids that can be reduced only by surgery. When surgery is necessary, we do a hemorrhoidectomy, which requires a several-day hospital stay. The operation entails surgically removing the hemorrhoid and sewing the tissue back up. But rubber-band ligation has largely replaced hemorrhoidectomies over the past 10–15 years.

**Source:** Interview with Thomas A. Stellato, M.D., general surgeon and assistant professor of surgery, Case Western Reserve University.

## KIDNEY STONE PREVENTION

Small daily doses of magnesium oxide seem to forestall the formation of calcium-oxalate lumps, by far the most prevalent kind of kidney stone. The magnesium apparently flushes out the excess calcium that is the basis of most kidney stones. This simple therapy brings relief to thousands of sufferers of this painful condition, formerly treated with restricted diets, water guzzling and surgery.

**Source:** Stanley Gershoff, MD, dean of Tufts University School of Nutrition, and Edwin L. Prien Sr., MD, a urologist at Newton-Wellesley Hospital in Massachusetts, quoted in *American Health.*

## NON-SURGICAL KIDNEY STONE TREATMENT

Kidney stones may no longer require major surgery. With a new procedure called *percutaneous ultrasonic lithotripsy* (PUL), a doctor makes a small puncture over the kidney and inserts a tube. Instruments are inserted through the tube to break up and remove the stones. Advantages: Less pain, a briefer convalescence and a 97% success rate. In the works: A technique using shock waves (transmitted through water) to break the stones into sand-fine fragments. The particles would then pass out of the body on their own.

**Source:** Joseph Segura, M.D., a urologist at the Mayo Clinic, Rochester, MN.

## WHAT YOUR DOCTOR MAY NOT KNOW ABOUT GALLSTONES

Gallstone attacks occur randomly and cannot be prevented with a low-fat diet, new evidence indicates. Yet many physicians continue to prescribe such diets despite the futility of following them.

**Source:** Study by Michael Mogadam, M.D., Georgetown University, reported in *Medical World News,* New York.

# WHEN NOT TO WORRY ABOUT GALLSTONES

Gallstones may best be left alone until they act up. Current practice: To remove them as soon as they are detected. A recent long-term study of 123 males with gallstones showed that over a 15-year period, only 16 developed problems and only 14 required surgery. About 15 million people have gallstones.

**Source:** William A. Gracie, M.D., University of Michigan, reporting in *The New England Journal of Medicine*, Boston, MA.

# WHAT HORMONES ARE AND WHAT HAPPENS WHEN THEY GO AWRY

Hormones affect many different actions in many parts of the body, and their smooth functioning is crucial to the maintenance of good health. However, there are many misconceptions about hormones—what they are, what they do, what constitutes a hormone imbalance and how to tell if you have one. Most imbalances are fairly obvious and are therefore easy to diagnose and treat. Some, however, are asymptomatic, and it's these that we have to be on the lookout for.

### What Hormones Are

Hormones are substances secreted by various glands in the body. . . the pituitary, thyroid, islets of Langerhans, adrenals and gonads (ovaries and testes). Microscopic in size, they are carried by the blood stream. They affect many body tissues, regulating their functions, which must interact in a harmonious fashion to be effective. Example: Thyroid hormone sets the metabolic rate in many tissues.

### Hormone Imbalances

A hormone imbalance occurs when the normal feedback mechanism between the pituitary and the gland it regulates goes awry. Most common: The gland itself malfunctions and no longer responds to pituitary control. More rare: A pituitary malfunction, which occurs in the case of brain injury or tumor. Exception: The glands that are not under pituitary control may also cease to function. Example: The islets of Langerhans in the pancreas can produce too much insulin, which might mean a tumor. Or not enough is produced, because for some reason the body needs more than they can produce. Or they may stop functioning altogether because of disease, as in certain types of diabetes.

About 95% of all endocrine disease is caused by thyroid disorders and diabetes, the two most frequent hormone imbalances. If they go undetected and untreated, which often happens when the disease is asymptomatic, serious illness or death can result.

*Thyroid disease:*

• Hyperthyroidism (overactive thyroid) is most common in young women. In this disorder, the thyroid is usually unhinged from pituitary control, and something is driving it wild. Symptoms: Increased sweating, weight loss despite excessive food intake, goiter, rapid pulse, fine skin and hair, tremor, rapid mood swings and (in some cases) bulging eyes. Treatment: A drug to block thyroid production, radioactive iodine to destroy part of the thyroid or an operation to remove part of it. This disorder is easy to spot and reacts well to treatment.

• Hypothyroidism (underactive thyroid) is caused by a failure of the thyroid gland to make enough thyroid hormone despite pituitary stimulation ("primary hypothyroidism"). However, in some forms of hypothyroidism, the failure is at the level of the pituitary ("secondary hypothyroidism").Symptoms: Slow thinking, pasty skin, slow speech, dry coarse hair, constipation, reduced appetite. Treatment: Thyroid hormone replacement therapy produces a dramatic cure. Common misconception: That an underactive thyroid can cause obesity. This is virtually impossible. Reason: The thyroid regulates the interaction of body metabolism and appetite. If the thyroid is underactive, appetite will not be great enough to create obesity. About 99% of people with an underactive thyroid are not overweight. Dangerous: Thyroid hormone to treat obesity. An excessive amount can induce hyperthyroidism, causing severe side effects such as an overworked heart, muscle breakdown and psychological changes.

• Asymptomatic hypo- and hyperthyroidism. There's a recent awareness that as many as 10% of depressed patients have underactive thyroids. In a number of manic patients or agitated depressives, there can be a transitory increase in thyroid function. Also: Certain drugs given for mood disturbances, such as lithium, can cause hypothyroidism. Unresolved dilemma: Which comes first, thyroid malfunction or the mental disorder. Treatment: Correction of the thyroid imbalance may, in some cases, bring about relief from psychotic behavior. Research is still being done in this area. Hyperthyroidism frequently goes unrecognized as the cause of heart disease in aging people. The symptoms are masked, and the elderly don't have the reserves to cope with the strain excess thyroid hormone makes on the heart. Strongly recommended: The elderly with cardiac abnormalities, and manic or depressive patients, should be tested for thyroid abnormalities.

*Diabetes:*

The early signs of diabetes, such as excessive urination, thirst and fatigue, may not be present. Most dangerous: Gestation diabetes. Every pregnant woman has an increased need for insulin during the second half of pregnancy. But 2%–3% of pregnant women can't produce enough to meet the demand. This type of diabetes, almost invariably asymptomatic, can endanger the life of the child. Recommended: All pregnant women should be tested for diabetes around the 28th or 30th week of pregnancy. Also: People over 40 should have regular diabetes screenings, especially if they are overweight or have a family history of diabetes. Many middle-aged people contract asymptomatic diabetes, which can cause an increase in heart disease and in cataracts and other eye problems. These are potentially rectifiable illnesses once the diabetes is detected.

**Source:** Interview with Norbert Freinkel, M.D., Kettering professor of medicine and director of the Center for Endocrinology, Metabolism and Nutrition at Northwestern University Medical School and director of the Endocrine Metabolic Clinic, Northwestern University-McGraw Medical Center, both in Chicago.

# WHAT EACH GLAND DOES

• *The pituitary* (in the brain) is the control tower for most of the body's hormonal functions. In addition to regulating the way the kidneys handle water, its hormones stimulate correlating glands throughout the body to produce their own hormones. The pituitary controls all major glands except the insulin- and adrenalin-producing glands.

• *The thyroid* is in the neck. Its hormone controls heart and pulse rate, reaction to heat or cold, hair and skin texture and food metabolism.

• *The islets of Langerhans* (in the pancreas) control the body's production of insulin, glucagon and somatostatin. Insulin, which regulates sugar metabolism, is this gland's major secretion.

• *The adrenal gland,* just above the kidneys, consists of the adrenal cortex and the adrenal medulla. The adrenal cortex makes cortisol and adrenal hormone, which control sugar and protein metabolism, and aldosterone, which controls salt metabolism. The inner core of the adrenal, the adrenal medulla, makes adrenalin and noradrenalin.

• *The gonads* control the functions of the sexual organs. The ovaries produce estrogen and progesterone, and the testes produce testosterone.

# CHILDREN'S DISEASES THAT ENDANGER GROWN-UPS

Childhood diseases afflict many adults. About 5%–10% of the cases of measles, mumps and chicken pox in the US are among adults. The rate is even higher for rubella (German measles). Reason: These diseases were never completely eliminated from the population. New cases are constantly imported from other countries by travelers. Caution: Adults are in greater danger than children from these diseases. Many doctors don't look for them in adults and frequently try to treat the diseases as allergies. Also, a childhood disease is likely to be much more severe in an adult than in a child.

**Source:** Center for Disease Control, Atlanta.

# VACCINES FOR ADULTS

More than half of American adults fail to take advantage of available vaccines. Important: Don't count on your doctor to keep track for you.

Recommended:

• Tetanus and diptheria immunity: Important for all adults. Requires an initial series of three shots (usually given in childhood) and boosters every 10 years.

• Measles vaccine: Should be given to any adult born after 1956 who has not had either a documented case of the disease or an injection with live-virus vaccine. Caution: The killed-virus vaccines available between 1963 and 1967 are ineffective. If you're unsure, it is advisable to have a live-virus baccine administered.

• Rubella vaccine: Should be given to all adults who were not immunized as children. Most in need: Women likely to become pregnant. (Rubella severely damages developing fetuses.)

• Hepatitis vaccine: A good idea for those who are routinely exposed to blood and blood products.

• Influenza vaccine: Should be given annually to everyone over 65. Others at high risk because of poor health or frequent exposure to people sick with the disease should also consider vaccination.

• Pneumococcal pneumonia vaccine: For everyone over 65 and others at high risk. This vaccination is relatively new, effective and vitally important. (Pneumonia is a major cause of death among older people.)

Additional protection (against malaria, polio, meningitis, etc.) may be necessary if you plan to travel outside the US. Contact your state's health department for instructions appropriate to your destination.

**Source:** Interview with Steven Wassilak, M.D., medical epidemiologist, division of immunization, Center for Disease Control, Atlanta.

# HOW OFTEN TO HAVE TETANUS SHOTS

Tetanus booster shots are necessary only once every 10 years for healthy adults. Exception: If you're badly cut while working in dirty surroundings and haven't had a booster within five years, the doctor will probably give you one.

**Source:** *Cosmopolitan.*

# SCREENING MUST

Huntington's chorea now can be detected even before its symptoms (nervousness and memory loss) appear. Result: Adult offspring of Huntington's parents can screen themselves to determine whether they're likely to pass the disease on to their offspring.

**Source:** *New Scientist.*

# BRAIN-DAMAGE ALERT

Brain damage can occur even without a direct blow to the head. Signs of trouble: Problems with memory and concentration. Or the victim becomes unstable, lethargic or easily fatigued without knowing why.

**More information:** National Head Injury Foundation, 18A Vernon St., Framingham, MA 01701.

# AFTERMATH OF VIRAL ILLNESSES

A viral illness can leave the patient with abnormal muscle functions long after the actual disease has disappeared. The patient may experience lingering exhaustion and fatigue, muscular pain and persistent feelings of unsteadiness.

**Source:** *The Lancet.*

# HOW ALLERGIES CAN CAUSE HEARING PROBLEMS

Hearing loss caused by allergies is now being treated. Often allergic reaction inflames and swells the nerve fibers of the inner ear or plugs the delicate middle ear with mucus. Patients lose hearing without discovering the cause.

Treatment: Tests are given to determine the allergy. (Common culprit: corn.) Next, anti-allergy drugs are administered, and small amounts of the allergy-causing substances are injected into the body to build an immunity.

Result: More than half those treated in one study temporarily regained normal hearing within 30 minutes after taking anti-allergy drugs. This might be viewed as one of the therapeutic tests implicating allergy. With continued treatment, the regained hearing ability can become more long-lasting. For others, normal hearing returned within months.

Those with unexplained hearing loss should consult a specialist with extensive interest and experience in problems involving both allergy and otolaryngologic allergy in the same patient.

**Source:** Leonard Girsh, M.D., director of allergy and clinical immunology, Medical College of Pennsylvania, Philadelphia.

# MORE ABOUT ALLERGIC DEAFNESS

Allergic deafness occurs when the Eustachian tubes swell in reaction to some food or household substance. Common culprits: Wool blankets, dust, pollen, pet dandruff, and molds or mildews in milk, wheat and corn. The condition is usually curable: The patient avoids the substance or is desensitized with injections.

**Source:** *Omni,* New York.

# TINNITUS RELIEF

White noise, the soft static between FM stations, can offer relief to people with tinnitus (chronic ringing or clicking in the ears). Latest development: A combined hearing aid and white-noise emitter.

**Source:** Research at the University of Oregon School of Medicine, Eugene.

# A BABY'S CRYING CAN MAKE YOU DEAF

A baby's screams can be literally deafening. The howls of an 11-month-old child were measured at 100–117 decibels at six inches (the average distance between an infant and the mother's ear when she's holding the child). This is equal to the noise of a jackhammer, and more than enough to cause a temporary hearing loss.

**Source:** Study at the University of Minnesota, reported in the *New England Journal of Medicine,* Boston, MA.

# HEADSET WARNING

Personal stereos needn't be at maximum volume to damage your ears. At just one-half the maximum level, headsets transmit sounds between 85 and 111 decibels—enough to impair hearing after a long period.

**Source:** Research by Dr. Hubert L. Gerstman, chief of the Speech, Language and Hearing Center, New England School of Medicine, Boston.

# HELPING THE HARD OF HEARING

Always speak in full view of a nonhearing person. Don't talk while rocking in a chair, chewing gum or eating.

If the person has a hearing aid, move closer and speak normally. If not, raise your voice without shouting.

To get attention, gently tap the person's shoulder or come into full view before speaking.

When in a group, avoid whispering or covering your mouth while talking. Never speak about hearing-impaired people in their presence. (They might pick up more than you assume.)

Be sensitive to facial expressions. They'll tell you if you're getting through.

**Source:** *For Your Good Health.*

# HI-TECH HEARING AID

Artificial-ear implants convert spoken words into electrical impulses, to be transmitted directly to the brain. They were recently introduced by Kolff Medical (manufacturers of Barney Clark's mechanical heart). Cost: $8,000–$12,000.

# DIAGNOSING DYSLEXIA

Dyslexia may not be diagnosed until its victim is an adult. Reason: Mild forms of dyslexia (reversing letters and numbers, forgetting names of common objects) can be overcome by mental adjustments and tricks. Sufferers don't know they have a problem until they encounter a situation where the tricks do not work. The person may need tutoring and special aids to be able to function in that new situation.

# HOW TO DEAL WITH DYSLEXIA

Dyslexia, the inability of the brain to process written words properly, can be especially detrimental to students and office workers. But if it's recognized early, dyslexia can now be helped greatly, if not completely overcome. The symptoms:

• Reversal of letters when spelling.

• Illegible handwriting.

• Difficulty remembering right from left, up from down.

• Confusion over time.

• Trouble finding the right word.

• Trouble remembering words.

Dyslexia has nothing to do with intelligence. Among the sufferers: General George Patton and Leonardo da Vinci.

If you suspect your child is dyslexic, have a test done early, though testing before a child enters the second grade isn't always definitive. Early treatment is essential because a child with dyslexia often develops emotional problems. If the school can't provide it, outside tutors can be located through the Orton Dyslexia Society (724 York Rd., Baltimore 21204) and through several other organizations.*

Helping adults with dyslexia is more difficult because comparatively few therapists specialize in their problem. There's no reason for a company to reject a dyslexic for a job that doesn't require writing skills. Dyslexics are often articulate in speaking.

While public school systems frequently pay the cost of helping a dyslexic child, adults have to foot the bill themselves. Group therapy can cost as much as $40 for tutorial sessions that last four weeks. But since tutoring takes many months, and possibly years, fees can become substantial.

*The Association for Children with Learning Disabilities, 4156 Library Rd., Pittsburgh 15234, and the Learning Disabilities Hotline at Albert Einstein College of Medicine in New York, (212) 409-2233. In addition, large teaching hospitals often have departments that deal with communications problems.

**Source:** Interview with William Ellis, president of the Orton Dyslexia Society.

# SOME TRUTHS ABOUT STUTTERING

The causes of stuttering remain obscure. Best theory: A combination of genetic and environmental factors. One person out of every 100 stutters (2.1 million Americans). Four times as many men are afflicted as women. Stuttering was once thought entirely psychological. But stutterers are not more neurotic than the rest of the population. Most victims do not stutter when they sing, whisper, affect a foreign accent or speak to small children or pets.

Ways to respond: Never finish a sentence for a stutterer. Never ask for a repetition. Do not show impatience. Worst: To turn away.

Half of the children who stutter outgrow it by adolescence.

**More information:** The Stutterers' Association, Teachers College, Columbia University, 525 W. 120 St., New York 10027.

## TIP FOR STUTTERERS

Often, the problem is that you're paying too much attention to the act of speaking. Try holding a small object in each hand while you practice talking. Focus your attention on the weight in your hands. That diversion can aid your speaking.

**Source:** *Talk-Power* by Natalie H. Rogers, Dodd, Mead &Co., New York.

## COLD PREVENTION

One of the most effective cold prevention measures is to maintain an indoor relative humidity of 45% or above. The membranes of the nose, throat and lungs are less vulnerable to irritation and viral infection. Use a gauge to check the humidity, and turn on a steam vaporizer to increase the humidity level, if necessary.

**Source:** *Sports Medicine Digest.*

## COLD WATCH

Hand-to-hand contact spreads colds more than does sneezing, coughing or kissing. It's possible to "catch" a cold by shaking hands—or even by grasping a doorknob up to 72 hours after it was touched by an infected person. Cold-prevention tactics: If someone in the house has a cold, encourage all family members to wash their hands often. Promote air circulation in the house. Keep hands (both yours and other people's) away from your face.

**Source:** Research by Jack M. Gwaltney Jr., M.D., University of Virginia, Charlottesville.

## YOU CAN GIVE YOURSELF A COLD

You can catch a cold from your own germs, viruses your body has harbored in an inactive state for months. The bugs become active only when your immune system weakens, as in a period of high stress.

**Source:** Harold Muchmore, M.D., Veterans Administration and University of Oklahoma, quoted in *Science Digest*, New York.

## THE LATEST ON COLDS

Common colds usually run their course—with or without your doctor's help—in about a week. General prescription: Rest and plenty of fluids (two quarts a day for adults).

When to call your doctor: The first day, if you have a fever over 103°F., suffer from shortness of breath or wheezing, or develop a bad pain in the chest, head, stomach, ears or glands in the neck. Call the second day, if your sore throat is getting worse and your temperature is above 101°F. Call the third day if sore throat and a 101°F. fever have persisted. If, after a week, you still have some fever and a sore throat, see your doctor.

**Source:** Department of Family and Community Medicine, University of Missouri, Columbia.

## PROPER WAY TO SNEEZE

Stifling a sneeze may increase pressure in the nasal cavity and push up mucus into the eustachian tube, causing an ear infection. Since the sneeze is nature's way of clearing irritants from your nose, it's much healthier to cover your nose and mouth with a handkerchief and let it go.

**Source:** *American Health*, New York.

## TWO COMMON REMEDIES THAT DON'T WORK

• Taking aspirin to bring down a fever when you have a virus actually weakens your body's defenses. Interferon, a protein produced by the body to fight off the virus, works less effectively when the fever is brought down.

**Source:** American Physical Fitness Research Instiute.

• Two aspirin at the first sign of fever may actually prolong the illness we're trying to control. Reason: A heightened body temperature makes white blood cells more mobile—and more effective in killing germs.

**Source:** *Prevention*, Emmaus, PA.

• Although most physcians say the folk remedy of using alcohol to lower a fever works if done correctly. . .if the fever's not too high. . .if you just sponge the patient, as opposed to immersing him in alcohol. . .there's just too much of a chance of something going wrong.

Examples: Alcohol splashed in the eyes can cause painful corneal abrasions. . . alcohol can be absorbed through the skin, leading to alcohol poisoning, especially in infants. . .too much alcohol evaporating from the skin causes shivering—making the patient even more uncomfortable.

Better, safer, cheaper: Sponge bath with tepid water—80°–90°F—that feels barely warm to the touch. Or: 15–20 minutes in a bathtub filled with water of the same temperature.

Guidelines: Infants up to three months: see a doctor for any fever. . .4–12 months, tepid water sponge baths for fevers up to 101°. If higher, see a physician immediately. One year and up, tepid baths for fevers of 101°–103°.

**Source:** Normal Scott, M.D., pediatrician, Kaiser-Permanente Health Maintenance Organization, Denver, CO.

## ANTIHISTAMINES CAN PROLONG A COLD

Discontinue antihistamines when a cold shifts to the chest. They help relieve upper respiratory conditions but can aggravate lower respiratory ones, such as bronchitis and asthma. By reducing mucus production, antihistamines make bronchial secretions stickier. This plugs the bronchial tubes more and makes it harder to clear them with coughing.

**Source:** John H. Dirckx, M.D., writing in *Consultant*, New York.

## BED-REST WARNING

Bed rest may be good for a cold—but only to a point. It's also important to move around a bit. Even some moderate exercise won't do any harm. Point: Muscle atrophy begins within 24 hours of total bed rest.

**Source:** Study by NASA.

## TREAT A COLD WITH BOOZE FUMES

A California general practitioner swears by this cold remedy: Take a thick mug and fill it with boiling water. After about two minutes, throw the water away. Put in two ounces of brandy or bourbon, and then fill the mug almost to the top with boiling water. Cup your hands over the top of the mug to make a nose cone. Place your mouth and nose inside the cone. Blow on the surface and inhale the fumes for 15 minutes. You should feel the vapor penetrating your sinuses. Drink the mixture if you want to. Take a cold pill to keep your sinuses open overnight and repeat the treatment in the morning. If you start this at the first signs of a cold (before nasal passages are blocked), your cold should vanish in 24 hours.

**Source:** Dr. Robert K. Julien, Turlock, CA.

## COLD STOPPER

An interferon-based nasal spray can ward off the common cold. This could be particularly significant for elderly people, in whom colds can sometimes be life-threatening. About 25% of the volunteers who have used the spray have developed a mild "stuffy nose" symptom, but this is a side effect common to all nasal sprays.

**Source:** Schering-Plough, Galloping Hill Rd., Kenilworth, NJ.

## HIGH-TECH KLEENEX

Killer Kleenex will help stop the spread of the common cold. Now in clinical trials, the tissue is suffused with an antiviral compound. Impact: Viruses are killed before they can spread nose-to-hand or hand-to-hand—the most common routes.

**Source:** Research by Elliot Dick, M.D., University of Wisconsin, in *American Health*.

## COLD VS. FLU

A cold is characterized by a sore throat, sneezing, a runny or stuffy nose, and mild fatigue. Flu symptoms include fever (rare in a cold), severe head and body aches, and extreme fatigue. Chest pain and cough: Moderate with a cold, sometimes severe with flu.

**Source:** *Ladies' Home Journal*, New York.

## FIGHTING THE FLU

Annual shots are only 70% effective. Reason: Vaccine is made from last year's antibodies, and influenza virus alters its structure each year. Who should receive shots: Those with asthma, chronic bronchitis, cardiovascular or kidney problems and immunity weaknesses. Who should avoid shots: Healthy young people, most pregnant women (shots can provoke a mild flu) and anyone allergic to eggs, the vaccine's culture medium. Help for the un-inoculated: *Amantadine hydrochloride*. It's a prescription drug that works against Type A flu (most common and not severe). It can prevent infection or ease symptoms once flu strikes.

## WHEN ASPIRIN MAKES ALLERGIES WORSE

A mild food allergy can become severe if the offending food is eaten right after you've taken aspirin. Since aspirin increases the stomach's absorption ability, the allergen enters your bloodstream in much larger amounts than it normally would.

**Source:** *British Medical Journal*, London.

## WHO'S MOST LIKELY TO BE ALLERGIC TO YELLOW FOOD DYE?

People allergic to aspirin have a 15% chance of also being allergic to a common yellow food dye called tartrazine. Found in some orange- and lime-flavored drinks and drink mixes, colored gelatins, instant puddings, lemon-drop candies, cake mixes, salad dressings and "cheese food" snacks, the dye can cause a runny nose, hives or even bronchial asthma attacks in sensitive people. Consumers should check food labels for FD&C yellow No. 5, the official FDA designation.

## FOOD ALLERGY ALERT

Food allergies may play a role in chronic nasal congestion, post-nasal drip, chronic cough, asthma and recurrent pneumonia. Most common culprit: Milk. Others: Soy, peanuts and pork.

**Source:** *Annals of Allergy.*

## THE ALLERGY/EXERCISE CONNECTION

Severe allergic reactions have been reported by some persons who exercised right after eating certain foods, including celery, shellfish and fruit. The same persons reported no problems if they fasted for two hours before exercising.

**Source:** *Employee Health & Fitness.*

## WHAT TO DO IF YOU'RE ALLERGIC TO YOUR PET

Owners who find themselves or a member of their family sensitive to a cat or dog needn't always give it up. A new system developed by the American Society for the Prevention of Cruelty to Animals helps cut down the sneezing and itching that accompany such allergies. The key: Many scientists believe that animal allergies are caused by saliva adhering to the pet's hairs and not by the hairs themselves. The regimen:

1. Brush the animal two or three times a week with a soft, non-irritating brush.

2. Wipe down the animal once a week or so with a wet towel to remove saliva and loose hairs.

3. Shampoo the animal once every couple of weeks (less frequently if the allergy

subsides). Use a final rinse with fabric softener to eliminate static electricity. Proportions: One tablespoonful of softener per one quart of water.

Cat owners can use diluted fabric softener in the toweling step instead of step three.

**Source:** Interview with Charles Schaubhut, D.V.M., a staff veterinarian with the Henry Bergh Memorial Animal Hospital, New York.

## YOUR CAR'S AIR CONDITIONER CAN MAKE YOU SICK

Summer sneezes may be caused by your car's air conditioner. In a study of allergy and asthma sufferers, 18% said symptoms got worse when they drove with their air conditioner on. Findings: Different fungi are circulated by auto air conditioners, including some that can trigger breathing problems. Recommended: Have your mechanic clean the air conditioner and capsule before the hot season.

**Source:** Research by Prem Kuman, M.D., associate professor of medicine, Louisiana State University, Shreveport.

## OFFICE ALLERGIES

More than 35 million Americans suffer from allergies or asthma that's often triggered by dust and mold found in office rugs, furniture, draperies, books, files and air conditioners. Hay fever alone accounts for a loss of more than three million work days annually. Preventive measures: Use plastic or synthetic fabrics that retain less mold. Clean heating or cooling system ducts and filters once a month, and. . .when they're first turned on, leave the area until the trapped dust is completely blown out.

**Source:** *Nation's Business.*

## COPY-PAPER WARNING

Carbonless copy paper can cause severe allergic reactions. It poses a health hazard to one in 10 people. The problem occurs when the microscopic balls of liquid embedded in the paper burst during use, releasing a hydrocarbon gas. Caution: When handling the product, keep hands away from face. . .and wash frequently.

**Source:** Dr. Joseph Trautlein, associate professor of medicine, Pennsylvania State University College of Medicine, PA.

## LIFE-THREATENING INSECT BITES

Allergic reactions to insect stings are life-threatening to many people. Offending insects: Hornet, honeybee, yellow jacket and wasp. Antidote: A vaccine made from insect venom immunizes a person against the same type of insect. Who should take the vaccine: Anyone over 40 who is allergic to at least one insect venom. Those between 15 and 40 who have severe reactions to stings. Those bitten who suffer a reaction from a sting and have not taken the vaccine need an immediate shot of adrenalin. Special kits are available at drug stores with a doctor's prescription.

## HAY-FEVER CURE

Hay-fever relief will soon be available with the Rhinotherm, a device that blows hot, humid air into the nasal passages. In double-blind trials, researchers treated allergy sufferers with three 30-minute doses of the hot air at two-hour intervals. A week later, 75% of the patients were still free of hay fever symptoms. A month later, more than two-thirds were still without symptoms.

**Source:** *New Scientist*, New York.

## TWO NEW KINDS OF DRUGS

Nasal congestion caused by seasonal allergies can be relieved by two categories of prescription drugs. The first, nasal steroids, are inhaled twice daily and work over a period of a few days to decrease congestion. Side effects are minimal. The second, nasal cromolyn, available under the name Nasalcrom, blocks the release of chemical mediators leading to allergic reactions. Side effects: Minimal.

## WIDE-AWAKE ALLERGY PILLS

New drugs will fight allergy symptoms such as sneezes, runny noses and watery eyes—without putting the patient to sleep. How they work: A tiny molecular variation keeps the new drugs from crossing into the central nervous system.

## ASTHMA SUFFERERS AND SULFITES

Eating at restaurants can be hazardous to asthmatics' health. To preserve color and freshness, restaurants often spray raw vegetables with sulfites. But sulfites trigger allergic asthma attacks in about 10% of sufferers. Additional danger: Sulfites are also added to wines to inhibit the growth of undesirable organisms during fermentation.

**Source:** *Medical Tribune.*

## MSG STRIKES AGAIN

Severe asthma attacks can be set off by monosodium glutamate, the common flavor enhancer used in Asian restaurants. If you're susceptible, ask the waiter to omit MSG from your meal.

## ONCE-A-DAY DRUG FOR ASTHMA RELIEF

Asthma sufferers will find relief with a once-a-day capsule being marketed by G.D. Searle & Co. The drug, Theo-24, is also suitable for bronchitis and emphysema patients. How it works: The capsule contains hundreds of tiny beads of theophyline. They settle throughout the gastrointestinal tract and act as miniature time-release systems.

## ASTHMA AND VITAMIN C

Asthma symptoms may be eased by vitamin C. A 500-milligram dose stimulates the body to dilate swollen bronchial tubes.

**Source:** Research by the John B. Pierce Foundation Laboratory, New Haven, CT, in *Prevention.*

## IF YOU'RE CAUGHT WITHOUT YOUR MEDICINE

Strong coffee can help asthma sufferers who are caught having an attack without their medicine. In a new study, caffeine was found almost as effective as theophylline (the most common asthma medication) in opening bronchial passages and allowing asthmatics to breathe while they're having an attack.

**Source:** Pilot research at the University of Manitoba, Winnipeg, Canada, in *The New England Journal of Medicine.*

## BEST COLD-WEATHER SPORT FOR ASTHMA SUFFERERS

Exercise-induced asthma can be provoked by a combination of heavy exertion and cool temperatures (typical of an early-morning jog). Symptoms: Wheezing with a cough, shortness of breath. Target population: Sports enthusiasts between 40 and 65. Treatment: The same medications that work in allergic asthma. Prevention: Wear a mask or scarf over the mouth and nose when exercising in cold weather. Switch from sports such as basketball, soccer or marathon running (long periods of stress) to swimming, tennis or golf (short energy bursts).

**Source:** *World Tennis.*

## FACTS AND FALLACIES ABOUT DENTAL CARE

• Bad teeth don't cause headaches, bursitis or anything like that. But jaw and tooth pains may be "referred" pains that originate in other areas.

• A tooth knocked out in an accident can be saved. When a child falls and loses a tooth, pick it up, don't stop to clean it. Wrap it in a wet cloth, and bring it and the child as quickly as possible to the dentist. Reimplantation works best with children (sometimes works with adults, too).

• Playing the trumpet or trombone can correct a bad bite. However, playing flute or piccolo can make it worse. Saxophone can work either way.

• Pain perception is less in the morning than in the afternoon, according to recent research. Suggestion: Schedule dental appointments early in the day.

• If you don't want to pay for a crown for a badly decayed tooth, ask for a filling with reinforcement pins. That does the job almost as well at a fraction of the cost.

• Toothbrushes. Use two or more in rotation, so that they can dry out properly. Soft nylon is best. Natural bristle brushes take longer to dry. If not used properly, they can damage gum tissue because bristles are too firm and coarse. Angled brushes may help in reaching some areas. Caution: Too vigorous brushing can wear grooves in tooth enamel. When used correctly, a toothbrush will not abrade tissues or teeth. And hardness of the bristles is not as significant as the way the brush is used and the time spent brushing.

• Dental floss. Unwaxed floss is better because it absorbs particles.

• Flushing devices (such as Water Pik): If used with too much pressure, devices can damage tissue, force debris into periodontal pockets, and cause inflammation and infection. Recommendation: Use at half the recommended pressure.

# VERY, VERY, VERY AESTHETIC DENTISTRY

The concept of aesthetic dentistry has been around for a long time, but only in the last few years—with the advent of tooth bonding—have many smile-improving techniques become universally available.

Until recently, there wasn't much a dentist could do to create teeth that were beautiful as well as healthy. Now dentists can close the spaces between teeth, cover stains, repair chips, and create caps and dentures that look real. And it's all done quickly and relatively inexpensively.

### Bonding

Bonding is still new. How it works: The tooth is roughened with a mild acid. Next, a liquid material is painted on in layers and set by an intense white light. Then a tooth-colored bonding material of a puttylike consistency is sculpted onto the tooth. This material will not set until an intense white light is applied to it.

The first bonding materials set by themselves and were difficult to shape before the hardening began. By using the light, the dentist has time to create an aesthetically pleasing look, setting each layer at his convenience.

What's new in bonding: Porcelain laminates. Previously, we used a composite material of plastic and barium glass, but porcelain has big advantages. The composite could chip and stain. Porcelain doesn't chip at all, it doesn't absorb stains, and it offers more durable color and brightness.

### Crowns

For a long time, gold crowns were the standard for rehabilitation and durability. Next, we tried using plastic on the surface to cover the gold. But the plastic absorbed odors and water. . .and stained and wore away. Porcelain over the metal was better and is considered the ideal crown or bridge replacement today. (However, with the metal underneath, the color can be compromised, and the crown may look somewhat outsized and less like a real tooth.) All-porcelain caps were more delicate and aesthetically pleasing but were not strong enought to hold up well over time. A compromise between durability and looks has always been necessary.

We now have what we call *cast ceramic* for crowns. Ceramic is associated with procelain, but it has more glass in it. The process, developed by Corning Glass, uses ceramic material that we can cast the same way we cast gold. It's almost as strong as metal and looks much better.

This technique is very new, and it will take about five years for most dentists to become familiar with it. If you want cast-ceramic crowns now, you may have to search for a leading-edge dentist.

### Bridges

The newest thing in bridges is the Maryland bridge. Let's say you're missing a front tooth. Instead of grinding down and ruining the teeth on either side of the space in order to attach a bridge, we can now bond metal to the backs of the adjoining teeth so that it doesn't show and attach a porcelain tooth in between. This prevents the destruction of good teeth. Problem: For people who have strong bites or large spans of missing teeth, the Maryland bridge is not advisable.

The Maryland bridge is well-established in dentistry today—almost everyone is doing it.

### Dentures

Many years ago, we made the teeth for dentures and their base material small, on the theory that it would make them less noticeable. Actually, we should have done the opposite. Those dentures cause the classic denture look—a face that seems fallen in, with lines around the lips. What causes it: The bone that holds a tooth also holds out the face. When the tooth is extracted, that bone moves to fill in the hole left by the tooth, depriving the face of skeletal support. Today, we realize that the denture should be used to support the face. A person wearing dentures should look the same as he or she did with teeth. Dentures can even be used to improve the appearance of someone whose face was too small or badly shaped before.

Also, today's false teeth are aesthetically beautiful. Made of procelain or a more resilient plastic, they come in different shades and can be constructed with slight irregularities so that they look as alive and healthy as good natural teeth.

### Other Techniques

• Implantology, a new field, has arisen because of the problems with denture adjustment. Dentures may look good, but they are no more comfortable today than they ever were. Implantologists lock metal onto the bony structure underneath the gums. Little struts come out that look like teeth, and a bridge is cemented to these struts. When the patient has too much bone loss for a permanent bridge, a removable bridge that won't come out while chewing is attached to the struts. Problems: It doesn't work for everyone, and some implants have a limited life span. However, implants are definitely the wave of the future. They're improving all the time. Implantology is a new concept. Ask your dentist or local dental association for a referral.

• Oral (orthognathic) surgery: If someone's jaw sticks out or his face is misshapen, the jaw can be broken and then reset to look normal. This procedure is best performed by an oral surgeon rather than by a plastic surgeon.

• Prevention: After age 40, most people lose teeth because of periodontal conditions. We've learned to recognize gum problems early, and periodontics is one of the fastest-growing specialties. There are a number of new techniques, including bone replacement.

### Finding a Good Aesthetic Dentist

Always go to a dentist who thinks in terms of prevention . . . one who teaches you how to brush and floss properly and who shows concern about the future of your teeth.

It can be difficult to find a dentist who is artistically talented, as well as technically competent. Some feeling for aesthetics is essential to make teeth look cosmetically pleasing. The best way to find someone is through a personal reference. If someone you respect has had extensive bonding or crown work done and the teeth look natural, you've probably located a good aesthetic dentist.

Cost: This varies extensively, according to the dentist's expertise, as well as the part of the country in which you live. Bonding runs $150-$600 per tooth. Crowns cost $400-$1,200 per tooth. When you deal with aesthetics, it's more time-consuming and more expensive. But keep in mind that dentistry today is as much an art as a science.

**Source:** Irwin Smigel, D.D.S., the founder and president of the American Society for Dental Aesthetics.

## NO-DRILL DENTISTRY

Something we've all been waiting for is now just around the corner. . .made possible by a chemical, GK 101-E, that actually dissolves the decayed part of the tooth in minutes. (The patient then simply rinses his mouth and spits out all the decayed material!) The new technique removes only the decayed portion of the tooth; conventional drilling removes healthy tooth as well. No danger to hard or soft tissue of the mouth or gums. Reason: The dissolving substance is bio chemically targeted for diseased dental tissues. Already in use in Japan.

**Source:** National Patent Development Corp., New York.

## SEALANTS MEAN NO MORE TOOTH DECAY

Improved dental sealants prevent tooth decay—these improved formulas are 100% effective in protecting teeth as long as the plastic film is retained. . .and more than 80% of the films last seven years or longer. Background: Sealants developed back in the 1960s gave the concept a bad name— basically because they just didn't work very well. But studies run on the new generation of sealants indicate supereffectiveness and durability. Important: Even if you drink fluoridated water—and over 50% of US residents do—you're still not totally safe from cavities. Fluoride seems to work best on the smooth surfaces of teeth—but crevices and pits of molars are still highly vulnerable to decay. The sealant's thin coat of plastic on uneven surfaces prevents the entrapment of food and bacteria that produce decay-causing acids. Best bet: Fluoridated water and sealant. Cost: About $6 or $7 per tooth—and not all teeth need the protective coating.

**Source:** James Bawden, D.D.S., University of North Carolina, Chapel Hill.

• Sealing is most effective when done as soon as the permanent back teeth emerge in childhood. But it can still be worth doing for teenagers or adults who are troubled by cavities.

**Source:** *Harvard Medical School Health Letter*, Cambridge.

## FIGHTING CAVITIES BY EATING CHEESE

Eating cheese before dessert—an old French custom—helps fight cavities. The cheese prevents dental bacteria (plaque) from breaking down sugar into the acid that destroys enamel. Most effective: Aged cheddar, Monterey Jack, Swiss.

**Source:** Charles Schachtele, D.D.S., professor of destistry and microbiology, University of Minnesota, in *McCall's*.

## LOOK, SON, NO CAVITIES

Older people get fewer cavities because they "immunize" themselves against tooth decay. We're always swallowing tiny amounts of *Streptococcus mutans*, a bacterium that decays teeth. As we age, the strep eventually sets off an immune response, and the antibodies attack the bacteria in the plaque deposited on teeth. Under testing: A vaccine to produce the specific antibody.

**Source:** Roland Arnold, an oral biologist at Emory University, Atlanta, GA.

## GOOD NEWS FOR CHOCOLATE EATERS

Chocolate lovers will be pleased to know that chocolate is not as dangerous to teeth as other candies. Anti-decay factors in cocoa counter the damaging action of the sugar. Cocoa tannins seem to inhibit plaque formation, and the fat in cocoa may protect the teeth by forming antibacterial coating.

**Source:** National Institute for Dental Research, Bethesda, MD.

## FRUIT JUICE ALERT

Fruit juices can be just as bad for your teeth

as soft drinks, such as Coke. Both drinks can cause cavities. Although fruit juices have more nutrients, they contain natural sugars that are harmful to teeth.

**Source:** Swedish study, reported in *Executive Fitness*.

## HIGH-TECH TOOTH CARE

There's a toothbrush that cleans without water or toothpaste (pretreated with a special toothcleaning agent—two flavors!). Great for travel to countries in which it's ill-advised to sample the local water.

**Source:** Halbrand, Inc., Willoughby, Ohio.

• Portable dental spray squirts a spinning jet of water between teeth and gums. Squeeze bottle, requires no electricity.

**Source:** CJM Products, Huntington Beach, CA.

• Professional dental pick for home use removes impacted food. Curved edge can scrape away plaque.

**Source:** Dental Concepts, Inc., Bronx, NY.

## WHEN YOU CAN'T SEE YOUR DENTIST

If you lose a filling (or a cap or some bridgework) and can't see a dentist immediately, temporary repairs can be made with dental emergency "glue." Available over the counter (for about $2), a kit consists of zinc oxide powder and oil of cloves. In a crisis, you mix the two, then reset the filling. The glue should be good for several days. Caution: Don't use the glue if there's a throbbing pain or swelling, signs of infection that may be aggravated by the zinc oxide.

## BITE STRATEGY

Poor bite is often misdiagnosed as a migraine or pinched nerve. People with faulty bite often unconsciously grind their teeth to align them better. Result: Headaches, earaches and pains in the jaw, neck and shoulders. Treatments: Spot grinding by a dentist to even the bite. Exercises to relax the jaw muscles. A plastic device that fits over the upper and lower teeth to protect them from grinding, help readjust the bite and ease pressure on jaw muscles.

## WISDOM TOOTH WISDOM

Extracting impacted (unerupted) wisdom teeth before they can cause trouble has been a common practice in preventive dentistry. Some new studies suggest that this expensive oral surgery is premature in many cases. Reason to keep impacted wisdom teeth: Given time, many will erupt perfectly normally by themselves. There is little evidence to support the fear that impacted wisdom teeth cause later crowding of lower front teeth. As patients grow older, they may need their wisdom teeth (even impacted ones) to hold bridgework.

## NEW PROCEDURE HELPS REPAIR BONE DECAY

Bone decay caused by periodontal disease, an infection of the gums that afflicts 75% of adults, can be repaired with bone tissue from human cadavers. Procedure: Specially treated cadaver bone is ground into powder, then made into a puttylike material. This is used to fill in the spaces around the teeth where jaw bone has deteriorated. Result: The bone begins to repair itself through the production of new tissue.

**Source:** Procedure developed by researchers at the Harvard School of Dental Medicine and the Brigham and Women's Hospital in Boston, reported in *Science Digest*.

## IF YOU WEAR BRACES

People who wear braces on their teeth may need more calcium. When teeth are moved, it creates gaps in the jawbone that must be filled. New bone requires calcium. Sources: Green leafy vegetables such as asparagus, broccoli and turnip greens, milk, calcium supplements.

**Source:** David Ostreicher, D.D.S., orthodontist, professor of preventive dentistry at Columbia University, College of Physicians & Surgeons, New York.

## TIP FOR DENTURE WEARERS

Removing dentures at night can lead to aching jaws, headaches and insomnia. Reason: Jaws adapt to closing over teeth. If you sleep without your dentures, you may "overclose"—which strains the jaw joint and muscles. Recommended: If you have morning-after pain, try leaving dentures in at night (but remove them for four hours during the day).

**Source:** An Army study of 200 denture wearers, cited in *American Health*, New York.

## DENTURE ADHESIVES ALERT

Denture adhesives can actually be more harmful than helpful to users. Karaya gum, a common ingredient, is highly acidic and eats away the enamel of natural teeth. Constant use may dissolve bone tissue and promote fungus infections in the mouth. The good news: Properly fitting dentures don't require adhesives in the first place.

**Source:** George Murrell, D.D.S., University of Southern California, Los Angeles.

## WHY YOU SHOULD BRUSH YOUR GUMS

Brushing the gums with a soft toothbrush can help reduce inflammation from wearing full dentures. Best method: Circular brushing for two and one-half minutes twice a day.

**Source:** *Special Care in Dentistry*, American Dental Association, Chicago.

## BEST WAY TO STOP BAD BREATH

Mouthwash does not kill the germs that cause bad breath, according to the Federal Drug Administration. What does improve bad breath: Brushing your teeth and tongue often and using dental floss to clean between the teeth and under the gums. If halitosis persists, see a doctor.

**Source:** E. L. Attia, M.D., otolaryngologist, McGill University, quoted in *American Health*, New York.

## ANOTHER REASON TO EAT BREAKFAST

Bad breath can be caused by skipping breakfast—even if you brush your teeth. Reason: Chewing stimulates the flow of saliva, which freshens the mouth. And food passing over the tongue (the source of most bad breath) removes bacteria buildup accumulated overnight.

**Source:** William Lawson, M.D., professor of otolaryngology, Mount Sinai School of Medicine, New York City, in *Mademoiselle*.

## EDIBLE BREATH FRESHENERS

Try chewing celery and carrots, which help rid the teeth of bacteria and make your mouth cleaner. Bad-breath foods: Meat, stringy vegetables and sticky sweets, which cling to your teeth and feed oral bacteria.

**Source:** *Vogue Magazine*, New York.

## BEST MOUTHWASH

Bad breath is cured best by mouthwashes containing zinc. The source of most mouth odor is sulfur compounds. The zinc mouthwashes negate these compounds for at least three hours. Contrast: Nonzinc mouthwashes attack bacteria. Point: Check the labels of mouthwashes for zinc.

**Source:** Joseph Tonzetich, Ph.D., professor of oral biology, University of British Columbia, Vancouver.

## TRUTH ABOUT A COATED TONGUE

A coated tongue may not be attractive, but neither is it necessarily a sign of disease. The coating comes from the millions of dead cells even a healthy tongue sloughs off daily.

**Source:** Samuel Dreizen, M.D., Department of Oral Oncology, University of Texas Health Science Center, Houston.

## A SIMPLE EYE EXAMINATION CHECKS MORE THAN VISION

The eyes permit a look directly inside the body, enabling a doctor to see clues to literally hundreds of different systemic illnesses. The eyes can act as an early warning system for diseases that may not otherwise be apparent. Examples:

• High blood pressure: The ophthalmologist sees changes in the eyes than can include blood vessel spasm or narrowing and microscopic hemorrhages within the retina. Sometimes there is swelling of the optic nerve in the back of the eye, indicating severe high blood pressure that requires emergency treatment.

• Diabetes: A patient might experience some blurriness of vision and sudden nearsightedness. This change occurs because high blood sugar affects the water content of the lenses, causing them to swell. Distance vision improves and near vision deteriorates. Once the sugar problem is corrected, vision often returns to normal. Examination of the retina can reveal vascular changes, some of which can respond to laser therapy. This could prevent visual disability in the future.

• Heart valve infection: This is most characteristic in patients who have run a low-grade fever over a period of time and may have a history of childhood heart disease or rheumatic fever. How it happens: From a wound or infection somewhere else in the body, the bloodstream is temporarily seeded with certain bacteria that can settle on a heart valve, especially if it was previously damaged. The bacteria slowly grow like vegetation on the valve. The symptoms can be very subtle, including headaches, sweating and low-grade fever. Occasionally little infected blood clots with bacteria on them travel to the eyes. Called Roth spots,

these might be the only clue to a heart-valve problem that could be cured with intensive antibiotic therapy.

• Strokes: Episodes of amaurosis fugax (temporary blindness) can be evidence of an impending stroke or an indication of atherosclerosis of the carotid artery (the large artery in the neck).

• Brain tumors and other neurological problems. Some can come to light as a result of eye problems. Example: A taxi driver had been getting into a number of accidents and couldn't figure out the reason for it. A thorough eye exam revealed that he had a visual-field defect indicative of a certain type of brain tumor. The tumor was pressing on the optic nerve, causing loss of peripheral vision. He was unaware of the loss because it had come on so gradually.

• Thyroid disease: This disease can cause swelling and increased prominence of the eyes. Sometimes only one eye seems to bulge, or there may be a too-wide stare or an eyelid lag.

• Inflammatory diseases: Rheumatoid arthritis and certain back diseases occasionally cause severe inflammation of the eyes. The eyes may turn red and be very dry, sandy and scratchy.

• Hereditary defects: On occasion, metabolic disorders can be seen in the eyes. It may be possible to examine an entire family to see who is at risk for a particular genetic disease.

• Infectious diseases: Long-term syphilis and other abnormalities in the bloodstream may affect the eyes. As a medical student, I saw the tragic case of a perfectly healthy-looking young man admitted to the hospital with a diagnosis of leukemia. I refused to believe the diagnosis—until I looked in his eyes and saw a splinter hemorrhage. That made the problem all too believable.

### Eye Examination

The Society for the Prevention of Blindness recommends a complete eye exam (not just a vision test) every two years for everyone. That should include: A vision test . . . a glaucoma examination . . . the taking of a medical history. . .and a medical examination of both the surface and the interior of the eyes (which frequently necessitates eye drops to dilate the pupil).

Don't be frightened if the ophthalmologist recommends a medical checkup. Very often there are minor or unimportant findings that require confirmation of your general health.

**Source:** Interview with B. David Gorman, M.D., adjunct ophthalmologist and coordinator of resident education at Lenox Hill Hospital, NY.

## DO-IT-YOURSELF EYE TEST

Adult home eye screening is a test to monitor your vision between visits to the optometrist. Object: To catch any of several eye diseases in their early, treatable stages (particularly important for people who are over 35).

**Source:** Minnesota Society for the Prevention of Blindness, St. Paul, MN.

## CATARACT SURGERY UPDATE

Cataract surgery can now be performed in the eye surgeon's office. This outpatient procedure reduces recovery time, is less expensive and restores vision immediately in 75% of patients. No need for thick eyeglasses or contact lenses either.

## HELP FOR GLAUCOMA SUFFERERS

New ultrasound worked in 81% of cases of secondary glaucoma where surgery had failed. The ultrasound waves create tiny lesions that reduce fluid and pressure without harming the retina. Limit: The treatment can only arrest the disease, not reverse existing damage.

**Source:** Dr. D. Jackson Coleman, American Academy of Ophthalmology, New York Hospital—Cornell Medical Center, in *Medical World News.*

## VITAMIN THERAPY FOR DRY EYES

Chronically dry eyes will soon be helped by direct applications of a vitamin A ointment. Preliminary tests show that the ointment can reduce dryness and irritation, increase tear production, and actually improve impaired vision.

**Source:** Scheffer Chuei-Goong Tseng of the Massachusetts Eye and Ear Infirmary, Boston.

## WINNING THE FIGHT AGAINST BLINDNESS

A leading cause of blindness can now be treated. Ten million Americans suffer from macular degeneration, an incurable retinal disorder that most ophthalmologists used to think was also untreatable. But recent success has been reported using a combination of good lighting, high-powered lenses (over ordinary glasses) and off-center viewing techniques. Bottom line: Up to 95% of macular degeneration sufferers can regain functional eyesight.

**Source:** Paul B. Freeman, M.D., Pittsburgh, a specialist in low-level vision.

## TRUTH ABOUT PUFFY EYES

Puffy eyes are not always a sign of sleep deprivation. During the night, fluid sometimes accumulates in the tissues around the eyes and causes swelling. During the day, blinking flushes the fluid back out.

## SPORTS ALERT

Racquet sports, particularly squash and racquetball, can and do cause serious eye injuries if players don't wear protective goggles of some sort. Least effective: Open goggles without lenses. Best: Polycarbonate lenses that have been tested to stop a .22 bullet at 20 feet in a lab test.

**Source:** *Harvard Medical School Health Letter.*

# EXERCISE MAY BE DANGEROUS TO YOUR EYES

"Nautilus eye" is a superficial infection picked up from the pads of exercise machines such as the Nautilus system. The sweat on the pad facilitates the growth of bacteria that cause conjunctivitis. The eye becomes infected by direct contact or by touching the pad and then your eye. Suggestion: Bring a towel to use as a barrier between the pad and your skin.

**Source:** *Glamour.*

# HELP FOR THE NEARSIGHTED

Behavioral optometrists believe you can prevent myopia—or keep it from getting worse—through changes in environment or lifestyle. Ideas: Take a break from close work every 20 minutes to gaze into the distance. Keep your work space evenly lighted. Maintain good posture, so both eyes are equidistant from your work.

**Source:** Dr. Richard Kavner, a behavioral optometrist.

# ALL ABOUT CONTACT LENSES

As contact lenses become more and more sophisticated, the options for wearers seem endless and the differences confusing. To choose the right lenses, you must take into account your budget, lifestyle, and the degree of vision correction you need.

The different kinds of contact lenses available, their special features, and their pitfalls:

• Hard lenses: These are the oldest kind of contact lenses. They are made from rigid plastic and fit over the cornea of the eye. Hard lenses must be removed each night before bed and are soaked overnight in a sterile solution. Lenses are tinted both to enhance your eye color and make a dropped lens easier to find. Hard lenses can be worn 10–14 hours per day and must be removed for sleeping. Although they should be professionally cleaned and polished once a year ($15–$35), hard contacts can last for many years without needing replacement. Cost: $150–$250.*

• Gas-permeable firm lenses: A variation on hard contact lenses—part plastic and part silicon. This contruction allows the gas-permeable lenses to "breathe," allowing a freer flow of air to the eyes. This is healthier for the eyes and also permits a longer wearing time (14–18 hours per day). Like hard lenses, gas-permeable lenses are especially good for patients with astigmatism (an egg-shaped cornea that focuses distorted images on the retina of the eye, causing blurred vision). The care and replacement schedule is similar to that of hard lenses. Gas-permeable lenses are the choice of most optometrists when a rigid lens is needed. Cost: $200–$300.

• Soft lenses: These are larger than the hard ones and are made from a spongelike plastic that can be tinted. Modern soft lenses are extremely durable and are far stronger than the original soft contact lenses. People who play contact sports sometimes find it easier to wear soft lenses, since hard ones can pop out of the eye with a rough blow. Soft lenses cover the entire cornea and reduce discomfort from dust or grit in the air—a boon to city dwellers. They must be removed every night and sterilized either with a special machine that heats them or with a chemical disinfectant solution, depending on the care your doctor prescribes. They can be worn all day with ease. The life span of soft lenses can be as long as two years. New on the market: Bifocal soft lenses. They are not suitable for everyone, but some wearers find them very convenient. Ask your optometrist to test you for them if you're interested. Cost: Regular, $200–$350; bifocal, $250–$450.

• Extended-wear soft lenses: These are soft lenses that transmit more oxygen than daily-wear lenses. They can be worn all day and night without removal. The ads claim you can wear them a month between cleanings, but I have my patients remove and clean them once a week. (It extends the life of the lenses and keeps the eyes healthier.) They can be tinted. Although they can be made for astigmatic eyes, extended-wear lenses are particularly appropriate for severely nearsighted people or for cataract patients because they eliminate the distortion and magnification that very thick glasses produce. Or they can be simply a convenience—for example, they would be ideal for a fireman, who may not have time to put in lenses when the firebell rings in the middle of the night. Extended-wear lenses must usually be replaced every one and a half to two and a half years. This replacement does not require refitting, however. Cleaning involves the same sterilization processes that are used for soft lenses, although on a less frequent schedule. Cost: Regular, $350–$450; astigmatic, $400–$500.

After examining you and fitting your contact lenses, most doctors suggest a service contract that offers replacement lenses at reduced fees.

Although you may wear your lenses every day, I recommend that you also keep an updated pair of spectacle glasses handy to wear in case of an emergency.

### Where to Go

Be wary of the discount commercial establishments—they deal in quantity, not quality. Their emphasis is on product, not on service. Physical changes can take place in the eyes as a result of wearing contact lenses. These should be carefully monitored and adjusted for.

My earnest recommendation: Never look for bargains in parachutes or in eye care!

*Prices should include examination, fitting, cleaning equipment and follow-up eye care.

**Source:** Interview with Robert Snyder, OD, an optometrist in private practice, Beach Haven, NJ.

## CONTACT LENS OF THE FUTURE

Eyedrop contact lenses that are washed out at night and replaced in the morning are on the horizon. Breakthrough: a promising new optical technique that controls the light-bending properties of a liquid without changing its thickness. Result: Once perfected, eyedrops that work like contact

The drops are placed in the eye, then "programmed" with an electronic remote control.

**Source:** Dr. Seymour P. Kern, Newport Beach, CA, reported at a Research to Prevent Blindness conference in Washington, DC.

## DISPOSABLE CONTACT LENSES

Disposable lenses are coming soon—for the contact wearers. These inexpensive, ultra-thin (as light as plastic wrap) lenses come six to a pack. The idea: Throw them away every month or two—cost will be about the same as (or less than) cleaning one pair with chemical solutions. Saves the bother and risk of not getting them really clean.

**Source:** Wesley-Jessen, Chicago; Ciba Geigy, Ardsley, NY; Bausch and Lomb, Rochester, NY.

## WHAT THE "PILL" HAS TO DO WITH YOUR CONTACTS

Going off the Pill may necessitate a change in contact lenses. Reason: The Pill can alter the shape of the cornea. When the Pill is discontinued, the cornea may return to its original shape. Eyeglasses wearers: No change is needed.

**Source:** *McCall's.*

## CONTACT LENS IRRITATION

A number of people don't wear contact lenses because their eyes get irritated. But the eyes may be reacting to a chemical in some wetting solutions rather than to the lens. About 10% of people become intolerant to this agent. Remedy: Change wetting solution.

**Source:** *Western Journal of Medicine.*

## SUMMER CARE OF CONTACTS

Extended-wear contact lenses need special

care during summer activities. They're fine for ocean swims. (But keep your eyes closed under water to keep the lenses in place.) Take the contacts out before entering a chlorinated pool (they'll absorb chemicals) or a stagnant lake (bacteria could lead to infection). In dry, air-conditioned rooms, lubricate them often. On airplanes (the driest of all), rewet them every half hour.

**Source:** Dr. Spencer E. Sherman, associate professor of ophthalmology, Mount Sinai School of Medicine, in *Glamour*, NY.

## EXTENDED-WEAR LENSES

Don't wear extended-wear lenses for more than one week without cleaning, suggests Dr. Melvin Schrier, New York optometrist. On the seventh day, clean them and sleep without them that night. Don't enzyme them for more than 15 minutes. Lens saver: A brief daily massage through closed eyelids seems to deter the buildup of protein deposits that damage the lens and make it uncomfortable to wear.

## IF YOU LOSE A CONTACT ON A CARPET

Contact lenses lost in a carpet. Place a nylon stocking over the nozzle of a vacuum cleaner and carefully vacuum the area. The lens will be pulled up onto the stocking.

## BEST EYEGLASS CLEANER

Use a piece of damp newspaper. There is less chance it will scratch the lenses than cloth or tissue.

**Source:** *Shortcuts*, edited by T. Augello and G. Yanker, Bantam Books.

## MOST EFFECTIVE SUNGLASSES

Ordinary sunglasses may fail to protect your eyes, even if they feel comfortable and reduce glare. Reason: They don't screen out ultraviolet light, which has been linked with cataract formation. Most at risk: People with light-colored eyes, contact lens wearers and recent eye-surgery patients. For these groups, sunglasses with ultraviolet-ray filters are best.

**Source:** Dr. Richard Gibralter, ophthalmologist, Manhattan Eye, Ear and Throat Hospital, quoted in *Ladies' Home Journal*.

• The best sunglasses for very sunny days are the mountaineer's variety. They feature leather sidepieces and optical-grade plastic lenses, which offer shatterproof protection from ultraviolet rays.

## DAY OF THE WEEK YOU'RE MOST LIKELY TO SUFFER A HEART ATTACK

Sudden heart attacks in otherwise healthy executives occur most frequently on Monday. A long-term study showed that 75% of those felled at work and nearly 50% of those who died at home were Monday victims. Cause: Monday blues due to stresses of returning to work. To lessen the pressure: Enjoy some relaxation time during the week and don't cram all the fun into the weekend.

**Source:** *Health Talk*.

## WHEN CHEST PAIN MEANS HEART ATTACK AND WHEN IT DOESN'T

Chest pain is psychosomatic almost half the time, according to a recent study. Key: If the pain is sharp and stabbing, or it's on the left side of the chest, it's likely caused by psychological stress. But a heavy, gripping sensation in the central chest is a typical heart attack sympton, especially if it lasts five to six minutes. Consult your doctor in either case.

**Source:** Study by Dr. Christopher Bass, King's College Hospital, London.

## WHAT YOUR EARLOBES SAY ABOUT YOUR HEART

Your earlobes can tell you if you're a high

risk for heart disease. Check them in the mirror. If you notice a diagonal crease, you may be more likely to have clogged coronary arteries. See your doctor.

**Source:** Joe Graedon, writing in *Medical Self-Care.*

## HEART DISEASE DETECTION

A new, highly refined ultrasound machine spots plaque buildup long before a stroke or heart attack. The device can see constructions blocking the arteries. By detecting problems early, doctors can persuade patients to change their diets and unhealthful habits before they need surgery.

**Source:** *Discover,* New York.

## PREDICT HEART ATTACKS YEARS IN ADVANCE

A simple test tells you whether you are a "high risk" candidate for heart disease—even before any evidence of disease exists. It predicts potential trouble with higher accuracy than any single test currently available. How it works: Determines the body's predisposition to clog arteries with cholesterol by measuring the levels of two substances that control cholesterol in the blood. Apolipoprotein A-1 (APO A-1) binds cholesterol to artery walls. (Absence of this binding substance would totally rule out cholesterol buildup, regardless of the quantity of cholesterol in the blood.) Apolipoprotein B (APO A-B) prevents cholesterol from binding to the arteries. (Absence of APO A-B could enable a trace of cholesterol to prove fatal.) What it means: If the test indicates that you have a high ratio of APO A-1 to APO A-B, you are classified at high risk for heart disease. (This ratio is genetically determined; it can be measured at any time—even prenatally.)

**Source:** Tago, Inc., Burlingame, CA.

## GOOD AND BAD NEWS FOR WOMEN ONLY

• Women who work outside the home are less likely to develop heart problems. Working women have much higher levels of HDL, a protein that clears unhealthful cholesterol out of the blood.

**Source:** Study at the University of Texas Health Science Center, San Antonio, reported in *Management Focus.*

• Estrogen therapy, often used to prevent or treat osteoporosis in older women, can be dangerous. Recent studies show that estrogen users are 50% more likely to develop cardiovascular disease. Most vulnerable: Women with a history of heart problems, high blood pressure, high cholesterol, diabetes or smoking.

**Source:** *Internal Medicine News,* New York.

## STRESS AND THE HEART

Why do many calm, apparently healthy people suffer heart attacks and sudden death? Recent research suggests they may be "hot reactors"—people whose cardiovascular systems go haywire when subjected to stress. Typical reactions: Increased blood pressure, cardiac output and blood vessel resistance. It is comparable to trying to drive a car at high speed with the brakes on. Who's affected: One in five adults, many of whom are not tense or hard-driven Type A personalities. Under development: A simple way to detect hot reactions to stress, which could then be unlearned.

**Source:** Robert S. Elliot, M.D., chairman of the department of preventive and stress medicine, University of Nebraska School of Medicine, writing in *Hospital Practice.*

## NEW THINKING ON TYPE A PERSONALITIES

Type A behavior, long considered the cause of nervous-system and heart problems, may in fact be the result of an overly sensitive nervous system. Recent studies found that coronary patients taking Inderal showed fewer Type A traits (impatience, hostility and rapid speech patterns). And another study found that Type A patients showed greater increases in blood pressure while undergoing surgery, when there is little conscious awareness.

**Source:** Dr. David S. Krantz, associate professor of medical psychology, Uniformed Services University of the Health Sciences, Bethesda, MD.

## WHY CYNICS ARE CANDIDATES FOR HEART DISEASE

Type A personality has long been associated with increased risk of cardiovascular disease. But recent research shows that hostility, and more particularly, cynicism is the active problem. Anyone who's constantly cynical runs an increased risk of heart disease. Reason: The cynicism translates into mistrust, which often produces a significantly larger release of epinephrine in cynical people than occurs in more trusting individuals. Cynical behavior is difficult to modify, but doctors can prescribe a beta blocker medication to reduce the harmful effects of the epinephrine.

## ANGER IS BAD FOR YOUR HEART

Angry people are more prone to heart disease than less hostile personality types. After calculating the "hostility scores" for 255 male doctors who took the Minnesota Multiphasic Personality Inventory 25 years ago, a researcher compared the results with current health records of the subjects, who are now between 45 and 50. More than 12% of those who had high hostility ratings now suffer from heart disease. Less than 3% of those with low hostility ratings are heart patients.

**Source:** Redford B. Williams, Jr., M.D., Duke University.

## PSYCHOLOGICAL COUNSELING FOR TYPE A BEHAVIOR

• Type A behavior, a risk factor for heart attacks, can be treated effectively through a combination of psychological counseling and medical advice. When a group of patients who had experienced recurrent heart attacks received dual therapy, the heart attack rate was only 7% within three years. With practical counseling only, patients suffered a 13% recurrence rate.

**Source:** Meyer Friedman, M.D., writing in *The American Heart Journal.*

• Psychological counseling reduces heart disease by 50%. Counseling aimed at modifying the aggressive, hard-driving, competitive, Type A personality is as important to lowering the risk of heart attacks as modifying diet, stopping smoking or increasing exercise, according to a recent study. Patients who received counseling in addition to advice concerning diet and exercise had 50% fewer heart attacks than patients who received no counseling for their Type A behavior. Moreover, 80% of those in counseling were able to handle stress more effectively, slow down their lives and improve self-esteem by the end of the three-year study.

**Source:** Susan Beauchamp, research director, American Physical Fitness Research Institute, Los Angeles.

## SLOWING DOWN

Ways to modify that dangerous Type A behavior: Walk and talk more slowly. Reduce deadline pressure by pacing your days more evenly. Stop trying to do more than one thing at a time. Don't interrupt other people in midspeech. Begin driving in the slow lane. Simply sit and listen to music you like while doing nothing else.

**Source:** *Treating Type A Behavior and Your Heart* by Dr. Meyer Friedman and Diane Ulmer, Alfred A. Knopf, Inc., New York.

## PREVENTIVE MEASURES MAY NOT BE WHAT YOU THINK

Heart disease is a major concern for millions of Americans. In response to what seems to be a national obsession, new (and often conflicting) information is published almost daily on the causes and cures.

Some of the risk factors most publicized are greatly exaggerated.

And some of the preventive measures recommended are too extreme, prohibitively expensive or just plain unprofitable.

### Risk Factors

• High cholesterol, along with smoking and hypertension, is considered to be one of the three major risk factors. People with high cholesterol and a low HDL* fraction are apparently more susceptible to heart attacks. Problem: A large proportion of heart attack victims and people with arteriosclerotic heart disease have relatively normal levels of cholesterol and HDL. High cholesterol and low HDL can be altered 15%–20% with diet, exercise and medication. But altering a cholesterol level that's within normal range is difficult, if not impossible. Also: The drugs used to lower cholesterol are highly unpleasant. It's unclear whether lowering your cholesterol will lower your risk anyway.

• Hypertension is alterable. People who have it are more likely to get arteriosclerotic heart disease and coronary artery disease. As with high cholesterol, however, a large number of heart attack victims don't have hypertension.

• Smoking is a very strong risk factor. The evidence is unequivocal on this one. Smoking definitely increases the risk of developing heart disease and reduces the longevity of heart attack victims.

• Genes are not commonly listed as a major risk factor, but their influence is highly significant. Many heart attack victims have relatively normal cholesterol and no hypertension, and they don't smoke. Most of this group have bad family histories. If your father and uncles died of heart attacks at age 40, you may be in big trouble. And there may not be much you can do to alter this risk factor.

• Obesity, strangely enough, is not one of the major risk factors. However, insurance company statistics do show that very overweight people don't live as long as normal-weight people. Although heart disease may be one reason, respiratory illness, diabetes and other diseases are contributing factors.

• Salt intake may not be a factor. Statistical studies have shown that in areas where the water is soft (contains increased levels of sodium), there is increased evidence of hypertension. but these studies are remote, and the link between salt intake and heart disease is tenuous. It can't hurt to reduce your salt intake. But it may not help, either.

• Stress and the Type A personality are probably minor risk factors. Whether type As (continually wound up) can be changed, or want to be, is questionable. If possible, reduce stress. It's easier than changing your personality.

• Hormones protect women, who apparently peak with heart disease 10–15 years after men. This difference is presumably hormone-related. In a number of studies (discontinued 10 years ago), men were given female hormones to see if they were thus protected against heart disease. The studies were unsuccessful because the men developed impotence, breasts and skin changes.

### Prevention

• Diet. It makes good sense to reduce your weight to low normal if possible, especially if you've already had a heart attack. Weight loss will lower cholesterol and decrease hypertension. Also: Since major lesions in arteries are related to cholesterol and fat deposits, these deposits may be decreased if you're not taking in extra calories. Don't go on a fad diet like the Pritikin Diet. This diet is very fat-restricted, quite unpalatable and no better than any other sound diet. Besides, there's no proof that it works. Pritikin's claims of success are all anecdotal, and you can find people who are pleased with anything. Do go on a moderate reduced-calorie diet that includes all the major food groups.

• Exercise. Most studies have shown that mild or moderate exercise makes for very little change in cardiac status. What exercise does do: It trains you to perform more before getting angina pains. In terms of heart rate/blood pressure, the patient will get the angina at the same point—it just takes longer to get there. Other benefits: Exercise tones the heart and peripheral muscles. It improves the quality of a cardiac patient's life. When I put my heart patients on a running program, I don't get calls like. . ."Can my husband carry this package up the stairs?" If he can run five miles, he can carry a package. Cardiac patients who exercise feel healthy, and the resulting high spirits and sense of well-being can only increase longevity.

• Marathon running. No formal studies have been done of the effects of very strenuous exercise on cardiac status. As a marathoner myself, I like to think it helps. We train our cardiac patients to run up to five miles a day, and some run marathons. They do quite well. It's conceivable that running 70–100 miles a week and staying bone thin might be protective, because whatever the runner is metabolising is going into the machinery that keeps the muscles moving. There's no fat left over to clog the arteries. Also: Most doctors throughout the country report very few deaths in cardiac-patient heavy-exercise groups. Marathoners as a group have a low incidence of heart disease. Contradiction: A group of South African ultra-marathoners out running were killed by a drunken driver. The autopsies showed that two or three of them had significant coronary artery disease.

*HDL is high-density lipoprotein, one of the breakdowns of cholesterol that can be measured in the bloodstream.
**Source:** Interview with Edward J. Berman, M.D., chief of cardiology at Gardena Memorial Hospita, Gardena, CA.

# FIRST-LINE TREATMENT FOR ANGINA

Diet therapy may be a first-line treatment for people with angina (chest pain caused when not enough oxygen reaches the heart). Recent studies suggest that a low-fat, low-calorie diet makes the heart work more efficiently. Other benefits: Weight loss, cholesterol reduction and the toleration of strenuous exercise.

**Source:** *Lancet,* London.

# COLD-DRINK WARNING

Angina, or heart pain, can be caused by overexertion, stress or exposure to cold air.

Recent studies have shown that cold drinks can raise heart rate and blood pressure, which increases heart strain. Result: Angina. Caution: Individuals who suffer from angina should be aware that cold liquids may be detrimental to their hearts.

**Source:** *American Heart Journal.*

# BEATING NOCTURNAL ANGINA

Nocturnal angina is all but eliminated by this new, drug-free method: Tilt the bed at a 10-degree angle. Lie with the head up and the feet down. The angle reduces the return blood flow to the heart, preventing the troublesome chest pains that hit heart patients at night. (Usually this return flow is cut back with drugs such as digitalis and diuretics.)

**Source:** Experiments made with heart patients in Israel as reported in *Lancet,* London.

# BONUS FOR ANGINA SUFFERERS

Diltiazem, a prescription drug presently available in the US for use as a calcium blocker, has recently been found to block the development of plaque in blood vessels even if cholesterol levels are high. Many people are presently on this medication in an attempt to block angina, and the newly recognized added benefit may be a substantial bonus.

**Source:** *Medical Tribune,* New York.

# BLOOD-PRESSURE CONFIDENTIAL

Blood-pressure readings are often deceptively high when taken in a hospital or doctor's office. Reason: The patient's system reacts to anxiety over the test or the doctor's presence. In an Italian study, 47 of 48 patients' pressure rose after the doctor appeared. (In one case, the systolic reading went up by 75 points.) Solution: When three or four measurements were taken over a period of 10 minutes, the last was likely to be accurate.

**Source:** *New Scientist,* New York.

## TWO DRUGS THAT MAY IMPAIR YOUR MEMORY

Two high-blood pressure medicines can impair verbal memory. Inderal (propranolol) and Aldomet (methyldopa) have been found to cause memory loss in both hypertensive patients and patients with normal pressures. Such impairment was not observed in hypertensive people taking only diuretics.

## CAFFEINE, CIGARETTES AND MEDICATIONS DON'T MIX

Caffeine and nicotine can interfere with high blood-pressure medications. Drugs (such as Inderal) used to treat high blood pressure work by reducing the amount of adrenaline in the patient's system. Caffeine and nicotine stimulate the production of adrenaline. Solution: Avoid cigarettes and caffeine-laden products. . .or consult your doctor.

## NEW AND EASY WAY TO TAKE YOUR MEDICINE

Hypertension medication is now able to be delivered through the skin by transdermal clonidine patches that deliver the medication at a steady rate for seven days. The patches, similar to Band-Aids in appearance, have been successfully tested. The medication is no different from that administered orally. . .it's just more convenient for people who forget to take their medicine or just don't like to.

**Source:** *Drug Topics.*

## FACTS ABOUT ONE KIND OF HEART ATTACK

Myocardial infarction (MI)—a type of heart attack—in women under 50 years of age (very rare) is associated with cigarette smoking, hypertension, angina, diabetes, Type A blood and a family history of MI. Surprise: Neither obesity nor a nervous disposition seems to be a factor.

**Source:** *Journal of the American Medical Association,* Boston, MA.

## STROKE WARNINGS

Strokes are often preceded by warning signs. Reacting quickly can help prevent the stroke or reduce its damage. Danger signals that warrant an immediate doctor visit: Sudden weakness or numbness in the face, arm or leg that lasts a few seconds or minutes. Sudden, temporary dimness or loss of vision, especially in one eye. Sudden, temporary double vision. Temporarily impaired speech or loss of speech due to difficulty in moving the tongue or jaw. Temporary dizziness or unsteadiness. Unexpected headaches or a change in headache patterns.

**Source:** Dr. Edward Cooper, professor of medicine, University of Pennsylvania, chairman, Stroke Council, American Heart Association.

## WHAT YOUR DOCTOR SHOULD BE DOING

Ask your doctor to listen with his stethoscope for a bruit—a high-pitched murmur over the neck that could signal turbulence in the flow of blood through the carotid artery that leads to the brain. In about 60% of the cases where a bruit is detected, the artery may be narrowed by atherosclerosis, which raises the danger of stroke.

## A MAJOR CAUSE OF STROKE

Brightmode ultrasound is used noninvasively to examine the carotid arteries in the neck area for evidence of plaque buildup. Plaque commonly occurs in people with high cholesterol levels and is a major cause of strokes because it may chip off or clog the blood pathway to the brain. If identified, the plaque can be removed surgically.

**Source:** *Internal Medicine News.*

# STROKE CLUBS

When stroke victims join the nearest stroke club, their improvement is remarkably better. The positive attitudes fostered by the group play an important role in overcoming depression and cause stroke patients to push to regain control over their limbs. There are about 300 clubs in the US. Contact a local American Heart Association chapter.

**Source:** *Journal of the American Medical Association.*

# HELP FOR HEART DISEASE

Coronary artery bypass surgery is the fastest-growing major operation in the United States.

First popularized in 1961 at the Cleveland Clinic, the procedure involves taking a healthy vein (usually from the leg) and grafting it into an obstructed artery near the heart. The graft literally bypasses the blocked section and allows a free flow of blood to the heart. A double bypass operation repairs two blockages with two grafts. Triple bypass surgery repairs three blockages.

### What Bypass Surgery Accomplishes

Angina attacks are usually caused by a clogged artery. After physical exertion, the patient feels chest pains, shortness of breath, a tingling sensation (often in the left arm) and/or a variety of other uncomfortable symptoms.

Bypass surgery offers relief to angina sufferers who do not respond to drug treatment with nitroglycerin, beta blockers or calcium blockers. It does not cure the arteriosclerosis that underlies angina, but it can put back the progress of both diseases 5 to 10 years. Patients must still fight the buildup of plaque in their arteries with a low-fat diet, abstinence from smoking, exercise and, sometimes, medication. It's unclear why some people are more prone to this buildup than others, but the sclerosis can affect the new grafts as well as the natural coronary arteries.

Problems: Like any major surgery, a bypass operation carries risks. A poor heart muscle, for example, can cause complications. The patient's age and general health and the extent of the heart disease all must be taken into consideration before bypass surgery is recommended. It is not the preferred treatment for everyone.

### Angioplasty: New Alternative

Safer—and cheaper—than bypass surgery is a new technique for opening up the obstructions in coronary arteries by attacking them internally. Developed within the last two years, angioplasty is only a semisurgical procedure, much less traumatic to the patient's system. How it works: A plastic tube with a small balloon attached is inserted into a narrowed artery. The balloon is then inflated to break up the plaque and widen the passage.

Still confined to major medical centers and teaching hospitals, angioplasty has its risks, too. If the balloon can't disperse the plaque or if there are complications during the procedure, bypass surgery must be performed on an emergency basis. Whenever angioplasty is scheduled, a surgical team is put on standby, ready to move in at once if necessary.

**Source:** Interview with Raymond Matta, M.D., a cardiologist on the staff at Mt. Sinai Medical Center in New York City.

# HOSPITAL VS. HOME CARE

Heart care at home may be just as effective as hospital coronary care units in treatment of simple heart attack victims. In a British study, there was no significant difference in the mortality rate over a six-week period between the home patients (13%) and the hospital group (11%).

**Source:** *Journal of the American Medical Association*, Chicago, IL.

# POST-CORONARY SEX

Post-coronary patients can resume normal

sexual activity without risk in 80% of cases. The remaining 20% need not abstain—just adjust their lovemaking style to their ability to tolerate exercise.

**Source:** *Sex Over Forty.*

## REHABILITATION MUST

Exercise rehabilitation programs to improve heart function in individuals with heart disease have proven to be effective even when the patients were also taking beta-blocking drugs to slow down their heart rate.

**Source:** *American Heart Journal.*

## CORONARY SURVIVORS

Two-thirds of all people who suffer heart attacks survive them. But one survivor in five dies within a year. Danger signs for attack survivors: Rales (a crackling sound caused by an accumulation of fluid in the lungs), inefficient pumping of the heart, arrhythmia (irregular heartbeats), and a history of chest pain and shortness of breath. Each condition is a signal of increased risk of another heart attack. A combination of the conditions is most dangerous. Good news: Each of the problems can be treated by drugs and/or surgery.

**Source:** Study by Dr. Arthur Moss, University of Rochester, reported in *Discover.*

## WHY A PET CAN HELP YOU TO LIVE LONGER

Heart patients live longer when they have pets. Dogs are especially good. Theory: A pet can cut through the depression, anxiety and loneliness that aggravate heart disease.

**Source:** Grace T. Mayes in *Parade.*

## STOPPING HEART ATTACKS WHILE THEY ARE HAPPENING

A simple injection may soon be available to stop heart attacks in progress. In recent trials, an injected drug called tissue plasminogen activator (t-PA) dissolved blood clots and stopped attacks in six of seven men. Added benefits: Unlike other clot dissolvers, t-PA causes neither excessive bleeding nor allergic reactions.

**Source:** Clinical trials at Washington University Medical Center, St.Louis, and the University of Louvain, Belgium, cited in *Self,* New York.

## THE ABCs OF ANTACIDS AND OTHER STOMACH MEDICINES

Most stomachs produce acid 24 hours a day in intermittent bursts (usually after meals). As part of the evolutionary refinement of the human physiology, this process probably served our prehistoric ancestors well. The acid acted as a built-in food sterilizer. Although that function is not crucial today, most people live comfortably with their stomach acid and suffer only brief upsets now and then. However, for about 10% of the population this acid causes chronic problems because their systems make too much of it or don't drain it away fast enough, or because the linings of their stomachs are very sensitive to it. The result may be frequent and painful irritation of the stomach, the uppper intestine or the esophagus (heartburn). Worst problem: Ulcers.

The classic treatment for these acid-related digestive problems is antacids to neutralize the gastric juices and diet to prevent excessive irritation. (Spicy foods, alcohol, coffee, tobacco, aspirin and stress can all be irritants.)

### Ulcer Treatment

A breakthrough for ulcer treatment has been the development of Tagamet, a drug that stops the production of stomach acid. On the market since 1976, Tagamet has revolutionized the care of ulcer victims. Ranitidine is even more potent and has few side effects. Another new ulcer drug, Sucralfate, sticks to raw areas like a bandage, protecting the sores from irritation as they heal. Its side effects are minimal.

**For Indigestion**

Short of ulcers, most stomach upsets can be treated with simple antacids. The basic neutralizers are sodium bicarbonate, calcium, magnesium and aluminium salts.

Sodium bicarbonate—the baking soda your grandmother used to take—is found in such over-the-counter antacids as Alka-Seltzer, Rolaids and Bisodol powder. The problem for people with high blood pressure is the high sodium content of these products. Alka-Seltzer combines sodium bicarbonate with aspirin, which is fine for many people. It can be counterproductive, however, for those whose stomachs are irritated by aspirin.

The calcium-based antacids (Tums, Equilet and Titralac) are best for occasional mild indigestion.

In general, liquid antacids are more potent and quicker acting than antacid tablets. However, magnesium-based antacids (such as Phillips Milk of Magnesia) have a laxative effect and are not terribly effective for stomach upsets.

Aluminum-based antacids (Amphojel, Alternagel, Basaljel and Robolate) are also mild, but they have a binding action (good for people who tend to diarrhea).

Combination antacids, the obvious compromise, make up the majority of products on the market. Maalox and Mylanta have more magnesium and tend to cause loose stools. Aludrox, Gelusil and Riopan, heavier on aluminum, are weaker, but they cause less diarrhea. Gaviscon, a magnesium-aluminum combination, has a special foaming action. It floats on stomach juices and prevents the acid from coming into contact with tender digestive linings. Gaviscon is especially useful in stopping heartburn.

Some antacids also contain simethicone, an antiflatulent (Simeco, Maalox Plus, etc.).

The most potent antacids are extra-strength preparations such as Maalox T.C. and Mylanta II. Doctors use these products to treat severe digestive-tract problems because patients may need as much as seven ounces of antacids a day. When such heavy doses are called for, taste becomes important. If someone really gags on the medicine, he won't take it regularly. Antacids now come in various flavors such as peach, watermelon and mint. Suggestion: Chilling them helps to inhibit the taste.

Chronic use of antacids can interfere with the body's absorption of minerals and other medications. People with persistent stomach problems—or those over 40 who suddenly develop digestive upsets—should be under a doctor's supervision.

**Source:** *Bottom Line/Personal* interview with Bruce H. Yaffe, M.D., a gastroenterologist in private practice in New York.

## HEARTBURN PREVENTION

Avoid excess fat, alcohol and acidic foods such as coffee, citric juices and tomatoes. Stop smoking, and lose abdominal weight, which causes pressure on the lower esophagus. Eat more foods that are high in protein. Foods to avoid: Gas-producing foods, such as onions and cabbage, and foods like peppermint and chocolate that reduce esophageal pressure.

## A BETTER ORANGE JUICE

Reduced-acid orange juice is now available in frozen concentrate under Minute Maid's label. A boon to people whose stomachs will not tolerate the acidity of regular orange juice, the new product has as much vitamin C as other frozen orange juices.

## ULCER MYTH

Although milk products may soothe your stomach for a short time, they actually worsen symptoms in the long run. Reason: The protein and calcium content stimulate acid secretion. Other false ulcer friends: bedtime snacks, frequent small meals.

## SOME FACTS ABOUT BLAND DIETS

• Bland diets aren't necessary for all people with duodenal ulcers. A study of ulcer patients given chili powder in large amounts over a four-week period showed no adverse effect on healing. Conclusion: Bland diets play little role in healing ulcers. Ulcer patients should be able to eat almost any food that doesn't cause pain or discomfort. Still to be avoided: Cola, coffee, alcohol, aspirin and tobacco.

**Source:** *British Medical Journal*, London.

• Ulcer relapses are less likely in patients who eat a bland, high-fiber diet. Bonus: Constipation, a problem in many ulcer patients, is prevented by the same high-fiber intake.

**Source:** *The Lancet, London.*

## SIMPLIFIED ULCER TREATMENT

Cimetidine (Tagamet) or ranitidine (Zantac) are both successful in curing 80% of all ulcers. But new studies show that a single nighttime dose is as effective as the two to four daily dosages presently being recommended. Nighttime acid secretion seems to be the culprit. And . . . suppressing it with 300 milligrams of ranitidine or 800 milligrams of cimetidine, taken before bedtime, is easier for the patient to remember and also reduces medication cost.

**Source:** *Lancet.*

## DRUG COMBINATION TO AVOID

Peptic ulcer sufferers should not take antacids at the same time as cimetidine (the generic name for an anti—ulcer drug). Both antacids and cimetidine ease the ulcer condition when taken at the proper times. The best routine: Take cimetidine an hour after using antacids, near bedtime and an hour before taking antacids at mealtime.

**Source:** A study done at the George Washington University Medical Center.

## HIATUS-HERNIA ALERT

Chest pains, heartburn, difficulty in breathing or swallowing and other symptoms that mimic heart attacks may sometimes be due to acid irritating the esophagus, associated with a hiatus hernia. The condition is suffered by as many as 20% of all US adults and 60% of those above 60. A hiatus hernia occurs when a section of the stomach protrudes into the chest cavity, allowing stomach acids to back up into the esophagus. Causes: Strenuous exercise or anything that increases abdominal cavity pressure. For relief: Eat smaller meals. Avoid tight clothes and irritating foods, such as coffee, chocolate and alcohol. Don't eat for several hours before bedtime, and elevate the head of the bed.

## CHRONIC CONSTIPATION REMEDY

Severe chronic constipation is a common adult disorder, particularly among women. Problem: Sufferers treat themselves with laxatives, but the cause may actually be lack of muscle tone in the colon. A better remedy usually is a high-fiber, high-fluid diet coupled with medication to help improve the colon muscles. Bottom line: For incapacitating constipation, see a doctor.

**Source:** *Lancet.*

## LAXATIVE CONFIDENTIAL

Laxative abuse can damage the internal wall of the colon and destroy intestinal muscle tone, leading to dependence and colitis. Most dangerous: Chemical stimulants (senna, phenolphthalein, castor oil) and saline laxatives (magnesium hydroxide, magnesium sulfate, sodium sulfate). Better: Bulk-forming agents (such as Metamucil and Mitrolan), which encourage your own system to do the work. Best of all: A daily diet rich in whole grains, unrefined bran, and vegetable and fruit fibers.

**Source:** *Prevention, Emmaus, PA.*

## LAXATIVE SIDE EFFECTS

Laxatives based on bulk, such as Metamucil, are commonly prescribed for constipation.

Most people assume that there are no side effects from these laxatives. But psyllium, the active ingredient, can cause nasal congestion, sneezing and asthma.

**Source:** *Journal of Allergy and Clinical Immunology.*

## NEW LOOK AT IRRITABLE BOWEL SYNDROME

Irritable bowel syndrome may be simply the result of social conditioning. Persons who complain about physiologic problems—including gastrointestinal trouble—often are rewarded emotionally by their families and friends. Other possible causes: An exaggerated response to stress, psychological disorders and insufficient fiber in the diet.

**Source:** *Medical World News, New York.*

• Irritable bowel syndrome, a common digestive complaint often associated with times of stress, can be helped with psychotherapy. A recent Swedish study found that when patients received only conventional medical care for one year, their average condition deteriorated. But patients who received both medication and psychotherapy showed significant improvement over the same period.
**Source:** *The Lancet, London.*

## A VERY COMMON PROBLEM

Chronic diarrhea, gas and other stomach complaints are often linked to lactose intolerance—the inability to digest milk. One of every four adults suffers from this problem. Reason: Their bodies don't make enough lactase, the enzyme that breaks down milk sugar in the intestinal tract. Among the offending foods: Milk, ice cream, chocolate, soft cheese, some yogurts and sherbet. Lactose is also used as a filler in gum, candies and many canned goods.

## ONE WAY TO BEAT LACTOSE INTOLERANCE

People with lactose intolerance can enjoy

milk again without cramps and diarrhea. Lact-aid, a form of the enzyme lactase, is added to the milk the day before use. It not only predigests the lactose but also aids in calcium absorption. Milk with this additive is sold in several parts of the US.

**Source:** *Journal of Pediatric Gastroenterology and Nutrition.*

## HELP FOR SOME

Adults who can't digest milk should do better with yogurt, according to a recent study. Reason: Yogurt bacteria produce the enzyme lactase, which, in turn, digests the milk sugar lactose. This spares the eater from diarrhea, flatulence or cramps.

**Source:** *The New England Journal of Medicine, Boston.*

## A GOOD DESSERT FOR ALMOST EVERYONE

Tofutti, a frozen dessert made from a powdered soy base, makes a good ice-cream substitute for those with lactose intolerance. It contains no lactose, butterfat or cholesterol, and it has only 128 calories per four-ounce scoop (less than half the calories of a premium dairy ice cream). Best flavor: Banana pecan.

## THE TRUTH ABOUT PAINKILLERS

Despite the recent innovations in pain relief, the best drug for most pain is still aspirin. It works as well as or better than many pills that claim to be stronger, including Darvon (propoxyphene), Clinoril (sulindac) and Motrin (ibuprofen).

We know by now that all aspirin, whether buffered or not, works the same. (In fact, nearly all brands are made by one of two manufacturers: Dow or Monsanto.) Most brands, whether popular or generic, dissolve at about the same rate. Most brands, whether buffered or not, can severely damage the stomach lining if taken in excess. If aspirin works for you but bothers your stomach, you might try an enteric-coated tablet, such as Encaprin or Ecotrin. They are designed to dissolve in the small intestine rather than in the stomach.

Brand names can make a difference. One study found that up to one-third of aspirin's pain relief is the result of the placebo effect, based on the patient's seeing a familiar name on the tablet. Bottom line: If you have a favorite nonprescription pain reliever, keep using it. If you believe in it, it's probably worth the premium.

Acetaminophen (Tylenol, Datril, Anacin-3) is about as good as aspirin for relieving pain and fever. This drug is also useful for avoiding stomach irritations and ulcers. (Aspirin works better with arthritis, however.)

Drawback: Heavy long-term use of acetaminophens can result in liver damage. Tylenol may be a liver hazard if it's mixed with barbiturates, anti-anxiety agents (Valium and Librium) or alcohol.

Most potentially dangerous: Combination painkillers, such as Vanquish or Extra-Strength Excedrin, that include more than one analgesic. These may increase the risk of kidney damage, and combination painkillers have been banned in several countries.

The next step up is Dolobid (diflunisal), a new nonnarcotic analgesic. It may be a better mousetrap, a chemical cousin to aspirin that gives relief for up to 12 hours rather than four. In a well-controlled study, Dolobid was found to be as good as or better than Tylenol with codeine or Darvocet-N 100 for relieving post-operative dental pain—and without risk of addiction.

Drawback: Like aspirin, Dolobid can irritate the digestive tract. It's a poor choice if you're allergic to aspirin or have kidney problems.

Codeine is used for relieving moderate pain. Although the chance of physical addiction is very low, steady users can develop a tolerance and psychological dependence. People with alcohol problems or other drug problems should be especially cautious about this.

### Heavy Hitters

For severe pain, your doctor may prescribe a heavy narcotic such as Percodan, Demerol or Dilaudid. To minimize side effects, avoid taking these on an empty stomach. They also don't mix with alcohol, sleeping pills, muscle relaxants, antihistamines and some antidepressants.

Some doctors prescribe Phenergan (promethazine), an antihistamine, along with a narcotic. This duo will cause extreme drowsiness, so turn the Phenergan down. Also avoid combination painkillers (Compal, Maxigesic, Mepergan or Stopayne) that contain promethazine. In addition to making you sleepy, they may increase your pain.

If you develop tolerance to a narcotic, there's a way to get off without going cold turkey. A blood-pressure drug called Catapres (clonidine) acts as a "parachute" to help kick a habit gently, without serious withdrawal symptoms. Although Catapres hasn't been approved for this use by the FDA, it's a tremendous improvement over the old way, and many doctors will oversee your using it.

The future: Upjohn is developing a new compound that will relieve severe chronic pain without risk of addiction or respiratory side effects. Now known as U-50, 488, it acts to augment the body's supply of endorphins, which are natural pain-killing chemicals.

**Source:** Interview with Joe Graedon, author of *The New People's Pharmacy*, Bantam Books, New York.

# THE PAINFUL FACTS ABOUT OVER-THE-COUNTER ANALGESICS

The ads are often more effective than the products, and they drive up prices. Buzz words: Gentler, faster, tension-relieving, stronger. Fact: Only two nonprescription painkillers are proven to work—aspirin and acetaminophen (known to most people by the trade name Tylenol). Both are equally fast and effective in relieving pain, milligram for milligram. (A standard tablet of each is 325 mg.) The same is true for bringing down fever. Big difference: Cost.

Extra strength formulas of any of these products simply have more aspirin or acetaminophen per tablet, at a much higher cost. Caution: Twelve standard aspirin or acetaminophen tablets (3,900 mg) in a 24-hour period is the maximum dosage an adult should take without a doctor's supervision.

### Drawbacks

Problems with aspirin: Some people find aspirin irritating to the stomach, and a tiny number are allergic to it. People with ulcers shouldn't use aspirin. Heavy users (arthritis patients, for example) may need enteric-coated aspirin to keep the drug from hurting their stomachs. (It dissolves in the small intestine, not in the stomach.)

Problems with acetaminophen: Unlike aspirin, it does not reduce inflammation, an important part of arthritis treatment. Overdoses can cause liver damage.

### Other Products

Bufferin and other buffered aspirins give no faster pain relief than plain aspirin, according to the FDA. Nor is the claim to being gentler to the stomach adequately documented. Anacin, advertised as giving fast relief for muscle-tension headaches, is now a combination of aspirin and caffeine. (It has had other ingredients in the past.) Caffeine's role in pain relief is not certain, but it relieves headaches by constricting blood vessels. It is, however, more likely to cause tension than to alleviate it.

Excedrin combines aspirin, acetaminophen and caffeine. Vanquish and Gemnisyn are similar combinations. There is no evidence that the combination of aspirin and acetaminophen is any stronger than either alone.

**Source:** Interview with Bruce M. Yaffe, M.D., an internist in private practice in New York.

## CAFFEINE/ASPIRIN MYTH

Caffeine enhances the effectiveness of aspirin if you use enough of it. Earlier studies had concluded that caffeine does not boost the pain-killing properties of aspirin. Recent tests used 65 mg of caffeine per standard tablet (double the amount of the previous studies), which was found to increase pain relief by 40%.

**Source:** Study by the Rockland Research Institute, Orangeburg, NY.

## ASPIRIN ALERT

Aspirin temporarily dulls the central nervous system, even when taken in small doses. Take this into account when engaged in an activity that demands vigilance.

**Source:** Study at Stony Brook School of Medicine, Stony Brook, NY, reported in *Prevention*, Emmaus, PA.

## SAFER OVER-THE-COUNTER PAIN RELIEVER

Ibuprofen, the newest over-the-counter pain reliever, appears to be less dangerous in accidental overdoses than either acetaminophen or aspirin. A child who took 33 times the recommended adult dose of ibuprofen recovered with little after-effect.

**Source:** Harold M. Silverman, Ph.D., author of *Consumer's Guide to Poison Protection*, Avon Books, New York.

## THERAPY FOR PAIN RELIEF

Your new book tells all about your very special method of relieving pain... *myotherapy*. Why do you call it that?

The word simply means muscle therapy. A lot of the pain that people suffer—whether from illness, injury or stress—involves muscles. The approach I use was pioneered by Dr. Janet Travell, John F. Kennedy's physician. She identified tender muscle spots that she called trigger points. These control pain in various parts of the body. (More than 70% of her trigger points correlate with acupuncture points.) To treat pain, she injected a saline and procaine solution into the appropriate trigger point.

Since then, we have developed the system further, discovering many additional trigger points. We have also learned that these points can differ from person to person. Big difference: We treat pain by applying physical pressure to the trigger points rather than using drugs or needles.

What kinds of pain do you treat with your therapy?

We have had great success with back, shoulder, knee, leg, foot, and jaw pain, headaches, and even the discomfort of arthritis and hemorrhoids.

What are trigger points and where are they found?

No one is sure exactly what these spots are or how they are created. We do know that when the proper point is put under pressure, muscle pain is relieved. Trigger points are not always found at the actual site of the pain. Jaw pain, an acute problem for many women who are anxious or under stress, can be lessened through pressure points in the seat muscles (gluteals) and the groin. Lower back pain is thought to be connected with the spine, and is also relieved by finding trigger points in the same seat muscles and groin. The trigger points causing shoulder pain are often found in the arms, chest muscles, upper back, neck and armpits. Trigger points are always painful to a firm touch.

I believe trigger points are formed by damage or stress to muscle fiber—from an accident, an illness or occupational stress. Dentists and violinists, for example, must stand for long periods at an unnatural angle. This can bring on back pain and neck pain. When a person is under extreme emotional stress, the trigger points flare up and cause pain.

Can people relieve their own pain?

Yes, although sometimes you need a second person to reach the trigger points. If you have lower back pain, for example, you can lie face down on a flat surface while a friend feels for trigger points in the back-pocket area of your seat muscles. Method: The friend leans across you and probes for the trigger points with an elbow. When he finds a spot that hurts like hell, he should press on it steadily for five to seven seconds. (Never let him push harder than you're willing to accept, because it is counterproductive.) Then he should look for three or four other similar spots in the same area and repeat the pressing. After three pressings, roll onto your opposite side and pull the knee up to the chest. This stretches the worked muscle. Then stretch the leg out about eight inches above the other leg. Next, lower it to rest for three seconds. Repeat this procedure four times, and always to both sides, even if only one hurts.

For long-term relief, you must build up your muscles with exercise.

What kind of exercise can keep you fit and pain-free?

Calisthenics are absolutely essential to fitness, whatever aerobic exercise or sport you choose. You should never begin any physical activity without a 10-minute warm-up. A good warm-up gets the heart going and the blood circulating. Warm muscles are pliable and less prone to injury.

Hiking in hilly country is terrific exercise. Avoid doing any aerobic exercise on a hard surface. Aerobic dancing, for example, should never be done on a cement floor (shin splints and calf muscle spasms are almost guaranteed). Don't run or jog on pavement—keep to tracks, trails or cross-country runs. Running on a hard surface causes lower back pain and knee injuries, regardless of the shoes you wear.

**Source:** Interview with Bonnie Prudden, author of *Pain Erasure the Bonnie Prudden Way,* Ballantine Books, New York.

## WESTERN EXPERIENCES WITH ACUPUNCTURE

In a study of twenty patients with chronic pain syndrome, five reported complete pain relief after a series of acupuncture sessions, and nine others experienced partial relief. The group also showed less depression following the treatments. Conclusion: Acupuncture probably increases levels of endorphins and met-encephalins, natural "opiates" that suppress pain and elevate mood.

**Source:** Research by the departments of psychiatry and anesthesiology, University of Texas Health Science Center, Dallas, reported in *The Lancet,* Boston, MA.

## RELIEF FROM CHRONIC PAIN

Computerized, self-operated painkilling pumps will soon be on the market, allowing patients to self-administer painkilling drugs at home. The pumps will be programmed by the doctor to administer only the prescribed dosage at proper intervals. This lessens the possibility of accidental overdosing. In addition, because they inject the medication directly into the bloodstream, the pumps may bring faster relief from pain.

**Source:** Richard L. Bennett, Ph.D., assistant professor of anesthesiology, University of Kentucky Medical Center, Lexington.

## WHY PAINKILLERS CAN BACKFIRE

Painkillers that are taken for a headache can, ironically, cause the same symptoms they're taken to cure. What happens: Three to four hours after the headache remedy is taken, its level comes down in the bloodstream . . . and the headache returns, sometimes even worse than before.

**Source:** *Internal Medicine News*, Rockville, MD.

## CURE FOR TURTLE HEADACHES

Turtle headaches (from burrowing under the covers during the night) are often caused by cold bedrooms—even in the summer, if the air conditioning is on. Prevention: Use an electric blanket.

**Source:** Janet G. Travell, M.D., Washington, DC, in *Journal of the American Medical Association*, Chicago, IL.

## TIPS FOR PARTY GOERS

A few of the best-loved party refreshments ruin good times for some people by giving them headaches. The culprit: Tyramine, an amino acid that can also act as a stimulant and tongue loosener. If parties start your temples throbbing, look out for tyramine-containing foods like aged cheese, chicken livers, chocolate and pickled herring. Drinks that have it include beer, champagne, red wine and sherry.

## FOODS THAT GIVE YOU HEADACHES

• MSG is not the only culprit. Look out for tyramine-containing foods like aged cheese, chicken livers, chocolate and pickled herring. Drinks that have it include beer, champagne, red wine and sherry.

• Ice-cream headache is a brief, but intense, pain in the throat, head or face that results from biting into ice cream. The pain is a physiological response of the warm tissues of the mouth to the sudden assault by cold. The pain is sometimes felt throughout the head because cranial nerve branches in the area spread the pain impulse along a broad path. Prevention: Allow small amounts of ice cream to melt in the mouth before eating successive large bites.

**Source:** *Freedom from Headaches* by Joel R. Saper, M.D., and Kenneth R. Magee, M.D., Simon & Schuster, New York.

## PREVENTING MIGRAINES

Limit your intake of caffeine, which can bring on attacks if consumed in excess of 500 milligrams per day (the amount contained in four cups of brewed coffee). Be sure to count other sources of caffeine too. Skip foods that are rich in tyramine (aged cheese, Chianti wines), sodium nitrate (cured meats) and sodium glutamate (used widely in prepared foods). Don't take oral contraceptives or estrogen.

**Source:** *US Pharmacist*, New York.

## HYPOGLYCEMIA ALERT

Hypoglycemia (insufficient blood sugar) may trigger migraine headaches. Mechanism: Hypoglycemia dilates the cranial blood vessels extensively. Susceptible persons should avoid activities that might alter their normal blood sugar levels—skipping a meal, fasting, sleeping too late, or eating a heavy dose of carbohydrates.

**Source:** *RN*, Chicago, IL.

## GOOD AND BAD NEWS ABOUT A NEW DRUG

Migraine frequency was reduced nearly 50% by the drug verapamil (brand names Calan and Isoptin). And there were fewer side effects than the propranolol (Inderal) or methysergide (Sansert). Drawbacks: (1) Verapamil must be taken frequently. (2) Its use may mask early warning signs that can alert migraine sufferers to abort attacks with another drug.

**Source:** *Journal of the American Medical Association,* Chicago, IL.

## NEW MIGRAINE TREATMENT

Recurrent migraine headaches may be prevented in many cases by using a new treatment, calcium-channel blockers. These drugs are currently used to prevent coronary artery spasms. Researchers believe they may also be effective in preventing spasms in arteries near the surface of the brain, where migraines often begin. Bonus: Side effects seem to be minimal.

**Source:** *Journal of the American Medical Association,* Chicago, IL.

## HEADACHE RELIEF WITHOUT DRUGS

Relief from incapacitating tension, vascular and migraine headaches is possible without drugs, using a self-administered form of acupuncture known as acupressure.

The technique: Exert very heavy thumbnail pressure (painful pressure) successively on nerves lying just below the surface of the skin at key points in the hands and wrists. As with acupuncture, no one's sure why it works.

Pressure points to try:

• The triangle of flesh between the thumb and index finger on the back of your hands (thumb side of bone, near middle of the second metacarpal in the index finger).

• Just above the protruding bone on the thumb side of your wrist.

## DRUGLESS HEADACHE CURES

(1) Eat a cheese sandwich. (2) Take a hot shower, followed by a cold one—until you shiver. (3) Place crushed ice in the mouth and throat (not for the elderly or ill). (4) Massage the lower part of the big toe and beneath all the toes. (5) Breathe into a paper bag (stops hyperventilation). (6) Ask a partner to press your "trigger" points (temples, back of the neck, below your shoulder blades). (7) Rotate a hairbrush in small circles, starting above your temples, and working it down over your ears to your neck.

**Source:** *Spring*

## BACKACHE'S SILLY SOURCES

Backache may be caused by discomfort and tension arising from poor everyday living habits, Dr. Hans Krause has found. Examples: Gobbling food, sleeping on a sagging mattress, wearing uncomfortable clothing, using appliances in a restrictive way or simply sitting too long.

### Dressing

• Clothing should never be tight! This applies to pajamas and nightgowns as well as to everyday dress.

• Avoid narrow-toed shoes. They tense the leg muscles, which in turn affect the back. Heels should not be too loose or two tight. Either extreme produces ankle sway which works its way up to the back and neck. Women's high-heeled shoes shorten the hamstring and calf muscles, causing the tension that frequently leads to backache.

• Toes of socks and stockings should not be tight. You should be able to wiggle your toes freely.

• Too high or too tight a collar can cause a stiff neck. Wear collars half a size larger and, if your neck is short, stick to soft, narrow collars.

• Narrow shoulder straps of brassieres can cause shoulder and upper back pain, especially if they are pulled too tight.

### Sleeping

• Wide shoulders require bigger pillows for those who sleep on their sides.

• Foam rubber pillows force the neck into a rigid position. Use a feather pillow.

### Sitting

• Never sit in one position for more than an hour or two. Get up and move around.

• On car trips, stop frequently to limber up.

• While reading, avoid strain by keeping the page at a comfortable distance. It's also important to have enough light.

### Telephoning

• To use muscles more evenly, office workers should shift the telephone from one side of the desk to the other each day.

• Instead of tensing when the phone rings, make it a practice to shrug the shoulders before reaching out to pick up the receiver.

**Source:** *Backache, Stress and Tension* by Hans Krause, New York.

## BEST BACK INJURY PREDICTORS

Strength tests are better predictors of back injuries than X rays (which show only bone alterations, not sprains or future disk problems). Isometric strength tests, in which a person slowly increases the force exerted on a set of handles, are easy, quick (15–30 minutes) and safe (no injuries in over 3,000 tests). Employees hired after these tests had one-third fewer injuries than those hired after traditional medical exams.

**Source:** *Plant Engineering*, New York.

## ALTERNATIVES TO PAINFUL MYELOGRAM

Myelogram, a technique to diagnose lower back pain caused by disk problems, is painful and expensive and usually requires an overnight hospital stay. Alternatives: Nerve and muscle conduction studies, electromyograms and CAT scans can replace myelograms in many cases, saving the patient much time, money and discomfort.

**Source:** B. O. Khatri, M.D., writing in *Archives of Neurology*, New York.

## DRUG THAT MAY MEAN NO MORE BACK SURGERY

*Chymopapain*, a new drug, may cure back problems without an operation. It is injected to dissolve protruding and swollen tissue, thereby removing pressure on the nerves. This procedure eliminates the need for surgery and is at least as safe.

## HOW TO PREVENT BACKACHES

To prevent back problems: Keep your weight down. Sleep on a firm surface. Don't smoke. Exercise to build strong back and stomach muscles. When lifting heavy objects, always squat first, and lift with your legs and thighs.

**Source:** American Academy of Orthopedic Surgeons, Chicago.

## CHIROPRACTORS VS. ORTHOPEDISTS

Chiropractors outperform orthopedists in relieving many kinds of back pain. This was the opinion of 500 back and neck pain sufferers. Exception: For patients who are suffering from acute disk pain, orthopedists and rehabilitation specialists are more effective.

**Source:** *Omni*, New York.

## SELF-HELP THERAPIES FOR BACK PAIN

The best self-help therapies for acute low-back pain are bed rest, cold therapy, acupressure, posture realignment, stress reduction and individualized personal habits.

**Source:** A survey of 492 back sufferers, cited in *Back-Ache Relief*, Times Books, New York.

## FOUR EASY EXERCISES TO STRENGTHEN YOUR BACK

Strengthening the back and stomach muscles is the best protection against a back injury. Four simple and fast exercises that will help accomplish that:

(1) Flexed-knee sit-ups. Lie on your back, with knees bent and arms at your side. Sit up slowly by rolling forward, starting with the head.

(2) Bent-knee leg lifts. In the same position as the sit-ups, bring one knee as close as you can to your chest, while extending the other leg. Alternate the legs.

(3) Knee-chest leg lifts. Work from the bent-knee sit-up position, but put a small pillow under your head. Use your hands to bring both knees up to the chest, tighten the stomach muscles and hold that position for a count of 10.

(4) Back flattening. Lie on your back, flex the knees, and put your arms above your head. Tighten your stomach and buttock muscles and press the lower back hard against the floor. Hold this position for a count of 10, relax and repeat.

Cautions: Don't overdo the exercises. Soreness is a sign to cut back. Never do these exercises with the legs straight. If you have back trouble, consult your doctor before starting this, or any, exercise program.

**Source:** *American Journal of Nursing*, Chicago, IL.

# RELIEF FOR "TAIL-BONE" PAIN

Pain of the coccyx, the "tail bone," is hard to live with and has been even harder to treat. Evidence shows that a three-inch-wide belt worn around the body just above the bone prevents ligaments from pulling on this sensitive area. If worn constantly for three months, the belt gives many patients significant relief.

**Source:** Galaxy Systems, Los Angeles.

# INVERSION-THERAPY DOUBTS

Hanging upside down in a special device is supposed to ease back ailments and stretch short or tense muscles. Doctors and therapists have been reporting a high suc-

cess rate among people undertaking this inversion therapy. But some professionals are leery of the procedure and of certain back-strengthening exercises. They recommend more study before these procedures are adopted universally. Safer: A horizontal home traction unit sold in medical supply stores.

**Source:** *Medical World News*, Houston, TX.

# THE WAR ON CANCER

A diagnosis of cancer is no longer a death sentence. Actually, cancer is probably the most treatable chronic disease in the US— three million Americans who were diagnosed with cancer five years ago are still alive. For most cancers, patients who survive five years have an 85% chance of surviving 20 years.

### New Cure Rates

In some cases, even in common tumors, the improvement has been nothing short of spectacular. With the aggressive lymphomas, such as advanced Hodgkin's disease, cure rates are up from 5% in 1973 to 70% today. With testicular cancer, the most common cancer in young men, the rate is up from 10% in 1973 to 70% today.

Other encouraging five-year survival rates: Thyroid, 92%. Endometrium (uterine), 87%. Melanoma, 79%. Bladder, 72%. Prostate, 67%. Uterine cervix, 67%. Larynx, 66%.

Some improvements, such as those in testicular cancer and the lymphomas, are due to specific advances in cancer therapy. Others, such as those in stomach cancer, are due to environmental factors. In the 1930s, stomach cancer was one of the leading causes of cancer death. Today, US death rates for stomach cancer are among the lowest in the world. Suspected reason: The easy availability of refrigeration starting in the 1930s led to lower consumption of smoked and preserved meats and to year-round availability of vegetables.

New scientific discoveries are also providing hope for the future. In liver cancer, for example, it's been discovered that the hepatitis virus is a strong risk factor. A recently developed hepatitis vaccine is being given to high-risk people, such as health workers, which should lower the incidence of liver cancer. Discovery of the role of viruses in cancer, as with the human tumor cell lymphoma leukemia virus (HTLV-III) that was found to cause AIDS, is giving impetus to the hope for prevention. The goal of the National Cancer Institute: To decrease cancer mortality by another 50% by the year 2000. The big initiative over the next 10 years is finding drugs that prevent cancer.

### More Upbeat Statistics

• Lung cancer. Lung cancer is the most common form of cancer in men. Since 1953, lung cancer rates have gone up 172% for men and 256% for women. Smoking alone contributes to 30% of all cancer deaths. In addition to lung cancer, smoking has been associated with cancer of the voice box, head and neck, esophagus, bladder, kidney, pancreas and stomach. Treatment: Overall, only 9% of lung cancer patients live five years or more after diagnosis. However, for one type of lung cancer, we've had a 33% five-year survival, the best ever reported. Problem: Lung cancer metastasizes very quickly. As yet, there is no way of detecting it early enough. Some types are very resistant to treatment. To protect yourself: Stop smoking, of course. If you're determined to smoke, studies have shown that smokers who consume a lot of carotene (in carrots and other yellow vegetables) and vitamin A have lower lung cancer rates.

• Colon and rectal cancer. Although these cancers are second in incidence to lung cancer and there have been no real changes in treatment, five-year survival rates are up from 43% to 51%. Surgery is the most effective treatment. Many victims fear a permanent colostomy, but only 15% of cases detected early will need one. To protect yourself: Cut down on animal fat and increase dietary fiber. The decreased incidence of this disease may be due to changes in eating patterns. Have yearly rectal exams after age 40 and yearly stool blood tests after age 50. Early detection boosts the five-year survival rate to 75%.

• Breast cancer. There is substantial improvement here, too. A woman with breast cancer today has about a 73% chance of being alive in five years. It was 63% in 1975. Also, in many cases less mutilating procedures (particularly removing just the lump itself or part of the breast) in combination with radiation therapy provide the same five-year survival rate as radical mastectomy. To protect yourself: Monthly self-examination by all women . . . and regular mammograms for those over 40, depending on age and risk factors.

• Cancer in children. Although there were only 6,000 new cases in 1984, making it a rare childhood disease, cancer is still the chief cause of death by disease in children between the ages of three and 14. However, leukemia is no longer the death sentence it once was. With improved chemotherapy, survival rates have risen from 5% in the 1960s to 50% today. The latest statistics show that with leukemia, once five-year survival is reached, relapse is unheard of. Survival rates for other childhood cancers vary considerably, depending on the site, but the overall death rate of children with cancer is about half the 1950 rate.

**Source:** Interview with Gregory A. Curt, M.D., medical oncologist, Division of Cancer Treatment, National Cancer Institute, Bethesda, MD.

# CANCER CURES ARE BOOMING

Reason: Breakthroughs in early detection, surgery, radiation, chemotherapy and experimental immunology. Many cancers once considered fatal now have survival rates of 75%–95% when caught early.

Good resolutions: Adults over the age of 40 should have annual exams to look for cancer of the thyroid, mouth, skin and lymph nodes. Men must be alert for cancer of the prostate and testes, women of breast and ovaries. Ask your doctor about home tests for cancers of the colon and rectum.

# ANOTHER VITAMIN C MYTH

Vitamin C has flunked again as a treatment

for advanced cancer. In a study of 144 cancer patients, those receiving daily doses of the vitamin survived no longer than those receiving only placebos. Note: Linus Pauling, Nobel Prize winner and vitamin C advocate, disputed the findings, saying the vitamin's effectiveness was undermined by the patients' previous chemotherapy.

**Source:** *Medical World News,* New York.

# CARCINOGENS IN EVERYDAY FOODS

Why do cancer-causing agents occur naturally in some foods?

Plants, like any other living creature, need a defense system. They synthesize their own pesticides in large amounts to defend against animals and insects. There is an enormous variety of these chemicals. . . and new ones are being discovered regularly. The amount of natural pesticides we regularly ingest is about 10,000 times the level of man-made pesticides. In my opinion, the man-made pesticide residues in our diet don't represent a significant cancer risk relative to natural pesticides.

What foods are these natural carcinogenic pesticides found in?

A few are mustard, horseradish, black pepper, mushrooms, some herbal teas, celery, parsnips and parsley. Alfalfa sprouts also look suspicious. By introducing plant strains that resist insects and fungi, plant breeders may be creating plants that contain even more natural carcinogens. In addition to these natural pesticides, molds also make a great variety of carcinogens. These are found in mold-contaminated foods such as corn, grain, nuts, peanut butter, bread, cheese, fruits and apple juice. Some of these toxins, such as aflatoxin (found in peanut butter), are among the most potent carcinogens known. Many, or even most, of these plant toxins may be new to humans in the sense that our diet has changed drastically in recent history.

What a long, depressing list! Is that all the bad news, or is there more?

Oh yes, there's more, some already familiar. All burned and browned foods, including cooked food, contain carcinogens. We ingest more each day from fried hamburgers, browned muffins, roasted coffee, etc. than a two-pack-day smoker inhales, although the risk from eating these things could be much less than breathing in cigarette smoke. Also, high fat intake has been associated with colon and breast cancer, and high alcohol intake with mouth, esophageal and other cancers. There is preliminary—but not conclusive—evidence that heavy coffee drinking is also associated with cancer.

With so many foods on the list, what can we do to lower our risks?

I personally don't hesitate to eat a peanut butter sandwich, for instance. The risk is so low as to be negligible. However, there is no doubt about the risk of smoking cigarettes, which causes 30% of all cancer in the US. It also may be wise to cut down on charred meats and burned foods. Studies suggest that it's prudent to increase the consumption of fiber-rich cereals, vegetables and fruits and decrease the consumption of fatty foods and alcohol. There is evidence that a balanced diet may protect against lung cancer in smokers. In several studies in Japan and the US, smokers who have a diet rich in green vegetables are less likely to get lung cancer than smokers who don't eat them.

Are there any foods you should eat to help prevent cancer?

The human diet contains a great variety of both cancer-causing and cancer-preventing agents. Research on aging has indicated that our oxygen metabolism may be involved with cancer, a disease which seems connected to the body's fundamental, destructive aging process. A major source of the damage may come from molecules called oxygen radicals, which damage DNA. All animals have many defenses against oxygen radicals (called antioxidants). Man evolved from shorter-lived animals. We have a lower rate of oxygen consumption and perhaps increased levels of some antioxidants. Many antioxidants protect us against oxygen radicals. A few are: Vitamin E, beta-carotene, selenium salts, glutathione, vitamin C and uric acid. Some researchers on aging have recommended dietary changes and supplements (some of those mentioned above plus others) to prevent and retard aging. The evidence isn't yet in on whether these regimens really work, and some supplements, such as selenium, are very toxic at high levels.

It is important to recognize that nature is not benign, and no human diet can be entirely free of carcinogens. The foods I mentioned are only representative examples. What we can do is eat a balanced diet and eliminate the known risks such as smoking. Biological research is progressing remarkably rapidly, and we should know much more about the causes of aging and cancer very soon.

**Source:** Interview with Bruce N. Ames, Ph.D., chairman of the biochemistry department at the University of California at Berkeley.

## CANCER PREVENTION DIET

Eating less fat and more fiber has been reconfirmed as the best dietary defense against cancer. The American Cancer Society now joins the National Cancer Institute and the National Academy of Sciences in similar recommendations.

Besides cutting down on all fats (animal fats in particular) and eating more whole-grain foods and fresh vegetables and fruits for fiber, the guidelines also suggest eating: Less salt-cured, smoked or charcoal-broiled meat. More fruits and green vegetables (rich in vitamin C). Plenty of foods with beta carotene (a kind of vitamin A), such as asparagus, cantaloupe, carrots, spinach and tomatoes. More vegetables in the cabbage family—broccoli, brussels sprouts, cauliflower, turnips, watercress—and, of course, cabbage. They contain chemicals that inhibit cancer.

Bottom line: Research suggests that 35% of new cancer cases in the US could be prevented by proper diet.

## WHAT DOCTORS DON'T KNOW ABOUT CANCER CAN SAVE YOUR LIFE

When it comes to cancer (or any other serious disease), the patient's sense of helplessness is his worst enemy. In our society, we depend too much on science and technology to heal us, giving over total control of our bodies to doctors. Being a passive victim in the hands of the medical establishment can be an extremely stressful experience. The effects of stress have recently been implicated as playing an important role in immune-system response. And certainly nothing is more stressful than learning you have cancer and going through the ordeal of cancer treatment.

Ten years ago, I was diagnosed as having cancer and was given a 10% chance to live one year. I was an uncooperative patient, always wanting to know what the doctors were doing and why. If I didn't agree with a procedure, I refused it. I now think this active participation, which made me feel in control, along with the stress-management techniques I employed, played a large part in my survival. And research now indicates that cancer patients with key psychological skills live longer and more satisfying lives.

### Your Beliefs Can Be Powerful Allies

Cancer has traditionally been a dreaded word, synonymous with death. Times have changed, however, and today, 50% of all cancers are curable. With many, the cure rate is much higher.

The body produces billions of cells and routinely identifies and kills cancerous ones. Once the major cancer-removal job is done by surgery and chemotherapy, your body can take over. But you must free up energy to mobilize your body to fight cancer. How to do it:

• Express your feelings. Patients who express anger and sadness survive the longest. Expressing your feelings reduces stress and releases energy. Suppressing feelings uses up valuable energy that should be mobilized to fight the cancer. Example: In a study at Johns Hopkins, patients with metastatic breast cancer who survived more than a year were those who expressed their depression, anxiety and sense of alienation. They were also judged by their doctors as being poorly adjusted to the disease and as having negative attitudes toward their doctors.

• Avoid blame, guilt and self-criticism. You are not being punished for wrong-doing. The question "Why me?" should be replaced with "What can I do about it now?"

• Seek support. Discuss your situation with a therapist, family member or support group. Important: Talk with a former cancer patient who has been pronounced cured or has survived for years with the disease. This can be a powerful combatant of negative feelings.

• Take positive steps to help yourself. Recognize that your life has changed, probably forever, and that your old ways of coping are no longer viable and may even be implicated in your illness. What must change: Gratification from compulsive goal-seeking The cancer patient must start to develop a sense of self-worth that comes from within rather than from outside goals such as success, money or sexual conquests. Also: Express love and learn to say no. Every moment is precious. Why waste it on trivia or worrying about whether an extra phone call will bother your doctor.

• Speak the unspeakable. The relatives and friends of cancer patients often feel certain subjects are taboo. This leads patients to suppress their feelings in order to protect their loved ones. But when patients and the people they're close to talk openly about their feelings, it can be an enormous relief and source of strength.

### Techniques That Help

There are a number of specific exercises that can help reduce stress and fight the illness. Relaxation techniques enable the patient to experience the replacement of stress-producing thoughts with positive, health-facilitating ones. Examples:

• Autogenic (self-control of the body) techniques teach the patient to speak to himself in calming language and to control some of his own bodily functions.

• Imaging is somewhat similar to self-hypnosis. It involves imagining that you are healthy or that your cancer is melting away.

• Stress inoculation involves exposing yourself gradually to a stressor through frequent mental rehearsals. This helps you remain relaxed when you face the situation in reality.

### Actively Choosing Treatment

By actively choosing your treatment, you reduce the stress of feeling like a passive victim. Example: I felt emotionally and physically debilitated by the side effects of chemotherapy. I'd slipped into thinking that I had to take these drugs for my doctor. To combat this, I reminded myself I was taking those drugs because I wanted to—they were powerful allies of my body.

The doctor-patient relationship can be crucial in allowing the patient to retain a sense of control. You must choose a doctor who you feel has some concern for you as a human being and who takes your values and life goals into consideration when medical decisions are made. Your doctor should give you information about treatment plans and alternatives and be open to negotiating alternatives with you rather than assuming a "take it or leave it" attitude. Example: A woman with breast cancer should choose a doctor who is open to less extreme "lumpectomy" procedure over one who always insists on radical mastectomies.

### Special Diets and Cancer

Although I don't believe that any diet, per se, can really be touted as "curing" cancer, following a special regimen can help a patient to fight cancer.

The very act of choosing a rigorous diet and sticking to it gives you a sense of control over your body. Each time you prepare a meal you are, in effect, taking a specific step to fight the disease.

And eating nutritious, more easily digested foods such as whole grains and fresh fruits and vegetables rather than too much meat, processed foods and excessive fats not only fortifies your body but also frees up sources of energy to fight the cancer—energy that might have been diverted to digesting a steak or a piece of pie.

**Source:** Interview with Neil A. Fiore, Ph.D., a psychologist who works for the University of California and has a private practice in Berkeley.

## FIGHTING BACK

A will to survive does activate your immune system, according to studies of breast cancer patients. Passive patients who responded to their illness with feelings of fatigue and helplessness also had less active white blood cells (the cells that destroy cancer cells). Patients who were most distressed by their disease had the best chance of being alive a year later.

**Source:** Sandra Levy, Ph.D., a psychologist at the National Cancer Institute, Bethesda, MD, speaking to the American Psychological Association.

• Patients who fight cancer respond better to treatment than those without hope. The fighters also suffer less frequent and less severe side effects.

**Source:** American Physical Fitness Research Institute, Los Angeles.

• Angry cancer patients do better in fighting their disease than those who are apathetic, depressed or silently hostile, according to recent studies. Fact: Depressed patients have less active immune systems— and the immune system is responsible for stemming ( or not stemming) the spread of cancer.

**Source:** Studies at Yale University and the University of Pittsburgh School of Medicine.

## CANCER COUNSELING

Dr. Carl Simonton, a pioneer and leading practitioner in the field of psychology and cancer, has started a program for training patients to build up their psychological defenses against the disease. Every month, his center in Texas runs a five-day seminar in which each cancer patient, along with a "support" person, is taught "mental imaging" techniques. For example, patients are asked to picture the drugs or the radiation treatments killing the cancer cells in their blood streams and the white blood cells carrying the dead cancer cells away.

The psychological techniques Dr. Simonton prescribes are not meant to replace conventional medical treatment, but to supplement it. The treatment deals with the patients' reactions to stress and other emotional factors and helps them learn the techniques of psychological self-awareness and self-care.

Dr. Simonton treats patients with all types of cancer. Children may not attend the seminars, although they seem to do particularly well with the "mental imaging" technique when their parents work with them.

**Source:** Carl Simonton, Ph.D., Cancer Counseling and Research Center, Azle, TX.

## CAUSE OF PATIENT DEPRESSION

Depression among cancer patients is often caused by drugs used in chemotherapy. It's not always brought on by simple worry, as previously believed. Boston researchers now suspect that several cancer drugs interfere with the production of noradrenaline, and this in turn affects mood and emotion.

## PROTECTION AGAINST BREAST CANCER

A special heat-sensitive "bra" will be the first product women can use at home to detect cancer and other breast diseases at their most critical point—when they first appear. (This new product can alert a woman to trouble even before a lump can be felt.)

How does it work? First, a physician makes a color-coded picture of the breast area on thin, heat-sensitive film. This "thermograph" is the normal reference image. Then, periodically, the patient slips on a bra made from the same heat-sensitive material, and any alteration in the color pattern will prompt a call to the doctor for further evaluation. (Most breast diseases will cause a variation in the heat-generation patterns produced by breast tissue; cysts will show as "cold" spots, cancerous growths as "hot" areas.) Completely safe: No radiation or penetration of the body is involved.

**Source:** BCD Products, Inc., New York.

## WHO WILL DEVELOP BREAST CANCER

Known carcinogenic patterns are of little value in determining which women will develop breast cancer. It occurs in one out of 11 women, and accepted risk factors are relevant in only 30% of cases. All women should be considered high risk. They should do breast self-examination. Starting by age 40, they should have an annual mammogram.

**Source:** American Cancer Society, New York.

## BEST WAY TO SCREEN FOR BREAST CANCER

Breast imaging techniques such as thermography and ultrasound, are still unproven for screening early breast cancers. Only reliable screening methods: Monthly self-examination and regular X-ray mammography.

**Source:** The American College of Radiology, cited in *The Harvard Medical School Health Letter*, Cambridge, MA.

## SCREENING: NEW METHOD

Light scanning (also known as diaphanography) will become a widely available alternative to X rays for detecting breast cancers. The technique: A low-intensity light is shined through the breasts. Abnormalities are then projected as colored images on a screen. In a recent study of 500 patients, 83% of those with cancerous biopsies tested positively with light scanning—the same accuracy rate as with mammography.

**Source:** Study at Dartmouth-Hitchcock Medical Center, NH, reported in *Good Housekeeping*, New York.

## CURE MAY BE JUST AROUND THE CORNER

British scientists may have found a cure for breast cancer. A drug called 4-hydroxyandrostenedione (4HAD) actually appears to kill breast tumors, instead of merely stopping their growth as do conventional cancer drugs. Reason: 4HAD, now undergoing tests, blocks production of estrogen, without which breast tumors cannot survive.

**Source:** *New Scientist,* London, Eng.

## SURPRISING TRUTH ABOUT DRINKING AND CANCER

Alcohol consumption does not affect a woman's chances of developing breast cancer. Previous research had indicated that cancer was almost twice as likely to strike drinkers as nondrinkers.

**Source:** Study by the Division of Reproductive Health, Centers for Disease Control, reported in *The Lancet*, Boston, MA.

## ANOTHER SMOKING HAZARD

Heart disease and lung cancer are not the only hazards of smoking. Women who smoke triple their risk of getting cancer of the cervix. Apparently cervical cells are exposed to the carcinogenic components of smoke that have been absorbed by the blood.

**Source:** *Journal of the American Medical Association,* Chicago, IL.

## SEXUAL ACTIVITY AND CERVICAL CANCER

Chances of cervical cancer are greatly increased by early sexual activity and also by having numerous partners. The reason is still unknown, but scientists theorize that venereally transmitted organisms are to blame. Evidence: The disease is almost never found in nuns. Amish, Mormon and Seventh Day Adventist women have 50% less cervical cancer than the national average. Recommendations: Postpone sexual activity as long as possible. Limit the number of partners. Use barrier contraceptives (condom and diaphragm) to protect your cervix. Have an annual Pap test.

**Source:** Robert Yule, M.D., consulting pathologist at Christie's Hospital, Manchester, England.

## TALCUM POWDER ALERT

Talcum powder can cause ovarian cancer in women. Particles enter the vagina, work their way up to the ovaries and are absorbed—a contributing factor in the outbreak of cancer.

**Source:** *Harvard Medical School Health Letter,* Cambridge, MA.

## FOR MEN ONLY

Without prompt treatment, 29% of men who have testicular cancer will die from it. But virtually all could be cured if treated within a month of the onset of symptoms.

Recommended: Give yourself a testicular self-exam once a month. The exam takes only three minutes. It is best administered after a warm bath or shower, when the scrotum is most relaxed.

Technique: Examine the testicles separately, using fingers of both hands. Put your thumb on top of the testicle underneath. Roll the testicle gently. (If it hurts, you're applying too much pressure.)

A normal testicle is firm, oval and free of lumps. Behind it you'll feel the epididymis (sperm storage duct), which is spongier.

Danger sign: A small, hard, usually painless lump or swelling on the front or side of the testicle. When in the slightest doubt, see a doctor.

**Source:** George Prout, M.D., chief of urology, Massachusetts General Hospital, in *Prevention,* Emmaus, PA.

## PROSTATE CANCER DETECTION

NMR imaging, performed with high-pow-

ered magnets, is an exciting new way to differentiate between benign and cancerous prostate enlargements. Older men suffering prostate enlargement (many cases are cancerous every year) can be checked without biopsy. NMR works especially well deep in the pelvis, where other methods can't detect cancer until it has spread.

**Source:** *Science News,* Marion, OH.

## NEW TREATMENTS FOR PROSTATE CANCER

Prostate cancer surgery often leaves men both impotent and incontinent. However, a new surgical technique eliminates both problems in virtually every case. Secret: The preservation of nerve bundles that are severed in conventional surgery.

**Source:** Technique developed by Patrick C. Walsh, M.D., chairman, department of urology, Johns Hopkins University School of Medicine, reported in the *Journal of The American Medical Association,* Chicago, IL.

• Use of a pituitary-blocking agent plus an androgen-blocking agent has in preliminary studies resulted in a 100% response in patients with advanced prostate cancer. By blocking all of the body's male hormones with these agents, surgical removal of the testicles and the prescription of female hormones can often be avoided.

**Source:** Fernand Labrie, M.D., Laval University, Quebec. reported in *Oncology Times,* New York.

## ABOUT MOLES

Some moles that grow on the skin after birth are likely to get bigger and turn into melanomas (skin cancers) before a person reaches age 70. Most dangerous: Moles that are about a quarter of an inch in diameter. Precautions: (1) Self-examine large moles every month to be sure they aren't growing. (2) Have them checked by a physician every six months. (3) If a mole is getting bigger, have it removed before it can become a melanoma.

**Source:** *US Pharmacist,* New York.

# MELANOMA WARNING

Blondes are seven times more likely to suffer malignant melanoma (a severe skin cancer) than people with black hair, a British study showed. Other melanoma links: Fair skin, heavy freckling, atypical skin moles, exposure to sunlight.

**Source:** *The Lancet*, Boston, MA.

# THE SUN AND SKIN CANCER

By now, we've all been repeatedly warned about the damaging effects of too much sun. But those still desperate enough for a tan to bake their bodies at noon haven't really absorbed the bad news. Although you may think you already know how harmful the sun is, it's probable that the facts are really even worse than you have believed.

The sun is responsible for 95% of all skin cancer, which is the most common form of cancer in America. It afflicts one out of every four to seven people, with 500,000 cases reported every year.

Americans are developing it at ever younger ages, due to the increase in leisure time spent in the sun. Nineteen years ago, the average age of my patients was 65. Today it's in the late 50s, with an increasing number of even younger people. So, I'd like you to know the new discoveries about how to avoid skin cancer that you probably don't already know. In addition, there's an exciting new treatment—chemosurgery—that has the highest cure rate and causes less disfiguration.

### Prevention

The most frightening aspect of skin cancer is not knowing whether you've already been overexposed to the sun. Skin cancer is cumulative, and if you've been a sun addict for years, there's no way to predict at age 40 whether or not you'll develop it at age 60. All you can do is start taking precautions now.

Some little-known facts:

• Your risk of burning is greater at higher altitudes, since the thinner atmosphere filters out fewer rays. Use a sunscreen when skiing or mountain climbing.

• Sitting in the shade does not guarantee protection. Sand, snow, concrete and water can reflect more than half the sun's rays onto your skin.

• Many common drugs increase your sensitivity to the sun...antihistamines, tetracycline, sulfanilamides, some diuretics, antidepressants, antihypertensives, anticonvulsants and oral contraceptives. If you're on medication, check with your doctor or pharmacist before going out in the sun.

• Dark-skinned (and black-skinned) people get sunburned too. Although light-skinned people are the most vulnerable to the damaging effects of the sun and have the highest rate of skin cancer, a dark complexion is no guarantee against developing it.

• Although clothing and tinted window glass may reduce the sun's intensity, they do not entirely eliminate the burning rays. Helpful: Tightly woven clothing and a large-brimmed hat.

• Melanoma, the most virulent and deadly skin cancer, is also associated with overexposure to the sun.

• Ultraviolet light may have a generally negative effect on the immune system. Preliminary experiments with mice indicate that it lessens their resistance to disease.

• Artificial tanning machines are harmful and increase your risk of skin cancer.

### Sunscreen Savvy

• A sunscreen with a sun protection factor (SPF) of 15 or greater should be used by everyone, regardless of skin type. It should normally be reapplied every couple of hours, and also reapplied after swimming or perspiring heavily.

• Some people are allergic to certain sunscreen ingredients, especially PABA. If you develop a reaction, change brands.

• Products approved by the Skin Cancer Foundation: Coppertone Super Shade, Total Eclipse, Bain de Soleil Ultra Sunblock, Sea & Ski Block Out, Pre-Sun and Chapstick Lip Balm.

• To protect against both types of ultraviolet rays, use a broad spectrum sunscreen. Reason: Ultraviolet B (UVB) rays are the burning ones, whereas ultraviolet A (UVA) rays have been thought to be associated with tanning only. But UVA rays have recently been shown to cause premature aging and may also be implicated in skin cancer. A broad-spectrum product contains both PABA to protect against UVB and benzophenones to protect against UVA.

### Skin Cancer Detection

With early detection, skin cancer is almost always curable. The rule: Have your body examined once a year, especially if you're in the high-risk group (already extensively exposed to the sun in the past). We say, "Get your birthday suit checked on your birthday."

Skin cancer signs:

• Any skin growth that increases in size and appears pearly, translucent, tan, brown, black or multicolored.

• A mole, birthmark or beauty mark that has changed in any way or is irregular in outline.

• Any open sore or wound that does not heal in two weeks or continues to itch, hurt, scab, erode or bleed.

### The New Treatment

Standard techniques use guesswork when removing cancerous tissue. The surgeon removes whatever seems to his eye to be cancerous, sends it to the lab, and waits for the biopsy report. There's no certainty that all the cancer has been removed.

Chemosurgery (also known as the Mohs method or microscopic control surgery) provides an almost 99% chance for cure. With chemosurgery, the patient waits in the office while the surgeon examines the tissue microscopically, pinpointing the exact location of any remaining tumor. If more cancer is found, the procedure is repeated, thereby tracing the cancer to its roots.

Advantages of chemosurgery: Less disfiguration, since only cancerous tissue, not normal tissue, is removed. The highest rate of cure, especially with cancers that have previously resisted treatment. Disadvan-

tage: Since the method is time-consuming and requires highly specialized training and personnel, only a few medical centers in the US are currently equipped to do it.

**Source:** Interview with Perry Robins, M.D., associate professor of dermatology and chief of Mohs surgery at New York University Medical Center.

## ABOUT COLON CANCER

People with active jobs get less colon cancer, a new study reports. Researchers divided patients' occupations into three categories: Sedentary, moderate- and high-activity. Those in such sedentary jobs as bookkeeping and computer operating had a 60% greater risk of colon cancer than high-activity workers, including auto mechanics and plumbers. More job activity appears to stimulate contractions that move waste material (assumed to contain carcinogens) through the colon. The faster waste is removed from the body, the less risk of colon cancer, researchers said.

## DIET AND COLON CANCER

A high-fiber diet isn't the only way to help prevent colon cancer. Other prevention methods: Daily milk (for calcium), daily sun exposure (20 minutes for a day's worth of vitamin D) and regular exercise.

**Source:** *American Health*, New York.

• Anti-cancer food. Fifty-percent of all colon cancers and polyps are directly related to diet and nutrition. Dietary changes can cut your risks: Stay on a life-long diet of at least 32 grams of fiber per day. Get this by eating oranges, grapefruit, apples, leafy green vegetables, carrots, tomatoes, whole grain products.

**Source:** *Seminars in Oncology*, New York.

• Seventh-Day Adventist vegetarians have a 40% lower risk of intestinal cancer than the general population.

**Source:** Memorial Sloan-Kettering Cancer Center, New York.

## COLOSTOMY MYTH

Treatment for colon or rectal cancer usually results in a colostomy. Fact: Advanced surgical technique has generally eliminated the need for colostomy in treating cancer of the colon. In rectal cancer, only one of seven surgery patients requires a colostomy. Bottom line: Early treatment of these cancers could increase the five-year cure rate from 44% to 75%—saving 40,000 lives each year.

**Source:** Sidney J. Winawer, M.D., chief of the gastroenterology service, Memorial Sloan-Kettering Cancer Center, New York City.

## HOW LONG CAN YOU EXPECT TO LIVE?

Longevity myth: With improvements in diet and disease prevention, it's now possible to achieve a "longevity breakthrough" well beyond 100 years. Fact: There is no evidence that maximum potential lifespan has been extended beyond the 85–100 years that's now normal in many developed societies.

**Source:** *Journal of American Geriatrics Society*, Philadelphia, PA.

• Women are now expected to live to the age of 86 and men to 74. Until recently the Census Bureau was predicting life expectancy up to the year 2000 at only 70 for men and 78 for women. Reason for the new figures: An unexpected decline in deaths from some major diseases over the past decade, including heart disease, stroke, diabetes and pneumonia among those over 65.

**Source:** *Perspective, New York.*

## KEYS TO LONGEVITY

(1) Commitment. To get involved in whatever you're doing. . .(2) Control. To feel you have influence in confronting life's contingencies. . .(3) The ability to meet challenge. To view change as a natural part of life, an opportunity rather than a threat.

**Source:** Dr. Suzanne Kobasa, in a study at the University of Chicago.

## PRIMER ON LIFE EXTENSION

Scientists now think that it is no longer a question of whether we will be able to extend human life, but when. Aging is a more limited and mechanical process than had been thought, and some of the hottest new biomedical research is uncovering the mechanisms by which animals—and people—age.

Specific hormones, enzymes and genes are responsible for promoting or inhibiting various aspects of aging. Scientists are trying to understand how these substances work on a physiologic level, so that they can learn to manipulate them and intervene in the aging process. Some of this manipulation has already been tried in the laboratory—with impressive results. Life spans of some animals have been doubled. And there are many experiments in which longevity has been increased 20%, 30% or 40%.

Why has life extension become a hot area of interest now as opposed to, say, five years ago?

Until recently, aging research was a kind of fringe or quack area of biology. It was the kind of thing that retired physiologists would go into. Several things helped boost the field, however. The discovery of DNA (the basic hereditary material) provided the basis of today's aging research. And new genetic engineering techniques have helped, too. Also, the explosion of the over-65 population has given impetus to gerontology as an important specialty. With the establishment of the National Institute on Aging in 1976, the area was stamped as legitimate. Before the NIA, one had to bootleg research on aging by borrowing money from other grants. Now there is money coming into the field directly.

What is the aging process? How does it work?

Aging is a developmental process, like growth and maturation. Although we have bits and pieces of the puzzle, no one knows yet exactly how it works as a system. Most of the theories can be grouped under a genetic umbrella. In fact, one of the hopeful things we have discovered is that aging is regulated by a small number of genes. (The more dispersed the regulation system through the genes, the harder it would be to manipulate.) We've been able to identify one group of key genes—that's the major histocompatibility complex.

Is that the "supergene"?

Yes. The name refers to its broad immune system responsibilities. It regulates DNA repair and enzymes, such as P-450, which detoxify pollutants in the environment. Remember, the immune system is the pacemaker of aging—it declines with age, eventually turning upon itself and becoming self-destructive. The fundamental cause of aging, however, remains at the level of the genes. They, of course, act via the immune system.

What is the most significant work going on in the field at the moment?

Dr. Takashi Makinodan of the Veterans Administration Hospital in Los Angeles has found that weekly injections of a drug called 2-mercaptoethanol (2ME) into aged mice may break certain cross-links that develop with age in genetic material. Cross-links are probably responsible for the general rigidification of the body, including loss of skin elasticity and hardening of the muscles, arteries, etc., with age. Cross-linking refers to molecules that actually become linked together to form a rigid structure instead of freely moving units, as in younger tissue.

Anything else?

Yes, there's interesting work going on with hormones produced by the thymus gland (thymosin). These hormones may be used to beef up the body's natural defense network and to slow or even reverse some of the immune deficiencies of aging. Nobel Prize laureate Sir Macfarlane Burnet has speculated that the thymus gland (located in the middle of the chest) may be a primary pacemaker for aging. It shrinks as we grow older, and because it's the master gland of the immune system, this shrinkage may be responsible for the falloff in immune capacity, which, I've already mentioned, is closely linked with aging. Small quantities of thymus hormones may slow aspects of the aging process over time. The

key would be to mass-produce the substances so that more tests can be performed.

What about "free radicals?" Why are they damaging?

"Free radicals" are naturally occurring substances in our bodies, our food and the air we breathe that attack cell membranes, destroy DNA and the DNA repair mechanisms, initiate cross-linking and generally promote aging. Examples of free radicals are singlet oxygen, superoxide and hydrogen peroxide. The body produces its own enzymes to attack these free radicals, but Dr. Denham Harman of the University of Nebraska has shown convincingly that supplementing the diet with substances called free radical scavengers will substantially increase life span in animals. (Free radical scavengers are also called anti-oxidants because they act on substances that oxidize tissue—the way oxygen causes iron to rust.)

What are free radical scavengers?

You're already familiar with some of them. Vitamin C is one. Vitamin E is another. The element selenium and several sulfur-containing amino acids such as cysteine are also anti-oxidants. Many people are surprised that BHT, the food preservative, is also a powerful free radical scavenger. It has been shown to increase life span in experiments with mice by as much as 30%. The supplements I just mentioned are part of my diet regimen and are all anti-oxidants.

**Source:** Interview with Roy L. Walford M.D., who directs the immunology and aging research laboratory at UCLA Medical School. He is also a member of the White House Conference on Aging and Chairman of the National Institute on Aging, Task Force in Immunology.

## HAPPINESS DOESN'T END AT 55

In our youth-oriented culture, the idea that older people are less satisfied with life is generally accepted. This is not true. Older people tend to expect less, and, therefore, they usually adjust more easily to changes. They are more inclined to look on the bright side of situations.

**Source:** Results of a survey of 9,000 workers of all ages made by Anna Herzog and colleagues for the University of Michigan.

## AGES OF GREATEST HAPPINESS

The greatest happiness usually comes not in youth, but in old age. Men generally are happiest during their middle sixties, women, during their seventies. Unhappiest time: Early fifties for men, late forties for women.

**Source:** *Pathfinders* by Gail Sheehy, William Morrow & Co., New York.

## BEST RESISTERS OF AGE

Our personalities needn't grow old. Although the machine we call our body changes, even breaks down, the thing inside that says "I" can remain quite constant. Who resists age the best: Creative people.

**Source:** Observations of British poet Stephen Spender.

## EARLY RETIREMENT CONTROVERSY

• Retirement is not responsible for a decline in health, contrary to the prevailing belief. The Veterans Administration recently examined 200 retired men aged 55-70, along with 409 men of comparable age who had continued to work. Result: The retired men were no more likely to suffer from health problems than were the working men.

**Source:** Report in the *American Journal of Public Health, New York.*

• Early retirement could shorten your life. A survey showed that men who retired at 62 died younger than those who worked until 65. At age 74, the survival rate for the later retirees was 13% higher. Trap: Boredom often leads to overeating, oversleeping and inactivity, which, in turn, increase vulnerabililty to heart attack.

**Source:** A government study of 64,000 people born between 1900 and 1910, reported in *American Health, New York.*

## SEX AND AGING

Contrary to general belief, sex remains a vital part of most people's lives into their seventies and even beyond. A survey of 4,246 men and women aged 50–93 found that:

• More than 75% of married couples in their sixties have intercourse. Average frequency: Once a week.

• More than three-quarters of single men (widowed, divorced or never married) remain sexually active in their seventies. So do half the single women that age.

• Six out of 10 married couples in their seventies still have regular intercourse. Average frequency: Three times a month.

• Common ailments (arthritis, diabetes, heart disease) cause little decline in sexual activity.

**Source:** *Love, Sex and Aging: A Consumers' Union Report* by Edward M. Brecher and the editors of Consumer Reports Books, Little, Brown and Co., Boston.

## AGING AND THE MIND

Forgetful older people may be the victims of a self-fulfilling prophecy. In fact, recent research suggests that people's ability to make complex judgments and solve problems increases well into their eighties, assuming they stay healthy.

What older people lose: Abstract reasoning abilities (used in situations such as playing chess). But even here the decline is generally slight and slow.

Who loses the least: People who are socially involved, mentally active, and flexible in dealing with new experiences. Key: You'll stay sharper if you reject the stereotype of a helpless old age.

**Source:** Research by John Horn, psychologist, University of Denver, reported in *The New York Times.*

## HELP FOR FADING MEMORY

Short-term memory tends to fade as you age. But you can stay sharper longer by avoiding vitamin deficiencies (particularly of $B_{12}$). . . limiting yourself to no more than two alcoholic drinks a day. . . keeping your blood pressure down. . . staying mentally active through reading, writing, crossword puzzles, etc.

**Source:** *The Washingtonian, Washington, D.C.*

• Egg-yolk extract may help people with mildly impaired memories, according to recent research. The substance (active ingredient: lecithin) apparently makes aging brain cell membranes more flexible by displacing cholesterol deposits. Another use for the extract: Easing the withdrawal symptoms of alcoholics and drug addicts.

**Source:** Research by David Samuel M.D., head of the Center for Neurosciences and Behavioural Research, Weizmann Institute of Science, Rehovot, Israel, in *Medical World News, New York.*

• Walking helps to keep your mind young, according to a recent study of 200 elderly people. After a four-month program, the subjects all showed improvement in reaction time, short-term memory and reasoning power.

**Source:** Study by the Veterans Administration.

## SENILITY'S EARLIEST SIGNS

Poor memory and decreased concentration. These may be related to poor nutrition. It was observed that individuals without good diets and adequate vitamin intake were the first to suffer these mental insufficiencies.

**Source:** *Journal of the American Medical Association,* Chicago, IL.

## UNDERSTANDING AGING

Contrary to popular myth, the psychological problems caused by the stress of the aging process can be treated successfully. With properly supervised medication and psychological intervention, many disorders in thinking and behavior to which aged people are subject can be minimized and, frequently, reversed.

Stress factors that contribute to problems of aging: In addition to the normal declines in intellectual function and memory that are to be expected, elderly people also must cope with the increased likelihood of physical illness, loss of family and friends and often a general loss of esteem in the community. These factors produce tremendous stress of the kind that frequently leads to mental confusion and depression. Organic Mental Syndrome (OMS) is a state in which the elderly person becomes disoriented and suffers intellectual impairment of a fairly constant kind. The important thing is to recognize that some kinds of OMS are reversible. It should be determined at the outset which sort the elderly person has.

A confused state of long duration is not necessarily irreversible. There are many long-standing conditions that can cause such confusion. The reversal or amelioraton of these conditions will, most of the time, lead to reversal of the elderly person's symptoms. Most common causes of reversible OMS:

• Medication. This can cause problems because of the drug itself or because the person has taken an overdose, as elderly people frequently do. Just about any kind of medication can cause confusion of this sort. Elderly people are extremely susceptible to drugs. Reasons: The liver and the kidneys, which excrete drugs, don't work as efficiently in old people as in younger ones. Drugs remain in their bodies longer. Fat, which stores drugs, is present in a higher ratio in the bodies of old people. Cardiac function is not as good in an old person, so not enough blood gets to the brain. Result: Drugs build up unpredictably in the body and cause confusion. It is vital to carefully supervise any medication old people take.

• An undetected illness. This includes heart conditions, abdominal problems, cancer and diabetes. Undetected diabetes is a particularly common cause of confusion in persons of any age, including children. Even a minor infection, such as an upper respiratory infection that would make a younger person merely sick, can cause OMS in an old person. Other causes: Thyroid abnormality, alcoholism, nutritional deficiencies and anemia.

• Disorientation. The simple fact of being put in a hospital for any ailment can lead to a state of confusion in an old person.

Common effects of OMS: Old people very often become paranoid as a result of their confusion. It's very hard for old people to admit to themselves that they've misplaced an item, or that they don't know what's going on, or that they've forgotten something. As a result, they make up stories. "The building superintendent stole my watch." "My daughter stole my dress." Paranoid states of this kind are eminently treatable. In fact, this is the easiest OMS condition to reverse. It responds very quickly and very well to low doses of a major tranquilizer. The side effects are very few, but careful supervision of old people taking this drug is still important. Buildup in the system can lead to over-sedation.

Depression is a very common cause of confusion in the elderly. It can be treated with a high degree of success by an anti-depression medication such as Elavil. Possible complications of antidepressant drugs: They can be dangerous to old people with cardiac problems. A good many old people are easily over-sedated by them. They also sometimes cause orthostatic hypertension, a condition in which the blood pressure doesn't rise quickly enough when a person moves from a sitting to a standing position. This can result in fainting or falling. Other possible side effects: Constipation, urinary retention, dryness of mouth and glaucoma.

What to do when an old person shows symptoms of OMS:

• Avoid arguments and head-on confrontations with them. Old people who insist that someone is stealing from them will continue to protect their stories. It's useless to tell them it's not true or to imply that their confusion is caused by mental deterioration. It is far better to be understanding and to begin establishing more structure in the old person's life. Check up on the elderly on a regular basis, or arrange homemaker visits.

• Don't assume that they can continue to take care of themselves. Old people who show signs of confusion should not, for example, be permitted to ride a bus alone. And don't fall into the error of refusing to acknowledge that the old person has become confused or is showing signs of disordered behavior at home. Very often, not only the old people deny they have a problem—their children or other relatives deny it as well.

• Arrange for a thorough physical examination. If the symptoms are especially severe, that should include a neurological workup with a brain scan. But don't stop with a physical or allow a general practitioner or anyone else to decide there's "no more to do" for the old person. The next step should be a geriatric center, which specializes in medical and psychological problems of the aged. Aim: To determine whether the OMS is reversible. A neurological exam and psychological testing can usually determine that very quickly.

Where to go for help:

• Hospitals. Most of them have geriatric centers. Any hospital should be able to refer you to a geriatric internist and psychiatrist.

• Social agencies for the aged. Virtually all have resources that can help in arranging treatment by geriatric specialists. They can also help arrange for home care or visiting nurses and provide information about what benefits are available from Medicaid and

Medicare. They can give information about the many benefits available in areas such as housing. Many benefits are available for elderly people, despite the recent government cuts.

• Day hospitals. These are places where elderly people can spend the day in activities that help increase reality-orientation or in other supervised recreation. Day hospitals can enormously ease the burden of caring for a confused elderly person.

• Senior citizens centers. These are important resources, like the day hospitals, which can provide the day-to-day structure that elderly people need in their lives. It's important that the elderly person who shows signs of confusion not be allowed to sit home staring at the four walls all day. (This is also true for elderly people who are not confused.) Senior citizens centers are equipped to handle confusion if it is not too severe.

**Source:** Inteview with Michael Levy, M.D., a psychiatrist in private practice, New York.

## ALUMINUM AND ALZHEIMER'S DISEASE

What exactly is Alzheimer's disease?

Alzheimer's disease is a progressive degenerative disease referred to as "senile dementia." First identified as a specific neurological disease in 1906, today, Alzheimer's disease has been estimated to be the fourth leading cause of death among the elderly. The disease frequently starts with simple memory loss and ends by depriving its victims of speech, thinking, memory, perception and the ability to process visual and auditory impulses. Eventually, the ability to walk and eat are also lost, and death most frequently comes as the result of pneumonia.

How is aluminum implicated?

An elevated level of aluminum has been found in the nuclei of the nerve cells affected by Alzheimer's disease. This is not a haphazard accumulation of aluminum throughout the brain but a concentration of it in the specific areas that the disease has damaged. In areas of the brain not affected by the disease, there is no abnormal elevation of aluminum. The aluminum seems to produce damage that prevents normal utilization of calcium ions, which are essential for neuronal function. So it's not necessarily true that aluminum is toxic in itself. Rather, aluminum apparently prevents normal metabolism of calcium and possibly of other essential nutrients.

What do we do about it all?

In our research we are trying to determine whether protecting the Alzheimer's disease victim from aluminum will either slow down or arrest the progression of the disease. We've postulated the existence of a protective barrier against aluminum in the body that Alzheimer's disease victims lack. We must assume that you and I, since we're all exposed to aluminum, have natural protection against it. But it might be the other way around . . . people might get Alzheimer's disease first and then become vulnerable to aluminum as a result of the disease. The answers aren't yet in. Ours is a long-term study, and we're far from drawing conclusions.

What information do you have now?

Some researchers have concluded that Alzheimer's disease is caused by aluminum. This is not the case. Although the specific cause of Alzheimer's disease has not yet been determined, we do know many factors are involved, including genetic and environmental ones. Aluminum is an environmental factor. All that can be said with certainty is that aluminum figures prominently in the chain of events leading to the development of Alzheimer's disease.

Can people be protected from aluminum?

We began to look at ways to protect people who already have Alzheimer's disease from aluminum. This is difficult, if not impossible. Aluminum is the most common metal in the earth's crust, and we are in contact with it through our water, grain, meat, milk . . . you name it. It's in the food chain. You can reduce the amount of aluminum you ingest by avoiding aluminum-containing man-made substances such as antacids, baking soda, aluminum foil, aluminum pots, deodorants, etc. But these are minor factors. Simple and clear: After every meal, the level of aluminum in the blood serum of every human being becomes elevated. There is no way to avoid the aluminum in what we eat.

Have pollution and technology increased the level of aluminum we ingest, maybe dangerously?

There's a legitimate concern as to what extent we have increased the amount of aluminum in the food chain. For example, some fertilizers contain aluminum. And acid rain increases the aluminum in the soil because aluminum is readily soluble in acid. But remember that when Alzheimer described the disease in 1906, there was no acid rain or aluminum pots. Actually Alzheimer's disease has always existed . . . The symptoms of "senility" have been noted since antiquity. Eventually, we may have to take a hard look at how we purify our water, bake bread with baking soda, use fertilizers, and so on. But we'll need more evidence before that.

What can people do to reduce their risk of getting Alzheimer's disease?

I don't believe in alarmist approaches. It's foolish to think that if you throw away your aluminum pots and stop using baking soda, aluminum foil or aluminum-containing antacids, you'll be safe from Alzheimer's disease. Nothing could be farther from the truth. Some people even speak against aluminum-containing deodorants, although there's no evidence that aluminum can be absorbed through the skin. However, someone who is developing Alzheimer's disease would probably be wise to cut back on these things, since it's possible that a lot of aluminum might accelerate the progress of the disease. But the general population should follow common sense. If it's just as easy to wrap food in plastic and take non-aluminum antacids, you might as well.

Are there any other preventive measures people can take?

It seems to me that there might be some value in zinc, which has been used experimentally to prevent some of the damage done by aluminum. This doesn't mean one should take in too much zinc, but rather eat a well-balanced diet that includes normal amounts of zinc. (The US recommended daily allowance is 15 milligrams.) Apparently overindulgence in alcohol helps aluminum from the normal diet to enter the brain. So, cutting down on alcohol may be helpful. The old rule about moderation is a good one—avoid extremes.

**Source:** Interview with Leopold Liss, an M.D., in neuropathology and professor of pathology and psychiatry at Ohio State University, Columbus OH.

## EXERCISE HELPS THE ELDERLY

Exercise keeps the joints from becoming stiff and immobile and may even strengthen the bones themselves. Reason: The pull of muscles on bones often stimulates the bones to acquire calcium. Best exercises: Flexing and stretching. Gently bend, extend or rotate the neck, shoulders, elbows, back, hips, knees and ankles. Best aerobic exercise: Walking. Also beneficial: Swimming, dancing, riding and using an exercise bicycle.

**Source:** *Consumer Info Center, Pueblo, Co.*

## HOW MUCH WATER SHOULD YOU DRINK?

An aging body needs at least six glasses of water every day. Reason: A young adult's body is 60% water, but this amount decreases with age. Results: Skin dries out, and the kidneys do not flush wastes as well. Drinking more water means the skin has less chance of becoming dry. And the water dilutes the salts and minerals that pass through the kidneys, helping to prevent the formation of kidney stones. Suggestion: Have a glass of water with every meal and another before going to bed. Take the other two glasses during breaktime. Substitute water for that second and third cup of coffee.

## SUGAR ALERT

Sugar is also tougher on your body as you grow older. Healthy people, ages 22–30, have twice the insulin-binding abilities of people ages 40–59. Result: Older people become more glucose-intolerant.

**Source:** *Diabetes, New York.*

## FOSTER GRANDPARENTS: SUPPORT SYSTEM FOR TROUBLED KIDS

The inspired matching up of retired older Americans who have time on their hands with handicapped children who need patient, regular companionship and guidance is a legacy of the 1960's federal poverty program.

Volunteer citizens bring their tender, loving care and attention to young clients—who need it as much as medicine, food and shelter. This fills an urgent need at short-staffed institutions, whether for the mentally retarded and emotionally disturbed, the pediatric wards of general hospitals, rehabilitation centers for the physically handicapped or correctional facilities, day-care centers or schools.

Many of these volunteer efforts are organized by the institutions themselves or by local social-service agencies. Volunteers receive orientation and training before they start, and supervision and counseling are available on the job. Tasks vary from feeding and dressing a child, playing games, reading stories and working on specific physical therapies, to simply offering un-threatening companionship for a few hours a week.

For many of the children served, the foster grandparent represents the only meaningful adult relationship in a troubled life. Watching a youngster learn to trust another human being or master a skill can be very rewarding.

The government-sponsored Foster Grandparents Program, given a boost by First Lady Nancy Reagan's 1982 book, also offers financial assistance to low-income senior citizens who sign up. Eligible people must be at least 60, in good health, and below a particular income level (around $5,000) which differs from state to state. For 20 hours of "grandparenting" per week, each volunteer receives a $2-an-hour stipend, transportation, a daily meal, an annual physical examination and some insurance coverage. Administered by ACTION,* the federal volunteer service agency, the program reaches almost 55,000 children.

**Source:** *For information on the government program: Write to ACTION, Washington, DC 20525.

# AGING PARENTS

Before letting them move in with you, consider. . .who will bear the brunt of the extra work? Is that person willing? Are there any old family feuds that could flare up? On the other hand, grandparents are often revitalized by their grandchildren. And the children enjoy contact with an older person as confidant and guide rather than authority figure. If you can't take your parents in, remember that regular, supportive contact is more important than money, whether they live independently or in a nursing home.

**Source:** Stanley Cath, M.D., Family Advisory and Treatment Center, Belmont, MA, cited in *Levinson Letter*, Cambridge, MA.

# HELP IN CARING FOR AN ELDERLY PARENT IN ANOTHER CITY

As our population becomes older and more mobile, a growing number of middle-aged people are trying to care for elderly parents or relatives who live a considerable distance away. Even if the relative is nearby, the busy "child" simply may not have the time or skills to devote to caretaking. Government services are little or no help, since they're focused mainly on the indigent, not on the older person who has been prudent enough to plan ahead. People who have any kind of means generally prefer to pay for what they need.

A number of private services have gone into business in response to this need. Usually run by social workers, they find and coordinate services for the elderly who want to remain at home but are no longer able to care totally for themselves.

### How They Work

Agencies provide what they call "case management." This includes the following:

• Assessing the individual situation, either in the home or at their office. The assessment determines what is needed. This can include anything from helping balance a checkbook once a month to supervision of 24-hour-a-day nursing care.

• Finding the right staff to do what is needed. As professionals in the field, these agencies know where to locate reliable housekeepers, homemakers, cooks, nurses, physical therapists, companions and medical assistants. They interview and check references on whoever is hired. Even out-of-the-ordinary needs can be filled.

• Supervising whatever arrangement is made. This is one of the most valuable services provided. You can hire help on your own to care for a parent, but there is no guarantee that the person you hire will fulfill his or her responsibilities.

Good supervision should consist of:

• Managing money.

• Submitting bills to lawyers and families.

• Checking on whether the client is getting regular exercise and recreation.

• Checking medication.

• Determining the need for psychological or other consultation.

• Making sure medical appointments are kept.

• Assessing menus, taking into account good nutrition and individual taste and eating habits.

• Handling anything else that comes up.

The case manager should do basically what you would do if you could. She also should take a personal interest in your parent, treating him or her like a human being and taking individual needs, feelings and preferences into account.

Example: One of our clients loved classical music but was too ill to go to concerts any longer. We made sure that recordings of his favorite music were played for him regularly.

### Costs

Private case management isn't cheap, especially considering that the cost is in addition to homemaking, nursing or whatever else is needed. Agencies generally charge about $50 an hour. An initial assessment runs $100–$350. If a medical doctor accompanies the social worker to the home, for instance, the bill will be in the higher range. Monthly case management can run from $500 to $1,000 for supervision of a round-the-clock situation. Some agencies bill on a flat-fee basis rather than hourly. If less service is needed, the bill will be lower.

When calculating costs, take into account fees of approximately $6–$18 an hour for homemaking or nursing, depending on the level of care needed, plus case management.

### Evaluating Agencies

What to ask:

• Will the agency do an assessment in the home? (Some do only a phone or office in-terview with you.) A home assessment is important, to see how the elderly person relates to the environment and to determine if any structural changes can be made to improve safety or comfort.

• What is your gut feeling about the case manager? Experience and a caring attitude can be more important than fancy credentials.

• Will the agency be on call 24 hours a day? Will it give you a home phone for after-hours emergencies?

• Does the agency have access to and familiarity with the latest medical home-care equipment, such as heart monitoring?

• Will the case manager visit your parent's home at least once a week?

• Can the agency have a private ambulance summoned if necessary, or is it dependent on public services?

• Will the agency give you and your family regular reports and tell you about anything else that might relieve your anxiety? Will it give you advice on how to deal with your sick relative?

• Is there an M.D. on its staff who can consult with the family physician? Does it have access to psychiatric consultants and other medical consultants?

• Will the agency tell you when it thinks the time has come for nursing-home care? At a certain point, your parent's home can become more of a jail than a home.

### How to Find a Good Agency

This is the hard part. A recent Brown University study counted 22 such private agencies in seven states. These don't even begin to fill the need. Indications are, however, that new services will be springing up in response to the burgeoning demand.

Our agency will help you find a social worker or agency in any area of the country to assess an elderly parent's condition and arrange for necessary services. There is also a national consultation service in Maryland that makes such referrals.*

Other sources:

• The local Congressional office in your parent's district is a good place to start and should give you a few leads.

• Geriatric lawyers offer a new specialty for protecting the assets of the elderly. Ask your own lawyer for a referral, or try a few trust and estate lawyers. Geriatric lawyers are trust and estate specialists.

• The local university may have a gerontology program, which gives a new master's degree in the care of the elderly. You might find an individual or agency through such a program.

*Aging Network Services, Suite 821, 7315 Wisconsin Ave. West, Bethesda, MD, 20814.

**Source:** Interview with gerontologist Gloria A. Scherma and psychiatrist Kenneth L. Caccavale, M.D., directors of Multi-Comprehensive Consulting Service, Inc., a private agency providing case management for the elderly, located in New York.

## HOW TO FIND A GOOD NURSING HOME

Most families postpone as long as possibile the decision to use a nursing home. Once the decision is reached, the process of selecting a good facility is so painful that often they move too fast. Good advice: Give your parent time to get used to the idea. Meanwhile, investigate every possible choice thoroughly.

How to begin: Get lists of not-for-profit, community-based homes from your church, fraternal order, state agency on aging, American Association of Homes for the Aging (Suite 770, 1050 17th St., NW, Washington, DC 20036), or American Health Care Association (1200 15th St., NW, Washington, DC 20005).

Costs: If your parent's resources are small, Medicaid may provide financial support for nursing home care. Homes offering complete care in metropolitan areas usually charge $50–$80 per day (depending on the amount of care required). Some require a large advance gift or admission fee. (Health insurance sometimes covers nursing homes.) Patients paying their own way may be eligible for Medicaid assistance after their savings run out. Check the rules in your state.

### Evaluating a Nursing Home

1. Accreditation, license, and certification for Medicare and Medicaid should be current and in force.

2. Best to arrive without an appointment. Look at everything. The building and room should be clean, attractive, safe, and meet all fire codes. Residents should not be crowded (ask about private rooms; sometimes they're available at a reasonable extra cost). Visit dining rooms at mealtime. Check kitchen, too. Visit activity rooms when in session. Talk to residents to find out how they feel about the home.

3. Staff should be professionally trained and large enough to provide adequate care for all residents.

4. If the home requires a contract, read it carefully. Show it to your lawyer before signing. Some homes reserve the right to discharge a patient whose condition has deteriorated even if a lump-sum payment was made upon admittance. Best: An agreement that allows payment by the month, or permits refunds or advance payment if plans change.

5. Find out exactly what services the home provides and which ones cost extra. Private duty nurses are not included. Extras like shampoo and hairset, can be exorbitant. (A box of tissues can cost a dollar.) Make a list of the "extras" your parents will need for a comfortable life. Try to supply some of them yourself.

Before you decide on a home, you and your parent should have a talk with the administrator and department heads. Find out who is in charge of what, and whom to speak to if problems arise.

**Source:** Sheldon Goldberg, Am. Assn. of Homes for the Aging.

## MORE ON HOW TO PICK A NURSING HOME

Placing a troubled, dependent relative in a nursing home is a heart-wrenching ordeal. To ease the way, know when a nursing home is the only answer. Deciding factors: When there is a loss of control of bodily functions, a loss of memory or an inability to perform the basic activities of daily life, such as shopping, cleaning and dressing. People do not age physically and emotionally at the same rate.

Never coerce a person into a nursing home. Rather, open the decision for discussion. When possible, have the person accompany you when you shop for the proper home.

The nursing homes with the best reputations, highest staff-to-patient ratios and longest waiting lists are non-profit. That is, they are run by churches, fraternal orders and charities. Hitch: Only about 25% of all homes are non-profit.

The majority of nursing homes are for profit, or proprietary. Other differences among homes:

• Health-related facilities emphasize personal, not medical care. These are generally non-profit homes.

• Skilled nursing facilities are for patients with serious mental and physical disabilities. Most of these places are proprietary.

Non-profit homes usually charge a flat, high monthly fee with no extras for added services. Proprietary homes ask a lower monthly fee with extra payments for services. Always be certain that you understand the rates and service charge.

Many proprietary homes don't take Medicaid patients. The amounts paid by the state and federal health plans aren't always enough to cover the costs. Patients without any money should be placed in a non-profit home.

To select a home, start by asking the patient's physician, relatives and friends who have gone through a similar experience for information. Also, get information from the state departments of health and social services.

Begin the search long before it becomes necessary to find a home. Caution: Many emotional problems among the elderly occur during the waiting period because of the stress of being in limbo.

Since this is an emotional experience, take a close friend with you when you inspect nursing homes. The person will look for things that you forget.

What to seek in a home:

• Good location. The right home is close enough for convenient visits. Avoid places in run-down or dangerous neighborhoods. Best: A residential area with gardens and benches.

• Well-lit, cheery environment. Doors to the room shouldn't have windows. This is a home, not a hospital.

• The home's affiliations with hospitals and associations. And, find out how many patients are on Medicaid. If the number exceeds 50%, the home is not likely to provide adequate care.

• A professional staff. There should be a full-time or regularly visiting doctor with specialized knowledge in geriatrics. The total number of registered nurses, licensed practical nurses and nurses' aides should be at least 40% of the number of beds.

• The residents. Nothing speaks better for a nursing home than active, vital patients. Observe the staff to see if they treat residents with respect. Talk to the residents and ask for their complaints. Bad signs: If more than 3% of the residents are in the hospital at one time. If patients are still in bed or in bedclothes at 11 A.M. If many residents are catheterized to avoid linen-changing. Ask what happens when a patient is hospitalized. Is the nursing home bed still available afterwards?

• Handrails in hallways and bathrooms.

• Smoke alarms in public areas and each room. Ask to see the latest fire inspection report and note the date.

• The dining room should be clean, bright and inviting, with no dirty trays around. Are special diets adhered to ?

• The residents' rooms should be comfortable and attractively furnished. Be sure the room can be personalized with pictures, plants, knick-knacks. Drawers should be lockable.

• Happy patients are those plugged into the outside world. Newspapers and large-print books should be readily available. The home should show movies, bring in entertainers and provide outside trips. Other necessary activities: Gardening, workshops, education courses, lecture series and discussion groups. Find out about religious services and provisions for voting.

• Special services should include visits by a licensed physical therapist and workable therapy equipment that the patients can use. Visits by other specialists: Speech therapists for stroke victims, audiologists, dentists, psychiatrists, optometrists and podiatrists.

What to watch out for:

• Patients who are sedated to keep them quiet.

• The home asks for a large sum of money up front.

• Doctors who hold gang visits (they see 40–50 patients during each call).

• You are denied visiting rights to the kitchen, laundry and library.

• The Patient's Bill of Rights isn't displayed.

Before you leave: Stand in the home and feel the ambience. Ask yourself if you would like to live there. Return to the place several times. Arrive at least once unannounced. The best time to visit is 11 A.M. or 7 P.M.

To monitor nursing homes for abuses: Put small pen marks on the patient's body and bandages to check frequency of bathing and bandage changes. Visit at mealtime. Get weekly weight checks of the patient to be sure nutrition is adequate. Learn the names of the nurses and aides on all shifts to determine who's responsible for the patient's care.

**Source:** Texans for Improvement of Nursing Homes, Houston.

# 10. Discovering the Best in You

# Discovering the Best in You

## HOW TO HELP YOUR BRAIN

The brain works best in a cool room (65° Fahrenheit). Also helpful: (1) Diffused light (either natural or artificial light reflected from the ceiling and walls). (2) Upright posture, with the back bent slightly forward.

**Source:** *The Brain Book* by Peter Russell, E.P. Dutton, Inc., New York.

## SOME PLAIN TRUTHS ABOUT YOUR BRAIN

A popular misconception concerning human potential is that only 10% of the brain is ever utilized. This leads to the logical assumption that 90% of the brain is idle, waiting to be activated. Common belief: If people could only learn to stimulate and direct that latent brainpower, they could accomplish the work of a genius.

Plain truth: The brain does not lie 90% fallow awaiting the proper inspiration. That statement about 10% of the brain being in use is perpetuated by purveyors of the human-potential movement. The brain cannot be increased tenfold through application and drive. It's an illusion that vast multiples of brainpower are available. Although additional skills requiring greater application of the brain can be learned, they require special methods of application.

### Some Truths and Fallacies

• The quest to master such skills as deductive reasoning, musical achievement, martial arts, meditation or creative expression requires an enormous investment of time and effort. Fallacy: The messianic, utopian concept that relies on tapping the power of the unused brainpower. Fact: This leaves out the most important ingredient—the work effort.

• Innate abilities are important. There are several forms of intelligence, which include the verbal, logical, spatial, musical and interpersonal abilities, as well as the body abilities of athletes and dancers. The brain has many capacities, but most people have innate abilities in only a few of these areas, not in all. Fallacy: You can become an accomplished master in anything you attempt if only you can persuade your brain to cooperate.

• The brain works in ways that are far from understood. The exact function of the "unused" brainpower isn't clear. Indeed, the precise—or even approximate—amount of unused brainpower isn't provable in any way. Little of the brain is a wasteland—each portion has its purpose. Example: Memory is apparently spread around the brain mass, and any bit of a memory can reconstruct the entire experience. Thus the brain has the tremendous ability to reduplicate itself. If parts of the brain are damaged or destroyed, the remaining portions can often take up much of the load without serious impairment of human activity. In this way, most of the brain is in use all of the time. It is not lying idle.

• The brain has a built-in rate of forgetfulness. While a person strains to fill the brain's neurons with new information, the brain is busy actively unloading previously stored information. Needed: A sophisticated, realistic awareness of those factors in order to achieve personal growth.

### Personal Growth

• Personal growth is a positive commitment that is aided by in-depth reading and conversations with those who have done it. Search out people who are skilled in a field in which you wish to advance. Learn about the dedication required and the attitudes that will help to make your effort fruitful.

• Never forget the level of application demanded. Depressing cycle: Beginners start out wildly enthusiastic, eager to master a chosen endeavor, such as playing the violin or unraveling the secrets of Zen. But they have been oversold on self-development without effort, and they quickly become discouraged at the first patch of difficulty. Do experimental trials before making a total commitment. Try a class, session, an interview or book. Be certain you are ready to give yourself to the project.

• Be aware that such achievement requires personal commitment. You must have the fortitude to overcome discouragement, persevere when the spirit is weak and stay with it despite long odds. And—this is not just inspirational verbiage. Many creative people develop blocks from the fear of defeat or failure. The term "writer's block," for example, describes a creative person who has temporarily lost the courage to take the risks that writing entails. Similarly, a "negative attitude" is a defense employed by people hoping to avoid the pain of failure by rejecting their chances of success.

A positive mind-set is best: You are then more likely to be courageous. And it will be easier to find a purpose and the strength to accomplish the objective.

### Bottom Line

All people who are accomplished in a given field share one vital quality—the willingness to work hard. That quality is learned and trainable. Requirement: The willingness to disbelieve those who claim that everything is simple once that mythical 90% of the brain is activated.

Postscript: Some people do not want to make the effort to grow. They are content with what they are, character faults and all. That's all right! Knowing your limits and accepting yourself are also part of realizing your potential.

**Source:** Interview with Martin G. Groder, M.D., a practicing psychiatrist and business consultant in Chapel Hill, NC.

# WORKING FROM BOTH SIDES OF YOUR BRAIN

Have you ever felt "of two minds" about something? There's a valid reason for it. Try this mini-quiz:

1. Without looking at your watch, do you know about what time it is? (a) Yes. (b) No.
2. Do you believe in intuition, hunches and horoscopes? (a) Yes. (b) No.
3. Are you goal-oriented in almost everything you do? (a) Yes. (b) No.
4. As a student, did you prefer (a) algebra or (b) geometry?
5. Would you rather (a) do the talking or (b) listen?
6. Do you prefer your activities to be (a) planned in advance or (b) spontaneous?
7. Are you well-organized, a maker of lists and schedules, etc.? (a) Yes. (b) No.

If your answers are predominantly *a*'s, you are very likely left-brained. Conversely, if most of your answers are *b*'s, your are right-brained. What does this mean?

### The Split-Brain Theory

In 1981, the most exciting news in the scientific community was neurosurgeon Roger Sperry's proof of the split-brain theory, for which he was awarded a Nobel Prize.

Sperry's proof confirms that the two hemispheres of the human brain house separate, though sometimes overlapping, skills. (The two halves communicate through a central connector, the corpus callosum.)

The left brain is logical, verbal and linear, while the right brain is visual, emotional and intuitive. You use your rational left brain to add a line of figures or to make a speech. You use your more spontaneous right brain to imagine yourself on a tropical island as you drive in rush-hour traffic. You shift back and forth between the two hemispheres, depending on the tasks you are performing.

Sperry also proved that individuals tend to prefer one side of the brain to the other. The degree of preference or dominance (known as "brain bias") profoundly affects each person's thinking style, physical and mental abilities, personality and job performance. As people develop and learn to depend on the skills of one half, they tend to neglect the other. Bottom line: Although you cannot change your brain bias, you can develop the abilities of the less-preferred half through exercise and practice. You can increase your brain power by learning to use both sides of your brain.

### Thinking Styles Mirror Brain Bias

One thinking style is not better or smarter than another, any more than right-handed people are more dextrous than left-handed. But your ability to function in the work world is indisputably related to your thinking style and your sensitivity to the styles of others.

Example: A left-brained secretary, typically tidy and efficient, might be driven crazy by a messy, absent-minded ad executive who stares out the window all day. This boss might see the secretary's efforts to impose neatness and order as an irritating waste of time. The secretary, though, would undoubtedly see the exec's daydreaming as unforgivable when he should be clearing his desk. In truth, the left-brained secretary is unable to work efficiently in a cluttered, chaotic environment, while the right-brained ad exec comes up with his best ideas while staring out the window. These co-workers need each other and would get along better if they understood each other's brain bias. The secretary's need for structure and the boss's for flexibility are as real—as physical—as the need for well-fitting shoes or a bright reading lamp.

By learning to recognize the characteristics of brain bias, managers can place their staff in positions that will better suit their talents and temperaments.

### Group Bias

Like individuals, companies, organizations and groups exhibit brain bias as well.

American business (and Western society as a whole) has traditionally valued the skills of the left hemisphere: Logic, speech, attention to detail, efficiency, order. But the most effective managers successfully combine left-brain abilities with creativity, warmth, and the talent to perceive an overall situation—skills from the right hemisphere.

Although the computer has taken over many of the more tedious leftbrain tasks, the spontaneous associations, sensitivity to others and inventiveness of the right brains cannot be replicated. American management (like the much-lauded Japanese) is learning to rely more sincerely on right-brain skills. A study of executives who acknowledged the validity of insights and hunches—right-brain talents—showed that those with the greatest reliance on intuition had the highest profit records.

Some of America's most successful companies are enrolling workshops devoted to whole-brain thinking. Sophisticated tests, including biofeedback, are used to measure brain bias. Exciting new techniques help the individual to develop his or her less-preferred side and to recognize when and how to switch to the "task-appropriate" hemisphere.

For the left-brained, increased access to the right brain leads to improvements in memory, creativity, communication and social skills. The right-brained sharpen their verbal and organizational skills when they learn to "switch left."

### Examples of Switching Techniques

Your mind wanders in meetings (right-brained). Switch left by taking notes or planning a question to ask. Use your right brain to imagine yourself in the speaker's position. Why does he think that point is important? Where did she get her data? You'll find your interest renewed.

You are facing a problem. Use your left brain to define the problem as clearly as you can. Write it down in simple language. Then free your right brain with "internal brainstorming.'" Let your ideas about the problem flow, and jot down or tape your associations, no matter how wild. Include your feelings. Do not stop to judge your thoughts. Later, using your left brain again, evaluate your ideas one at a time, focusing on the useful ones. Finally, employ your whole brain to recognize a solution and to fill in the details.

Additional exercises for problem solving: Imagine the extreme opposite of the situation. Assume the role of someone else. Reverse your objective. Suppose that all your information is wrong.

Learning abilities thrive on challenge, risk and variety. Without these elements, people stagnate.

**Source:** Interview with Jacquelyn Wonder, communications and creative management consultant, Denver corporate seminars.

## NEW THEORY OF INTELLIGENCE

Intelligence is more than verbal and mathematical abilities, according to a new theory. Hypothesis: The brain has six intelligence domains—musical ability, spatial skills, bodily talents and personal abilities, as well as language and logical reasoning skills. These different domains can work separately or they can work together. Note: Different "intelligences" seem to wax and wane at different times during a person's life.

**Source:** *Frames of Mind: The Theory of Multiple Intelligences* by psychologist Howard Gardner, Harvard Unversity, Basic Books, New York.

## TRUTH ABOUT IQ SCORES

IQ Scores and achievement are closely linked in men—but not in women. In one study, two-thirds of the women with genius-level IQs (170 or above) were housewives or office workers.

**Source:** *What's the Difference? How Men and Women Compare* by Jane Barr Stump, William Morrow and Co., Inc., New York.

## AGING ISN'T ALL BAD

Intelligence doesn't necessarily decline with age and neither does an individual's learning ability. Crystallized intelligence—the ability to make judgments and solve problems by using one's accumulated information—actually increases over the years. Memory loss due to age is usually con-

fined to unimportant matters, such as phone numbers. The key factor is mental alertness. People who stay socially and mentally active suffer no decline in mental powers.

**Source:** John Horn, psychologist, University of Denver, University Park, Denver.

## TV AND TEENAGERS

The more junior-high and high-school students watch television, the worse they do on standardized tests. The correlation applies in writing, math, reading and science exams. However, researchers found no comparable relationship between fourth-graders' TV habits and test performance.

**Source:** Study by Illinois State Board of Education.

## HOW TO EXPAND YOUR THINKING POWER

Over the past few years, there have been important developments in our understanding of effective thinking and how to teach it.

Because of the well-publicized decline in Scholastic Aptitude Test scores and other indicators of educational achievement, most of this effort has been directed at students. But there's every reason to believe that many adults suffer from the same kinds of difficulties as schoolchildren. Research shows that the means are now available for adults, as well as children, to improve their reasoning skills

### Reasoning Power

When we think of reasoning, we think of *formal* reasoning—that is, mathematical, logical or symbolic thought. But one of the most important areas in which people need skill is *informal* reasoning. In fact, 99% of our reasoning is informal, the kind you would use to figure out what house to purchase, what stock to invest in, what job to take, to whom you offer a job and so on.

Yet our research shows that four years of high school, four years of college and even four years of graduate school do little to sharpen one's informal reasoning skills.

A characteristic pitfall of informal reasoning is incompleteness. People fail to take advantage of the information they have to investigate an issue throughly. Most people neglect to argue both sides of a case or to develop more than one or two lines of an argument. In informal reasoning, since every line of argument is only probable, not absolute, you need to develop several lines to be convincing.

Example: We did research into how people think about everyday issues such as the litter-reducing effect of a 5¢ deposit on bottles. People commonly give the most obvious response: Litter will be reduced because people will return the bottle to get the 5¢. And that's about it. Or they get a little more sophisticated with: If you return the bottles all at once, it's not such a burden. But these responses aren't sufficient to sort out the issue thoroughly. One overlooked issue, for instance, is that the majority of litterers aren't at home. They are at outdoor picnics or in parks. It's much more of a burden for them to save the bottles than to toss them.

Another pitfall is overlooking counter examples. People are prone to sweeping generalizations. We've done research on statements such as *Art is creative,* a natural, conventional belief. The catch is that there are lots of counterexamples, such as dime-a-dozen ocean scenes or clown paintings. Thinking more acutely will lead to the conclusion that art isn't necessarily more creative than anything else, unless it's original or very unusual.

## Creative Thinking

In this area, there's a gap between understanding and practice. People are full of sensible advice about what to do in difficult situations. They know you should be thorough, use what you know, look at both sides of the question, challenge your own assumptions, try to imagine a different approach to break the mind-set you're in, put the problem aside for a while and come back to it and so on. There's one catch... most people seldom follow their own advice.

## Tricks of the Trade

It's not true that simply knowing a little about how to think well guarantees that one will think well. Forces in human psychology tend to undermine our best thinking. One of the simplest is the effort required. Carefully critical or creative thinking requires more work, exacting a price in terms of effort expended and frustration encountered, even though the result may be better.

Also, your personal bias in favor of a particular conclusion may prevent you from exploring the other side. Just to think in another direction is almost painful because it seems to put at risk everything you've invested so far.

If you pay attention to what you already know about thinking, you'll improve your reasoning skills:

• Using analogies and metaphors. Deliberately ask yourself, What am I assuming? If art is creative, for example, does that mean business is noncreative? This will lead you to think about the real meaning of creativity.

• Not getting bogged down in a particular line of reasoning. Deliberately step outside it. Suggestion: Take 10 minutes to think of the problem in a completely different way. If that doesn't work, you've lost only a little time.

• Paying more attention to the aesthetic aspects of the problem than to the pragmatic ones. The aesthetic and pragmatic are really the same thing seen through different windows. By looking through the aesthetic window, you get a fresh hold on the problem. Example: If you're designing an inventory system, it shouldn't only be functional but should also solve certain difficulties in keeping track of things in an easy, elegant way.

• Looking at how you're being conventional. Break that conventional set. Watch out for cliches. Avoid timeworn and obvious answers.

• Being self-conscious. It's a myth that self-consciousness is a barrier to effective thinking. Be aware of the way you do things. Do you brush aside problems, or do you take them seriously? Do you look for opportunities to think about something a little longer, or do you pass them by? Don't be put off by the initial awkward feeling that self-consciousness will give you. As with any skill, the more you practice, the easier and more natural it becomes.

• Opening up to ideas. Don't dismiss suggestions with "That's just common sense" or "I already do that." Common sense isn't always common practice, and if you think you already do it, you probably don't. Research on actual behavior tells us that people don't accurately perceive whether or not they follow their own advice. Typically, they don't.

If you want to take a course in thinking, look for one that requires a lot of small-group work over a substantial period of time. The one-shot workshop typically washes out in a couple of weeks. The extended program that meets for six to 20 weeks and keeps at the objectives in a persistent, fresh and involving way can really remake a person's pattern of thinking.

Courses are common, but quality differs widely. Investigate of course carefully, including the teacher's credentials, before taking it.

**Source:** Interview with David N. Perkins, Ph.D., senior research associate in education, Graduate School of Education, Harvard University, Cambridge, MA.

## NEW MIND DRUG

Drugs to influence memory, alertness, learning ability and other aspects of human mentality are the most exciting area of new pharmaceuticals research. Most of these "mind" or cognitive activator drugs are still in early testing stages, but overwhelming evidence suggests that deterioration of critical mental processes (like memory) can be stopped—and even reversed.

How cognitive activators work: The basic effect of most of the new drugs is to dilate blood vessels in the brain, thereby increasing the availability of oxygen to cerebral nerve cells. Key: The brain requires vast amounts of oxygen to function op-

timally. (Although the brain accounts for only 2% of our overall body weight, it is responsible for 20% of the body's total oxygen consumption.) This is why an aging-related disorder like hardening of the arteries can have such a devastating effect on memory and alertness.

Cognitive activator drugs are now in development in several countries around the world. One of the most promising is pyritinol.

Increased alertness is pyritinol's almost immediate effect. Although "alertness" may seem difficult to assess, it can be measured on electroencephalograms, the spiky line graphs of brain activity.

Improved endurance and resistance to exhaustive stress are other effects of pyritinol. Animals that had been given pyritinol prior to the commencement of testing on exercise wheels performed better than an untreated control group. Another animal experiment revealed pyritinol's marked protective ability against alcoholic intoxication. Subjects maintained coordination, muscle tone and alertness.

Even more important, pyritinol has been shown to improve short-term memory and immediate retention in healthy human volunteers. The drug enabled them to look at a page and quickly absorb and recall the information. (Heightened capabilities persisted for up to four weeks.)

Pyritinol is manufactured in West Germany by E. Merck.

## VISIT WITH DR. NORMAN VINCENT PEALE

*Editor:* As I passed your church the other day, I saw the notice of your upcoming sermon: "Have a wonderful time living." And I thought, what does "wonderful time" mean? And what does "living" mean?

*Dr. Peale:* "Wonderful" means something happy, pleasant, exciting, satisfying. And living, of course, is the act of survival, from cradle to grave. But there are gradations. Some people merely exist their way through life. Some have pain all the way and never find themselves. So, it's what level you're living on that counts.

To me, "living" would be vigor, enthusiasm, vitality, joy—everything that is positive in nature. I've seen people who are crippled in wheelchairs and who at the same time rise above that because their spirit is victorious. With an indefatigable spirit, you can have a wonderful time living.

*Ed.:* But perhaps you're raising our expectations too much. Isn't it unreasonable to expect every day to be wonderful? There's an awful lot of the day that has to be mundane and ordinary, at best.

*Dr. Peale:* It all depends on the attitude with which you wake up. A man I once knew —he used to write for the old *New York Herald Tribune*—was a philosophical sort of character. When he got out of bed, he projected his day as far as he knew it, and he resolved to do everything that day as best he could. He would be contented and happy, no matter what came along. Then, when he went to bed, he'd go through his day— his "little world," as he put it—and drop out all the unpleasant things. He'd say, "I commit them to oblivion."

*Ed.:* I'm not sure I'd find that so simple.

*Dr. Peale:* You can't always do it. But if you make the effort, you can take the sting out of anything.

The main thing is to keep your attitude up, no matter what. I'm not a Pollyanna, but I go on the theory that everybody is greater than anything that happens to them. If you've got a sound concept of what life is all about—that is, a mixture of laughter and tears, pain and pleasure—you'll be all right.

*Ed.:* Given the mixture, what can we reasonably expect from life?

*Dr. Peale:* You expect the best, and usually you get the best, but anybody's a fool who thinks he won't have a lot of trouble mixed in. Maybe the best day of all is when you have some trouble or pain and overcome it.

You see, life is a mixture of opposites— negatives and positives, good and bad, dark and light. But you can draw out the positives and make them work for you. Every day you'll meet a scoundrel or a fool, but every day you'll also a meet a delightful person. Once, in Rome, I was at the foot of the Spanish Steps. The crowds were surging around, and there was a little boy eight or nine years old with a daisy in his hand. He was studying this flower, totally oblivious to all the confusion around him. And he didn't just tear it apart, either. He'd just lift up a petal and look underneath. So, I'd say he had a wonderful day, and he certainly contributed to mine.

*Ed.:* Speaking of opposites, it seems that people's strengths often turn out to be their weaknesses. If a person is forceful, he forgets he has a softness as well.

*Dr. Peale:* That's true. But the way I see it, even your negatives can be turned around. Years ago, someone said: We become strongest at our weakest place. When a piece of metal breaks, that's its weakest place—the spot where it broke. If you want to put it back together again, you apply heat and weld it. Now, even if that metal broke again, it would probably do so at a different point, because the weakest place is now the strongest one.

If a person has a weakness in his makeup, and he really works on that weakness, in the end he can make it his strongest element. Which is part, I'd say, of living a wonderful life.

**Source:** Interview with Dr. Norman Vincent Peale, who has presided at the pulpit of Marble Collegiate Church in Manhattan for more than half a century. His most popular book is *The Power of Positive Thinking*, Prentice-Hall, Englewood Cliffs, NJ.

## LOOKING AT JOY, PLEASURE AND LIFE

To take full pleasure from life, you must be spontaneous. Most of us are raised to dredge up the past and prepare for the future, rather than simply to enjoy today. And that's a mistake.

When we go to a party, some of us look over our "partner's" shoulder to check who else is coming in, to see where we could be having more fun. We miss so much. When my students ask me, "What are we going to do?" I tell them, "We're already doing it." The only reality is the present. Yesterday is gone, and we can't predict tomorrow. If we lose *now*, we've lost the essence of living.

### To Enjoy Relationships

As you embrace the moment, so you must accept people as they are. Nothing kills a relationship faster than the expectation that you can change someone. It's impossible. Trying to change someone else is a lost cause. The best you can do is to become more tolerant and flexible yourself, to encourage an atmosphere for change, and then hope for the best.

When you meet someone you want to share your life with, stop a moment. Ask yourself: Is this person enough just the way he or she is? If not, watch out. Don't expect strong, silent types suddenly to become demonstrative just because you love them.

Remember that you can never own people, even (and especially) a lover. You have to merit those you care about and work at the relationship. It's a forever process.

When you give, give freely. If you expect people to give the same back, measured by the cup, you'll always be disappointed. If they respond, that's great. And if they don't, that's all right, too.

### The Importance of Honesty

At the same time, you need to be honest with the people you care about. I knew a case where one spouse's insistence on squeezing the toothpaste tube in the middle, a classic little problem, became an "irreconcilable difference" that led to divorce. Get rid of petty irritants. Don't suffer in silence until you finally explode. Say what you mean and feel. If the other person turns out to be hopeless in the tube-squeezing department, work out a compromise. (You might buy two tubes, one for each.)

Honesty needn't be cruel. Good rule: Be as tactful with your spouse and children as you are with friends and distant relatives. We're wonderful in courtship. But later we get careless. Love is not a license for rudeness.

We also tend to use our families as alibis when we fall short of our own goals. Stop underestimating these people. They're much more flexible than we assume. We can make our dreams real if we want them enough—and share them with the people we love. But if you never say, "Let's go to Nepal!" you'll never get there.

Of course, you're taking a chance. If your family picks up the challenge, you'll still have to work to achieve that goal. No fairy godmother will simply wave her wand and give you your heart's desire.

Many years ago, I dreamed of building a big institute to study the dynamics of human relationships. A very wealthy woman finally said she'd endow the school if I'd be president. Suddenly I was faced with my dream...and I didn't take the reality. I decided I wasn't ready to sit behind a desk. It was a good decision—but if I hadn't been confronted with it, I still might be moaning about the institute that I never really wanted.

### Living with Risk

Above all, you must accept that life is, by definition, always in flux. Everything is perpetually in a state of change. There is no real peace out there, no wall high enough to protect you. You must be your own anchor and have the courage to risk. Every moment is a risk. When you accept that, you'll be filled with the invigoration of your own power.

The biggest risk of all is to love. We're scared to death of expressing ourselves. When you meet people on the street, don't be afraid to greet them—your tongue won't fall off. Hug people—your arms won't fall off. I'm not ashamed to show that without love, I would die of loneliness. It's a gamble to be vulnerable. But you never really lose because the risk itself reminds you how richly you are living.

**Source:** Interview with Leo Buscaglia, author of *Loving Each Other*, Holt, Rinehart and Winston, New York.

## WHAT MAKES A PERSON HAPPY?

Twenty-five years ago, men defined happiness as a steady job with a future, while the typical woman looked to a secure marriage with children. But a recent survey found that difference has blurred. Women depend more on work for their satisfaction than they used to, and men depend more on family life. Bottom line: A sense of well-being is conditioned more by society than by any basic difference between the sexes.

**Source:** Study by psychologist Joseph Veroff, Ph.D., reported in *Vogue*, New York.

# ALL ABOUT HAPPINESS

Sometimes happiness seems like a terribly elusive goal. We tend to forget that it doesn't come as a result of getting something we don't have, but rather of recognizing and appreciating what we do have. Some steps on the pathway to happiness:

• When you think about time, keep to the present. My research suggests that thinking too much about events far in the future or in the distant past leads to unhappiness. Very often those who are future-oriented tend to score very high in despair, anxiety, helplessness and unhappiness. As much as is practical, focus on the here and now.

• Don't dwell on past injustices. You'll be unpopular company. No one wants to hear about how you got a raw deal in your divorce or how your boss doesn't appreciate you. Bill Bradley once said that one of the biggest problems a basketball player could have was to keep on replaying the game in his head after it was over. This is also true of life. If you keep doing instant replays, you'll lose your chance to enjoy the present.

• Check your goals. Many of us get so wrapped up in the means that we forget about the ends. Ask yourself from time to time: "Why am I doing this? Am I working hard because I love my work, or because I think money will buy happiness?" Maybe you'd really like peace of mind or recognition or job satisfaction. These can be more immediate, attainable goals. If you're working yourself to the bone because you think money will eventually buy contentment, maybe you can discover that you don't really need a million dollars. Making enough money to buy a small country retreat might do the trick.

• Drop your bucket where you are. Legend says that an explorer's sailing ship was be-

calmed in the mouth of the Amazon River. Thinking they were in the salty ocean, he and the crew were dying of thirst. Out of the sky a voice commanded, "Drop your bucket where you are." They did so, pulled up fresh water, and were thus saved. Lesson: Take advantage of what you already have. There are interesting, stimulating adventures waiting in your own backyard. Get to know your own children, for example.

• Develop the habit of noticing things. An active mind is never bored. While I walk to work every morning, I always try to pick out a house to look at carefully—one I haven't really paid attention to before. Make a resolution to notice new things each day—about nature, people, or anything else that interests you. Ask questions. Don't assume you know all the answers or that showing curiosity will be considered prying. Most people love to talk about themselves or their interests. Example: Talk with old people about their childhoods. You may have the fascinating experience of finding out about another world.

• Make some time for yourself. Everyone needs at least 20 minutes a day for quiet reflection—just-thinking time. If you think while walking or running, leave the radio home. Let your thoughts drift to who you are, how you feel, what you're doing, how your life is going.

• Exercise. It's good for the mind. I don't mean jogging 10 miles a day. But a brisk walk, maybe during your self-reflection time, will put you in a better frame of mind. And it's important to do it regularly, as part of your daily routine, just as you shower and eat at certain times.

• Establish a regimen for yourself. This will give you a feeling of control. If you can stop smoking, lose weight, exercise, stick to a schedule, etc., you'll gain a sense of mastery. Anything that proves you can affect your own life will give you a positive sense of self.

• Listen to the old saw about accepting what you cannot change. As we get older, we have to accept our limitations. At some point in life, we all must recognize that we'll never be president of General Motors, a

Nobel Prize winner, a *Time* cover subject, a perfect "10," or whatever else we thought was crucial to happiness. At this point, you have to be able to say sincerely, "So what!"

• Learn to like yourself. The best way to think positively about yourself is to think positively about others. They will then reflect back to you how wonderful you are, which will make it a lot easier. Our sense of self is a reflection of other people's responses to us. Exercise: Pay three sincere compliments a day to others. You'll soon see how much better this makes you feel about yourself. The key word is *sincere*. Finding things you really like will change how you think about people, which will, in turn, make you a lot more likable.

• Don't wear too many hats. Focus on one thing at a time. Make policy decisions ahead of time about situations such as taking work home. Set time aside for your family, your self, your golf game, etc.—for having fun. If you set your priorities in advance, you avoid the anxiety of making moment-to-moment decisions. These priorities don't have to be carved in stone, but they'll help you cope. Also: If you stick to your plans, you don't have to feel guilty because you're having fun and not working.

• Keep your sense of humor. A good laugh goes a long way in making almost any situation bearable. It also lightens the impact of life's inevitable tragedies.

**Source:** Interview with Fredrick Koenig, Ph.D., professor of social psychology, Tulane University, New Orleans, LA.

## HAPPY PEOPLE ARE UNSELFISH

To prove it, make a list of 10 people you know well. Write *H* for happy or *N* for not happy after the name of each. Then go down the list again and write *S* for selfish or *U* for unselfish beside each name. Odds: You will find that most people you rate as happy will also be considered unselfish.

**Source:** Surveys by psychologist Bernard Rimland at the Institute for Child Behavior Research in San Diego, as reported in *Psychology Today*, New York.

## SMILING TROUBLES AWAY

You may be able to alter your mood with a grin or a frown. Reason: Facial expressions lead to changes in the involuntary nervous system, reinforcing the appropriate emotion. For better empathy: Mimic the expression of the person you're dealing with.

## WHY LAUGHING IS GOOD FOR YOUR HEALTH

A good guffaw is more than a great tension reliever. It also can: Aid digestion, lower blood pressure, stimulate the heart and endocrine system, activate the right brain hemisphere (your creative center), strengthen muscles, raise pulse rate, soothe arthritic pain, work out internal organs and keep you alert. No joke!

**Source:** William F. Fry Jr., M.D., professor of psychiatry, Stanford University, quoted in *American Health.*

## TO STOP UNWANTED THOUGHTS

The average person has more than 200 negative thoughts a day—worries, jealousies, insecurities, cravings for forbidden things, etc. (Depressed people have as many as 600.) You can't eliminate all the troublesome things that go through your mind, but you can certainly reduce the number of negative thoughts. Here's how:

1. When a negative thought begins to surface in your mind, pause. Just stop what you are doing for a few seconds. Don't say anything—talk will reinforce the bad feeling.

2. Take five deep, slow breaths. By taking in more oxygen, you flush out your system and lower your level of anxiety. If you do this correctly, you will approach a meditative state.

3. Concentrate on a pleasant, relaxing scene—a walk on a breezy beach, for example. Take two to three minutes for a minor trouble, up to 10 minutes for a serious upset.

Best: Use this technique continuously until the upsetting thoughts begin to decrease. Then practice it intermittently.

**Source:** Interview with Elior Kinarthy, Ph.D., professor of psychology, Rio Hondo College, Whittier, CA.

# DEALING WITH LONELINESS

Virtually everyone is lonely from time to time, but chronic loneliness is a matter of more serious psychological dimension. Most people have no trouble describing what loneliness feels like. Emptiness, tightness in the throat, anxiety or feelings of "deadness inside" are among the phrases that recur when people talk about their lonely feelings. The trouble people do have is in locating the sources of their loneliness. The most common error: People who feel lonely blame themselves for their condition. In fact, it is usually some situation or external problem that causes the loneliness, rather than some inner psychological mechanism. No one is "genetically" lonely or "naturally lonely."

Social forces have a good deal to do with being alone, the most common cause of loneliness. Being alone is in good part the product of the high divorce rate and the fact that wives outlive husbands. It is also a product of our culture's emphasis on "self-sufficiency" and independence.

Popular fallacy: That old people are the most lonely members of our society. Just the opposite is true. They are the least lonely. (Research shows that young people are the most lonely and also the most unhappy, the most often bored and the lowest in self-esteem of the entire population.) Old people are the least lonely because we become wiser and psychologically sturdier as we age. It's also possible that the unhappy, lonely people die off sooner, leaving the more optimistic, cheerful ones to survive and be counted. Another fallacy: Women need men more than men need women. Fact: Indications are clear that men tend to be more dependent on women. One reason: Women are far more skilled than men at establishing intimacy and at creating nurturing relationships.

## What to Do About Loneliness

• Recognize that there are ways in which you may have become accustomed to dealing with loneliness that can in fact exacerbate it and be harmful in other ways. Examples: Solitary drinking, taking tranquilizers or other drugs, or watching television. The last is a particularly insidious (because ostensibly harmless) diversion that, like many other escapist solutions, can reduce your capacity to be alone and introspective. (It's no accident that in a study of high school students, the ones who had the lowest social status and self-esteem were the ones who watched television most often.) Television tends to serve as a substitute for social life, not a route into it. It's potentially more harmful than smoking a little marijuana on occasion.

• Learn the benefits of solitude by undertaking some of its more active forms, such as journal writing, letter writing or reading. Such activities contribute to your sense of personal strength and your level of awareness, and they enhance your sense of creativity. These are all vital contributions, since low self-esteem is a central factor in loneliness. It's important to learn the positive benefits of being alone. It's a mistake to spend time with people to cope with feelings of emptiness. Surrounding yourself with people you don't like is just as bad as stuffing yourself with food you don't need in order to cope with loneliness. They are narcotics, not solutions to the problem of the void you feel.

• Remember that the way in which you perceive being alone is the decisive factor in whether you feel lonely. People who equate loneliness with being alone are the ones who end up actually feeling lonely in solitary circumstances. There are, after all, many peole who have been living alone all their lives, yet are among the least lonely people.

• Consider how to establish more intimate ties with other people. This is, above all, the prime factor in avoiding feelings of loneliness. Such feelings reflect the fact that you have insufficient or inadequate personal ties in your life.

**Source:** Interview with Carin Rubenstein, Ph.D., senior editor of *Psychology Today* and co-author (with Phillip Shaver) of *In Search of Intimacy*, Delacorte Press, New York.

## SINGLE DOESN'T MEAN LONELY

Most older single people aren't as lonely as is commonly thought. In a recent survey, only 2% of unmarried men and women over 50 said they were "almost always" lonely. Another 14% were "often" lonely, and 35% felt that way "sometimes." But 50% were "hardly ever" lonely.

**Source:** *Love, Sex and Aging* by the editors of Consumer Reports Books, Consumers Union, Mount Vernon, NY.

## HOW OFTEN DO PEOPLE CRY?

Many men (55%) cry at least once a month, and 73% of them feel better afterward, a recent study found. Women cry five times as often, and 85% of them feel better. Most common crying time: Between 7 P.M. and 10 P.M., while watching a movie or visiting with friends or relatives.

**Source:** *What's the Difference? How Men and Women Compare* by Jane Barr Stump, William Morrow & Co., Inc., New York.

## HOW DO YOU GET OVER THE BUMPS IN LIFE?

• Letitia Baldrige, president, Letitia Baldrige Enterprises: "I call on Claire Boothe Luce's phrase, which I learned while working for her in Rome—*No good deed goes unpunished*. It gets me through the bumps in life because I know I'm going to get a slap in the face after having done someone a favor."

• Dr. Harold B. Ehrlich, chairman, Bernstein-Macaulay: "For me the phrase would be *No decision is irrevocable*. The only irrevocable decision is death."

• Robert Half, president of Robert Half International, Inc.: "My shock absorber is to say the word *Smile*. Even if I have to force the smile. . .it works. You have to smile to say the word. Then I try to get outside and walk, smiling at people as I pass them.

• Dave Johnson, manager, New York Mets baseball team: "I say to myself, *Things always happen for the best*. Regardless of what has occurred. . .and how bad it may seem at the time. . .it works out that everything really does happen for the best."

• Robert MacNeil, The MacNeil/Lehrer Newshour: "Since I was about 20, the phrase I have said to myself in difficult moments is *Think how this will look to you five years from now!* It reduces the situation to a comfortable perspective."

• Milton Margolis, president, Host Apparel: "I always say to myself, *Don't take yourself too seriously.*"

• Archbishop John J. O'Connor, Roman Catholic Church, New York Diocese: "I always say Mother Teresa's own prayer—*Give God permission*. When I wake up early in the morning, I always ask God to keep me from preventing anyone from doing any good that day."

• Joseph Papp, Off-Broadway producer, New York: "My helpful phrase is *Nobody's perfect.*"

• Pauline Trigere, fashion couturier: "I swear in the four languages that I know—and if I knew four more languages, then I would swear in those, too."

## HOW TO SELF-INDULGE

It's been a grueling week. Meetings, deadlines, pressure, crises—and now, finally, Friday is almost over. M. feels the tension begin to melt. His eyes focus on some distant point outside his office window. This week should be Mozart or Mendelssohn? he wonders. A concerto for flute or for violin? Jean-Pierre Rampal or Itzhak Perlman or maybe Rosalyn Tureck playing Bach? He smiles at the decision that lies ahead.

M. is getting ready to self-indulge. Every Friday he pops into a record store and buys a classical music tape as a gift to himself for making it through the week.

It happens that M. can afford to order the entire Columbia Masterworks Library in a single stroke. Obviously, he can also buy his tapes on Monday or Wednesday or by mail order. But that is not the point: M. is not methodically pursuing a hobby or building a music collection. He is practicing artful self-indulgence. That is why he chooses to savor his purchases, one by one.

Artful self-indulgence is a ritual. It is theater (because the anticipation is as satisfying as the performance itself). It is a reward for good behavior bestowed by the person who knows you best—you.

The difference between artful self-indulgence and spoiled-brat hedonism lies in moderation and self-knowledge. For example, the person who pigs out on a quart of Haagen-Dazs mocha chip is usually following a false messiah. It is rare to find salvation in an act so gross, guilt-producing and common as eating too much ice cream. On the other hand, the person who rewards herself with a Shiatsu massage once a month may enjoy a sense of physical peace that nourishes her for weeks.

I've found that practioners of this art, or survival skill, fall into two broad categories: Those who self-indulge by buying and those who self-indulge by doing.

### The Buyers

B. buys accessories: A streamlined coffee maker that plugs into the car cigarette lighter, state-of-the-art earphones for his stereo, a fancy carrying case for his floppy disks, you name it. B. is convinced that each accessory is absolutely necessary to the usefulness of his existing machines or appliances. That belief gives him psychological permission to self-indulge.

R. buys stationery. She likes choosing paper to match her subject and her moods. She buys everything from lined pads at the dime store to monogrammed notepaper from Tiffany's. When she's depressed, she buys antique postcards. She doesn't call her habit self-indulgence. She calls it "buying myself a clean slate."

W. buys courses. At the moment, it's a writing seminar. Before that, it was an all-day conference on "Selling Yourself." Next, he's considering either conversational Chinese, "The Wines of California," or flying lessons. He says he sets aside a strict percentage of his paycheck for these courses—not to earn college credit or Brownie points with the boss, but to "keep on growing."

A. is a hardware-store freak. She buys tools and gadgets; the more obscure their function, the better. She buys electrical supplies—and hooks, screws, nails and every manner of fastener. Nothing delights A. more than having precisely the right item for any fix-it job. Her idea of lip-smacking self-indulgence is spending Sunday afternoon hanging a 40-pound picture on a hollow wall.

### The Doers

Most of us reward ourselves after an exhausting day by flaking out in front of the TV set or going to sleep right after dinner. But there's another breed of humans who treat themselves well by going into action. I don't mean your ordinary 12-miles-a-week jogger or daily-health-club fanatic. I'm talking about people who give themselves an occasional well-planned, very special treat. Here are a few virtuoso self-indulgers:

*The New York Times* recently featured an investment banker who goes hot-air ballooning, a computer consultant who plays "Ultimate Frisbee," a croquet player, and several race walkers, boccie players, rock climbers and parachute jumpers. But they didn't name my personal self-indulgence: Motor scootering. Despite the known hazards of New York City traffic, I find a ride around Central Park or a run up and down Riverside Drive to be among the most refreshing activities available to an urban dweller.

E. gets his jollies by making weekend brunches. He spends many day-dreaming moments during the work week planning his invitation list and a unique menu. Although he sees the creativity as self-indulgence (and a costly one if he chooses something like a caviar omelet party), he says, "I have fun twice: Once while I'm cooking and then while I'm with my friends."

B. considers her volunteer work as self-indulgent as anyone else's luxuries because it gives her so much pleasure. B. is a black woman who owns her own business. On weekends, she is a Big Sister to a 13-year-old black girl. Together they go to the movies, to the beach, to museums, shopping, bike riding, whatever. And they talk. When a school holiday coincides with a work day, B. takes her Little Sister to the office with her. "I want her to form an image of her own future possibilities," she says.

H. writes in his journal. He doesn't expect ever to get published, but that's not his goal. His goal is to slow down his life, to observe and to record his feelings and experiences before everything blurs in his memory. Since he started writing in his journal, he says, he has become much more sensitive about noticing the things around him and understanding himself and the people he loves.

To each, his or her own. Happily, artful self-indulgence is a private transaction between you and your passions. So, if you can afford it and it makes you feel good and it doesn't hurt anyone—go to it!

**Source:** Letty Cottin Pogrebin is an editor at *Ms.* magazine and the author of *Family Politics,* McGraw-Hill, New York.

# THE POWER OF POSITIVE IMAGING

Over and over again, I've seen that when people begin to think positively about what they want to accomplish and how to do it, the chances are very good that they'll reach their goals.

One of the most important elements of positive thinking is positive imaging. That is, creating a picture in your mind in which you actually visualize yourself doing whatever it is you want to do. These pictures—and the suggestions they generate—can have a powerful effect.

When they apply: Visualization can work for virtually any personal or professional goal. Sports figures have long used visualization techniques to improve performance. Even health problems can be alleviated through effective imaging. All it takes is a defined goal, a logical process of achieving it and an attitude that says, I truly want to meet that goal.

### Breaking Barriers

Consider the four-minute mile. It appeared to be insurmountable, the Mt. Everest of track. Nobody seemed able to break that four-minute mark. Roger Bannister did it, however, in 1954...and within 15 years, 274 men had run a four-minute mile or better. Bannister's accomplishment changed the mental image of the race for those who followed.

There are many similar stories. I know a top golf pro who had never stroked a putt until he heard—in his mind's ear—the thud of the ball dropping into the cup. And baseball players visualize themselves at the plate, watching for the pitch and taking the perfect swing. Through the process of concentrating on a realizable goal and "seeing" it reached, they fulfill their true potential.

### Finding Direction

Obviously, putting positive imagery to work is like using any other tool. First, set reasonable goals. Second, believe you're capable of reaching them. Third, work at changing your thought habits.

I once met a young man raking leaves on a golf course. He told me he wanted to get somewhere in life. But he didn't know where he wanted to be, when he wanted to get there...or even how to get there. My advice to him... Go think about it, and then write down and show me what you want, when you want it and so forth.

This young man later told me he aspired to be a foreman at a nearby factory. He showed me his timetable. He had developed his plan, but he still had one obstacle to overcome—he didn't think he had any ability beyond that foreman's job. But positive imaging proved him wrong, and now he runs that factory!

### Mind over Matter

This type of imaging works. I have no doubt about it. I once knew a 97-year-old man, the oldest practicing physician in New

York. He was one of the healthiest people I've ever known. How did he stay so healthy? He encouraged his organs to do their jobs and do them well. Every morning this man jumped out of bed and paid homage to his body, starting with his brain and working down. He'd thank God for his wonderful stomach, kidneys, liver and so on. And then, he'd tell these organs how much he appreciated the fine job they were doing. He venerated his physical organs and visualized them doing well.

He was living proof that you can improve yourself by seeing yourself as vigorous and vital. But it wasn't just the veneration of his organs that kept him so healthy. His appreciation of his body helped him conduct his life in a manner that was supportive of his health.

### Images and Expectations

Developing images of your own performance is only one side of the coin. You also have the opportunity to help yourself and others by applying mental imagery to the people with whom you work. Perhaps there's someone in your business with whom you're always at odds. You've developed an enemy relationship with this person. You don't like each other.

Solution: Think of this person as someone you like, someone who can work with you. Create in your mind an image of the relationship restored. Put aside your negative feelings and begin to treat this person as a valued friend and associate. You won't see immediate results, but over time, you'll find that this person is responding to you in a more positive way. The lesson: Be aware of your expectations of others. People are likely to deliver what you expect them to.

The mind is a powerful tool, and you'll be pleasantly surprised by the results of positive imagery. You won't always accomplish everything you visualize, but you'll do much better than you would believing you'll never reach your goals.

**Source:** Interview with Dr. Norman Vincent Peale, author and lecturer, New York.

## ZEN IN DAILY LIFE

*Zen* translates loosely into *mind.* By being mindful of our daily life we can relieve the alienation and anxieties of the world around us. In a general sense, Zen is a way of living attentively, joyously and spontaneously.

Many of the Zen lessons used for meditation can be applied to daily life. Since these lessons are very general in meaning, they can be applied to everyone's life. The following lessons are ones that I find useful.

• *Ichi go ichi e: Concentrate on each moment as though it is your last.* Even commonplace behavior such as walking is important. To get the most out of your life, you must be aware of what you are doing. Example: If you have a meeting with a client, take advantage of the time and do your best. You may not get another chance that is as good.

• *Onore hige sezu: Believe in yourself.* If a challenging opportunity comes along, don't immediately feel you are not able to do it. Don't think of failure, but instead, try hard to succeed. Example: You are given a new task at work that involves talents you have never used before. Don't say you don't have the skill; instead, bring together all your abilities and try your best to do it.

• *Iken no uketori kata: Be a good listener and take opinions, advice and criticism from all sources.* You never know when you will hear something useful. Good ideas come from many sources. Forget your ego and listen. Example: If a project that you're directing is not going well, ask the people around you what they think. One of them may give you fresh perspective or even a solution

• *I no naka no kawazu taikei shirazu: A frog in a well can't know the ocean.* This is a traditional Japanese saying. Let's say that you are a frog living in your own well. The well seems like a fairly large universe. In fact, it is quite limited. . . bounded by walls and containing a finite amount of water. Now, along comes another frog, who tells you of a boundless body of water full of strange plants and fish. The frog asks you, "Do you know about this place called the ocean?" You would answer, "Of course I know about the ocean. After all, I've lived in the water all my life."

We are all specialists, having intensively studied or practiced one art or discipline (law, medicine, business, etc.). We also like to think of ourselves as being quite worldly and well-versed in the different ways people live. With this attitude, we are actually closing ourselves off in our own little world. Once we circumscribe our view of the world by our knowledge and past experience, we close the door on being able to learn and grow.

• *Gassho: Step back and appreciate your life by considering all the good aspects at once.* We all have pressures in life from our careers, our families, etc. Despite the tedious and unpleasant aspects of life, there is happiness to be found. Think about all the good things you have at once—your health, your home, your children—and you will take a more optimistic view of the world.

• *Setsu do motsu: Always leave setsu (space) to enjoy what you are doing and to dwell on what you have accomplished.* Leave time to ask yourself, "What is missing?" with regard to your training or your life. Think calmly about what needs to be done to improve. In order to accomplish this, you must allow for *setsu* and be flexible. Example: Bamboo can be bent back almost double upon itself and still spring back to its original shape because of the bands that separate each section of the stalk. These bands are like *setsu*. They allow the plant to be flexible in life and avoid being broken.

• *Fu gen jikko: Actions speak louder than words.* You must take responsibility for your life. If something is important to you, don't just talk about it—do it!

Strive for a strong mind and spirit (*Kokoru*). Take care of yourself, both mind and body. Concentrate on all aspects of being human, and you will become a better person.

**Source:** Interview with Shihan Tadashi Nakamura, founder and chairman of the World Seido Karate Organization, New York.

## LEARNING THE VIRTUES OF ENDLESS PATIENCE

Endless patience is a discipline that takes time, practice and, yes, patience to learn. It means having enough patience for a crucial project even when it is unclear how much will be required.

Goal: To undertake long, complex, open-ended personal and business ventures and bring them to a conclusion without being consumed with unnecessary anxieties and worries.

Problem: Most people are easily overcome by petty concerns and spend many wasted hours fretting. Result: They pay a huge emotional price in turmoil about things over which they have little control.

The route to mastering endless patience starts with understanding the concept of risk taking. Most ventures have, at best, a 50% chance of success. People tend to forget this. They pray to Lady Luck that every project will turn out well. Then they are disappointed—and shocked—at the failures. They must learn to wait patiently to see which projects will survive and which will go under.

Trap: Blind faith, whose followers fervently believe that they will succeed. They hang on to any undertaking, no matter how clear the signs that it will fail. Contrast: People with endless patience are willing to pay the price to achieve the goal only as long as it is feasible. When feasibility dies, the practioner of endless patience knows it is time to quit.

Secret weapon of achieving endless patience: A calm, analytical state of mind. The mystical writer Carlos Castaneda give this explanation of what makes a good warrior-hunter-stalker: "The warrior never frets."*

To avoid fretting: Identify the real problems. Make sure that everything humanly possible is being done to solve them. Then, sit back and stop worrying. Insight: Your patience does not expire until the project succeeds, dies or is killed.

Most innovation has a long portion of the exponential curve, in which there is hardly any incremental value during long months or years. Then it might suddenly swerve upward and keep climbing. Impatient people do not hang in long enough to witness this upturn.

Helpful analogy: Practicing endless patience is similar to setting out in unknown territory to find diamonds. You know from research that the diamonds are out there. You are even familiar with the type of ground in which they may be located,

*The Eagle's Gift* by Carlos Castaneda, Simon & Schuster, New York.

though you lack a map marking their site. You plan for the expedition, anticipate your problems and set out in the hope of succeeding.

Endless patience prevents you from fretting over a missed turn, sprained ankle or minor setback. You press on toward your goal without agonizing over small annoyances or uncontrollable events. You may find the diamond field—or you may at some point decide the search is no longer feasible. Either way, you will have exercised the correct approach.

Patience must also be exercised in short-term dealings with people and situations. Understanding the basic concepts of endless patience ends much unproductive behavior.

Another way out: Develop the practice of focused attention. Concentrate on the problems that cause you real concern. Puzzle out ways to solve these problems, and then relax.

**Source:** Interview with Martin G. Groder, M.D., a psychiatrist and business consultant who practices in Durham, NC.

# OBSTACLES TO SUCCESS

There are certain obstacles that we all have to deal with before we find success. The problem is in recognizing the obstacles. All too often, ambitious people delude themselves into thinking that the path to success is clear. Then, they wind up stumbling without really knowing why.

Ironically, the lack of a clear goal is the most common obstacle to success, even for people with large amounts of drive and ambition. Typically, they focus on the rewards of success, not on the route they must take to achieve it.

Remedy: Whenever possible, write down your goals, forcing yourself to be specific. Periodically make a self-assessment. Take into account your education, age, appearance, background, skills, talents, weaknesses, preferences, willingness to take risks and languages spoken. Ask for feedback from others. Don't try to succeed at something for which you have no talent. Try out your

goal part time. If you dream of owning a restaurant, work in one for a while.

### Failure and Fear

Sooner or later, everyone who's ambitious will experience a failure. Many don't recognize, however, that failure is necessary. There are many secret payoffs for failure: The humble poor are never accused of exploiting others. They can feel morally superior to money-grubbing, power-hungry moguls. They're comfortable as part of the culture that supports being a cog in a machine. They get righteous satisfaction from complaining about the system.

To understand failure, evaluate honestly what stands between you and success, both in the outside world and within yourself. Find a mentor who will be open with you about his or her own struggles with such blind spots. Read biographies of people who overcame their own fears to become successful.

Without realizing it, many people fear the *Peter Principle*, which says they'll rise to their level of incompetence and will be exposed as inadequate. Others are so afraid of failure that they become paralyzed. They forget that if they never try anything worthwhile they've already failed.

What everyone must realize is that if you take risks, there's no way to avoid failure. You can't succeed without struggle. But if you're able to learn from what went wrong, you can do it right the next time.

Other obstacles to success:

• Inability to let go. People often stick with a dead-end job out of pride, stubbornness or unwillingness to admit that they made a mistake. Sometimes, the comfort of the familiar is just too seductive. To start letting go: Take small, safe steps at first. Start talking to friends and associates about possible new jobs. See what's available during your vacation. Shake things up at the office by suggesting some changes in your current job. Take some courses and learn new skills.

• Lack of self-esteem. This is an enormous stumbling block. But, in fact, you may be judging yourself by excessively high standards. Example: An architect who started his own firm realized he was a total loss in math and engineering, and that his only talent was design. If he'd felt inadequate about his deficiencies, he might not have gone into business at all. But as a realist, he simply concentrated on his own area of expertise and hired experts to fill in on the technical end.

• Procrastination. If you delude yourself by thinking something will be easier to do tomorrow, you can avoid looking at why you aren't doing it today. Like alcoholism, procrastination is a subtle, insidious diesease that numbs the consciousness and destroys self-esteem. Remedy: Catch it early, but not in a harsh, punitive, self-blaming way. Look at what you're afraid of and examine your motives. Example: You may not really want to leave your low-level job, but feel you ought to because your spouse is anxious for more money and status. Once you can acknowledge the real cause, you can escape the depressing downward spiral.

• Shyness. If you're shy, the obvious remedy is to choose an occupation that doesn't require a lot of public contact. But even shy salespeople have been known to succeed. As long as they're talking about product lines and business, a familiar spiel can see them through. Casual socializing seems hardest for the shy person. Remedies: Don't put enormous pressure on yourself to socialize if it makes you uncomfortable. Concentrate on getting ahead by doing a terrific job rather than by being Mr. or Ms. Charming. Or, take a Dale Carnegie course. They *are* helpful.

• Unwillingness to look at yourself. If you're not willing to assess yourself honestly, success will probably forever elude you. People tend to avoid self-assessment because they feel they must be really hard on themselves. How to look at yourself: Realize you've probably taken the enemy into your own head—you've internalized that harsh, critical parent or teacher from your childhood. Instead, evaluate yourself as you would someone you love, like a good friend whom you'd be inclined to forgive almost anything. Example: Anwar Sadat was raised with the teachings of a harsh, judgmental religion. While in prison he read about another religion, which had a loving, forgiving, supportive God. This made all the difference in his life.

**Source:** Interview with Tom Greening, Ph.D., clinical supervisor of psychology at the University of California at Los Angeles and a partner in Psychological Service Associates.

## CURE FOR SHYNESS

Shy people are too preoccupied with themselves, new research reports. How to improve: Stop focusing on your perceived inadequacies and feelings of anxiety and pay more attention to other people. That way you're concentrating on other people's cues—what they say and do—rather than worrying about how you appear to others.

## DEVELOPING YOUR WINNING POTENTIAL

I used to work in a mental institution where I discovered that motivating some of my patients to speak normally was like getting your coffee table to talk. They have a formula for losing. This started me thinking about whether successful people have a formula for winning.

They do. And there's nothing mysterious about the formula. It's something all of us can learn by bringing out our own winning potential.

Imagine that in every possible area crucial to success there's a scale ranging from 1 to 10. Schizophrenics are at 0 or 1 on the scale, average people are at 5–6, and winners are at 9–10.

How it works: In the area of positive thinking, for example, schizophrenics I treated thought that everyone was out to destroy them, and they spent their time planning the demise of their supposed enemies. Average people often believe that others have insulted them or taken advantage of them. They spend their time blaming and hating those people. Winners, on the other hand, act positively and do something.

### The Winners' Scale

In a business setting, if something said to them sounds insulting, winners either assume it's their own fault—that they were communicating poorly—or possibly that they didn't hear what was said correctly, or that the others had incorrect information.

The key is that they take responsibility for the problem. Example: A politician I interviewed said that whenever he's in a confrontation, he makes an appointment and goes right to the "enemy" to discuss the problem. While the enemy may not become his friend, he's never as cutting or hostile again.

Sensitivity is another crucial measurement on the winners' scale. Schizophrenic patients weren't cruel and insensitive only to others but also hurt and humiliated themselves. Average people are kinder, but winners are considerate, thoughtful, caring and giving.

### Attitudes to Develop

The keys to developing your own winning potential:

• Take small steps. I once worked with a catatonic who hadn't moved in 30 years. In 31 days I got him to talk. But he did it in small stages. The first time he twitched his nose, I cheered. I was genuinely positive about it. Winners reinforce their own small successes. Example: The loser takes a course in computer programming, doesn't grasp it after the first week and gives up, assuming he's too stupid to learn the subject. The winner who doesn't grasp it after a week assumes he's doing well because he's figured out how to use the keyboard.

• Be willing to fail. Losers assume that winners never make mistakes, that they're just lucky. Often the opposite is true. Winners fail a great deal. One winner, the CEO of a famous company, says his failure rate is 70%. It's the old Babe Ruth story. The year he hit the most home runs, he also had the most strike-outs. Sometimes winners wind up succeeding simply because they stumble on the right answer by trial and error.

• Be kind to yourself. In a sense, you must become your own parent. Losers are brutal to themselves. Average people will lose $10,000 in business and spend years berating themselves for being fools and failures. Winners tell themselves. . .Well, I learned what I could from that venture. It's time to

move on. When you're feeling down on yourself, lift up your two index fingers, kiss them and plant a kiss on each cheek. Psychologically it works. You'll feel better.

• Listen to the beat of your own drummer. Ignore people who tell you to quit. Example: The inventor of tofutti, the current ice cream-substitute craze, spent all his spare time for years searching for the right formula. His wife got fed up and finally divorced him. Tofutti became a huge success (and its inventor is now happily remarried).

### Developing Self-Esteem

For those moments when you're not feeling good about yourself, try to realize that everybody else is probably frightened and feeling like two-year-olds. I've treated superstars, royalty, politicians and people on welfare. All of these people, no matter what their accomplishments were, felt insecure and scared as if they were swimming upstream.

Antidote for insecurity: Hard work. There's always room at the top. So get started. No matter how you feel about yourself, hard work will reinforce both your self-esteem and your chance of becoming a winner.

**Source:** Interview with psychologist and family therapist Irene C., Kassorla, Ph.D., author of *Go For It: How to Win at Love, Work and Play,* Delacorte Press, New York.

## CHECKING TO SEE IF YOU'RE ON THE RIGHT COURSE

Use your life goals as signposts to indicate you're on the right course. It's the overall direction of your life that counts, not the achievement of specific goals. Getting there isn't just half the fun—getting there is actually what we call living.

## SELF-CONFIDENCE STRATEGY

How to build self-confidence: Picture yourself a success and dress the part. Appraise yourself realistically—then add 10% to the estimate. In contrast, don't overestimate others. Don't conjure up obstacles for yourself, but learn to tolerate an occasional setback.

**Source:** *Fail-Safe Business Negotiating* by Philip Sperber, Prentice-Hall, Englewood Cliffs, NJ.

## THE TALL AND SHORT OF IT

Tall women are usually more independent than short women and more likely to strike out on their own. Short women, on the other hand, are more apt to marry and have children.

**Source:** *The Height of Your Life* by Ralph Keyes, Warner Books, New York.

## YOU DON'T HAVE TO BE LUCKY TO BE LUCKY

The luck you make for yourself has nothing to do with blind chance. Luck is what the Chinese call it: Opportunity. It knocks every day at your door. But it isn't enough to hear it knock. You have to greet it fearlessly and work with it.

Common obstacle to being lucky: Fear of failure. This fear causes people to put off new projects. Procrastination postpones the possibility of failure. Secret ingredient of luck: Willingness to confront the possibility of failure.

To make your own luck:

• Find an idea that offers a new and better way to satisfy people's needs. Start by analyzing your own needs and ways of filling them. You are your own best research laboratory.

• Move forward with your idea before your enthusiasm cools.

• Gather information from people who know most about the subject.

• Build a network of contacts who will help you get the idea off the ground. One contact invariably leads to another.

Characteristics of people who make their own luck:

• They are in touch with their gut feelings. As a result, they realize when a real opportunity is speaking to them. They go out of their way to be friendly. They know how to make contacts and use them.

• They do their homework. They lay the groundwork for their projects, gather facts and prepare in general.

• They take risks and aren't so enslaved by habit that they fear the unorthodox.

• They are skeptical. They never forget that a venture could fail. Insight: Being 100% sure of success is not confidence—it is foolhardiness.

• They take failure as a learning experience. They admit their mistakes and are undaunted by previous failures.

• They recognize that the capacity for change and growth exists within them. They know there is no such thing as bad luck that permanently imprisons you within an unsuccessful life style. The only villain who can do that is you.

**Source:** Interview with Bernard Gittelson, author of *How to Make Your Own Luck*, Warner Books, New York.

## SELF-DEFEATING BEHAVIOR AND HOW TO AVOID IT

Occasionally we all forget something crucial, come late to an appointment or manage to make a muddle of an important task. But when that type of self-defeating behavior becomes habitual, it signals to people that you're not dependable, that you're not willing to live up to your part of the bargain. Those messages, conscious or not, can have drastic consequences. . .loss of job, failure of marriage, etc. To understand why we are self-defeating involves a journey into the past. And to change a self-destructive pattern, we must be willing to do some serious self-evaluation.

### A Child's-Eye View
Children are naturally self-centered and aggressive creatures (as is obvious to anyone

who has watched small children fighting over toys). But in order to live in the world, the child has to curb his aggressive instincts. He may be furious at mother for toilet-training him, but restrains himself from hitting her because he also loves her. As we grow older we must learn to use aggression, as well as love to get on with our lives. Competition, the drive to succeed, both come from the aggressive impulse. Living happily in the world requires a very delicate balance between love and aggression, a balance many people never get quite right.

Unresolved aggression turns people into self-defeaters. They haven't learned to modify their aggression in work and love. Or, they've buried their aggression to the point that consciously they don't experience it as a problem, but it bubbles up unconsciously in all kinds of self-destructive ways.

### The Family Drama

We first learn competition in the family, by competing with siblings, who are symbolic stand-ins for the same-sex parent. We're really competing with the parent for what we perceive him or her as having—power, money, love, respect and so forth. Conflict: Feeling guilty about the competition and unconsciously not allowing ourselves to outdo the rival for fear of losing parental love or of inviting parental anger and aggression.

Defying parents' or society's expectations can also invite seriously self-defeating behavior. Example: A woman became a ballet dancer against her father's wishes. He thought dancing was tantamount to prostitution. She was a marvelous dancer but when she appeared in a ballet that demanded pirouettes, she could only perform well upstage, away from the audience. While pirouetting downstage toward the audience, she'd start to falter and finally fall when she reached the footlights. In this case the audience represented a judgmental father saying, "You're a whore."

Women have a more severe problem since they're trained to be nonaggressive and nurturing. To succeed in business, a woman must become competitive and exhibit behavior commonly thought of as masculine. Many career women become so frightened about losing their feminine identity that they trip themselves up before reaching their full potential.

### What to Do About It

• Examine your motives. If you find yourself exhibiting self-defeating behavior, maybe what you're really saying is, "I want out." Ask yourself: Am I successful on my own terms? Am I happy with my life? Wanting a different way of life from what is expected of you is a perfectly valid desire.

Example: Baba Ram Dass, Eastern-oriented spiritual leader, started out as Richard Alpert, son of the president of the New Haven Railroad. He gave up an executive position with the railroad because he was frightened by the power of his position. Alpert then became a psychologist and professor at Harvard until, along with Timothy Leary, he was dismissed for distributing LSD to students. A subsequent period of self-searching and drug taking was followed by his reemergence as Baba Ram Dass, after a spiritual pilgrimage to India; he became a guru sought after by millions. From his father's perspective, he could be considered a failure and a loony. In his terms, though, he's a smashing success.

• Don't sweat the small stuff. Realistically assess whether a particular behavior is truly self-defeating or merely annoying, and to what degree. If it's just a nuisance, like constantly losing your glasses, it may be better to realize you're making a big fuss over a minor problem and buy some extra pairs. Worry will make it worse. People who worry all the time about any behavior will do it more, not less.

• Become aware of what you're doing. This is difficult in our culture, which doesn't encourage self-reflection. Helpful: Keep a journal noting the various activities of your day and how you felt when doing them. Correlate the feelings in the journal with what was going on when you did something self-defeating. Once you start seeing a pattern, you can adjust for it.

• Pay attention. If things never go well for

you in a certain area and you don't know why, ask for feedback from a friend you trust to be objective. Your friend may have noticed a self-defeating behavior that you were totally unaware of. Also, listen to unsolicited feedback from others, without being defensive. If people in your life constantly complain about your lateness, for example, don't keep on giving what seem to you to be perfectly reasonable excuses. Look at the possibly psychic benefits you might be deriving from behavior that is ultimately self-defeating.

• Make a virtue out of your weakness. Almost any behavior can be turned to advantage if you acknowledge it and use it. The trick is to be conscious of what you're doing. Example: A sloppy dresser can present himself as an intellectual who is too concerned with really important matters to worry about looks. Albert Einstein wasn't known for his sartorial splendor.

• Seek professional help if the self-defeating behavior is a pattern that's out of your control and is adversely affecting your life. You may need therapy to root out the deeper causes and resolve the inner conflict.

**Source:** Interview with Simone F. Sternberg, Ed.D., a psychoanalyst and psychotherapist who is dean of students and clinical supervisor at the New York Center for Psychoanalytic Training.

# WHEN TO MAKE EXCUSES

Excuses often serve a positive function. They allow us to preserve self-esteem and reduce the stress of failure. . .maintain harmony with co-workers and friends when we foul up. . .acknowledge the validity of standards that we've violated. . .take risks that would otherwise paralyze us.

**Source:** C.R. Snyder, co-author of *Excuses: Masquerades in Search of Grace,* John Wiley and Sons, New York.

# LATENESS CAN BE CONTROLLED

Rarely is there such a thing as unavoidable lateness. The causes of lateness are many—

hostility, fear, contempt, self-destructiveness or the desire for attention. (The attention given to latecomers can be very gratifying and is thus a strong motivation for lateness. All eyes turn to the latecomer when he arrives, and he knows he has been the subject of discussion while the others have been waiting for him.)

Main misconception of latecomers: Their belief that they are late due to circumstances beyond their control. This is usually untrue. Simple fact: Some people are in the habit of being on time, and other people are in the habit of being late. Both types are easy to identify. The on-time people are not "lucky." They just know how to get somewhere on time.

### Dealing with Your Own Lateness

• Cutting it close. You leave just enough time to get there, and you're delayed because you miss a bus, or you have to stop for gas, or some other minor "unforeseeable" delay occurs. Solution: Assume that the worst conditions will prevail and plan your time with those in mind. Assume bad traffic, trouble finding a parking space, etc.

• Too many appointments. You can make them on time if each goes like clockwork, but they rarely do. Solution: Set your appointments with the expectation of the longest possible time for each appointment.

### Dealing with Lateness in Others

Study people's habits in regard to their lateness as you would study their habits in a poker game. How late is Jones, usually? Most latecomers have a predictable pattern. There are ten-minute-late people, half-an-hour-late people and very late people.

Best ways to cope with the chronic latecomer:

• Never arrange to meet him on the street, and try not to have him come to you. Instead, go to his place.

• Try not to meet for lunch where a reservation is involved. Go to his place and phone the restaurant from there.

• If you must meet a latecomer on neutral turf, be sure it's in a place where you can do paperwork or make phone calls while you're waiting.

• Don't deal with a latecomer by arriving late yourself. It isn't worth the discomfort. Eventually he will beat you at this game, and you will end up with a loss of self-respect.

Latecomers for social engagements: If you want to serve dinner at 8 with cocktails at 7:30, but some of your invitees are latecomers by habit, invite them for different hours. Invite the Joneses, who are on-time people, for 7:30. Invite the Smiths, who are usually late, for 7. Invite the Perrys, the worst offenders, for 6:30. They'll all probably arrive around 7:30.

In case the worst offenders surprise you by appearing considerably earlier than anyone else (on time!), tell them you purposely asked them to come early so you could have some time alone with them. If all else fails and you're still kept waiting at dinner, don't let the latecomers make an issue of their lateness. Cut off their apologies and excuses, and pleasantly but firmly divert the conversation to some other topic. This is the best revenge.

**Source:** Peter Shaw, a Ph.D. and associate professor of English at the State University of New York at Stony Brook.

## SIMPLE SECRETS OF SELF-IMPROVEMENT

Most advice about how we can change ourselves concentrates on self-image: Feel confident. Don't sell yourself short. Be relaxed. But some people change—or remain the same—because of repeated acts in a given pattern.

Shyness, for example, is strengthened every time the shy person falls silent after being interrupted. Self-confidence is eroded every time we fail to finish a project, even if we remind ourselves to feel confident.

There's a better way to improve yourself...change by doing.

Encourage friends to criticize you, and learn how to take criticism. Your critics may not always be right. But if you don't get the truth from others, you may never find it out.

Handling criticism:

• Let your critic finish what he has to say before you answer.

• Don't go into the reasons for your actions or behavior. This is really just a way of excusing them.

• Don't jest. It is insulting to the critic.

• Show that you have understood (whether or not you agree) by briefly repeating the criticism in your own words.

• Let your critic know that you understand how your behavior has caused inconvenience or made him feel.

• Don't open yourself to criticism for what you are—only for what you do.

**Source:** George Weinberg, Ph.D., author of *Self Creation*, Avon Books, New York.

## OVERCOMING INDECISION

Chronic indecision creates enormous stress on the individual. You are, in fact, divided against yourself. This conflict leads to tension, which in turn inhibits positive decision making. It's the most vicious of cycles. Examples:

In business, the indecisive manager is a disaster. He gains neither from success nor from setback. Afraid to err, he never learns from mistakes. His paralysis can sink a company.

In relationships we have the aging bachelor. Alienated from his own feelings, he's unwilling to commit himself to one woman. He's afraid to lose his precious freedom. But he never exercises that freedom, so he has lost it anyway. He forgets that freedom means making choices.

Some of us resort to pseudo-decisions—rushed and arbitrary stances that lack commitment or follow-through. But they aren't real decisions unless they are free, unconditional, total and personal...and lead to action relatively quickly...and engender no regrets, rage or emptiness afterward.

Although most people who suffer from indecision don't even realize it, the evidence is clear to those around them. Why do people waffle? Most often they're weighted down by self-hatred. They're terrified of taking responsibility for a decision because there is always the chance they will be wrong, unleashing still more self-hatred.

Another syndrome is rooted in the American Dream—the notion you can have it all without paying a price. But every true decision exacts a price: Giving up the options not chosen. So the dreamer remains inert, refusing to choose, like a child in a toy store.

To overcome indecisiveness, you must first combat self-hatred by ridding yourself of self-glorification. Realize that you have human limitations—and that one of those is making an occasional poor choice. At the same time, it's important to take stock of real assets such as talents, familial love, good health, etc.

To become a decision maker, you must accept what I call "The Big Fact": In very few instances is one decision actually better than another. Unless you're a surgeon deciding whether or not to operate, it probably doesn't matter what you choose. This is particularly true in relationships. After a romance fails, most people choose the same type of partner again and again. Their first choice wasn't bad. The real fault: Their lack of commitment—their failure to struggle and grow through communication.

If you're paralyzed by fear of failure, the best course is to meet the fear head-on. After you've failed a few times, you will be desensitized to it—and finally free to choose.

For a complex decision, it helps to assess your priorities. Consider what is most important to you . . . money, power, prestige, creative activity, pleasure, and so on. You can even assign point values to each category and then see how options stack up.

Make your important decisions when you feel your best. If you're rested and in a positive frame of mind, your decision will be freer. You will know you are making the best choice you can.

**Source:** Interview with Theodore Isaac Rubin, Ph.D., author of *Overcoming Indecisiveness*, Harper & Row, New York.

# HOW TO GET OUT OF A RUT

There's a hand-written sign next to an old dirt road in Georgia that reads: Pick your ruts carefully. You're going to be in them for the next 40 miles.

Unfortunately there's no warning sign for most of us when we land in a rut. Often we don't know how we got into what we're doing or why we stick with it. The one thing we do know is that we don't want to be stuck forever. And no matter how old you are or what kind of rut you're in, there is a way out. At least at first, you don't have to actually do anything. You just have to start thinking differently about who you are and what you want out of life.

### First Steps

Before escape is possible, a basic change in attitude is necessary. Most of the people who are stuck in ruts spend their lives complaining about their lot but never doing anything about it. The complaining makes them feel better (usually at the expense of everyone around them), but the end result is the same—nothing changes.

You must accept that no one is going to do anything for you. It is your responsibility, and yours alone, to change your own life. Start thinking constructively about what you want rather than moaning about what you don't have. If you're upset about your career, stop complaining and ask yourself: What do I really want to do? Where do I want to do it? With whom? Under what circumstances? What are my skills? (Include not only business experience but also hobbies, interpersonal skills and non-job-related skills.) What are my short-term goals? Long-term goals? Think long and hard and in great detail about what would make you happy. Don't be afraid to fantasize or hatch grandiose schemes. You may be able to make at least parts of your fantasy come true.

Exercise: Give yourself an imaginary $10 million and think about what you would do with it. Be specific. Then use your brain to see how much of your fantasy you can turn into reality. Sample fantasy: To live on a South Sea island and spend all my time sunbathing, fishing and picking coconuts. It may not be possible to move to the South Seas and loll about all day, but if you're living in a cold climate and really love the tropics, you might be able to get a job in Florida and spend all the spare time that you choose sunbathing and fishing.

### Rut-Removal Tactics

People automatically assume that their current job is a given that can't be changed. What escapes their notice is that sometimes you can get out of a rut right in the company where you're now employed. Examples:

• A bright young man of 35 was working in New York for a national firm. He'd been dreaming for years about living in California, and, as it turned out, his company had a branch there. Making the change was a little complicated because he was a high producer in New York and his boss didn't want to lose him. But he went to California and got to know the manager of that branch. Then he spoke to his boss, according to a carefully conceived plan, and explained how he would still be doing the company a lot of good in California. He also had a very promising replacement in mind whom he planned to train. His New York boss wound up supporting his move to California, and he's now very happy in the company's San Francisco branch.

• A senior vice president at a big East Coast bank was unhappy because he didn't spend enough time with his family. The family's hobby was sailing, but they often had to go without him since his weekends were spent working. He wasn't about to quit his job because, besides enjoying his work, he was in line for the bank presidency. The situation seemed impossible. Solution: He redesigned his job. He hired someone to take on his least favorite tasks and concentrated on his areas of expertise, thereby reducing his hours from 80 per week to 50. He started sailing with his kids on the weekends. Recently he got his biggest bonus—and he was truly worth it.

### Avoiding Extremes

If you've been in a rut for much too long without doing anything about it, midlife crisis can spark desperate measures. Too many people blindly flee either their job or their marriage, thereby destroying families, hurting children and wiping out the financial gains of a lifetime.

What people don't realize when they're establishing a marriage and career in their twenties is that 25–30 years later, they'll be different people with different ideas, hopes and dreams. If you recognize the inevitability of this process, which is really one of growth, you can factor change into your life. Don't develop tunnel vision about your work, no matter how much you love it. Keep learning and growing in other areas— socially, recreationally and professionally. You'll be less likely to wind up in a rut, and you'll have some means to get out of it if you're in one.

### If You Need a Drastic Change

• Start your own business. This does not have to be a total gamble. Overlooked clue to success: Research not only your venture but yourself. Too many people go into businesses they are personally unsuited for. Example: The couple who dreams of running a little hotel in the mountains won't make a go of it if they're shy, retiring types.

• Start communicating openly with your family. This hardly sounds like a prescription for drastic change. However, lack of communication is the primary reason for a marital rut. It can be an exciting, startling and totally new experience to find out what your spouse and children really think.

• Alternative to running off with your secretary: Consider going to a weekend marriage workshop, sometimes called a marriage encounter. This is a group of couples with an experienced leader. Spouses are taught how to be open with each other. It can be more effective than marriage counseling, which is often the last stop before the divorce.

**Source:** Interview with John C. Crystal of the John C. Crystal Center, New York. The Center offers intensive courses in creative life/work planning.

## 5 EASY CHANGES ANYONE CAN MAKE

To get out of a rut: Go to work by a different route or use another mode of transportation...unplug the TV for a month... take a child to a symphony concert or puppet show...take a bath instead of showering...skip the Valium (or martini) and try a walk in the woods.

**Source:** *The Psychology of Winning* by Dr. Denis Waitley, Berkley Books, New York.

## HOW TO BEAT BOREDOM

Boredom is often a form of emotional anesthesia self-imposed by those who do not want to experience their own feelings. It is also a method by which people keep themselves from changing and growing.

Boredom breeds more boredom. Hard truth: People are accountable for their own boredom. Blaming others or one's lot in life is no solution.

Ways out: Growth in areas such as the creative arts, work and study, and involvement with family and friends. This entails struggle, as bored people must use more of themselves than they have previously. And bored people must risk involvement even before a consuming interest materializes. Point: Involvement often sparks interest. Waiting for a bolt of lightning to ignite an interest results only in a continuation of apathetic boredom.

**Source:** *Dr. Rubin, Please Make Me Happy* by Theodore I. Rubin, M.D., Arbor House, New York.

## BIGGEST TIME WASTERS

Guilt: People spend hours moaning and worrying about mistakes they made like missing a bus or taking a wrong turn. This moping about something that has already happened and can't be changed not only uses up unproductive hours—it also incapacitates your mind for coping with the next project. Better approach: Accept accidents for what they are, pick up the pieces and go on about your business.

Disorganization: Not taking the time to work out a system for getting regular chores done or filing away important pieces of information can make simple tasks take twice as long. Keep an up-to-date, running shopping list. Put addresses and phone numbers into a book or a card file as you collect them. Schedule routine tasks to keep from wasting a weekend day just deciding what you should do first. (Too many choices will slow you down. Think of how much faster you get dressed on a trip when you only have one or two things to wear.)

**Source:** Barbara Platcher, Ph.D., executive director, National Association for Professional Saleswomen, Sacramento, CA.

## MAKING THE MOST OF A MIDLIFE CRISIS

The notion of a midlife crisis has developed only over the last 20 years. People used to stick with bad marriages, boring jobs and what Thoreau called "lives of quiet desperation." There was no real expectation of personal satisfaction. Several factors—a longer life span, increased mobility and the influences of the sexual revolution—have changed all that. Now people expect to live long, healthy lives that are both professionally and personally fulfilling.

Today, somewhere between age 33 and age 52, the majority of individuals in our society go through a midlife crisis. It involves questioning all the values they'd previously taken for granted. In a frantic desire to reject the past, a person undergoing midlife crisis often acts impulsively and destructively, squandering his hard-earned financial security or breaking up his family. But a midlife crisis can be a time for creative changes rather than destructive ones. Make the most of your own midlife crisis by understanding what it's all about and seeing it as an inevitable and positive part of your growth as a human being.

### Midlife Crisis Defined

A midlife crisis involves a period of self-examination sparked either by internal awareness of mortality or by an outside event, usually involving a loss of some kind. Typical: A divorce, loss of a job, death of a friend or family member, children leaving home. Or, there may simply be an awareness of change in oneself—the realization that life is half over. We see the first signs of aging and realize we're mortal. The awareness of mortality leads to an internal questioning process whereby we start to evaluate what we've done with our lives so far. The search for meaning begins.

Questions we typically ask ourselves: What do I want to do with the rest of my life? Do I really want to stay at my current job for the next 20 years? Am I really happy in my marriage? How would I like my life to be different?

There are many regrets to mull over. The childless regret never having had children. Parents regret not having spent more time with theirs—or not having more. Some people regret never having tried for the career they always dreamed of. Others feel that they missed opportunities to travel or find adventure.

### How to Handle Your Midlife Crisis

It's crucial to recognize that a healthy life involves balance. People tend to go to extremes. Some want money and success. Others will sacrifice anything to be loved. Midlife is the time to find the sense of balance within yourself. Suggestions:

• Stop measuring success by money. This is the current American mistake. Ask yourself what you missed in the making of the buck. Many people feel they lost contact with their children as they were growing up. It's important to realize when you've made enough and can begin to spend it. Use your goodies for yourself. It's not wise to leave them all to children, who generally tend to dissipate an inheritance they didn't work for.

• Don't dive into anything. It took you lots of years to get to where you are. . .and you don't have to make any instant decisions. Don't be the stereotypical midlife male who throws it all over to run off with a young girl, only to later regret his impulsive decision. Lifetime family and friendship networks are very important and should be preserved if at all possible.

• Learn to grow up. Changing your life doesn't have to be an either/or decision. Life is neither good nor bad. Today, it's one thing, tomorrow, another. Life involves balance plus movement. Keys to maturity: Keep moving. Stay active, and always be self-aware. Tune in to your thoughts and feelings—your entire being.

• Head off a crisis. Make changes before the axe falls. Example: The 45-year-old executive who sees that his new boss is a 34-year-old whiz kid and his co-workers are 25-year-old MBAs making a third of what he does. The tuned-in midlife exec sees the handwriting on the wall and gets out on his own terms.

• Change is not so much doing as undoing. If you've spent your life giving to others and sacrificing yourself, start seeing what you can give to yourself. If you've spent your life focused on yourself, start paying attention to others. Learn to undo whatever narrow force has been controlling your life so far. Then you'll be able to broaden your ability to experience and enjoy all of life.

• Don't be afraid to fantasize. The language of fantasy comes out of one's whole being and life experience. It's a beautiful language because it can lead to realizing that one's fantasies can possibly be achieved. When you really want something, your energies go in that direction. If you don't fantasize, you won't make a move. Example: My oceanfront house in Montauk came out of a fantasy I had during a fishing trip back in 1954.

• Don't break up your marriage over an infidelity. You may have to come to peace with your spouse's having had an affair. If he or she is a good husband or wife and loves the children, and something solid and good still exists between you, you don't have to break up. Expand your awareness instead. . .and give up the rigid notion that there can be only one true love forever.

• Learn to be open with your spouse. In a crisis that threatens a relationship you must learn to be open. With the average couple, neither one really wants to hurt the other, but boredom sets in and leads slowly to a crisis. The partners realize there's no more excitement, fun or laughs. How to create excitement: Trust each other with your inner thoughts and feelings. Share sexual fantasies. Join a therapy group for couples.

• Stop living by the "shoulds." Learn to be who you are rather than who you "should" be. People who live lives of quiet desperation are doing what they think (or someone else thinks) they "should" do rather than what they really want to do.

**Source:** Milton M. Berger, M.D., a psychiatrist and co-director of the American Short-Term Therapy Center, New York.

## IMPORTANCE OF LIKING YOUR JOB

Chinese proverb: If you would be happy for one hour, take a nap. If you would be happy for a day, go fishing. If you would be happy for a month, get married. If you would be happy for a year, inherit a fortune. If you would be happy for life, love your work.

• Liking your work shouldn't be considered an option or luxury. A compatible job lowers your risk of contracting serious diseases, including cancer. Chronic job stress weakens the body's immune system. If you feel trapped or really unhappy in a job, you should consider moving on—even if it means a cut in pay.

**Source:** Dr. Roy Walford, professor of pathology, UCLA School of Medicine, Los Angeles.

## WHY YOU SHOULD TAKE SICK DAYS

Sick days can be therapeutic, even when you're not physically ill. By taking an occasional day off to reduce stress or deal with a pressing problem, you may avoid severe burnout later on. How to use it: Read a book, watch a movie, take a long bath. The idea is to indulge yourself.

**Source:** New York psychologist Don Lewittes, quoted in *Glamour.*

## HOW TO LEAVE THE OFFICE AT THE OFFICE

As more homes begin to look more like offices, complete with telephone answering machines, beepers, computer terminals, tape recorders and coffee-making systems, it becomes difficult to make the break at the end of the workday.

Sometimes it isn't necessary to make the break. Work has its busy seasons and its peak periods. Then, and during ambitious times such as a start-up, it may not be appropriate to think of leaving the office behind every day. But that shouldn't always be the case. Balance is the goal to work toward.

### What to Turn Off
Make a conscious effort to change your mind-set when you are not at work. Clues that your head is still at the office: You chafe because the host is slow in moving you and other guests to the dining table. . .You make an agenda before going out to spend the afternoon with your child and stick to the agenda even when something more interesting intrudes. These are business mind-sets, not appropriate to non-office activities.

Give yourself a steady stream of physical cues to help you separate your office from your private world. Don't wear a watch on weekends. If you feel time pressures even when you're at home, don't use digital clocks in the car or home. They pace off the seconds and minutes too relentlessly for many people. Change your clothes as soon as you get home. And if you feel naked without your dictating machine or your briefcase with you at home, experiment with feeling naked!

Use your physical setting to help you keep work in its place. Tell yourself that you can work only at a particular place at home if you must work. Don't bring papers to bed with you. Don't spread them out over the couch, the dining table and the floor.

### Making the Shift
The key to making the shift from home to office or office to home is in the transi-

tion that happens each morning and evening. Working women especially have trouble giving themselves a 10-minute break when they get home because they're inclined to feel anxious about talking with the children or starting dinner. Take the break. It can make all the difference between experiencing the rest of the evening as a pleasure or as a demand for attention.

Rituals are a useful device for making the switch. Secretaries do this by tidying up the desk or covering the typewriter. Lyndon Johnson symbolically turned off the lights in the Oval Office when he left. For managers, some useful rituals are loosening ties or other constricting clothing, turning a calendar page or making a list of things to do for the next day. They all help make the break. The to-do list also helps curb the desire to catch up on tomorrow's tasks while you're at home.

### Unwinding Kinks

Resist the growing tendency to abuse the whole winding-down process by taking up activities that create problems of their own...compulsive sex...addictive exercise...overeating or overdrinking...recreational drugs. Better: Use the transition time as a period of discovery. Walk or drive home along a different route. Pick up something new at the newsstand instead of the usual evening paper.

The other side of leaving the office at the office is to leave home at home. It may be productive to use lunchtimes to buy paint, but that's not helpful in keeping the two worlds separate.

The goal of keeping the worlds more separate is to increase understanding of the difference between business friends and other friends. The stimulus of work can be addictive and can leave people feeling helpless when illness, a disability or retirement takes away the only stimulus they know. In the now famous quote of a hard-driving executive: Nobody ever said on his deathbed, "I wish I had spent more time at the office."

**Source:** Interview with Marilyn Machlowitz, Machlowitz, Ph.D., Associates, a management development firm in New York.

## VACATION MYTH

Not taking vacations isn't necessarily bad, contrary to popular belief. Many chief executives dislike vacations and rarely take them yet are stable, healthy and physically fit. They typically find the preparations needed to get away aren't worth the effort, and they view work involvements as activities that are more creative and pleasing than vacation activities.

**Source:** Study of 60 chief executives of major companies by William Theobald, professor of recreation studies, Purdue University, Lafayette, IN.

## BETTER TIME MANAGING CAN KEEP YOU HEALTHY

Beating the clock can cause ulcers, high blood pressure, heart attacks and even cancer. Managers who fret or fidget when they're forced to sit for only a few minutes are probably suffering from hurry sickness. They're more prone to disease and early death. Remedies: (1) Factor a time cushion into daily schedules. (2) Do things that must be done first and let less important matters wait. (3) Learn to say no to unwanted calls or visitors. (4) Broaden horizons with outside interests.

**Source:** *Creative Management*, New York.

## SHIFT-CHANGE WARNING

Frequent shift changes, from night to day and vice versa, lower productivity. Your body does not have time to adjust its internal clock to the new schedule. It becomes confused on when to sleep and when to wake, resulting in drowsiness on the job. Solution: Adhere to a normal 24-hour day and change shifts as infrequently as possible.

**Source:** Martine C. Moore-Ede, writing in *Natural History*.

## FACING YOUR OWN INCOMPETENCE

The Peter Principle: *In a hierarchy, individuals tend to rise to their level of incompetence.*

Many people who've read my book *The Peter Principle* have recognized only professional or technical incompetence. But it's more complicated than that. Incompetence has many faces and lurks in some heretofore unsuspected areas:

• Physical incompetence. A person who is professionally or technically competent may develop such anxiety over his work that he gets ulcers or high blood pressure. And that results in a poor attendance record. His boss and co-workers assume he's really very competent but just has health problems. In reality, he is physically incompetent to handle the strain of the job.

• Mental incompetence. This occurs when a person is moved to a level where he can no longer deal with the intellectual requirements of the job.

Example: Stu Pidd was the foreman of the lead sinker casting department. He was a pleasant, kindly person who did a conscientious job. When his company took on more products, he was promoted to supervisor. This job required decisions about the allocation of workers and equipment. Instead of simple orders, Stu received guidelines and policy statements from management. Lacking the ability to deal with these abstractions, he habitually misunderstood company policy and made illogical decisions, reducing his department's efficiency.

• Social incompetence. A person who is technically competent may be unable to get along with others. Or, problems may arise if he is promoted in an organization where a different class of social behavior is required when moving up the ladder. The Beverly Hillbillies syndrome then tends to set in.

Example: Mal Larkey was a salesman selling lead sinkers to the trade. When his company took on a line of tuning forks, he had to represent a whole different class of product to a tonier group of people. The dirty jokes and breezy manner that worked with the sinker customers didn't go over with the highbrow tuning-fork crowd.

• Emotional incompetence. A technically competent person may be too unstable emotionally to deal with a particular job. Creative types, who tend to be insecure, are particularly prone to this type of incompetence when promoted to administrative positions.

• Ethical incompetence. Richard Nixon is a good example. Despite his nickname, Tricky Dick, and even though he had been caught at deceptive practices in earlier campaigns, Nixon was still able to win the presidency in 1968. Only when the White House tapes revealed his dishonesty beyond a doubt was it clear that he had reached his level of ethical incompetence. His brand of manipulative persuasiveness, an asset in local politics, became a liability in the highest office in the land. Nixon Principle: If two wrongs don't make a right, try three.

### Why We Behave As We Do

The Peter Principle seems to be part of human nature. According to Abraham Maslow, the eminent psychologist, it's human nature to struggle onward and upward through varying levels of needs. First we take care of our survival needs. . . then our safety needs. . . then social needs. . . then esteem or ego needs. . . and finally self-actualization needs.* That's why an executive who has reached the top of the ladder in his own company soon gets the itch to start acquiring other companies.

The behavior our parents reinforce in us when we are children always encourages us to strive for bigger and better things. We gain approval for achievement and disapproval for failure. As adults, we keep striving because our developmental makeup says "You've got to have more."

The more recent neurological explanation of left-brain versus right-brain dominance is also relevant. Left-brain-dominant people tend to be the most linear in their thinking and therefore organize life step by step. Left-brain types often get into management, where they are good at control but dismal at stimulating creativity. They climb the hierarchical ladder because their natures are linear and methodical.

*Self-actualization: The process of realizing fully one's potential.

### Escaping the Peter Principle

Take your life and your job seriously. But don't take yourself seriously. Don't spend your life climbing and acquiring. Instead, combine accomplishment and satisfaction. A climber whose gaze is always focused on the next rung fails to appreciate the view from the rung he's on. Happiest: Those who climb to a level that they find fulfilling, stay there for a long period, and then move forward.

### To Avoid Your Level of Incompetence

Many organizations exert great pressure on employees to move upward, and an outright refusal of a promotion can be seen as disloyalty, incompetence or cowardice. It might even get you fired. You must approach promotion avoidance indirectly.

Worth trying: The dart strategy. When I was a happy university professor, I had to head off attempts to promote me to department chairman. Whenever the dean dropped into my office to ask me a question, I would reach into the desk drawer, take out a dart, and throw it at a target hanging on the office wall. I wrote down the number of hits, made a rapid calculation...and then proceeded to say no. I knew the dart strategy was a success when I overheard the dean say, "Peter is a genius, but he's a ding-a-ling." The attempts to promote me ceased. When they started up again, I took to strolling over to the window at department meetings and lighting my cigarette by focusing sunlight on it through a magnifying glass. That got me off the hook again.

**Source:** Interview with Dr. Laurence J. Peter, whose latest book is *Why Things Go Wrong, or The Peter Principle Revisited*, William Morrow & Co., New York.

## FIVE REASONS TO QUIT YOUR JOB

If you're clearly in the wrong job: (1) Why waste time failing? Admit you're licked and find a place to succeed. (2) Why ruin your self-image? The longer you stay, the more you'll feel like a failure. (3) Why wait for the axe to fall? If you know it's coming, don't torture yourself. (4) Why put failure on your record? Quitting is easier to explain than being fired. (5) Why bring others down with you? When managers fail, their subordinates suffer, too.

**Source:** *The Levinson Letter*

## WHY PEOPLE CHANGE CAREERS

Mid-life career changes are on the rise for women as well as for men. The average age for the change is in the late thirties. According to Nella Barkley, president of New York's John C. Crystal Center, people are thinking about the trade-offs in their lives much earlier and don't fit old stereotypes and patterns. Although many people are happy and successful in their professions, they're ready for new challenges and actively seek them. Reason: People in today's better-educated work force expect more from their jobs than a paycheck. They want to earn a living and fulfill themselves.

## 10 RULES FOR DEALING WITH PEOPLE

• Remember their names.

• Be comfortable to be with. Don't cause strain in others.

• Try not to let things bother you. Be easygoing.

• Don't be egotistical or know-it-all.

• Learn to be interesting so that people will get something stimulating from being with you.

• Eliminate the "scratchy" elements in your personality, traits that can irritate others.

• Never miss a chance to offer support or say "Congratulations."

• Work at liking people. Eventually you'll like them naturally.

• Honestly try to heal any misunderstandings and drain off grievances.

• Develop spiritual depth in yourself and *share* this strength with others.

**Source:** Time Talk.

# ALL ABOUT NERDS

Unlike wimps, nerds get attention by being obnoxious. They don't pay attention to the signals other people send them. They don't learn about themselves because they seldom stop to listen to others.

*How not to be a nerd:*

• Let people finish what they are saying.

• Don't always insist that you know more than other people about the subject under discussion.

• Slow down on advice-giving.

• Open up to new ideas.

• Let yourself change your mind once in a while.

When a nerd starts to realize that much of his behavior stems from anxiety about being accepted and loved, he is well on his way to being a nerd no longer.

**Source:** *The Secret of Charisma* by Doe Lang, New York.

# DALE CARNEGIE'S PERSUASION SECRETS

• Successful criticism. Most people begin their criticism with sincere praise followed by the word "but" and end with a critical statement. That's a trap. The other person feels encouraged until he hears "but" and then questions the sincerity of the original praise. Better: Use the word "and" rather than "but." By linking praise to a statement about higher expectations of performance, you're more likely to win the other person's willingness to accept, as well as respond to, your criticism.

• Friends. People spend most of their lives trying to get other people interested in *them.* The result is that they impress people but don't make many sincere, reliable friends. Secret: You can make many more friends faster by becoming genuinely interested in other people. The attention, time and cooperation of even the most sought-after people can be won by showing a genuine interest in their background and work.

• Win support for your ideas by making others think the idea is theirs. *Example:* Instead of urging customers to buy what you have, ask them to give you ideas on improving the product or service. This makes them feel part of the superior quality of the product. Then you don't have to persuade them —they'll feel the idea of buying was their own.

**Source:** *How to Enjoy Your Life and Your Job,* revised edition by Dale Carnegie, copyright by Dorothy Carnegie and Donna Dale Carnegie, Simon & Schuster, New York.

# INCONGRUOUS BEHAVIOR —HOW TO READ THE SIGNALS

People engaged in conversation are often nagged by thoughts contrary to their words. Nor can they always restrain these conflicts. They leak out through incongruous behavior, the sure sign that the speakers are not as comfortable, strong, truthful and sure of themselves as they sound.

There are many forms of incongruous behavior. They often center in the five major areas of nonverbal communication as delineated by Ray L. Birdwhistell* more than a decade ago. The five areas: Facial expression, hands, feet, posture and eyes. Another telling area: The manner in which the words are said.

Incongruity in communication occurs when these areas are not all in agreement with one another. It indicates that some kind of deception, including self-deception, is going on.

You can sharpen your perception of what is troubling a person who consistently practices incongruous behavior. (We are speaking here of people who are basically truthful but who have lapses that are deceptive.)

*Kinesics and Context: Essays on Body Motion Communication* by Ray L. Birdwhistell, University of Pennsylvania Press, Philadelphia.

Here's how:

• Study their lower limbs as they speak. That is where the tension and anxiety show. The person may claim to be relaxed, yet the legs are crossed tightly, and one foot thrusts so rigidly in the air that it appears to be on the verge of breaking off. Insight: People concentrate on hiding their tension from the waist up. Their real state is revealed in their legs and feet.

• Be aware of body segmentation, the assumption of closed positions, such as firmly crossed arms or legs, or both. Contrast: Someone who takes more open stances, such as moving the arms outwardly during conversation. Trouble sign: The person who cannot open body posture even when discussing such intimate subjects as friendship and trust.

• Listen to the voice. People often reveal their inner conflicts by fragmenting their sentences, failing to complete thoughts or skipping key portions.

• Hear the metaphors. A person who is talking of peace and harmony may be depending on metaphors related to war and turbulence.

• Be aware of the volume and rhythm of the voice and the dips in energy in the sentence structure. People tend to speak loudly to convince you of the truth of what they are saying. And they let their voices fall off when they feel they are saying things they do not necessarily want you to hear.

Any of these clues indicates that you are receiving edited versions of a speaker's thoughts, not the full report.

### Opportunity

When you spot the telltale signs of incongruous behavior, ask, "Is there something else you need to tell me?" This gives the person a chance to open up, a chance that would otherwise have remained masked behind the idiosyncratic behavior.

Some incongruous behavior is tied to cultural expectations. Example: People may say aggressive things with a smile. In many regions, this is a culturally accepted way for speakers to imply that they are only kidding (even if they aren't). It's more important to understand this type of coding than to con-

front it. If mixed messages like this are part of the local culture, don't be put off by them.

People who smile all the time, no matter what their message, are permanently incongruous. This suggests character-structure problems that need fuller investigation.

**Source:** Interview with Dr. Martin G. Groder, psychiatrist and business consultant in Durham, NC.

## THE POWER OF A SMILE

A smile will make people like you better whether they want to or not, a recent study suggests. Subjects' facial muscles were wired with electrodes while videotapes of Ronald Reagan were shown. When Reagan smiled, viewers consistently responded with tiny smiles of their own, even those who disliked his political views. Hypothesis: People are disarmed by heavy exposure to a smiling leader.

**Source:** Roger D. Masters, Ph.D., professor of government, Dartmouth College, quoted in *Success!*.

## HOW MAKING EYE CONTACT HELPS

Eye contact helps people in almost any walk of life. Examples: Salvation Army Santas claim they almost always get a donation if they make eye contact with pedestrians. Salespeople who use eye contact with customers generate more and larger sales. Hitchhikers stand a better chance of getting rides if they engage in eye contact with passing motorists. Managers and executives who use their eyes when talking with their staffs open communications. And parents often find eyes the most effective means of scolding children.

**Source:** Study conducted by the University of Utah, Salt Lake City.

## LOOKING SOMEONE IN THE EYE

Shifty-eyed people aren't necessarily deceitful. Often they're isolated loners who are uncomfortable with closer contact. If you have this problem: Try looking at people either just above their eyes or just below. This gives the inpression of warmth and openness, even when none exists.

**Source:** *Medical Aspects of Human Sexuality,* New York.

## WHAT SLIPS OF THE TONGUE REALLY MEAN

Most "Freudian slips" have no hidden motives or meaning, according to recent research. Why the tongue slips: A more familiar or simpler word replaces the intended one because of a failure in mental editing.

**Source:** James Reason, Ph.D., a psychologist at the University of Manchester, England.

## HOW TO SPOT A LIAR

When we lie, we feel varying degrees of discomfort. Some people feel actual fear—others, the mildest tension. But at least to some degree, our feelings are expressed in our behavior. We may control our words, our voice, our face or our posture. But we cannot control everything. To the astute observer we give ourselves away.

Sometimes the giveaway is only a "micromovement"—a brief, minimal change in facial expression. Example: I once offered a used-car owner $500. I watched his face and saw a fleeting smile. Although it lasted only a fraction of a second before he resumed his bland expression and proposed a higher price, I knew he was happy with the original offer. I didn't budge. He took the $500.

The voice is a rich source of information. People who are lying tend to talk slowly. (By definition, they're not spontaneous.) They speak in shorter sentences than usual. They realize that the more they talk, the more likely they are to slip up. In fact, they do slip up. Reason: Tense people are more error-prone in all areas. Liars tend to truncate words and sentences and to express incom-

plete thoughts. Their voices will be pitched higher than normal, another by-product of tension.

Because liars want to increase their distance from others, they cut back on gestures and eye contact. The less exposure, the better. They tend to sit sideways, rather than face to face. They rarely lean forward toward their listeners.

At the same time, liars are more self-conscious. They shift in their seats, adjust their clothing and scratch themselves. Often they bring a hand to the face—another way to reduce exposure.

A very reliable sign is body stiffness. Look for a rigid posture (whether the person is standing or seated), with strict symmetry of limbs.

Other non-verbal cues are less useful. Certain people—calmer types and men in general—smile more when they lie, since this is a channel they can control. But more anxious people tend to freeze and to smile less than normal when they lie.

A perspiring brow or flushed cheeks are primarily symptoms of high arousal. They may reflect anger, excitement, discomfort or fear. But if a flushed person also speaks in halting sentences and avoids eye contact, you would be wise to doubt his words.

It should be noted that these signals can appear in someone who is not lying. The person may simply be uncomfortable—either about saying something, or about saying it to a particular individual.

Once you suspect someone is lying, there are various ways to smoke him or her out. The key is to frame open-ended questions. Example: "What were you up to last night?" (not "Did you have a good time?"). Or ask him to repeat an obvious falsehood, saying, "I didn't hear that." He may get flustered enough to change his story. Another good ploy: Respond to an answer with silence. Just sit there and wait. The liar won't know whether you expect him to go on or not—a very stressful situation. The more stress you put on a liar, the more information you get.

But what if the tables are turned and you feel the need to lie? My advice is simple. . . use a letter rather than the phone, and the phone rather than speaking face to face.

But if you must lie to someone in person, avoid major changes in your behavior to mask non-verbal clues. Very few of us are good actors. The more alien your role, the more uncomfortable you'll feel—and the more obvious your lie.

**Source:** Interview with Albert Mehrabian, Ph.D., a professor of psychology at the University of California at Los Angeles.

## 4 CLUES THAT TELL YOU SOMEONE IS LYING

Look for the following signs of distress, fear or anger (typical reactions of people who are attempting to conceal something)... (1) Raised inner eyebrows. (2) Raised, knitted brows. (3) A narrowing and tightening of the red margin of the lips. (4) An asymmetrical smile. (The average persons tells a lie at least twice a day.)

**Source:** Paul Ekman, a psychologist at the University of California at San Francisco.

## OVERCOMING EMBARRASSMENT

Face up to the gaffe. Stop worrying about how silly you appear responding to your mistake. Look for the humor. Don't brood on the past or embarrassments will become inhibitions. Remember: Everyone has endured similar humiliations—even the people you fear are laughing at you now.

**Source:** *Cosmopolitan*, New York.

## FACE-READING

Large round eyes indicate bravery, and joined eyebrows reveal a mean and unforgiving nature, according to the ancient Chinese art of *siang mien*. Thin lips: Brutal, selfish (unless tempered by a rounded nose tip). Smooth, wide forehead: Clever, decisive. Cleft chin: A yen for the limelight. Large, long ears: Compassionate, understanding. Thin eyelashes: Sharp temper.

Wide space between eyes: Inner reserves of energy.

**Source:** *Secrets of the Face* by Lailan Young, Little, Brown & Co., New York.

## WALK TALK

A heavy step means you're down-to-earth but rarely spontaneous, says astrologist Maxine Fiel. A light step: Dreamy, optimistic. A long stride: Dynamic, forceful. A quick walk: Impulsive, alert. A slow walk: Comtemplative, careful. Bent forward: Goal-oriented, serious.

**Source:** *Mademoiselle*, New York.

## TIPS FOR MAKING FRIENDSHIPS LAST

Don't bother criticizing an insecure friend or relative, even in a constructive way. It won't do any good. For a person who lacks self-esteem, any value judgment, no matter how helpful or positive, is seen as an attack.

**Source:** *Medical Aspects of Human Sexuality*, New York.

• Never try to guess what's troubling a silent friend. Your assumption will probably be wrong and negative. Instead: Ask.

**Source:** *The Love Test* by Harold Bessell, William Morrow & Co., New York.

• To calm a friend who is furious at you, stay calm yourself. Moods are contagious, and it's hard to stay angry at someone who doesn't respond angrily. Keep your voice low and soothing. Good body language: An unwrinkled forehead. Relaxed eyebrows and mouth. Uncrossed arms, open hands.

**Source:** Arnold P. Goldstein, director of the Syracuse University Center for Research on Aggression, in *Vogue*, New York.

## BETTER ONE-TO-ONE CONVERSATIONS

We know it's been said before, but the surest way to improve your one-to-one conversations is. . .to become a better listener. Listening skills may seem simple enough, but many people (particularly men) need to work on them.

Live in the present moment. Resist all distractions. Don't let your mind wander to your bank balance or to after-dinner plans. Stay alert and concentrate on what your "partner" is saying—not only the words, but the emotions behind them. Then rephrase what you've heard in your own words (mentally or verbally).

Example: Your friend tells you he's gunning for a promotion but that his boss seems to be favoring a co-worker. Your response: "That sounds rough. Is it upsetting you?" This kind of reflection will not only help you understand. . .it will also make your friend feel you are trying to understand, and encourage him to share more with you.

(Such questions are especially effective for resuming a conversation several days later. You might lead off by asking your friend if the situation at work has changed. This lends continuity to a friendship. . . and shows you care enough to remember.)

If you follow this technique, you'll naturally become a more empathetic listener. You'll stop interrupting so much, a habit that discourages real communication. And you won't argue so frequently, since you'll be more concerned with grasping the other person's meaning than with scoring some rhetorical point.

Good listening is enhanced by appropriate body language. Consistent eye contact . . .leaning toward the person if seated. . . an occasional nod or smile. . .all can help show that you're an interested listener—if they're natural and timed correctly. But you can't fake it. If the gestures are forced or perfunctory, it will show.

Even the best listeners occasionally find themselves bored by some long-winded anecdote or complaint. How to handle it: Steer the conversation to a mutually interesting subject. Or. . .approach the old subject from a new angle.

Example: Your friend's complaints about his job have grown tedious. Your response: "Have you considered moving to a new company?"

When it's your turn to talk, think about the point you want to make before you start speaking. Then get to it in as few steps as possible. Important: Consider your audience. Make what you're saying relevant to the particular person you're addressing.

Beyond that, there are no simple tricks to enrich your conversations. Your talk reflects your life. If you are totally absorbed in your job, your conversations will inevitably stagnate as soon as they get beyond shoptalk. But if you approach life with curiosity and enthusiasm, your speech will range as wide as your mind. Especially useful: Reading outside your field. . .any subject that might spark discussion.

People tend to be more comfortable with others more like themselves. But it's the people outside your clique or specialty who may ask the freshest questions, even if less well informed. (Conversely, don't be afraid to ask a "dumb" question about a subject that's new to you.)

If your conversations seem bland, maybe you're suppressing honest disagreements. A dispute shouldn't hurt an exchange (or a friendship), as long as a certain etiquette is respected.

Useful: Give the other person credit for something before you disagree. Never say, "How can you think something like that?" Better: "That's a good point, but I see it differently. . . ." Or first point out areas of similarity: "We agree that world peace is vital—therefore. . . ."

Sometimes intense disagreements should be sidestepped. The old saw "Never discuss politics or religion" can be wisely applied—especially if you don't know the other person very well. An emotional argument can cut short a potential friendship.

**Source:** Interview with Mark Sherman, associate professor of psychology, and Adelaide Haas, associate professor of communications, State University of New York, New Paltz.

## CONVERSATION STRATEGY

"Stop me if you've heard this. . ." When a friend begins an anecdote already told several times, break in with a summarizing comment. ("Oh, yes, I remember your vivid description of. . .") Then follow up with a related question. You don't get bored or imposed upon, your friend isn't hurt and you can discuss the subject from a new angle.

## SAYING NO ISN'T EASY BUT IT'S IMPORTANT

People who think they can't say no don't realize that they actually do say no all the time—but in indirect and tortuous ways that aren't effective. Instead of refusing directly when confronted with a request they don't want to honor, they say things like "I'll try"—and then they fail to follow through. Or they begin to feel that the other person "owes" them, and somewhere along the line, they will try to collect. The other person will experience this as persecution. The the stage is set for a further round of psychological games.

The programming to say no starts very early. Some people decide, at a very young age, that compliance is the best way to respond to authority. They grow up unable to feel comfortable with saying no. (Others decide early on to respond to authority in a rebellious fashion. Often, they can't feel good about saying yes.)

Those who won't say no openly tend to be vulnerable to frequently recurring fears (such as the fear of rejection) and guilt. They may have a damaged sense of self-esteem, as shown by their need to please others—they feel the need to earn acceptance by being nice all the time. Result: They end up carrying around an accumulation of unacknowledged resentment at being "put upon."

People who don't know how to say no also don't know how to accept having others say no to them. Their own wildly disproportionate notions are projected onto other people. Result: When people say no to them, they experience it as an enormous personal rejection.

Learning to say no when you really want to is both healthy and necessary, even though society teaches us that "selfishness" is wrong and that it is virtuous to accom-modate others. The truth: If you don't take care of your own needs and wishes, neither can you take care of anyone else's needs effectively.

How to say no:

• Be clear about your preferences and feelings before answering a request. If you're not sure about what you want, set aside some time to consider your response. Say, "I'll think it over and let you know tomorrow."

• When you must say no, remember that you have importance for others, as they have for you. They need you, just as you need them. That importance can't be diminished by an instance of your saying no.

• Be aware that it's possible to say no without destroying the other person. There's always a feeling among "pleasers" (people who need to be nice to everyone) that if they refuse a request, the other person will fall apart. This is an illusion.

• Be consistent. Once you decide what you want to do in a given situation, be prepared to repeat saying no and to give additional information. Examples: "I won't do it because I don't have time." "If I say yes, I'll feel resentful or manipulated."

• Consider compromise. Compromise is not a dirty word, nor is it weakness. It's a useful way for two people to get the best outcome without either one suffering. Take time to explore the options. That doesn't mean changing your *no* to *yes*. It means looking for an alternative that might be acceptable to you.

• Practice saying *no* in your head. Whenever anybody asks you for something, try saying *no* silently, to see how it feels. This is particularly helpful in developing the sense of discrimination that is so necessary for "pleasers."

• Time bomb: When someone tries to persuade you to do something for them that you're really unwilling to do, be aware that if it's bad for you, it's bad for them. You end up with resentment and a muddied relationship.

• Learning to accept no from others objectively is a way to strengthen your own capacity to say no directly and without conflict. Learn to clarify what the other person's *no* means. That way you'll see it in better perspective. Example: If someone doesn't return your calls, phone the secretary. Find out if the person you want is just temporarily unwilling to speak with you or is uninterested in what you have to offer. The tendency to distort its meaning or exaggerate it, is what causes most of the emotional pain of having someone say no to you. If the no is a real rejection of you and objectively painful, it is better to acknowledge it than to keep putting yourself in the position of inevitable rejection.

**Source:** Interview with Gisele Richardson, president of Richardson Management Associates, Montreal, Canada. The firm specializes in assertiveness workshops and consulting.

# HOW TO SAY NO WITHOUT FEELING GUILTY

Many of us say yes more often than we'd like. Sometimes we feel we have to repay some actual or imagined favor. At other times we acquiesce out of fear of disapproval or out of some misguided idea of politeness. Whatever the reason, if you find yourself saying yes because you feel guilty about saying no, here are some practical measures to help you protect yourself.

### The Right to Stall

Many people fail to understand that they have a basic human right to say no. Frequently people with assertiveness problems are unsure of their feelings about a particular issue. A request is made of them: On the one hand, they want to help because the asker has done favors for them in the past; on the other, they don't have much enthusiasm for carrying out the request. But they will impulsively say yes because they lack the nerve to give a flat-out no.

Stalling is an enormously valuable tactic that gives you precious time to work up an honest rationale for a total refusal. Suggested stalling statements:

• I don't know. I need time to think about it—give me an hour.

• A lot of what you're saying makes perfect sense, but there's something about your request that makes me uncomfortable. I need some time to think it over.

### Other Helpful Tactics

There are other strategies by which the terminally guilt-ridden can stave off unwanted obligations. Humor is helpful. So is repeating the words, *I can't do that,* over and over. Flattery is another good tactic. White lies are sometimes necessary.

Strategy illustration:

While Loretta was at a co-op board meeting, the president asked her to serve as head of the decoration committee. Despite her initial impulse to say yes, she stalled: "It sounds like a good idea, and I'm sure I could do the job. But I have a few other obligations, and I need a day to think about it." A day later, Loretta called the president back and told him she was flattered that he wanted her for the job but that she just didn't have the time. He then attempted to pressure her by saying, "There's no one else who could do it as well as you." She came back with, "As a matter of fact, you're so artistic, you could do an even better job than I could. If you're too busy, why don't you try Jan or Nancy? They did a bang-up job on the landscaping last year." He then switched to guilt, pointing out that he'd done favors for her when she chaired a committee he was on. She teased him by pointing out that she thought she'd paid back that debt already, and she reminded him that she hadn't signed anything in blood. Finally he gave up good-naturedly.

### Saying No to Family

This is the hardest kind of refusal to deal with. You not only need the interpersonal skills to say no gracefully but you also have to rethink your real obligations to your family, so you can say no without guilt. Suggestions:

• Resist the hidden-bargain syndrome. Parents often operate under the assumption that since they've done all these wonderful things for their children to bring them up, the offspring owe them everything. Both young and grown children can be manipulated by this assumption. Remedy: Recognize that parents do nice things at least as much for their own benefit as for their children's sake. I do a lot of loving and giving to my own child, but primarily because it makes me feel good and gives me satisfaction. I am thus getting my payoff on the spot, through the act of giving itself.

• Recognize that a family member who acts hurt at a turndown is torturing himself. You're not responsible for other people's reactions.

Example: An elderly mother went to visit her son, who lived in an apartment too small for two people to stay in comfortably. When he told her he thought it would be better if he put her up at a hotel, she acted hurt. Remedy: The son must recognize that his mother is making herself unhappy by interpreting his hotel offer as a rejection. In truth, he has done nothing thoughtless or inconsiderate. He must point out to his mother that, despite her bad feelings, they would both be more comfortable if they stayed in separate accommodations.

• Don't sit on guilt. As soon as you feel it, share it. Guilt pushers are also guilt buyers, and they know better than anyone how awful it is to feel guilty. In the story above, the son could also tell his mother that she makes him feel terrible when she pushes guilt on him and ask her if that was her intention. Frequently, just pointing out a guilt manipulation makes the other back off. Once that's done, you're free to sit down and honestly discuss how making another person feel guilty hurts a relationship.

• Learn to say no to your children. Parents frequently feel guilty about poor parenting. They try to compensate by capitulating easily to their children's requests. More than anything, they want their children to like them. Often the parents themselves grew up in a restrictive environment, and they've vowed not to be as strict with their own children as their parents were with them. But children need structure and limits in order to learn self-discipline and independence. Helpful: Remind yourself that saying no to your child is an act of love, not of repres-

sion. You're doing your child a favor by teaching him how to grow up rather than remain a perennial emotional infant.

**Source:** Interview with Barry Lubetkin, Ph.D., a psychologist who is founder and clinical director of the Institute for Behavior Therapy in New York.

# HANDLING CRITICISM

Properly used, criticism enhances personal growth and relationships. Hitch: Even constructive criticism is not always presented in a good way. And learning to accept criticism is hard for most people.

Problem: Criticism is often prefaced with a dogmatic phrase such as "you should." This reveals the rigidity of the critic and makes those being criticized resist change. It also implies the erroneous concept that there is a right way and a wrong way to do things —with no acceptable middle ground.

Result: Critical statements are answered with equally critical rejoinders. Soon, each person is trying to top the other as the tone becomes increasingly personal.

There are ways, however, to avoid this familiar cycle. A checklist for giving constructive criticism:

• Target the behavior you want to criticize. Make your criticism as specific as possible.

• Save your critical comments for the appropriate time and place. Never blurt them out in public.

• Verify that the behavior you are criticizing is capable of being changed. If it cannot be, then say nothing.

• Avoid threats and accusations. Keep your comments brief and understandable.

• Do not allow a bad mood to color your words. Listen to your voice for signs of hostility or sarcasm.

• Offer to help in resolving the behavior you are criticizing.

Receiving criticism graciously is equally delicate. Prime lesson: Consider the consistency with which a specific criticism is offered. Regularly repeated criticism is probably valid. Other considerations:

• Avoid the inclination to defend yourself blindly against criticism. Instead, ask for more information and develop the skill of attentive listening.

• Request solutions to the criticism. Ask the critic, "What would you do in my place?"

• Summarize the criticism and your responses so that communication about the problem is clear. At the same time, plan a definable strategy for correcting the behavior.

**Source:** *Nobody's Perfect (How to Give Criticism and Get Results),* by Hendrick Weisinger, Ph.D., Warner Books, New York.

# BEST WAY TO APOLOGIZE

The one-minute apology: (1) Give it immediately—or as soon as possible—after making a mistake. The longer you wait, the harder it is. (2) Be specific as to what you are apologizing for. A simple "I'm sorry" isn't helpful. (3) Tell the person whom you wronged how you feel (embarrassed, sad, etc.). (4) Affirm yourself. Make it clear how unlike you this behavior was (so you can stop feeling guilty).

**Source:** Kenneth Blanchard, co-author of *The One-Minute Manager,* in *Success!*

# DEALING CONSTRUCTIVELY WITH ANGER

Recent evidence suggests that always getting your anger out and expressing what you're feeling perhaps isn't as cathartic as was once thought, though expressing anger is doubtedly preferable to sitting on your feelings. Even better: Learning how to manage your anger so you control it rather than letting it control you. Once you learn to deal effectively with anger, you'll have options. You can express anger when appropriate, stop it from bothering you when inappropriate, or channel it constructively. You won't constantly be at the mercy of this powerful emotion.

### Changing Your Behavior

Some of us have hot tempers that explode inappropriately, alienating friends, co-workers, bosses, spouses and our children. Others can be boiling inside but act timid when it comes to a confrontation. The trick: Expressing anger effectively.

If you have an explosive temper:

• Take time as soon as you begin feeling anger to identify its source. Sit down, close your eyes and visualize as clearly as possible the person you're angry at. See yourself dealing with that person in a reasoned, appropriate manner. As soon as you imagine yourself blowing up, stop and go back to the image of yourself being open, honest and direct—not shouting or being sarcastic or humiliating. This rehearsal will be useful in itself in controlling your anger response. By the time you confront the person, you'll feel less angry and be more effective.

• Do a daily anger assessment. Fill in a chart with three columns: What am I feeling? What am I thinking? What provoked it? The mere act of objectifying your anger will distance you from it and decrease the anger response. Now it's not emerging mysteriously from your system and taking you over. It's something you can rate. It has a beginning, middle and end.

If you're afraid to express anger:

• Visualization will help. See yourself confronting the person you're angry at and expressing your feelings directly and honestly, without retreat or apology. Once the time comes for performance, you'll know your lines well and be feeling comfortable with them.

• Pay attention to body language, so you don't undercut your message. People often smile, giggle, look at the floor or squirm around when they're expressing anger. Look at yourself in front of the mirror to practice what you think anger looks like and check out your body language. You might even ask a good friend to give you feedback.

### Changing Your Outlook

Tune in to the two types of personality: The requiring and the aspiring. The requiring type demands never to be put down and that the world always be fair. The aspiring type says it would certainly be nice if people never put him down, but he realizes that life is often unfair. You'll find yourself feeling much less angry if you recognize that good luck and bad luck are meted out randomly. Today may be your turn to get a bad break, but maybe tomorrow things will look up. Don't personalize unfairness. Angry people are apt to feel that they're being punished for something they did wrong.

How to be an aspirer:

• Eliminate the word *should* from your thinking. ("He should have treated me better, after all I've done for him.") When you're angry or upset, ask yourself: Does life always have to be the way I want it to be? Can I survive as a reasonably happy person even if I don't get what I want in this situation?

• Learn to accept what you can't change. Don't fool yourself that if you somehow magically do something different, the world will play fair with you. Example: You have a boss who always puts you down. You've tried everything to get him to stop, to no avail. You can't quit your job. Accept that he's got the problem, not you, and treat him as you would treat anyone you have to humor to get along with. Visualization exercise: He is putting you down. Instead of feeling helpless anger, you are merely disappointed, inconvenienced or sad. You realize that he is a disturbed person, so his behavior doesn't reflect on you.

• Don't invest all of yourself in one aspect of life. If your entire sense of self-worth derives from one area, you may experience enormous anger when it doesn't go well. Recommended: Make a list of how you spend your time. You may notice how many other things you do—and do well. Get involved in relationships and activities outside of that area to receive other ego boosts.

• Have a dialogue with yourself: Go back and forth between the part of you that puts up with bullying and the part that always responds with aggression and anger. Purpose: When people become angry, they're not aware of anything except the feeling of having to defend themselves. The dialogue will help you get in touch with why you need to defend yourself and why you need to stave off criticism. Your anger will be tempered by understanding.

• Find out where the anger comes from. Look at your anger assessment to see if your anger has a theme. Example: You always get angry when criticized by someone in authority. Think back over your childhood. In the past, someone caused you to feel helpless or hopeless because you were not allowed to express anger. You've carried into adulthood a storehouse of bad feelings that gets tapped every time you're confronted by authority. This realization won't necessarily stop you from geting angry, but your anger will be less corrosive once you understand it.

### Make Anger Work for You

• There's nothing wrong with seeking revenge, particularly if there's no other way of dealing with the situation. But make it classy. Don't get vitriolic or indulge in overkill. Be subtle, yet effective. Often, just thinking about bizarre methods of revenge will dispel your anger, and instead you'll find yourself laughing at your own ingenuity.

• Turn anger into positive energy. The physical feeling of anger produces almost the same bodily response as excitement or enthusiasm. The only difference is the label. Learn to use the energy that anger produces to do something for yourself. Recommended: Create an anger-option list with alternative ways to channel your anger. Whenever you feel irrationally angry and know that expressing it is a bad idea, substitute one of the items on your list. Examples: Make a phone call to a person who's been intimidating you, jog for a mile, put up shelves, shop for a new suit.

**Source:** Interview with Barry S. Lubetkin, Ph.D., clinical director, Institute for Behavior Therapy, New York.

# HOW TO MANAGE YOUR ANGER

Avoiding anger, or letting it off in some

harmless fashion, are both impossible. . . contrary to belief. Managing your anger is possible. Technique: Don't speak while angry—you're likely to be impulsive or lack judgment. Putting your feelings into a letter helps, but don't send it until you cool down. Ask a trusted friend to help decide whether your anger is appropriate. Sometimes, just talking eases the intensity. If you've really been mistreated, it's crucial to tell the other person clearly.

**Source:** *The Levinson Letter,* New York.

• Expressing anger is not always a release. Often it simply heightens the feelings. And repressing anger keeps it pent up, which is literally unhealthy. Best: Control your anger. How: Recognize it and identify it. Usually the object of your current anger is not the source of the problem. Determine how serious the problem is. Key: Let trivial upsets pass, and argue only over important matters. When arguing out your anger, never attack the personality or integrity of the other person. State your opinions clearly while keeping to the point. Worse: Sulking silently. This is merely another form of anger.

# HANDLING SOMEONE ELSE'S ANGER

Don't try to talk to people who are angry. Just listen. Let them blow off steam, and try to understand their feelings. Find a way to reopen talks later, when they have cooled down.

**Source:** *Supervisory Management.*

• Acknowledge others' anger quickly (ignoring it or laughing it off only adds fuel to the anger). Make it plain that you're concerned. Listen until they run down. Keep calm (don't take them too seriously). Find out what's really wrong. Strive for agreement on a solution with a timetable; then stick to it.

**Source:** *The Official Guide to Success* by Tom Hopkins, Warner Books, New York.

# THE BIG LITTLE THINGS IN LIFE

They seem harmless little quirks. The toothpaste tube is squeezed from the middle rather than the end. Or the milk is never returned to the refrigerator after breakfast. Yet at a certain point these bad habits of a spouse, lover, roommate or intimate friend become excruciatingly painful.

Why the exaggerated reaction? Main reason: There is already an alienation in the relationship that the bad habit confirms. Example: The person who takes extreme offense because the toothpaste tube is squeezed "incorrectly" feels that the offender does not care enough to be reliable or to be responsive to that person's needs and sensibilities. The careless act is interpreted as a deliberate effort to create pain or a willingness to inflict annoyance.

Often a probing discussion between the parties will uncover the major issues that led to the alienation. Remember, the problem is seldom the bad habit. That is only a manifestation of more serious difficulties. For many, professional counseling may be the only cure.

The ideal expectations of perfectionists cause them to fall prey to this condition. They regard those to whom they are close as minor gods or goddesses. The bad habit, however, is a visible sign of defectiveness which makes the other person unworthy of the perfectionist's feelings.

Perfectionism is sometimes healed by maturity as the sufferers realize there are no perfect people or situations. But severely afflicted perfectionists lose the company of other human beings, since their standards are impossibly high. They usually require psychotherapy. Problem: Often they find therapy unsatisfactory because the therapist is imperfect.

The one cause just discussed usually developed over time and grew from an ongoing relationship. There is another category, however, that earns the offender instant dislike. This occurs when the bad habit reminds a person of an important childhood figure who was a tormentor—a parent, sibling, relative or teacher. The habit summons up a traumatic recollection. It is hate at first sight.

The simple solution is to avoid the hated object. If that is impractical, psychotherapy enables the person to discover the memories that were repressed. This leads the way toward healing the fixation.

Simple prejudice spawns extreme reactions in some to the way certain people look and act. Those prejudiced against a race, creed, class or type seize on any identifying characteristic of that group as annoying. Example: People may be prejudiced against those with a different accent. The prejudiced claim the others are obnoxious because of the way they talk. Truth: It is not the accent that is the problem, but deep-seated prejudice.

Cure: If possible, cultural change and human growth. Sometimes discussion groups between conflicting groups can help breed tolerance.

**Source:** Interview with Martin G. Groder, M.D., a psychiatrist and business consultant who practices in Chapel Hill, NC.

# ALL ABOUT FORGIVENESS

To forgive another is the greatest favor you can do—for yourself. It's the only way to release yourself from the clutch of an unfair past. Beyond that, it opens the possibility of reconciliation, often a gift in itself.

In its simple essence, forgiving is a new way of remembering a person who has hurt you. When you are first wounded, you remember him only as a person who unfairly injured you. As you begin to forgive, you gradually see him as a weak, needy, silly and somewhat stupid person who tried to cope by being cruel to you. As your memory changes, your hatred gradually recedes and your healing begins.

When you've been unfairly hurt, you paint a mental caricature. If the person who wronged you is a bloated bag of undiluted evil, you feel all the more virtuous by comparison. Hatred can also make you feel strong. It's like a drug—at first.

Still, you need to forgive. If you try merely to forget, to erase a hurt like some cassette, the hatred comes back to haunt you. If you persist in passive hatred, it kills your joy. And if you seek revenge, you'll fail. You cannot even the score because two people in conflict never feel pain to the same degree. Revenge leads to further retaliation and (in retrospect) to guilt.

Forgiving doesn't make doormats out of people. You're not tolerating what was done or excusing the person who did it to you. You are holding that person accountable—and then seeking to go on with your life.

### How to Forgive

Every act of forgiveness grows out of unique circumstances. Guidelines:

• Take the initiative in forgiving. Don't wait for the other person to apologize. (That cedes control to the one who hurt you in the first place.)

• If the forgiven person wants to re-enter your life, it is fair to demand truthfulness. He or she should be made to understand, to feel the hurt you've felt. Then you should expect a sincere promise that you won't be hurt that way again.

• Be patient. If the hurt is deep, you can't forgive in a single instant.

• Forgive "retail," not "wholesale." It's almost impossible to forgive someone for being a bad person. Instead, focus on the particular act that hurt you. (It might help to write it down.)

• Don't expect too much. To forgive doesn't mean you must renew a once close relationship. (I knew one estranged wife who was afraid that if she forgave her husband, she'd have to go back and be beaten by him again.) Time and circumstances change. Healing yourself won't always end in a warm embrace. You have to begin where you are.

• Discard your self-righteousness. A victim is not a saint. You too will need forgiveness some day.

• Separate anger from hate. Anger is a great gift, a passionate desire to stop a wrong. You can forgive and stay angry. But hate and malice—wishing someone ill—are self-destructive. You can't forgive and still hate.

To dissolve your malice: Face your emotion and accept it as natural. Then discuss it, either with the object of your hatred (if you can do so without escalating the hatred) or with a trusted third party.

### Self-Forgiveness

The hardest act of all may be to forgive yourself. When we are genuinely guilty, we feel we deserve our own judgment. It seems outrageous to believe that the terrrible wrong we did is irrelevant to who we are. But it's the only way we can deal with the irreversible past.

Self-forgiveness allows us to be freer and to love better. When we're castigating ourselves, it's hard to help, care about and be glad for others.

Again, candor is critical. Admit your fault. Relax your struggle to be perfect. We all need an occasional guilt trip.

Then be concrete and specific about what is bothering you. Your deed was evil. You are not.

Ignore the grudge carriers. If you've fully acknowledged your wrong, you don't need to grovel.

To make self-forgiveness easier: Prime the pump of self-love. Do something unexpected (possibly unappreciated) for a person you care about. By acting freely, you'll find it easier to think freely.

**Source:** Interview with Lewis B. Smedes, author of *Forgive & Forget,* Harper & Row, New York.

# AVOIDING ONE KIND OF FAMILY SQUABBLE

When a parent dies, defer for a month the dividing of personal possessions. You'll be far more likely to avoid emotional squabbles.

**Source:** Avery Weisman, M.D., psychiatry professor, Harvard University, Cambridge, MA.

# HELPING HYPOCHONDRIACS

Try to be sympathetic without taking on responsibility. If you're bored, change the subject—but don't be rejecting. It's cruel to say, "It's all in your head." Pain is no less painful when imaginary. When a new complaint surfaces: Consider that it might be legitimate. Hypochondriacs are often ignored when they really need medical attention.

**Source:** *The New York Times Guide to Personal Health* by Jane Brody, Avon Books, New York.

# WHAT TO BRING A SICK FRIEND

When visiting a sick friend in the hospital, don't bring flowers, bring food. According to Dr. George Blackburn, director of nutrition at Boston's Deaconess Hospital, 10%–20% of hospital patients turn down hospital food to the point that their recovery is adversely affected. Caution: Before bringing food, check with the floor nurse about diet restrictions. Good food choices: Fruit juices (especially citrus), fruit, whole-grained breads, and of course, chicken soup. Let the patient's appetite be the guide.

**Source:** Cited in *American Health.*

# IMPORTANCE OF SADNESS

Showing sadness on a hospital visit is perfectly acceptable, even positive. Reason: It helps validate the patient's own feelings and reflects sincere sympathy. It doesn't pay to strain to cheer someone up. A person who's sick and away from home is entitled to feel unhappy. Recommended: Let the patient set the emotional tone for the visit.

**Source:** Ellen Martin, director of patient relations, St. Luke's-Roosevelt Hospital, New York, quoted in *McCall's,* New York.

# THE BEST KIND OF MEDICINE

Hot chicken soup is beloved by sick people. Yet the tender loving care that usually accompanies it may be at least as helpful to the patient. Levels of agents in the immune system that fight colds and viruses rose when subjects in a test saw a movie about Mother Theresa as she worked with the poor in India. Levels of these agents stayed high as the viewers later recalled times when they had been cared for by others.

**Source:** Research done by psychologists David McClelland and Carol Kirshnit at Harvard University as reported in *Psychology Today,* New York.

# 11. Having and Raising Healthy Children

# Having and Raising Healthy Children

## FERTILITY FACTS AND FIGURES

The peak of fertility comes at age 24 for women. The prime years for normal pregnancy and normal birth are 20–29. The of giving birth to a live child with some chromosomal abnormality are five for every 1,000 births at age 35. At 40, the figure jumps to 15 per 1,000 births. By 45, the chances of bearing a handicapped child zoom to 50 per 1,000 births.

**Source:** *Journal of the American Medical Association*, Chicago.

• One of 10 American couples has failed to conceive after at least one year of marriage without contraception. Reasons: A rise in pelvic inflammatory disease (often caused by veneral diseases). Delay of childbearing until the couple is older (and the woman is less fertile). Previous use of oral contraceptives (which delay pregnancies long after discontinued).

**Source:** *Journal of the American Medical Association*, Chicago.

• Genital-tract yeast infections (which affect both men and women) may be a leading cause of infertility. When husbands had active infections, women in one study had only a 5% pregnancy rate. In a second group, where the husbands' infections were eradicated, the pregnancy rate was 60%.

**Source:** Study at The New York Hospital–Cornell Medical Center, reported in *Vogue* magazine, New York.

## CAUSES OF DECLINING SPERM COUNTS IN U.S. MEN

Male reproductive problems account for 40% of infertility. Basic problem: A 50% decline in the average American male's sperm count since the 1960s. Causes: Tobacco and marijuana smoking. . . X rays. . . zinc and vitamin C deficiencies. . . exposure to toxic chemicals. . . stress.

**Source:** Sherman Silber, M.D., a fertility specialist at St. Luke's West Hospital, St. Louis, quoted in *Prevention* magazine, Emmaus, PA.

## NORMAL SPERM COUNTS AREN'T ENOUGH

Men with normal sperm counts can still be infertile if their sperm are unable to penetrate an egg. At one medical center, the new "zona-free hamster egg test" found that 20% of "normal" men had this problem. Bottom line: Since tests on women are relatively complicated, men should try the new test first.

**Source:** Study at the University of Nebraska Medical Center, Omaha.

## AGE AND MALE FERTILITY

A group of healthy men between the ages of 60 and 88 had the same testicular volume, ejaculate volume, sperm count or appearance, and testosterone levels as males under the age of 40. And sperm from older men doesn't appear to increase the risk of birth defects. What matters: When health deteriorates, sexual function and fertility will also deteriorate.

**Source:** *Medical World News* Houston, TX.

## WONDERS OF VITAMIN C

Doses of vitamin C apparently help men with a certain type of infertility problem. . . a clumping together of the sperm, called *nonspecific sperm agglutination*. In a test,

35 men with the ailment took 500 mg. of pure ascorbic acid every 12 hours. After only one week, the average percentage of sperm that agglutinated had dropped from 20%, which causes infertility, to 14%, a level within the range of fertility. Researchers now believe vitamin C can reverse infertility from this problem after three to four days of treatment.

**Source:** A study by Earl B. Dawson, M.D., and colleagues at the University of Texas Medical Branch, Galveston.

## VAGINAL-LUBRICANT WARNING

Commercial vaginal lubricants can cause fertility problems. They all contain a spermicical agent. Trap: Many people recommend using saliva instead, but that impairs the movement of the sperm. Best: Glycerin, petroleum jelly or raw egg white.

**Source:** *Fertility and Sterility*, Rochester, MN.

## JOGGING ALERT

Regular jogging causes infertility in some women. Running lowers the levels of estradiol and estrone, hormones that are needed for the reproductive process.

**Source:** *New England Journal of Medicine*, Boston, MA.

## TIME MAY BE ALL YOU NEED

Many infertility problems cure themselves over time. A Canadian study found that 62% of women with partially blocked Fallopian tubes eventually became pregnant without treatment. So did 60% of those whose husbands had low sperm counts and 44% who had ovulatory deficiencies. Bottom line: Unless the problem is severe—a man with no sperm production or a woman with both tubes completely blocked—couples should be wary of extraordinary treatments and just be patient.

**Source:** John Collins, M.D., quoted in *American Health*, New York.

• Infertility treatments may be overrated. This was the conclusion of a study at a clinic in Halifax, Nova Scotia. Of the couples treated, 41% conceived within a year—but so did 35% who were diagnosed as infertile but decided against treatment. Bottom line: Before undergoing extreme treatments such as hormones or surgery, a couple should consider letting nature take its course.

**Source:** *New England Journal of Medicine*, Boston, MA.

## EVERYTHING THAT YOU COULD WANT TO KNOW ABOUT SPERM BANKS

Sperm banks store human semen in deep freeze for future use in artificial insemination. Today, sperm banks create possibilities for family planning unimagined 20 years ago.

### Who Uses Sperm Banks?

One in seven married couples in the United States is infertile. These couples, as well as single women who want to have children, can turn to a sperm bank for semen from an anonymous donor. The world's largest sperm bank pays its donors (often medical students) $25 for each specimen deposited. It charges its clients $35–$45 for each specimen ordered. A woman may need to be inseminated several times before a pregnancy results.

For those considering artificial insemination, the first step is selecting a doctor they really trust. The doctor then coordinates with the sperm bank and performs the artificial insemination. Some sperm banks, particularly those affiliated with hospitals, have staff physicians who perform this service.

But sperm banks are not subject to federal regulation, and state laws vary widely. Since many physicians are unaware of the disparity between various facilities, it is important to know what to look for in a sperm bank.

### The Questions to Ask

• Does the bank have a full-time medical director, and is he a pathologist?

• Is there an affiliation with a university or hospital?

• Is the bank a member of the American Association of Tissue Banks? Does it follow the recommendations of the association's Reproductive Council?

• How are the donors screened? A complete physical description, personal and genetic histories, medical evaluation and laboratory analysis of the semen should be standard. The donor should be tested for such things as genetic disorders, damage resulting from environmental conditions, diseases such as AIDS and hepatitis, and sperm count and motility (ability to move). Some sperm banks subject a donor's semen to over 40 different tests. A blood donor, by contrast, is subjected to only three tests.

• Will you or your doctor receive a detailed description of the donor, including general information about his education, background and interests? Some banks supply only very limited information of questionable accuracy.

• Although donor anonymity should be scrupulously maintained, is there a coding system that allows you to check to see if sperm from the same donor will be available should you plan to have a second child?

• What is the bank's minimum acceptable sperm count? The average American sperm count is about 60 million motile sperm per milliliter. Banks vary in their criteria, and donor sperm may contain from 65 million to over 100 million sperm per milliliter.

### Saving for Posterity

Some men arrange for long-term storage of semen before a vasectomy, chemotherapy or exposure to hazardous waste, or numerous other situations. Essentially, they are purchasing fertility insurance, putting aside a deposit of sperm on the chance that they may want to father a child at a time when they are no longer fertile. Pregnancies have resulted from sperm stored for over 10 years.

A complete deposit of three to five cubic centimeters of semen may take two to three days of abstinence to accumulate. And it's important to ascertain that the fa-

cility's security system is adequate. One sperm bank was put out of business when the cooling system broke down and it suffered a "meltdown."

A client depositor owns the rights to his deposit, and he should sign a contract stating who, if anyone, should have access to the deposit in the event of his death. If his marital status changes, he should update the contract. A depositor must remember to pay his storage bill (approximately $10 a year), or he risks losing his deposit.

**Finding a sperm bank:** In a few areas, this is as easy as looking under Sperm Banks in the Yellow Pages. A list of selected members (free) and a booklet, *Standards for Tissue Banking* ($15), are published by and available from the American Association of Tissue Banks, 1117 N. 19 St., Arlington, VA 22209.

Interview with Joseph Feldschuh, M.D., medical director, Idant Laboratory, New York.

# FRESH SPERM VS. FROZEN SPERM

Many physicians use fresh sperm from donors with whom they have made private arrangements.

Advantages: It is cheaper to use fresh sperm than frozen, and it is more convenient for the doctor, entailing less paperwork. Donors can be paid in cash, and no records need be kept.

Disadvantages: A fresh donation—often made in an adjoining room while you wait to be inseminated—is rarely subject to the same rigorous testing that a frozen ejaculate is. Donor anonymity may be less well protected, and there is a possibility that a single donor's sperm may have been used frequently among one doctor's patients. Physicians generally have one donor for each "physical type"—one white male with brown hair and eyes, one blonde with blue eyes, one black male, one redhead, and so on. You may well find a much closer match among donors available through the largest commercial banks.

Myth: Fresh sperm is more effective than frozen. Fact: In a study of 192 couples, Dr. Jack Shuber of the University of Toronto found Idant frozen sperm to be equally effective.

**Source:** Interview with Joseph Feldschuh, M.D., medical director, Idant Laboratory, New York.

## NEW WAY TO MONITOR OVULATION

Infertile women have long depended on unreliable blood tests to monitor ovulation. Better: Ultrasound—high-frequency sound waves that produce a TV picture. Using ultrasound, doctors can determine the precise time to administer fertility drugs or artificial insemination. Results: In one study, five of 15 women with chronic infertility became pregnant.

**Source:** Study by University of Miami and Mount Sinai Medical Center, New York, reported in *USA Today*.

## ENHANCING FERTILITY

Missionary position is best. The woman lies on her back with knees drawn up. The man should penetrate as deeply as possible at orgasm. The woman should remain in her position for 15 minutes after sex.

**Source:** Michael Carrera, M.D., Hunter College School of Health Sciences, City University of New York, writing in *Glamour*.

## TRUTH ABOUT WOMEN WHO'VE HAD ABORTIONS

A single abortion or even several abortions do not decrease a woman's fertility. A Harvard study found that there was a higher rate of pregnancy among women who had had three or more abortions than among those with only one.

**Source:** *Medical World News*, New York.

## AN ALTERNATIVE FOR INFERTILE COUPLES

One out of every six couples is infertile. Adoption is the traditional solution. Artificial insemination by a sperm donor works in cases where the wife is fertile. However, a new development is gaining acceptance when it is the wife who is infertile: Surrogate mothering. Eight years ago, when I got involved with this procedure, there was only one such birth. Now it covers 27 states, and I have even represented couples from foreign countries.

Advances in medicine are breaking ground so quickly that we are already involved in research on alternative methods of surrogate mothering. But currently only a single method is being offered. How it works: Once an infertile couple has decided to have a baby by a volunteer surrogate mother, the husband impregnates the surrogate by means of masturbation and artificial insemination. There is no direct sexual involvement. The surrogate mother then carries the baby through the term of pregnancy.

### Who the Surrogates Are

Surrogate mothers come from all walks of life. We have had law students, nurses and Ph.D. candidates. Some are compensating for a previous abortion. Some have endometriosis,* a condition that can be alleviated by pregnancy. Some just like to be pregnant and feel more important when they are. Some are married and some are not. They are usually also interested in the $10,000 fee they get.

### The Legal Steps

If the surrogate mother is married, the father of the child files a paternity suit and claims the child as his own. That way the child bears his name, and he can take the child home from the hospital. If the surrogate mother is unmarried, there is no legal action, since the child can automatically bear his name.

Upon the birth of the child, the wife of the infertile couple files for adoption of the child. This is not a regular adoption but a *stepchild* adoption, since it is the husband's natural child. Some state legal systems equate surrogate mothering with "child buying." However, since a stepchild adoption requires no social service investigation, household profile or reporting of expenses or fees, there is no overtone that might be looked upon as illegal.

### The Fees

The infertile couple pays a total of about $22,000. It can run somewhat more or less, depending on how far they must travel to the sponsoring center and how far the surrogate mother must travel. The surrogate mother receives $10,000, $7,500 goes to the sponsoring organization, and the remainder of the fee covers medical screening, psychiatric screening, maternity clothes, life and health insurance, legal fees for the surrogate mother and travel costs.

The surrogate mother may meet with the infertile couple several times during the pregnancy. Since she is mothering the child solely for the infertile couple, she feels good about what she is doing, and we find it is beneficial for her to have a relationship with the prospective parents during the pregnancy. Often the couple is present at the delivery, the wife as a coach and the father as the natural father.

### Latest Developments

Eventually, we expect several variations of surrogate mothering to be available. One current experiment in California involves an *ovum transfer.* Again, artificial insemination of the surrogate mother takes place. But then the fertilized egg is washed out of the surrogate mother's womb before it becomes implanted in the uterine wall. (This is a simple doctor's office procedure.) The ovum is then implanted in the infertile wife's womb, and she can carry the baby through the term of pregnancy. This way, no one need know it is not her baby, and it would naturally bring her closer to the child.

*Reverse ovum transfer:* Here, although the couple is fertile, there is a medical reason why the wife cannot carry the child. She may have a partial hysterectomy or tend to have spontaneous abortions (miscarriages) in the second or third month. Here, the fertilized egg is washed out of the biological mother's womb after five or seven days and is then implanted in a surrogate mother's womb for the duration of the pregnancy. Thus, the baby is the biological child of the couple who could not ordinarily have a child.

*In vitro ovum transfer:* This can be done if the wife cannot conceive because her tubes are blocked. In this case, the egg of the wife is artificially inseminated by the husband's sperm in a test tube. The fertilized egg is then implanted in a surrogate mother who can carry the baby. (This procedure could also be done with the biological mother if she has a competent uterus.)

### Psychological Problems

A married woman may worry about accepting another woman's child or having another woman carry her husband's offspring. Or, she may also feel *This child is more his than mine.* However, by the time couples come to us, they usually have tried everything, and the rewards of having a child outweigh the concerns.

*The endometrium is the mucous membrane lining the uterus. Endometriosis is the presence of functioning endometrial tissue in places where it is not normally found.

**Source:** Interview with Noel Keane, executive director, Infertility Center of New York.

# POSTPONING PREGNANCY? SEE A DOCTOR FIRST

Waiting until your thirties to have children is often desirable, but you're asking for trouble if both partners aren't checked for physical problems before that time. These procedures should be included in a medical workup:

• Hysterogram. Dye inserted into the womb exposes deformities in the tubes, uterus or womb when X-rayed. Many types of abnormalities can be corrected by surgery.

• Laparoscopy. In this procedure, a telescope is inserted through the navel to spot abnormalities in the ovaries, tubes and womb. Hospitalization is necessary. Laparoscopies are often performed when a physician has reason to think there's a problem that hasn't shown up on a hysterogram.

• Temperature chart. Taken every morning for two months, a woman's temperature shows how well she's ovulating. If there are problems, medication may help.

• Sperm analysis. The physician will examine the number, volume, shape and motility (how they swim), and check for infections that may be asymptomatic. When sperm problems are the result of infection, they may be treated with medication. Alternatively, if a man has sperm abnormalities that a physician believes may get progressively worse, a couple may decide to have children soon rather than wait.

**Source:** Interview with Stanley T. West, M.D., a specialist in infertility, New York.

## MIDDLE-AGED MOMS

Older women may be better prepared emotionally and financially for childbirth than younger ones. Problems of giving birth past age 35 have been exaggerated.

Infertility is a very individual thing. Many women over 35 have no trouble getting pregnant. If no pregnancy occurs after four months of trying, consult a specialist.

Miscarriages are more likely among older women, but one miscarriage doesn't mean that a woman can't carry to term on her second try.

Older women may have more trouble with the placenta, which might peel away from the uterine wall or grow in the lower part of the uterus rather than in the upper part. The major symptom is bleeding, so, at the first sign of this, see the doctor.

The only genetic defect associated with older mothers is Down's syndrome, which can be detected by amniocentesis.

Although fibroids are most common in older women, many first-time older mothers have successful pregnancies and deliveries despite them.

Cesarean deliveries may be more common among older women because doctors think they are higher risks. Check your obstetrician's attitude on this issue.

## CHOOSING YOUR BABY'S SEX

The idea of choosing the sex of an unborn child has fascinated people since Biblical times. Motives aside, the reality is that we have yet to find a magic formula for predetermining a baby's sex. Although there are methods that claim success rates of 90% and more, they are not supported by statistics. Some may even jeopardize the

child's later health.

At best, parents can exert a *moderate* influence in this area. Using proven techniques of coital timing within the woman's menstrual cycle, you can increase your chance of having a boy from 50/50 to about 68/32. If you want a girl, the chance of success is 57/43.

What we can define more certainly is what doesn't work. Theories about influencing the sex of a baby with vitamin E, pre-sex coffee, hot baths, special positions for intercourse or the woman's having an orgasm before the man are all bunk. Also, there is no laboratory evidence to support the old saw that douches (baking soda for boys, vinegar for girls) have any effect. On the other hand, mild douches will do no harm. In general, baking soda might aid conception by lowering the acidity of a woman's vagina.

Equally pointless, but far more potentially dangerous, are faddish prepregnancy diets. There is not a shred of evidence that a high-sodium diet will help produce a boy or a low-potassium regimen, a girl. We *do* know that a balanced diet and proper nutrition before pregnancy are important to a baby's health.

In the early 1960s, Dr. Landrum Shettles developed a theory that conception two to 24 hours before ovulation favored male births. He proposed that earlier insemination (36 or more hours before ovulation) would more likely result in a female baby.

Although the "Shettles method" remains in some vogue, it is basically flawed. Shettles relied exclusively on data from artificial inseminations. More recent studies have conclusively proved the opposite sex trends for naturally conceived births. We now know that when intercourse takes place five or more days before ovulation, the probability of a male birth rises to more than 68%. When coitus occurs the day of ovulation, the likelihood of conceiving a girl increases to about 57%.

Aside from confusing people, the Shettles method encouraged many couples to delay intercourse until after ovulation had actually taken place. Result: A greater chance that an "old" egg would lead to miscarriage or birth defects.

*Ideal plan for couples hoping to conceive a girl:* Chart the woman's basal body temperature for several months. Upon reaching the cycle during which conception is planned, have intercourse one day before the projected rise in temperature (which occurs at about the time of ovulation).

Beyond that, there is little most people can do—for the moment. The future of sex selection may lie in sperm separation techniques, now in the testing phase. The pioneer is Dr. Ronald J. Ericsson, who exploited the fact that Y (male) sperm "swim" more rapidly than X (female) sperm. In Ericsson's technique (geared only to male babies), semen is placed on the top of a glass column containing serum albumin. Three hours later, the top portion of the serum is discarded. The remainder (with more Y sperm) is injected through artificial insemination. Ericsson reports a success rate of 77% boys out of 104 pregnancies.

Drawbacks: The procedure is costly (several thousand dollars) and often fails to result in conception for the first several tries. And there is no comparable technique to increase the odds of having a female baby.

The most drastic mode of sex selection is elective abortion following amniocentesis or the new ultrasound testing. Beyond its moral repugnance, however, this approach also poses a threat to the mother's health.

Bottom line: Don't plan to have a baby unless you'll be delighted with a child of either sex.

**Source:** Interview with Elizabeth M. Whelan, executive director of the American Council on Science and Health and author of *Boy or Girl?*, Bobbs-Merrill Co., Inc, New York.

## PREGNANCY TESTS: FASTER, EARLIER, MORE RELIABLE, AND CHEAPER

In three minutes, a doctor can determine with 99% accuracy whether a woman is pregnant—as soon as 20 days after conception. Cost: 75¢. Key: Sophisticated genetic engineering again . . . new testing agent is added to the patient's urine specimen—results can be read without a microscope. Current standard tests sacrifice at least one

attractive feature for another: Speed for early detection, low cost for accuracy, etc. Bonus: Simplicity—home version is nearly as accurate as the professional test. In the wings: A blood test using the same technique—detects pregnancy as soon as 10 days after conception. Projected cost: $3.00. Urine test, blood test available soon.

**Source:** Monoclonal Antibodies, Inc., Mountain View, CA, and Organon, a subsidiary of Akzona, Inc., West Orange, NJ.

## BOY OR GIRL?

Determine the sex of your unborn child through the use of a new 10-minute, over-the-counter urine test. It determines with 99% accuracy the sex of an unborn child after the sixth month of pregnancy. Cost: $19.95. Previous tests, requiring the withdrawal and study of amniotic fluid, were painful, potentially dangerous and expensive.

## GENDER TEST KIT WARNING

How reliable are the new over-the-counter gender test kits for pregnant women?

These tests often do not work. Of 12 I conducted with a kit on women in their late third trimester of pregnancy, none were clearly indicative. And of eight urine samples I sent to the manufacturer for interpretation, five were wrong. . . including a sample of my own urine, which was reported to indicate a female fetus!

The risk is serious. Besides the confusion, disappointment and psychological stress caused by the appearance of a baby of the "unexpected" sex, some women may choose elective abortion of a "wrong" -sex fetus.

According to the manufacturer, the Food and Drug Administration does not have to approve such a product before it is marketed. Along with home pregnancy tests, it claims gender tests fall into the "diagnostic product" category and therefore do not need FDA approval. However, the FDA has approved the home pregnancy tests and is looking into complaints about the gender tests.

Source: Interview with Bruce L. Flamm, M.D., an obstetrician-gynecologist, Kaiser–Permanente Medical Center, Anaheim, CA.

## WHY YOU SHOULD COUNT PRENATAL KICKS

Prenatal kicks provide an easy way for a pregnant mother to check her baby's health. Most unborn babies kick at least 10 and up to 125 times in a 12-hour period. In one test, only 36% of mothers whose babies kicked fewer than 10 times per day had normal deliveries...and the perinatal death rate of this group was 13 times higher than the national average. Recommended: Start counting kicks in the 29th week of pregnancy. If there are fewer than 10 per 12-hour period, or the last kick comes later each day, see your doctor.

Source: Study by Arnold Cohen, M.D., Albert Einstein Medical Center, Philadelphia, in Nursing Life, Springhour, PA.

## BETTER THAN AMNIOCENTESIS

Amniocentesis will be replaced by an ultrasound technique to sample cells of placental attachments. The sampling could identify birth defects as early as the sixth week of pregnancy. Amniocentesis results aren't available until the 19th or 20th week.

Source: Laird G. Jackson, MD, director of family genetics, Thomas Jefferson University Hospital, Philadelphia, in Medical World News.

## EATING FOR TWO

Pregnant women should not skip meals, particularly breakfast. Going without a meal can lower blood sugar and raise levels of fatty acids. These acids and other metabolic products pass through the placenta, where they could harm the fetus, especially late in pregnancy.

## NASAL CONGESTION AND PREGNANCY

About 10% of pregnant women develop stuffy noses. It usually begins in the third month and may last from several weeks to the duration of the pregnancy. Most likely sufferers: Women with previous nasal allergenic problems. Standard decongestants and antihistamines should be avoided unless cleared by a physician, as they might harm the fetus.

Source: Journal of Ear, Nose, and Throat, Williston Park, N.Y.

## SMOKING ALERT

Smoking during pregnancy decreases fetal mental development. Smokers bear lower birth-weight children, who tend to have shorter attention spans, hyperactive behavior and lower IQs.

Source: Obstetrics and Gynecology, New York.

• It's now common knowledge that pregnant women should stop smoking for the sake of their babies. But a recent study suggests that expectant *fathers* should follow the same rule. When Dad continued to smoke, the newborns showed significantly higher levels of thiocyanate (a tobacco smoke by-product) in their blood.

Source: Study at Cleveland Metropolitan General Hospital/Case Western Reserve University, reported in Glamour magazine, New York.

## GOOD REASON NOT TO SMOKE MARIJUANA

Pregnant women should avoid using marijuana. A review of the medical records of 12,424 women suggests increased occurrence of malformations and low birth weights among babies of marijuana users.

Source: American Journal of Public Health, Washington, D.C.

## LIQUOR AND PREGNANCY

Even moderate alcohol consumption by a pregnant woman can reduce her baby's weight and size, and it may take at least eight months for the baby to catch up with its peers. Just one or two drinks a day during pregnancy can have a greater long-term effect on a baby than smoking. An occasional drink may be harmless, but abstention is safest.

**Source:** Study at the University of Washington, Seattle.

## ARTIFICIAL SWEETENER WARNING

Aspartame (an artificial sweetener) may be dangerous to fetuses whose mothers ingest it. One person in 60 has a genetic intolerance to phenylalanine, an amino acid bonded in aspartame. Preliminary research suggests that if a pregnant mother with this condition uses the sweetener (NutraSweet or Equal), her child may have a lower IQ. Among potential dangers to adults: Brain damage and brain-tumor formations.

**Source:** Research by the Aspartame Resource Center, a branch of the Community Nutrition Center, Washington, DC, cited in *Vegetarian Times*, New York.

## TRUTH ABOUT PRENATAL FLUORIDE

Children whose mothers take fluoride supplements during pregnancy have fewer childhood (and adulthood) cavities. Additionally, the children are longer and heavier at birth.

**Source:** Frances Glenn, D.D.S., a Miami pediatric dentist, quoted in *American Health*.

## BEST EXERCISE FOR A PREGNANT WOMAN

Swimming is good exercise for pregnant women. The water suports the extra body weight, minimizes stress on body tissues, and helps build the stomach and lower back muscles that support the fetus. Caution: Diving, of course, can be harmful. Worthwhile: Ask your obstetrician if swimming is all right for you.

**Source:** *Working Woman*, New York.

## ANOTHER REASON TO USE A SEAT BELT

Pregnant women can better protect their unborn by wearing a seat belt. Seat belts give everyone a better chance of surviving an accident without injury, including pregnant women and fetuses.

**Source:** Richard Lehrfeld, M.D., in *Road & Track*, Newport Beach, CA.

## TRAVELING PREGNANT

Ask your doctor which shots can be harmful. Try to travel during the second trimester (the most stable period of the nine-month cycle). Avoid overexertion from sightseeing and exercise. Take the aisle seat on planes, buses and trains so you can get up easily. If you are going a long distance, walk around occasionally to restore circulation. Note: The general prohibition against medication during pregnancy applies to motion-sickness pills, too.

**Source:** American College of Obstetricians and Gynecologists, Washington, DC.

## PREGNANCY AND PLANE TRAVEL

A woman in advanced pregnancy should carry a doctor's certificate confirming her fitness to travel. Without the document, she may face embarrassing questions at check-in—and even be prevented from boarding.

**Source:** Barbara Reukema, instructor in aviation law, Southwestern University, Los Angeles.

## WORK HAZARD UPDATE

Pregnant workers and video display terminals. As controversy grows over whether the radiation from VDTs causes birth defects, a growing number of companies are temporarily transferring VDT workers into other jobs during pregnancy. Some other firms provide pregnant VDT operators with lead aprons to protect the fetus from any possible harmful radiation.

## THE GOOD AND BAD NEWS ABOUT BIRTH CENTERS

Birthing centers (independent obstetrical

care facilities run by nurse-midwives) are growing rapidly. Almost 100 are in operation around the country now, with 175 more scheduled to open soon. Main attraction: Reasonable fees. A complete birthing-center package, which includes prenatal care, ranges from $700 to $1,500. An obstetrician's fee plus hospital care starts at around $2,400.

**Source:** *Medical Economics*, Oradell, NJ.

• Birth centers offer parents more control over how their babies are born, and typically charge only half as much as a hospital for a delivery. Many insurers offer reimbursement for birth center services, and most states either already have or are drafting regulations for licensing and safety. Drawback: The centers are not as well equipped as hospitals to handle high-risk deliveries.

## SATISFACTION OF NATURAL CHILDBIRTH

Natural delivery, despite all its discomfort, appears to be more satisfying to women in retrospect than the pain-free birth experienced by mothers who were given a local anesthesia. In a survey of mothers at London's Queen Charlotte's Hospital a year after delivery, only 8% of those who received no analgesic during the birth process have unpleasant memories of the event. Of the mothers who had relatively painless deliveries, 16% felt dissatisfied with the experience. Most likely cause: More than half the deliveries under local anesthesia were forceps assisted.

**Source:** *The Lancet.*

## OLD TECHNIQUE THAT STILL WORKS

Breast stimulation may be better than drugs in strengthening uterine contractions during labor. Preliminary tests of 300 pregnant outpatients have made researchers optimistic about the effectiveness of this ancient technique of folk medicine. The method

allows patients to move around during labor and requires less monitoring than drug therapy. Most effective: Manual (rather than mechanical) stimulation.

**Source:** Peter Curtis, M.D., associate professor of family practice at the University of North Carolina, Chapel Hill.

## NOT SO NEW CHILDBIRTH METHOD

"New" childbirth method has the mother deliver while squatting—the same posture used throughout the world until modern times. Advantages: An easier and faster delivery (due to more efficient contractions) and less pain.

**Source:** *Vogue*, New York.

## POSTPARTUM DEPRESSION

Postpartum depression may be a nutritional problem more than a psychiatric condition. New theory: After delivery, a mother is stressed by hormone withdrawal and low blood sugar. Treatment: Intramuscular injections of vitamin $B_{12}$ every other day for two weeks. Also helpful: Extra B vitamins before delivery.

**Source:** *Foods for Healthy Kids* by Dr. Lendon Smith, Berkley Books, New York.

## WHY NEW MOTHERS MAY LOSE THEIR HAIR

New mothers who fear they are losing their hair are actually returning to a normal cycle. During pregnancy, hair that would otherwise be shed remains in a "resting" phase. After delivery (or quitting the Pill), this hair is shed, and women often experience heavy—but temporary—hair loss.

**Source:** *The New York Times.*

## PROBLEMS OF RETURNING TO WORK

Mid-career mothers often experience

alarm, depression, anxiety, confusion, rage and isolation when they leave their infants to return to work. The social, psychological and physical complexities of pregnancy are often underestimated. Older mothers want to be both selfless nurturers and successful career women, but they have few role models to observe and emulate. In making the transition back to the workplace, an understanding and helpful husband can be the most important support.

**Source:** Study by Robert E. Lee, M.D., *Journal of Sex & Marital Therapy.*

## WHAT A NURSING MOTHER SHOULD EAT

Nursing babies fall asleep faster and more deeply if their mothers eat a candy bar in the evening. Reason: Babies' sleep is induced by the amino acid tryptophan, which is produced by eating carbohydrates.

**Source:** Research by Michael W. Yogman, M.D., Children's Hospital, Boston, in *Moneysworth,* New York.

• Nursing mothers can make their babies smarter by eating oil-rich fish (such as salmon or mackerel). When mothers took fish-oil capsules, their milk contained more DHA, a fatty acid that fosters brain and eye development. Key: Babies' brains continue to form into early childhood.

**Source:** Research at the University of Oregon, cited in *American Health,* New York.

## EASY WAY TO MAKE SURE YOUR BABY GETS VITAMIN D

Breast-fed babies are more likely to avoid rickets (or the need for vitamin D supplements) if their mothers get even occasional sunshine. A recent study found that the vitamin D content in breast milk rose dramatically after the mother was exposed to midday summer sun for only 30 minutes. Even if the mother avoided further exposure, the vitamin level remained higher for up to two weeks.

**Source:** Study by the Wisconsin Perinatal Center, Madison, WI.

## GOOD NEWS ABOUT SOME COMMON CHILDHOOD DISEASES

Childhood diseases once common in the US are likely to be extinct soon. From 1980 to 1981, the incidence of measles was down 77% (to 3,032 cases). German measles: Down 47%. Mumps: Down 45%. Tetanus: Down 37%...only 60 cases. Whooping cough: Down 31%. Polio: Down 25%...only six cases. Reason: Stricter school-district enforcement of state-mandated immunizations.

**Source:** *Good Housekeeping.*

## NO MORE CHICKEN POX

A chicken pox vaccine will virtually wipe out the disease by the year 1990. Of 468 children who were test vaccinated (with a vaccine from a strain of live virus), none came down with chicken pox. In a nonvaccinated control group of about the same size, 39 cases were reported.

## LIFE EXPECTANCY OF KIDS BORN IN 1983

Children born in 1983 will live an average of 74.6 years—almost a year longer than those who were born in 1980. Boys' life expectancy: 70.9 years. Girls' life expectancy: 78.3.

**Source:** Metropolitan Life Insurance Co.

## WHEN NOT TO TREAT EYE PROBLEMS

Minor eyesight problems in children are best left untreated. Reason: Forcing eyeglasses on children who don't really need them creates conflict between parent and child. Going without corrective lenses won't aggravate a vision problem. In fact, astigmatism (but not nearsightedness) generally improves by itself as the child gets older.

Note: Children with major problems usually welcome eyeglasses.

**Source:** Dr. J. L. Kennerley Bankes, St. Mary's Hospital, London

## WHY A CHILD MAY BE NEARSIGHTED

Nearsightedness in children may be more a reaction to school pressures than an inherited visual problem. By emphasizing the acquisition of information in the classroom, educators encourage excessive concentration. This makes youngsters constrict their field of vision. Tension tends to restrict perceptual abilities, including sight. In a public school study, myopia was reduced by 50% among elementary school children when the teaching method changed from one dependent on frequent testing of skills to a more relaxed, multisensory approach to learning.

**Source:** Ray Gottlieb, a Los Angeles optometrist and vision trainer, writing in *Brain/Mind Bulletin*.

## CHILDREN AND EYEGLASSES

There is no evidence to support the myth that putting glasses on youngsters too soon will make the children dependent on the lenses and weaken their eyesight. A myopic (nearsighted) child's eyesight tends to worsen with time simply because his eyes are still growing. Children should have their eyes checked before they reach school age. Uncorrected vision problems can lead to delayed development and to stress at school.

**Source:** *Archives of Disease in Childhood, British Medical Journal.*

## AGE TO BEGIN WEARING CONTACTS

Contact lenses are often suitable for children as young as nine. Advantages: Unlike eyeglasses, contacts carry no psychological stigma, nor do they impede sports activities. Popular: Extended-wear lenses. They require less handling and therefore create fewer hygiene problems.

**Source:** Dr. Spencer E. Sherman, attending eye surgeon, Mount Sinai Hospital, New York, in *The Salk Letter*.

## EARLY TEST FOR DYSLEXIA

Dyslexia can now be detected before a child begins to read or encounters learning problems. The test, devised by Rutgers Medical School's Reading Disabilities Research Institute, monitors a child's eye while it follows a sequence of flashing lights from left to right. The dyslexic child will make more backward glances than normal.

**Source:** *Ladies' Home Journal.*

## THE END OF CHILDHOOD TOOTH DECAY

Tooth decay will be virtually nonexistent among children and young adults by the end of the century. Coming soon: Cloning of the gene that produces tooth enamel. Laser recrystallization of the mineral structure of decaying teeth.

**Source:** Dr. Harold Loe, director of the National Institute of Dental Research, Bethesda, MD.

## HOW TO CLEAN A BABY'S FIRST TEETH

Early oral hygiene can help babies avoid decay that would lead to problems with permanent teeth. Recommended: Clean the baby's teeth with moistened gauze wrapped around your finger. After three or four teeth have erupted, toddlers can use a baby's toothbrush—but without toothpaste (they swallow it).

**Source:** Stephen Goepferd, director of the University of Iowa's Infant Oral Health Clinic, in *American Health*.

## FOODS THAT HELP TEETH COME IN STRAIGHT

Tough foods may make your children's teeth grow in straighter. Squirrel monkeys (with teeth similar to ours) that ate hard food developed near-perfect bites. But those that ate soft foods suffered misaligned teeth and impacted molars. A tough diet helps up to age 11 or 12, when related bones stop growing.

**Source:** Study by Wright State University, Dayton, OH, reported in *McCall's.*

## PRIME SOURCE OF CAVITIES

Dentists are right—sugar is indeed a prime source of cavities in children. Researchers replaced sugar with natural fruit purees and sugar substitutes in the diets of 73 institutionalized children ages 5–17 for five years. Result: 53% of the children had no cavities. None were missing any permanent teeth.

**Source:** *American Journal of Public Health.*

## LATEST CAVITY FIGHTER

Sealing children's teeth with a coat of plastic resin can reduce cavities by at least 50%. The plastic is applied to the molars, the most likely starting points for decay. It dries into a hard shield against plaque or food particles and lasts up to seven years.

**Source:** Studies by the National Institute of Dental Research, reported in *McCall's.*

## WHY SOME KIDS NEED FLUORIDE SUPPLEMENTS

Fluoride supplements to fight tooth decay are recommended for children who live in areas with less than 0.7 parts per million of fluoride in the water supply. This includes about 40% of the US population. Supplements also help the teeth of breast-fed babies, since they usually drink little water, and human milk contains little fluoride.

**Source:** *Tufts University Diet & Nutrition Letter.*

## TEENAGERS' SPECIAL MOUTH PROBLEMS

Teenagers' mouths are especially susceptible to gingivitis—inflamed and often bleeding gums. Reasons: Adolescents' high hormone levels increase the number of blood vessels in the mouth. Prevention: A dental cleaning twice a year (to prevent plaque build-up) and reduction of sugary snacks. If unchecked, gingivitis can lead to periodontitis, a more serious gum disease.

**Source:** Dr. Jon Suzuki, University of Maryland, in *American Health.*

## FEAR OF DRILLING

When taking a child under six to the dentist, do not announce the visit until the day of the appointment (to minimize anxiety). Also: If there's going to be pain, be frank about it. Let the child know that it will last only a very short time. Follow the visit with an especially pleasant activity. Counterproductive: Threatening a child with a trip to the dentist as punishment.

**Source:** Barbara Melamed, professor of psychology, University of Florida, quoted in *USA Today.*

## KIND OF MUSIC PREMATURE BABIES LOVE

Premature babies appear to thrive on soft classical music. In one recent study, the weight of preemies increased faster than usual when doctors played Bach, Beethoven and Brahms. Less effective: Popular music or rock.

**Source:** Study at the University of California Medical Center, reported in *The Salk Letter.*

## HEAT AND BABIES' HEALTH

It is a great mistake to think that a newborn infant cannot be kept too warm. Over-zealous wrapping can cause dehydration and aggravation of fever, in some cases leading to convulsions, heatstroke and even death. A baby that has a high fever should not be wrapped or even covered if it is in a warm room. Sponge the infant with cool water to control fever and contact a pediatrician.

**Source:** *Archives of Disease in Childhood.*

## SPITTING-UP REMEDY

Infants who suffer from severe spitting-up problems (gastroesophageal reflux) can be helped. Recent studies suggest that keeping babies upright after eating—propped up in a molded plastic seat, for example—may aggravate the condition rather than help it. More effective: Placing babies face down in bed after meals.

**Source:** Research at LeBonheur Children's Medical Center, Memphis, reported in *New England Journal of Medicine.*

## MYSTERIOUS CAUSE OF RESPIRATORY PROBLEMS

Wood-burning stoves can cause respiratory problems in preschool-age children, according to results of a Michigan study. Reasons: Unclear.

**Source:** *Medical World News.*

## CHILDHOOD NOSEBLEEDS

Frequent nosebleeds in children are usually the result of rubbing the inside of the nose. To prevent nosebleeds: Clip the child's nails, insert a lubricant in the nose and use bedroom humidifiers in dry climates.

## DON'T IGNORE "GROWING PAINS"

"Growing pains" may indicate a health problem in your child. If they occur frequently, cause a fever, change the form of the body or are accompanied by weight loss—suspect trouble. Real growing pains take place during the night, between the knee and ankle. Aspirin, massage and heat will take care of most of the discomfort.

**Source:** *Salk Letter.*

## EARLY HEARING LOSS

Repeated colds and allergic reactions are experienced by one third of children in their first two years of life. Result: The baby doesn't hear as well as he should...which in turn hampers linguistic, mental and social development. Recommended: Have your baby screened for possible hearing loss, beginning at four months.

**Source:** Burton White, director of the Center for Parent Education, Newton, MA.

## *YOU* MAY BE THE CAUSE OF YOUR CHILD'S EAR PROBLEMS

A parent who smokes is more likely to raise children with chronic ear infections. When both parents smoke, their child is almost three times more likely to develop ear problems than a child in a non-smoking household.

• Persistent middle ear effusions (fluid buildup in the middle ear) are more common in children who are exposed to cigarette smoke. Exposure to three cigarette packs' worth of smoke increases the chance of infection four times. Children who are also predisposed to allergies or nasal congestion are six times as likely to have this problem.

**Source:** *Journal of the American Medical Association.*

## ANOTHER REASON NOT TO SMOKE

Children of smokers are more susceptible to coughing, wheezing and pneumonia than are children of nonsmokers. Also at greater risk: Nonsmokers who work closely with smokers.

## CAUSES OF BLOODY STOOL

Blood in a child's stool usually does not indicate a life-threatening condition. But consult your physician to be safe. The source of gastrointestinal bleeding in children is often temporary stomach irritation caused by aspirin. Other sources: Ulcers or rectal fissures. Often what appears to be blood in feces or vomitus is something else—for example, red jello, beets or even the antibiotic ampicillin.

**Source:** William Spivak, M.D., chief of pediatric gastro-enterology, Cornell Medical Center, New York, quoted in *A Letter from Dr. Lee Salk.*

## MONO ISN'T FOR TEENS ONLY

Mononucleosis can strike children of any age, not just adolescents. In young children, however, the disease manifests itself as a minor upper respiratory illness, not the exhausting condition associated with high school and college students.

**Source:** Dr. Stephen A. Spector, assistant professor of pediatrics, University of California at San Diego, quoted in *Parents.*

## SCOLIOSIS HOME CHECKUP

Scoliosis is the abnormal (side to side) curvature of the spine that affects some growing children. The curvature displaces bone structure, causing deformity and heart and lung problems. How to check: Ask the child to stand straight so you can see if the spine is normal. Then, as he bends over with his arms dangling, run your hand down his spine. Feel for any side-to-side movement of the spine. If you notice anything unusual, contact your doctor at once.

**More information:** Scoliosis Association, 1 Penn Plaza, New York 10119.

## LATEST TREATMENT FOR SCOLIOSIS

Curvature of the spine (scoliosis) now can be treated without surgery or bulky braces. ScoliTron, a device recently approved by the FDA, uses electricity to straighten the back. It sends short, painless impulses through the back muscles, causing them to contract, while the patient is sleeping. Note: Scoliosis afflicts one out of 10 children in this country.

**Source:** Intermedics, Inc., Freeport, TX.

## RITALIN DOES MORE THAN CONTROL HYPERACTIVITY

Hyperactive children who are treated with Ritalin (a stimulant) will reap the drug's benefit later on. Although stimulant therapy may not improve a hyperactive youngster's performance in school, studies show that the long-term benefits in behavior are significant. Hyperactive youngsters who have received at least three sustained years of medication have more self-esteem, better social skills and less aggressive behavior than similar children who have not been treated.

**Source:** Study by Dr. Lily Hechtman at Montreal Children's Hospital, cited in *The Salk Letter.*

## ADOPTED-CHILD ALERT

Adopted children are 10 times as likely to be hyperactive as other children. Possible reasons: Poor prenatal care and diet. The inability of an adoptive mother to nurse the baby.

**Source:** *Foods for Healthy Kids* by Dr. Lendon Smith, Berkley Books, New York.

## HEART DISEASE AND KIDS

One-third of schoolchildren face a high risk of premature heart disease. Signs: High cholesterol levels in the blood, high blood pressure, obesity, bad exercise habits and cigarette smoking. Although heart disease usually strikes at midlife, its seeds are planted in childhood, when lifetime habits are formed. Best: Give children a proper diet. Watch particularly that fat-and-sugar-loaded ice cream and pies and salt-laden chips and nuts are only an occasional treat. Of utmost importance: Establish good exercise habits. This is as vital to the child as eating, sleeping and going to school.

**Source:** Research by the American Heart Association quoted by Jane Brody in *The New York Times.*

## FITNESS AND U.S. CHILDREN

American kids don't exercise enough. A study of 8,800 youngsters in grades 5–12 showed that only half got enough exercise to develop healthy lungs and hearts. Possible reason: Inadequate physical education programs in school. Only 36% had daily gym classes, and only 47% of their gym time went to sports that can be continued into adulthood, such as running or swimming.

**Source:** A study by the US Department of Health and Human Services.

## ORGANIZED SPORTS ARE NOT FOR KIDS

Young children are neither psychologically nor physically suited for high-pressure organized sports. The average child doesn't attain metabolic or muscular maturity until the age of 15 or 16.

**Source:** Dr. Nathan J. Smith, writing in *Medical Aspects of Human Sexuality.*

## A LEADING CAUSE OF ATHLETIC INJURIES

Pushing young athletes can result in "overuse" injuries such as stress fractures, tendinitis of the shoulder, bursitis of the hip and tennis elbow. These injuries in children were unheard of before the advent of organized sports programs after World War II. Even now, doctors rarely see these problems in youngsters who play sports among themselves without special coaching. (Children do not push themselves too hard.) Most frequent cause of injury: Inappropriate or excessive training. Children are particularly susceptible to injury when they are tired or in pain. Remedy: Make sure that the coaches or trainers who work with your children are sensitive to this issue and that they have a proper perspective on what a sports program is really about.

**Source:** Dr. Lyle Micheli, director of sports medicine, Children's Hospital Medical Center, Boston, quoted in *The Ladies' Home Journal.*

## CORRECTIVE SHOE MYTH

Most corrective shoes for children are of little or no value, according to medical experts polled by *The New York Times*'s Jane E. Brody. Some 50%–90% of children are born with flat feet, bowlegs, pigeon toes or other "problems." The vast majority of children outgrow these conditions naturally if given the chance.

## NEW THINKING ON CIRCUMCISION

Circumcision, the most frequently performed operation in the US, is beginning to decrease in popularity. Currently, 80% of American males have been circumcised, although the American Academy of Pediatrics has said there is no real medical reason for the operation. Good hygiene, the Academy claims, can provide all the advantages of circumcision with none of the risks.

**Source:** Study by doctors at Johns Hopkins University cited in *Sex Care Digest.*

## BEST CIRCUMCISION METHOD

An electric cauterizing needle used in conjunction with a metal clamp to perform circumcision can be extremely dangerous. Infants may suffer severe penile burns. Best: If circumcision is to be performed, a physician should use the traditional scalpel and clamp, or electrocautery without a metal clamp.

**Source:** Dr. A. Barry Belman, Children's Hospital National Medical Center, Washington, DC.

## CIRCUMCISION MYTH

Circumcision is better with local anesthesia. A University of Iowa study shows that, contrary to popular myth, the operation is painful to infants. Those who are given anesthesia experience significantly less stress.

**Source:** *Mothers Today.*

## WHEN YOUR CHILD HAS TO GO TO THE HOSPITAL

Have a thorough talk with the doctor to find out what procedures are involved, how the child will feel and the probable length of stay. Explain to your child—simply but honestly—what's in store. Visit the hospital (with the child, if allowed). Try to meet medical and nursing staff. Find out if you can stay with the patient overnight. Pack your child's favorite clothes (if allowed) and toys. Make sure at least one parent is there throughout the child's waking hours. That way you can both keep an eye on what's happening and allay your child's anxiety.

**Source:** *Parents.*

## BAD-TASTING MEDICINE TIP

Bad-tasting medicine goes down more easily when you rub an ice cube over the youngster's tongue first. This temporarily "freezes" the taste buds to make the medication more palatable.

**Source:** *Practical Parenting Tips* by Vicki Lansky, Meadowbrook Press, Deephaven, MN.

## BEWARE OF SUGAR IN MEDICINE

Sugar in medicine makes it palatable to children. But it is harmful to their teeth if the medicines are taken regularly. Best: After taking sweet medication, children should rinse their mouths and brush their teeth.

## MEDICINES NOT TO GIVE YOUR CHILD

Alcohol-based medicines can make children nauseated, confused or sluggish. If taken intensively for an extended period, they can even lead to heart and respiratory problems. Trap: Alcohol is an unlabeled ingredient in many liquid antihistamines, cough syrups and anticolic medicines. Advice: Ask your pediatrician to preseribe a nonalcohol-based alternative.

**Source:** Dr. Jean Lockhart, director of the American Academy of Pediatrics, in *New Age Journal.*

## CHEWABLE VITAMIN ALERT

Chewable vitamins can cause serious overdoses in children who are allowed to eat them like candy. As few as 10 tablets may lead to stomach cramps and vomiting. Warning: Higher doses (especially of tablets containing iron) can result in permanent liver damage.

**Source:** American Academy of Pediatrics, Arlington, VA.

## WHERE THE FATTEST KIDS IN THE US LIVE

Children who live in the Northeast are more than twice as likely to grow up obese as those who live in the West. And they're three times as likely to be super-obese. The typical fat kid is also white and lives in a large metropolitan area. Theory: Environmental factors (such as a climate permitting year-round outdoor play) have a strong role in determining weight.

**Source:** Research by Dr. William Dietz and Dr. Steven Gortmaker, in *American Health*.

## WHY A FAT CHILD SHOULDN'T GO ON A DIET

• Fat children do better when encouraged to maintain their present weight, rather than to reduce it. Reason: If the child's weight remains constant, he'll grow naturally into it. But a strict diet could interfere with bone and tissue growth.

**Source:** *RN* magazine.

• Chubby children are more likely to become obese adults if they regain their baby fat before the age of five and a half. This "rebound" stage is the time when fat cells grow in size and number. Advice: Strict diets are a bad idea. But if children become plump at age three or four, encourage them to be more physically active.

**Source:** Research at the French National Institute of Health, in *American Health*.

## HOW A MOTHER CAN HELP HER CHILD DIET

Obese children lose the most weight when their mothers diet with them. Hitch: If the mothers attend the same weight-watching sessions as the kids, the diet program does not work as well for the child. Mothers must be involved, but at a distance.

**Source:** Dr. Kelly D. Brownell, University of Pennsylvania, reporting on a study of 42 obese children ages 12 through 16.

## WHY SOME KIDS MAY BE SHORT

Fear of obesity can lead to short stature and delayed puberty among children who regu-larly skip meals. A recent study found that 3% of high school students were short due to poor nutrition.

**Source:** *New England Journal of Medicine*.

## FOOD AND BEHAVIOR

Behavior problems among children have often been linked to chemical additives and vitamin deficiencies. But recent studies turned up two surprising villains: Wheat and milk.

When wheat was withdrawn from their diets, some problem children behaved normally—only to revert when they ate it again.

In another study, children with behavioral disorders were found to drink more than three pints of milk a day, as compared with less than half a pint in the non-offending group. Conclusion: When milk provides most of a child's protein, it can lead to an imbalance in amino acids, which in turn affects behavior.

**Source:** Study by Alexander Schauss, director of the American Institute for Biosocial Research, in *New Scientist*.

## TAMING YOUR BABY'S SWEET TOOTH

A baby's sweet tooth is natural, but it can be tamed by early eating experiences. Key: Avoiding baby foods with added sugar. Healthful sugar substitutes: Fruit juices plus water (for sweetened drinks). Fruits and vegetables (for candy and cookies). Unsweetened cereals (for presweetened ones).

**Source:** *American Health*.

## DON'T FEED HONEY TO BABIES

Hold the honey for babies under one year. Reason: Even "pure" or "filtered" honey contains tiny amounts of bacteria. Although harmless to older children and adults, these can lead to botulism in an infant. Symptoms: Constipation, lethargy, feeding trouble.

**Source:** *Vegetarian Times.*

## HOLD THE SALT

Infants who ate salty foods during their first 18 months tended to have a higher salt consumption at age 4. Conclusion: The taste for salt is acquired. If consumption can be cut early in life, that taste can be minimized—and with it, the risk of hypertension in adulthood.

**Source:** *Medical World News.*

## PEANUT-BUTTER HAZARD

Chunky peanut butter (which has pieces of peanuts in it) is potentially hazardous to younger children. Some children don't chew as well as others, and some have smaller passageways in the throat. Peanut fragments can get stuck. Safer: Creamy peanut butter.

**Source:** *Harvard Medical School Health Letter.*

## HOT DOG DANGER

Hot dogs can be dangerous for children. Hot dogs are just the right size to get caught in tiny throats. Better way: Cut the frankfurters lengthwise for all youngsters under 10.

**Source:** Time Tolls.

• More children choke to death on hot dogs than on any other food. Also dangerous: Cookies: Most lethal for adults: Steak, chicken, lobster.

**Source:** Research at John Hopkins University.

## HIGH BLOOD PRESSURE ALERT

A good breakfast can help prevent children from developing high blood pressure. Rea-

son: Children who skip breakfast often compensate later in the day by eating salty snacks, which then can lead to weight gain and hypertension.

**Source:** Robert Borgman, food science professor, Clemson University, Clemson, SC, in *American Health.*

## BABY-BOTTLE NIPPLE ALERT

Rubber baby-bottle nipples may contain unacceptable levels of nitrosamines, which are suspected carcinogens. Advice: Boil new nipples five or six times before use (using fresh water each time).

**Source:** US Food and Drug Administration, in the *Harvard Medical School Health Letter.*

## ACCIDENTAL POISONINGS

Two of every three poisoning cases involve children under age five. More than 500,000 children are victims each year.

Child poisonings are most apt to occur just before mealtime. Junior will consume whatever he can get his hands on. Children frequently eat poisonous indoor and outdoor plants. Example: Philodendron causes swelling of the tongue and severe vomiting.

**More information:** Send a stamped, self-addressed envelope to New York City Poison Control Project, Bellevue Hospital Center, 27th St. and First Ave., New York 10016, free.

## DIAPERING-TIME DANGERS

Changing diapers on a seven-month-old or older child can be dangerous, according to a survey by a Massachusetts poison control center. Starting at this age, tots have the strength and dexterity to grab the objects around them and put them in their mouths. Particularly hazardous: All the toxic substances that surround the changing table— powder, wipes, shampoo, ointment, oil, etc. (Keep a close watch on the open safety pins, too.)

**Source:** *Journal of the American Medical Association.*

## COMMON CAUSES OF POISONING

Poisons aren't limited to common household products such as cleaning agents or drugs. Cigarette butts, motor oil and some brightly colored berries also can be harmful to children. For further details, get the long list compiled by the National Capital Poison Center.

**More information:** Send a business-size stamped, self-addressed envelope to the National Capital Poison Center, Georgetown University Hospital, 388 Reservoir Rd. NW, Washington, DC 20007.

• Perfumes, colognes and aftershaves cause up to 10% of accidental childhood poisonings. Fatal ingredient: Ethanol (alcohol), which can be harmful even in small doses.

**Source:** American Red Cross.

## MOST DANGEROUS TIME OF DAY

Children are poisoned by household chemicals most frequently from 4 P.M. to 8 P.M. That's when they tend to be bored and their parents are busy with dinner activities.

**Source:** Whitehall Laboratories, New York.

## HOME SAFETY TIP

Red as a danger signal is a good lesson to teach children who cannot read. Once this lesson is learned, paint red the tops of all bottles or containers at home that hold harmful substances.

**Source:** *Parents.*

## WHEN A CHILD IS CHOKING

When a child is choking: (1) Place the child over your lap, head down, and try four to six slaps on the back (between and below the shoulder blades). (2) If the object is not dislodged, try four Heimlich procedures. Hold the child around the waist and thrust upward with a closed fist. (3) If that doesn't work, look in the child's mouth to see if you can remove the obstruction with your fingers. (4) As a last resort, try mouth-to-mouth resuscitation. Parent alert: Choking is the leading cause of accidental death at home for children age six and younger.

**Source:** *Clinical Pediatrics.*

## DOGS THAT SHOULDN'T BE TRUSTED

Evidence indicates that certain types of dogs pose the greatest risk to children who might be bitten by a pet. The danger: Dogs have a natural tendency to bite each other on the face and neck as a form of aggressive play. They might approach small children in the same spirit. Dogs most likely to exhibit the behavior include German shepherds, malamutes and huskies. To protect kids: Never leave a dog of any breed with a small child, even when the child seems safe in a playpen or crib. Explain to older children why they should use care when playing with a dog, even a familiar one.

**Source:** *Journal of the American Medical Association.*

## PLAY THAT COULD HURT YOUR CHILD

Tossing an infant playfully into the air can cause brain damage and even death. Also dangerous: Shaking a baby out of frustration, which can lead to whiplash and brain hemorrhages. Most vulnerable: Infants who are two months to six months old. But to be safe, parents should avoid shaking, throwing or swinging children under two years old.

**Source:** Dr. David Chadwick, medical director of San Diego Children's Hospital, San Diego, CA.

## TOY-RELATED INJURIES

A sled is safer if the crosspiece that steers it is jointed, rather than rigid. Most dangerous: Saucers and other novelty sliders with no steering mechanism, especially when they carry more than one child.

**Source:** *Parents.*

• Bicycles are the leading cause of toy-related injuries to children under 15. They necessitate 594,100 emergency room visits in just one year. Next: Impacting with or choking on small toys, 118,000. Others: Skates, 61,1900. Sleds, 16,600. Skateboards, 10,300.

**Source:** *Morbidity and Mortality Weekly Report.*

## CAR SAFETY SEATS

Children's safety seats reduce the chance of death in a car accident by 90% and the chance of disabling injury by 67%. Both the harness and shield designs are effective. Key: Find a model that conforms to the size and shape of the child. It should permit free arm movement and a full view. Make sure it's labeled "crash-tested safe" and meets the federal safety standards of January 1981.

**Source:** Study by Washington State Patrol, in *Mechanix Illustrated.*

## POOL SAFETY DEVICE

Floating pool alarm instantly senses if a child or pet falls in and sounds an alarm both at poolside and inside your home. Corrosion-resistant, 10 inches in diameter.

## WHEN PARENTS SUFFER FROM DEPRESSION

Children of parents with serious mental depression are three times more likely to suffer similar emotional distress than the offspring of more normal parents. They are also more prone to attention-deficit disorders, separation anxiety and behavior problems, including alcohol and drug abuse. Children of parents who both suffer depression are even more at risk. A recent study showed that the rate of major depression among children with one disturbed parent was 8.3% but rose to 12.2% with two ill parents. The incidence of all kinds of psychiatric disturbances among children with one depressed parent was 16.7% and with two such parents, 23%.

**Source:** Dr. G. Davis Gammon, child psychiatrist, Yale University, quoted in *The Journal of the American Medical Association.*

## CHILDREN AND STRESS

Children feel stress in the same manner as adults. Prime root of stress: Anxiety over school performance. Special problem: When a child who is naturally slower-paced is born to parents who are high achievers. They may expect too much. Other sources of stress: Insufficient playtime. . .minimal contact with the extended family (grandparents, aunts, uncles, cousins). . .peer pressure to keep up with fashions and trends. . .too much responsibility too soon. . .excessive TV watching.

## MEDICATION FOR VIOLENT KIDS

Violent children can be saved from institutionalization with daily lithium carbonate. This is the medication used for manic-depressives.

**Source:** *RN* magazine.

## THE SECRET KEY TO PERSONALITY

Being the first of many brothers and sisters, an only child, a middle child or the lastborn plays a major role in determining your personality. Understanding this role of birth order can help you know yourself and improve the way you deal with others at home or at the office. Although there are many exceptions, this is the general pattern:

• Only children may have a low sense of self-esteem in social situations.

• Firstborn children are expected by their parents and siblings to be serious and responsible.

• Middle children often become competitive.

• Lastborns are often carefree and fun-loving.

Birth order, of course, determines personality only in combination with other forces:

• Who runs the family?

• What do the parents expect from their children?

• How do children relate to their brothers and sisters?

On a practical level, if I were hiring the oldest of seven siblings, I wouldn't automatically assume that this person knows how to lead. I would ask about his role with his brothers and sisters.

### Interpretations

If he said he couldn't wait to get out and left home at 15, I wouldn't think that person would be a good manager. On the other hand, if he said he had been second-in-command after his mother, I would think he had already learned something about management. Birth order only suggests general patterns that help us understand personality.

### Only Children

Children without siblings may have parents who overprotect them. Everything is done for these chilren, and they never learn to do anything for themselves. At the other extreme are only children who are left very much on their own. Their problem is that they have no one to learn from.

Unless they have cousins or friends to play with, only children have no sense of the impact they make on kids their own age. Without feedback from playmates, only children may develop a low sense of self-esteem in social situations. Only children also tend to have a hard time at negotiating and often don't know how to handle conflict.

### Firstborns

Firstborns have a hard time because parents have a lot riding on these kids. The parents' self-esteem comes from the way the firstborn responds. As a result, firstborns aren't usually given much room to be on their own. (I often think it would be easier on firstborns if there were a "disposable training baby" that parents could use to practice their parenting on.)

Later, and often ironically, younger brothers and sisters look up to the firstborn to show them the way. One result: The attention from parents and siblings helps the firstborn develop a sense of responsibility, and that may be why firstborns have a high rate of achievement in later life.

### Second and Middle Children

By the time the second child arrives, the parents have had more experience and are usually more relaxed. Secondborns have an older brother or sister to learn from so they can say, *Oh, that's how folks react to that. I'm going to try something else.* From watching how their older siblings operate, secondborns can benefit socially. They're more easygoing and relaxed with others.

One problem secondborns may face is pressure if their parents have decided on only two children. The second is it—there aren't going to be any more. If secondborns feel this pressure, they may become more wary and defensive.

In two-children families, if the children have a disagreement, they don't have another sibling to turn to. The luxury of large families is the variety of relationships that can develop among siblings. However, if the three children are of the same sex and close in age, the middle child tends to feel lost or forgotten.

Middle children can become worry children with problems. The problems, of course, are rooted in their need for attention. Middle children get a lot of practice in seeking attention that can make them very competitive in later life.

In some cases, the middle child has a network of close friends outside the family and may well even "adopt" a friend's family.

### Lastborns

Lastborns are often treated as babies for their entire lives. It's a struggle for them to be seen by their brothers and sisters as an equal. Lastborns may also feel guilty if they surpass an older sibling in school or some other competition: I'm outranking my brother and I shouldn't.

But being the youngest can be enjoyable. Watching older siblings teaches lastborns a lot. Their parents aren't concerned enough to follow their every step, and a child can benefit from that benign neglect.

Lastborns often become high achievers because they've watched all the choices made by their older siblings and then selected the path that best suits them.

**Source:** Interview with Dr. Bunny S. Duhl, co-director of the Boston Family Institute, Brookline, MA.

## AN ONLY CHILD ISN'T SO BAD OFF

The only child is not as bad off as many people believe. A recent study at the University of Texas concluded that only children are happier in adulthood than are people with brothers and sisters. Reason: They develop greater self-esteem in childhood, which remains with them in later life. Although onlies are sometimes thought to be spoiled and selfish, the positive effects of this status outweigh the negative ones.

**Source:** *Amercian Demographics, Ithaca, N.Y.*

• Recent studies show that the size of a family matters far less than its social and economic status—and the presence of both parents in the home. Other findings: Compared to children with siblings, only children are just as popular with peers. . . express the same degree of general happiness in their adult years. . . are just as healthy, both physically and mentally. . . score higher in intelligence tests. . .have higher academic aspirations. . .reach higher levels of education. . .and attain more prestige on the job.

**Source:** Research by Toni Falbo, Ph.D., associate professor, University of Texas at Austin.

## DIFFERENT CHILD— DIFFERENT TREATMENT

Treating your children equally isn't always possible—or desirable. Don't be afraid to take into account the differences in your children—age, intelligence and maturity, for example—when granting privileges or setting rules.

## COPING WITH SIBLING RIVALRIES

Anyone who is not an only child can testify to the profound effect of the sibling relationship. Our research shows that it is a mistake to emphasize only the jealousy and rivalry. The same children who are at each others' throats one minute are also capable of great affection, concern and attachment to brothers and sisters. Even before the age of three, a child is capable of understanding the feelings of a baby sibling and showing empathy for the infant.

### Observations and Insights

There are patterns in families that may help parents better understand how sibling rivalry is triggered. Once mothers and fathers see what is happening, techniques for minimizing conflict between siblings make more sense. What we found in our research:

• In families where there is an intense close relationship between the mother and firstborn daughter, the girl is usually hostile to a new baby. A year later, both children are likely to be hostile to each other.

• Firstborn boys are more likely than girls to become withdrawn after a new baby's birth. Children who withdraw (both boys and girls) are less likely to show positive interest in and affection for the baby.

• In families where there is a high level of confrontation between the mother and first child before the birth of a sibling, the first child is more likely to behave in an irritating or interfering way toward the new baby.

• In families where the first child has a close relationship with the father, there seems to be less hostility toward the new baby.

• There is no indication that a child whose parents prepare him for the birth of a new baby with explanations and reassurances reacts any better than a child who wasn't prepared. More important: How the parents act after the new baby is born.

• Inside the family, girls are just as physically aggressive as boys.

• Physical punishment of children by parents leads to an increase in violence between children.

• Breastfeeding the new baby can have a beneficial effect on firstborns. Reason: Mothers who breastfeed tend to find distractions for the older child during feeding. This turns a potentially provocative time into a loving situation where the first child is also cuddled up with the mother, getting special attention while the baby is being fed.

### Dealing with Sibling Rivalry

• Don't blame yourself. Much sibling rivalry is unavoidable. There's no way you can blame a mother for an intense relationship with her firstborn child.

• Try to minimize a drop in attention to the first child. This change in attention is dramatic—not just because the mother is occupied with the new baby, but because she is often too tired to give the older child the kind of sensitive, playful focus he or she received in the past. Recommended: Get as much help as possible from the father, grandparents and other relatives and friends. The mothers we studied were exhausted. A month after the new baby came, half were still getting less than five hours' sleep a night. Also: Quarreling between siblings increases when the parents are under stress. Anything that alleviates the mother's fatigue, depression and irritability is likely to lead to a decrease in bickering and teasing among the children.

• Keep things stable. A child's life is turned upside down when a new baby arrives. Toddlers of around two and three appreciate a stable, predictable world in which the daily schedule of events—meals, naps, outings—can be counted on. In families where the mother tries to keep the older child's life as unchanged as possible, there is less disturbance.

• Talk to the older child about the baby as a person. Involve him or her in caring for the baby. In families where the mother draws the older child in as a helper for the new baby, there is less hostility a year later.

• Be prepared with distractions for the older child. An older child gets demanding the moment the mother starts caring exclusively for the baby, but mothers who are prepared with projects and helping tasks head off confrontations.

• Recognize and avoid favoritism. Our current study shows that mothers intervene three times as much on behalf of a second child, although the second is equally likely to have been the cause of the quarrel. (The first child's feeling that parents favor the second is realistic.) Parents tend to intervene on behalf of younger children because they see them as more vulnerable to abuse. But our studies show that older siblings tend to hold back because they know their aggression is disapproved of, while younger ones often physically attack brothers and sisters because they feel they can get away with it. Parents neglect to impose the same standards of behavior on the babies in the family.

• Be firm in consistently prohibiting physical violence. In the context of a warm, affectionate relationship, this is the most effective way to minimize sibling rivalry and to keep jealousies in check.

• Try to keep your sense of humor and your perspective when a new baby is born. Things will get better sooner than you think. By the time the infants in our study were eight weeks old, many of the firstborns were adjusting quite well.

**Source:** Interview with Judy Dunn, who co-authored (with Carol Kendrick) *Siblings: Love, Envy & Understanding,* Harvard University Press, Cambridge, MA.

# GROWING-UP MYTHS AND REALITIES

The study of human emotions is in its infancy, but a growing body of research has begun to dispel some harmful myths. These new insights can be helpful and reassuring to parents. Important new findings:

• Negative events in infancy do not irreversibly damage the mental health of the adult. Some repair is possible if the environment becomes more benevolent.

• The behavior of an infant does not provide a good preview of the young adult. A one-year old's tantrums don't foreshadow teenage delinquency, for example. Many infantile qualities disappear as their usefulness is outgrown. Adult behavior becomes more predictable after the age of five than it was before.

• Human beings are not saddled with a fixed "intelligence" or "temperament" in every situation. These qualities are related to context and can vary in different circumstances.

• A biological mother's physical affection is not basic to a child's healthy emotional growth. More important is consistent nurturing from primary care givers, related or not, female or male. The key is a child's belief in his own value in the eyes of the care givers.

### Charting Emotional Development

Developmental psychologists, long led by the Swiss theorist Jean Piaget (1896-1980), have been able to chart the stages of human intellectual growth with great success. They have found that our cognitive capacities (languages abilities, spatial skills, reasoning capacities, etc.) mature in a uniform, orderly sequence from infancy to adulthood.

A growing amount of evidence suggests that our emotional capacities also emerge in an orderly progression. But the interaction between biological factors—the growth of the brain and central nervous system—and developing emotional and cognitive skills is highly complex.

Studying human emotions poses many new problems. It is much harder to provoke, identify and measure a feeling than to test, for instance, whether a child understands the concepts "larger" and "smaller."

One problem is limited terminology. For example, because we apply the same "an-gry" to a two-year-old that we apply to an adult, it is easy to assume that the experience is the same for both. But we err in judging children's emotional reactions by adult standards. And words for feelings do not identify the *sources* or *objects* of our emotions.

### The Stages of Emotional Growth

*The first three to four months:* The emotional reactions a very young infant displays are associated with the events he or she encounters. The introduction of a stuffed toy might provoke a reaction of interest. The sudden slamming of a door might cause an infant to startle. Distress is a response to physical discomfort, relaxation, to gratification. All are familiar emotions to new parents. However, mothers can easily misinterpret their babies' facial expressions and actions. An infant's pushing the mother away, for example, may be seen as anger rather than as distress or fright.

*Four to twelve months:* As the infant's mental ability develops, new emotions appear. Fear of unfamiliar adults and sadness or anxiety at separation from a primary caregiver are examples of emotions that require the ability to compare the events of the present with the events of the recent past. The removal of a favored toy may provoke anger, as the baby is able to relate the loss to another person as its cause.

*One to four years:* With the recognition of standards, including self-generated goals, comes an increased repertory of emotional reactions. A two-year-old may show frustration when he is capable of imagining a tower of six building blocks but can balance only four of them before they tumble to the floor. Likewise, he will show satisfaction at a successfully completed task.

Late in the third year comes the understanding that one could have acted otherwise: Guilt. And by the fourth year, children can identify with people who lead them to feel pride in a parent's intelligence or shame at a sibling's dishonesty.

*Five years and up:* During the fifth and sixth years, a child begins to compare himself or herself with others on desired qualities. We then see the emergence of such emotions as insecurity and confidence. Problem: A child in a large peer group can compare himself with a pool of children and will find many children who have qualities superior to his own. He is therefore more likely to feel inferior if he is in a large peer group rather than in a small one. Better: Smaller classrooms with students of equal ability. Important: To be motivated, children need a reasonable expectation of success. Key: Reasonable goals.

*Adolescence:* The hormonal changes that occur in puberty permit a degree of sexual emotion not known in childhood. The adolescent also begins to examine his own beliefs for logical consistency and discovers many incompatible ideas. Example: Parents are all-knowing and always right, but my parents exhibit imperfections.

The ability to review ideas also allows an adolescent to recognize seemingly insoluble problems such as rejection by a lover or fatal illness. Result: A feeling of helplessness or depression. This may explain the popular misconception that teenagers are moody.

**Source:** Interview with Jerome Kagan, Ph.D., professor of developmental psychology at Harvard University and author of *The Nature of the Child,* Basic Books, New York.

## BABIES AND STRANGERS

When infants reach the age of six to eight months, most are upset by a stranger rushing toward them, especially if a parent is not right there. Reason: The baby has just come to realize that other people are separate individuals and doesn't know how to handle the stranger. Best: When approaching a baby for the first time, smile at the infant *from a distance,* talk in a low tone to other people in the room, and walk very slowly and casually. Don't rush up to the baby.

**Source:** Robert B. McCall, Ph.D., senior scientist, Boys Town Center for the Study of Youth Development, writing in *Parents,* New York.

## OLD WIVES' TALE THAT MAY BE TRUE

Slow walkers are slow learners, says an old

wives' tale. The trouble is, it may actually be true. Children who are slow to walk (or slow to walk and talk) have lower IQs. And they experience greater difficulties when they start learning to read. Surprise: Slow talking alone is not associated with low intelligence or with later reading problems.

**Source:** A long-term study of children done by Phil Silva, Rob McGee and Sheila Williams of the University of Otago Medical School, New Zealand.

## SUPERBABY MYTH

Some parents are trying to turn their babies into little computers in the belief that infants are like information sponges. Theory: Give children as much intellectual stimulation as possible and they'll grow into superadults. Trap: No amount of special training can turn normal babies into superpeople—and overdoing it may fail to give them breathing room . . . creating real problems in the future.

**Source:** *Psychology Today,* New York.

## A FATHER'S ROLE

Stay-at-home fathers contribute to precocity in babies. In one study, infants averaged six to 12 months ahead of schedule in problem-solving tasks when their fathers stayed home and mothers went off to work. Their social skills were comparable to those of the average baby 19 months older. Probable reason: The babies were getting love and attention from both parents.

**Source:** Research by Kyle Pruett at Yale University, quoted in *The Salk Letter,* Boulder, CO.

• Fathers who are active in raising their baby daughters are less likely to abuse the girls sexually later on. In a recent prison study, 30 of 54 abuser fathers had no contact with their daughters during the girls' first three years.

**Source:** Research by Seymour and Hilda Parker, researchers at the University of Utah, Salt Lake City.

## GIRLS WILL BE GIRLS

Baby girls who favor one hand over the other show faster intellectual growth than those who don't. But no such relationship was found in baby boys. Possible reason: Sexual differences in neural anatomy.

**Source:** Study at California State University in Fullerton, in *Science, 83*, Washington, D.C.

## WHAT HAPPENS AT AGE SIX

Boys and girls show similar traits up to age six, according to a recent study of 275 children. The researchers found no significant sex differences in timidity, aggressiveness, activity or intelligence. And both genders were treated similarly by parents. What did matter: Birth order. First-borns are generally pressured to achieve more, whereas later children get more unconditional praise and warmth.

**Source:** Study by Eleanor Maccoby, Stanford University.

## WHEN A CHILD WON'T SHARE

Toddler possessiveness can be a healthy sign. Reason: When a two-year-old guards toys before sharing them, the child is showing increased self-awareness—a natural stage of development. Bottom line: Don't insist that your toddler share toys right away. Support the child's possessiveness, then help negotiate.

**Source:** *Parents*, New York.

## BOYS AND DOLLS

Little boys who play with dolls will turn out fine. A recent study found that children's adjustment in first grade and beyond was not affected by whether they had played with sex-role "appropriate" toys. What did matter: Whether their toy play matched their mothers' sex-role expectations. Worst adjustment problems: When a boy played with "girl toys" (or vice versa) despite a mother's admonitions.

**Source:** Study by Michael Lewis, M.D., child-development researcher at the Rutgers Medical School.

## WHAT THE EXPERTS SAY ABOUT SECURITY BLANKETS

Most children give up a favorite blanket or stuffed animal by the age of seven. But some cling for years. Key: The less importance you attach to the blanket, the sooner the child will grow away from it. Steps: Start early (from the age of two) to build the child's self-esteem. Allow the child to make choices regarding meals, clothes, friends, books and games. If blanket-clinging persists, distract the child with a live pet or a new toy, book or game. Don't feel angry or guilty about the reliance on the blanket. Child psychiatrists agree that a security blanket is a natural and normal attachment for most youngsters. But if a child still needs it into adolescence, seek professional consultation.

## TODAY'S CHILDHOOD FEARS

Children's fears are changing. In 1939, fifth and sixth graders worried most about failing in school, not being able to find a job, and not having enough money. Today, kids are more concerned about deaths in the family, divorce, kidnappings, rape, robbery and nuclear war. To deal with childhood fears: Encourage verbalization. Provide information about the area of concern. Indicate how real the danger actually is. Suggest protective steps to be taken or report what preventive measures are already in place. Also teach your child to relax muscles and to recite "brave statements" while visualizing the disturbing scene. Such "rehearsals" in the presence of a supportive parent help the child gain mastery over the feared situation.

**Source:** Ruth Formanek, chief psychologist, Jewish Community Services of Long Island (NY), quoted in *US News & World Report*, New York.

## DR. SPOCK CORRECTED

Young children were barred from many a parental bed in the Dr. Spock era. Reason: Parents feared the experience might be too sexually suggestive. New thinking: Children generally crawl in with Mommy and Daddy when scared or sick at night. That may not be a bad idea—and they're usually willing to go back to their own beds after they've calmed down.

**Source:** Dr. Alvin A. Rosenfeld of Stanford University, quoted in *Ladies Home Journal*, New York.

## HELP FOR SOUTHPAWS

Left-handed children should be supplied early on with left-handed scissors and spiral notebooks with bindings on the right side. Also: Ask the teacher to seat the child at a left-handed desk. (Most schools are able to cooperate.) Aside from practical help, these measures will reinforce the child's self-esteem.

**Source:** *Working Parents*, New York.

## UPS AND DOWNS OF UNATTRACTIVE CHILDREN

Unattractive children usually develop other assets that enhance their personalities. Examples: Loyalty. A capacity for intimacy. The ability to share interests and feelings. Result: They often have an edge in the quest for success and happiness over the much more attractive children who have lived with undue emphasis on physical qualities. The most important trait: Self-assurance. The person who has this quality quickly overcomes any possible deficiencies in physical appearance.

• Physical unattractiveness and delinquency are often linked. Insight: We tend to treat ugly people like delinquents, so they act the role. Delinquency seems less common among the handsome. Suggestion: Be nice to unattractive people.

**Source:** Sociologist Robert Agnew, commenting on the results of a national study of adolescent boys.

## LIKE GRANDMOTHER LIKE GRANDDAUGHTER

High-energy, strong-minded women often rebel against their own mothers, but they still need a female role model. Readily available: One of the grandmothers. Usually it will be the powerful grandmother whom the granddaughter will choose—the one who is similarly strong-willed.

The skipped-generation effect is also involved. If the mother's mother was very strong, chances are the mother is weak because her will was broken early. The strong-minded daughter, in effect, overthrows her own mother to copy the behavior outlook of the maternal grandmother.

Insight: The daughter does not have to rebel against the grandmother, unless the older woman raises her. The grandmother has the advantage over the mother of not eliciting the day-to-day rebellion that is part of exercising daily authority over children.

This latching onto the grandmother occurs when the daughter is old enough to be verbal and has the capacity to differentiate between grownups. The older woman's days of struggle are behind her. Relative to the mother, the grandmother is calm and secure.

The grandmother needs to be available, but proximity is not as important as interaction. Sometimes all the grandmother and granddaughter need is a few weeks together once a year. Often the grandmother's house is a refuge where the granddaughter escapes the authority of her mother or of both parents.

The mother's reaction can range from accommodating and supportive to competitive and suppressive. Point: If the mother is jealous of a close relationship between the daughter and grandmother, that is her problem, not the child's. If the grandmother is a positive influence, she should be welcome. A child needs many affirmative adult role models.

This interaction is primarily a phenomenon of women. Although there is some role-modeling between grandson and grandfather, the line of descent in males is not as defined as in females. The women in a family are more available to one another and therefore exert more overt influence. Contrast: The males are generally less self-revealing to each other.

If you are really trying to learn what makes a certain woman tick and you cannot pick up the necessary information by knowing her parents, then look at her grandmother, especially on the mother's side. She will probably supply the insights as she presents the model that the granddaughter emulated.

**Source:** Interview with Martin G. Groder, M.D., a psychiatrist and business consultant who practices in Chapel Hill, NC.

# TRAPS IN ACCELERATED EARLY LEARNING

The first three years of a child's life are the most important for future development—to school age and beyond. Our studies bear this out, and modern middle-class parents know it, too. Result: A wave of expensive, elaborate early-learning programs. Children are rushed to swim by the age of three months, read by one year, and operate a computer at two.

Wanting your child to do better is very praiseworthy and understandable. But when you define *better* simply as *bright,* and you desperately reach out for almost any program that comes along, you're taking a great risk. Young children are heart as much as mind. Balance is the key. There's more to development than a surprising vocabulary. It's much easier to produce a bright, facile, obnoxious child than an unspoiled, likable, decent one.

In my view, none of these accelerated-learning programs are useful in the development of a well-rounded child. (An exception is Gymboree, a low-pressure exercise instruction program for parents and their babies.) At worst, they intrude on time and the child's need to develop social skills and motor skills.

In addition, too many parents come to value their children's achievement over the children themselves. Common results: Precocious, unhappy children who are socially incompetent.

There's growing evidence, in fact, that hurrying babies and young children intellectually often backfires in the future. David Elkind of Tufts University, a leader in the field of children's learning, has found that those who learn to read by the age of three are more likely to have reading problems later on. Key: Although these children learned the mechanics of reading, they understood little of its content. (In addition, Elkind found serious stress symptoms in three- to five-years-old early learners, including headaches and stomach aches.)

In the Harvard Preschool Project during which we studied several hundred families over a 13-year period, we defined a competent three-year-old by both intellectual and social criteria. These "model" children were imaginative, and they were good observers. They anticipated consequences better than the norm. They knew how to get attention in socially acceptable ways. Although they didn't hesitate to approach an adult when they needed help, they first tried to solve problems by themselves. In fantasy play, they often assumed the roles of grown-ups. They were good leaders, but they also knew how to follow.

Then we looked at their parents. Leading characteristics: As soon as the babies were ready to crawl (usually around seven months), the parents encouraged them to roam freely about the house. These children weren't penned up for long periods in playpens or jump seats. Instead, they were given full access to the living areas (which had been childproofed for safety)—to exercise their boundless curiosity, improve control over their bodies, and explore their new world.

These children didn't need expensive

educational toys. They received wonderful stimulation from Ping-Pong balls, plastic measuring spoons, plastic containers—any small manipulatable objects. Best books for the crawling set: Large ones with stiff cardboard pages. The literature is irrelevant; the point is to engage a baby's fascination with hinged objects.

### A Learning Environment

The best parents set up an interesting world for the child and then back off. They identify what the child is interested in rather than trying to focus the child's attention. It does no good to force learning on a child who is not interested at the moment. This only leads to boredom. Better: Wait for the child to come to you. During the crawling stage, that will happen an average of 10 times an hour—whenever the child feels excitement, frustration or pain. Then you'll have a motivated student. In half a minute, you can offer a new idea with a phrase or a toy—and accomplish more than an hour's drill with flash cards.

The best way to teach language skills is the same as it's always been... by simply talking, parent to child. Keep your talk concrete and in the present. Relate it to objects the baby can perceive... the sock you're putting on, the toy you're holding out. Never use baby talk. But keep in mind the child's limits. Most effective: Talking to children at or slightly beyond their apparent level of understanding.

Reading aloud can also be useful, but only if the child is receptive. Best opportunity: Just before bedtime.

### Most Important Advice

Let children develop at their own pace. They need their parents' assistance, but certainly not some rigidly choreographed approach to learning. You may not end up with a five-year-old violin prodigy, but perhaps you'll get something better. A well-rounded, delightful person—short run and long run.

**Source:** Interview with Burton L. White, director, Center for Parent Education, Newton, MA.

# DR. SEUSS WAS RIGHT

Pre-schoolers who learn to recognize rhymes become better readers later on, according to a recent study. And when low-scoring children were trained in sound recognition, their reading levels improved far more than those schooled in concepts and categories.

**Source:** Study at Oxford University, in *Psychology Today*, New York.

# A PLUS FOR EARLY WRITERS

Children who write at an early age almost always become good readers. Moreover, early writing helps teach children to structure and plan, to develop a concept of self and to become aware of others by considering their audience's point of view.

**Source:** *Growing Up Writing* by Linda Lamme, Acropolis Books, Washington, DC.

# STARTING-SCHOOL TIP

The first day of school usually proves unsettling for young children. Don't make things worse by painting too rosy a picture of what it will be like. Instead: Be honest. Tell your child it may be confusing, with teachers forgetting names and some children crying. Don't forget to point out, though, that things will soon improve.

**Source:** *A Letter from Dr. Lee Salk*, New York.

# WHAT'S IN A NAME?

Unusual first names have no bearing on a child's academic performance or social behavior. This was the conclusion of a recent study of more than 23,000 students. Previous research in the field had failed to consider a child's ethnic background.

**Source:** *The Chronicle of Higher Education*, Washington, D.C.

## BUDDING ENTREPRENEURS

Persistence is the most essential quality in children who display an enterprising bent. Example: Typical young entrepreneurs will try selling calendars and, if they don't make any money, they'll say the idea didn't work. They detach failure from themselves personally. . . and just go on to another idea.

**Source:** Marilyn Kourilsky, economist, University of California at Los Angeles, quoted in *Inc.*, Boston, MA.

## A GOOD REASON TO HAVE A PET

Childhood pet ownership and future career success may be linked. According to a recent survey among chief executive officers, 94% as children had either a cat or a dog. Findings: Pet ownership developed many of the positive traits that made for good managers—responsibility, empathy and respect for other living beings. And while just 53% of American households had either a cat or a dog in 1983, more than 75% of the CEOs had one of these pets or both.

**Source:** Peat, Marwick, Mitchell & Co.

## EARLY-TRAINING SURPRISE

In a follow-up look at a group of adults whose mothers had been interviewed on parenting practices when the children were five, two patterns emerged. The children who had been subjected to the strictest feeding schedules and toilet training have the highest need to achieve as adults. The youngsters whose mothers were most permissive about sex and aggression (allowing masturbation and fighting with siblings, for example) show the highest need for power as adults. Practices the researches expected to relate to adult characteristics did not show clear correlation in the study. How warm the mother was with the infant, or how long the child was breast fed, long assumed to be important to a child's well-

being, did not match up directly with specific adult traits.

**Source:** Study by psychologist David McClelland, Harvard University, reported in *Journal of Personality and Social Psychology*, Washington, D.C.

## YOUTHFUL CREATIVITY

Stressing success may make a child less creative. Reason: A child under too much parental pressure will try only the things he does well, rather than exploring new areas. Also critical: An ability to accept criticism and even to tolerate being laughed at.

**Source:** Dr. Joyce Brothers.

## MICKEY MOUSE VS. SPACE INVADERS

Video games don't stimulate a child's imagination as much as cartoons. Reason: The games restrict players to a concrete fixed-rule activity with someone else's fantasy material.

**Source:** Psychologist Jerome Singer, Yale University, in *Psychology Today*, New York.

## GIRLS ARE FALLING BEHIND

Today's computer culture is overwhelmingly male. Boys outnumber girls in computer camps by three to one. Video arcades are largely male preserves, with games oriented to boys' interests in war and sports. Girls need special encouragement from teachers and parents to avoid becoming second-class citizens in a computer-dominated job market.

**Source:** *Psychology Today*, New York.

## HOW TO TALK AND LISTEN TO YOUR KIDS

The beginning of wisdom is silence. Then comes listening. But it's not easy to hear what another person is really saying. Yet hearing is what children need most from their parents. To be an effective and caring parent, one needs to develop the ability to hear not just the words but the feelings those words try to convey. One needs to learn to listen with empathy.

### What Is Your Child Really Saying?

Example: A child comes home from school shouting, "I'm never going back to school. Do you know what my teacher did? She punished me because she caught me passing notes. She even called me names."

Many parents react to such an outburst with anger. They feel that their child has misbehaved and that they must discipline him so that he will not do it again. But this reaction is not helpful. It only makes the child who was angry at the teacher also get angry at his parent. When we hear only what the child did, not how it made him feel, we are unable to understand or be of help.

From their parents, children have a right to expect understanding, because what they need is help not with their behavior but with their feelings. A child who feels right usually behaves right.

Rule for parents: When a child is upset, no matter what the reason, even if he brought it on himself, the first thing he needs from his parents is a response that will take care of his disturbed feelings. How: By reflecting the feelings back to him. "You mean the teacher called you names in front of the whole class? That must have been very humiliating. No wonder you're so upset." Result: The child's anger will diminish and he'll be able to return to school.

Many parents may feel that this response doesn't teach the child anything, that he will misbehave again. But the teacher has already taken care of this behavior. The child does not need additional lessons in behavior. What he needs is his parents' understanding of his feelings.

### Empathic Listening

Empathic listening is the ability to put oneself in another person's place and understand where that person is coming from without imposing one's own point of view.

Only with an open mind can one listen empathically and hear even unpleasant truths. Problem: Listening with an open mind doesn't come naturally, especially when it concerns our children. Reason: We have a vested interest in them. They reflect on us. We're so busy trying to make them into the kind of adults we need them to become—beautiful, brilliant, athletic, popular, etc.—that we can't afford to listen empathically. Our first reaction is more likely to be "How will this behavior affect Jane's future?" than "My daughter Jane (whom I claim to love) is very upset."

We're also afraid to hear the truth from our children. What we fear: Feeling like a bad parent. Disruption of the status quo. Being forced to confront ourselves or them. Getting angry. Having to say no. Having to enforce limits. Being disliked. Feeling helpless.

### What to Do about It

It isn't dangerous to hear what our children are saying as long as we remember that we don't have to do anything about it. Most parents feel that when a child talks about a problem, they have to do something. In reality, the only thing a loving parent needs to do is to help the child feel better so that he can think rationally and use good judgment.

It's very important that we let our children solve their own problems in order for them to develop self-confidence, autonomy and a feeling of competence. When children don't feel competent, they become anxious. This is why it is not a good idea to solve children's problems for them. The only problem children can't help themselves with is their negative feelings. That's where they really need our help. Once these feelings are gone and the child feels good about himself, he'll be able to figure out what to do. When our child shares a problem with us, it's preferable to say, "I wonder what you can do about it," rather than, "I think you should do thus-and-such."

### The Secretive Teenager

When teenagers are not communicative,

parents need to ask themselves, "How do I talk to my child that makes it so difficult for him to talk to me?" We tend to blame our children, claiming there is something wrong with them. What's really happening: Every time a child has shared something really important, we have probably reacted negatively.

Today's parents say, "You can tell me everything." But do we really mean it? We usually get angry when children tell us things we don't want to hear. To mean it, we must be really prepared to listen empathically to information that may upset us. Example: Should your teenage daughter announce to you that she is pregnant, it would be more caring and effective to be able to respond with, "How terrible for you. I'm so glad you could share this with us. Can we be of help?" than to scream, "How could you have done this to us, after all we've done for you?"

**Source:** Interview with Alice Ginott, Ph.D., psychoanalyst and lecturer on communication in caring relationships.

# COMPUTERIZED CHILDREN

Encouraging your child to get more and more involved with the home computer is not a wise move. Even some of the most vigorous champions of teaching computer skills at earlier ages (such as Seymour Papert of the Massachusetts Institute of Technology, who invented the LOGO programming language for children) have suddenly developed misgivings. Papert said recently that the same computer whiz kids whom we now reward so handsomely with praise may turn out to be a generation of adult psychotics.

### New Babysitters

The problem: Computers are now being pushed on kids for many of the same reasons parents used TV—as a convenient, cheap babysitter. Dual-career couples and single parents find they can have a bit of peace at home (or time to do the work they brought from the office) if Johnny is off working on the terminal. But TV is now considered "bad". . .and computer work is now considered "good." Reality: Children are being encouraged to relate to a machine rather than to other human beings, just as they were with the TV screen. They're learning a narrow set of skills—and retreating from the more complex set of social skills that they vitally need for healthy growth.

The cycle: Parents who feel guilty about their neglect comfort themselves with the conviction that the computer is the savior, the key to their children's future. The kids accept the computer ("fall into the vortex," says one) because communication with the computer eases their loneliness and eliminates the pain and rebuffs that they experience in making and keeping up social relationships. Result: Technostress in the workplace and also in the home.

The symptoms of overuse of the computer:

• Edginess and crankiness—the result of mental fatigue.

• On and off communication patterns with parents and siblings. . .yes. . .no. . .yes.

• Impatience because. . .parents take too long to get to the point. . .the book has too many descriptive words. . .the situation is too ambiguous.

• Fewer friends, less time spent outdoors, less physical activity.

The conventional wisdom about the computer as a good teacher is that it doesn't give negative feedback. It keeps encouraging the computer worker to become more perfect, to stop making errors in the program, to work in a logical, deductive way. But. . .as youngsters develop their computer skills and focus their attention on the computer during more and more of their "leisure" time, they're also increasing the negative impact of such work:

• They don't learn as youngsters to deal with the inevitable negative feedback they'll get in real-life human relationships. As adults they may wind up being immobilized by criticism.

• Young children (4–6 years) begin matching their thinking style to that of the computer—which is logical and deductive. Computer thinking is really quite simplistic and "dumber" than the natural thinking of children of this age, which is metaphorical. Metaphorical thinking is at the base of true genius and creativity.

### Managing Kids and Computers

The rudest shock of all to the upwardly mobile, middle-class parents who are most likely to be computer fanatics for their children is that being a computer whiz may track their children into narrow technical work—not the usual high road to success in organizations. The social and psychological skills necessary to motivate and manage people are exactly the skills that computer addicts avoid learning

The solution isn't to throw out the computer. Instead:

• Put limits on computer use. . .just as limits should be put on TV watching. It's natural to lose a sense of time when working on the computer, so put a clock beside the terminal—and set an alarm to ring when the child must leave computer work.

• Train the child to recognize the signs of mental fatigue, such as taking deeper breaths or making more mistakes. Explain that when he feels those symptoms—or when the alarm rings—he must stop working on the problem. Teach children to state the problem they're working on—either by logging it on the computer or writing it in a notebook that they keep near the computer. Goal: Write the problem down so that the child doesn't have to keep it in his short-term memory and continue worrying about it.

• Allow for a 20-minute (at least) transition time between computer work and dinner or time for other family relationships. If this isn't done, the child will spend half the time at the dinner table thinking about what he just left on the computer instead of conversing with those around him. By the time he's ready to talk, dinner is over and everyone scatters again. Left alone, the child, looking for companionship, turns back to the computer—and still hasn't communicated with other members of the family.

### The Hardest Task

Don't let the computer substitute for time spent with your children. Though it seems silly to say it: Spend non-technological time with your children every day— not time spent watching TV, working on the computer terminal, working on the car, talking about new gadgets. Don't underestimate the value of simple playfulness and horsing around. And with older children, sit and talk for a few minutes each day— and not about objects.

Just as important: Your child can be very bright, yet totally uninterested in becoming computer literate. Don't press. . .and don't show your disappointment. Despite all the media publicity (much of it stirred by manufacturers of computers), not all children take to computers automatically. At least one child in three resists learning to use them—even for playing games. There's no reason to worry that such a child is scarred for life.

**Source:** Interview with Craig Brod, Ph.D., a psychologist who's made a specialty of treating technology-stressed adults and children in the high-tech area of northern California.

# HOW PARENTS CAN HELP THEIR ADOLESCENT

The transition to adolescence is a difficult time both for children and for parents. But parents can create an environment that will make it easier for everyone involved to weather this stressful preadolescent passage.

Entry into adolescence begins between the ages of 10 and 13. The process is earlier than it used to be and is much more condensed.

We look for the physical changes, such as body growth, hormonal functioning and appearance. But right before that, changes usually show up in feelings and moods, an increase in sexual drive and aggressiveness. Children eat a lot more and are more self-centered. They regress. Example: Boys tell toilet jokes.

Another symptom: Seventh-grade slump. Schools are often sensitive to dips in students' performances in the seventh and eighth grades. Parents need to be supportive but also must set limits so that the child doesn't go under completely. Be aware that there will be some slippage. That doesn't mean the youngster has sudenly become stupid or will never work again.

### Development Stages

Latency, the stage prior to adolescence, is is a period of mastering self, work, play and social relationships. In the uneasy transition to adolescence, youngsters are no longer involved in mastery. In fact, sometimes it looks as though it's all been lost. It hasn't been. The tasks of early adolescence are different.

The major task for the child is disengagement from parents. He experiences a conflict between the upsurge of drive and pullback to the early parental relationship. He acts older and then younger. He progresses and regresses.

The parent must disengage from the dependent child of the earlier period. The adolescent doesn't need as much nurturing and attention to his physical comfort. The parent must step aside in those areas and let the child do his own growing up.

The parent is heading toward middle age at the same time the child is heading toward adulthood. That's often painful.

### Mistakes Parents Make

Parents too often pull the child back into the nurturing, dependent status. The child may go along because it's hard to give that up.

Parents tend to enter adolescence with their children . . . by dressing like the child, getting involved with his friends, becoming a participant.

Neither of these attitudes helps the child, although he may enjoy it at the moment. Both are keeping the child with the parent at a time when he needs support in disengaging.

The healthy child will openly rebel at these and other ways by which parents hold on. This is preferable to the child's staying fixed in an earlier mode—looking like an adolescent but never engaging the most important adolescent task.

Expect some stress and conflict. No one disengages easily, whether he's 2 ½ or 12 ½ .

The parents of adolescents still have to be parents. Limits are still necessary, perhaps even more so. Let children know what you expect, but be reasonably tolerant. They are still not up to assessing the reality of the dangers of drugs, alcohol or herpes. Rules and regulations for social life are important.

### Strategies

There is a big jump in cognition at adolescence. A child is capable of much more abstract thinking and introspection. Despite all the turbulence, you have much more to work with. A parent can engage in a dialogue and work out compromises. A lot depends on the earlier relationship with the child.

Try to work on a rational level first. But remember: You are the parent. You have a certain awareness of the child's needs. Ask yourself: Why do I need to keep the child as a baby (which is not going to help him)? What do I need to be a parent who knows what's safe and what's reasonable? It's the ability to recognize one's own motivation that distinguishes parents who can handle their child's adolescence from those who can't.

### Different Growth Rates

Physical appearance becomes an important factor at this time. The child whose growth spurt comes early has a definite advantage. Those kids do better both academically and socially. Peer groups are important, and physically advanced children get more positive response.

The girl who doesn't get her period until after her friends or the boy who doesn't grow as quickly often needs more support from the parent. Such children see what is happening to their friends, and they get anxious, they worry, they act out.

Gender differences: By age 13, girls are two years in advance of boys. This makes it harder on boys because girls are more interested in them than they are in the girls. Parents sometimes become anxious, too.

### Change for Parents

During this transition, parents must shift. They have to find new sources of gratification away from their children and accept limitations. They can't control as closely as they did earlier.

The child will no longer tell you everything, which is actually positive. He won't be as responsive or as responsible.

Bottom line: The child has to change. But it's equally important for the parent to change as well.

**Source:** Interview with Pearl-Ellen Gordon, Ph.D., a child psychologist in private practice in New York.

## TEEN YEARS AREN'T ALL BAD

Most teenagers get along fine with their parents, despite their gripes. In a recent poll, 71% rated their relationship with Mom and Dad as good or excellent. . .and 84% said they confide in their parents. Most agree with their folks on politics, religion, moral issues and careers. Biggest complaint: Insufficient freedom and understanding.

**Source:** Survey by *Seventeen*, New York.

## HOW TO DEAL WITH TROUBLED TEENAGERS

Anyone with adolescent or young adult children who followed the trial of John W. Hinckley, Jr., must have felt a chilling identity with the young man's parents and wondered "Would I have recognized the depths of my child's problems?" or "Would I have known how to handle such a situation any better?" With that in mind, *Bottom Line/Personal* interviewed Dr. Anne deGersdorff, an analyst and chief psychologist at the Austen Riggs Center, a private psychiatric hospital in Stockbridge, MA, that specializes in treating young adults.

*How can parents tell if their teenage children are troubled enough to need professional help?*

Adolescence, which can last from puberty into the early 20s, is a difficult and moody time for everybody. Many healthy youngsters go through transitional problem periods and bouts of depression which are a normal part of growing up. Some disturbed young people act up enough to be referred for help by their schools or local police. More worrisome are the quiet, withdrawn students who keep up at school but don't really function at full throttle. Danger signs: A teenager with no friends and little or no peer involvement. Long periods of withdrawal and obvious unhappiness. Extended depression and passivity (just sitting around and watching television for weeks at a time, for example). Lack of interest in school or work with no motivation to participate in activities.

*Should adolescent suicide threats be taken seriously?*

Yes. Adolescents are melodramatic, and many of their emotional outbursts must be taken with a grain of salt. However, a suicide threat, whether made dramatically or not, should be treated with respect and considered a genuine call for help.

*What is the best way to approach a young person about getting professional help?*

Show your concern for his unhappiness and suggest that talking to someone outside the family about it might be useful. Assure your child that you want him to feel comfortable and free to talk with the therapist, and involve the youngster in the search for one. Don't impose your choice of a therapist on the child.

*What if you think your youngster needs counseling, but the child refuses to go?*

This situation is not unusual. By the time the family feels that a child is beyond its reach, communication has probably already broken down. The youngster will assume that you think he is crazy and that's why you want him to see a therapist. He has to prove he is not crazy by refusing to go. Better approach: Suggest that the whole family has a problem and might benefit from counseling. In truth, family counseling can help parents and siblings to manage living with a disturbed youngster whether that youngster responds to therapy or not.

*How do you find the right therapist for your child?*

You want a professional—either a man or a woman—with training in psychotherapy and experience in working with young people. A psychiatrist, psychologist or certified social worker (ACSW, CSW or MSW) could qualify. A psychiatrist is a medical doctor and can prescribe drugs, but many psychologists and CSWs work with hospitals and clinics and can make referrals for medication if they think it is necessary. Get recommendations from trusted physicians, friends, mental health clinics or social agencies. Three essentials: The therapist's training and credentials should check out; the young person must find the therapist easy to talk to; the therapist should be willing to talk with you *without* violating the confidentiality of the therapist-patient relationship. You and your child should interview several candidates before making a choice, and the child should have two consultations with the chosen therapist before making a long-term commitment.

*If the relationship between the child and the therapist is privileged, what rights do parents have?*

The relationship is privileged and should be respected. Your child must feel free to tell the therapist anything that is on his mind, without fear of anyone else's knowing about it. But you have every right to a general discussion of the problem to help in opening up communications with your child. Parents too often feel so guilty that their child is in trouble that they withdraw from his life just when he most needs their support and understanding. The therapist can help you with that understanding.

*What if you feel the therapy is not helping or is progressing in a way that disturbs you?*

Don't be afraid of your own common sense. If, for example, you feel your child is more disturbed than the therapist indicates, ask for psychological testing. It may point up problems to the therapist or, even better, reassure you.

If you question a course of action recommended by the therapist, you do have recourse. Request a consultation with another therapist (go back through the list of people you interviewed earlier). The consultant will interview the therapist, the patient and you, and give an evaluation of the situation.

Obviously, if your child's therapist resists either the testing or the consultation, you have grounds for changing therapists.

## FOUR SIGNS THAT MAY MEAN TROUBLE

A child's moodiness is usually a temporary condition that can be dissipated quickly with a little extra attention and affection. Signs that the situation might warrant professional help: 1) A dramatic change in behavior that persists more than several weeks. 2) Prolonged changes in eating or sleeping patterns. 3) Poor peer relationships. 4) A sudden change in communications (your child is hostile or won't talk to you).

**Source:** *A Child's Journey: Forces that Shape the Lives of Our Young* by Julius Segal, Ph.D., McGraw-Hill, New York.

## WHY KIDS SHOULDN'T GO TO ROCK CONCERTS ON SCHOOL NIGHTS

Rock fans who attend concerts on school nights will struggle in class the next day. Reason: After bathing their ears and brains with abnormally loud sounds, students will be able to hear only lower frequencies in a normal auditory setting. They'll be hearing their teachers as though pillows covered their ears. Their powers of concentration will be adversely affected, and they will not be attuned to the world in general.

**Source:** Paul Madaule, director, The Listening Center, Toronto, Canada.

## TEENAGE SMOKING

Since 1977, the number of high-school-age youngsters who use cigarettes has dropped 9%, but a recent survey of seniors indicates that 20% still do smoke. Young people smoke for different reasons than do addicted adults. Problem: The kinds of self-help groups that support adults trying to stop don't work with kids. Current best approach to teenage smokers: Life skills training that helps youngsters cope with peer pressures and other problems. When a teenager's self-confidence improves, he doesn't need to smoke to prove himself.

**Source:** *Changing Times*, Washington, D.C.

## DRUGS AND PEER PRESSURE

Peer pressure to try drugs and drink alcohol is experienced by school-children as early as fourth grade. About one-quarter say they are pressured by peers to try beer, wine, liquor or marijuana. Motivation: In the lower grades, to feel older. In the middle grades, to fit in. And in high school, to have a good time.

**Source:** A survey of 500,000 students by the *Weekly Reader*, Middleton, CT.

## WHY A CHILD BECOMES AN ADDICT

Addicts are made, not born. According to a study by the National Academy of Sciences, children are more likely to become drug or alcohol abusers if they are physically abused, lied to or humiliated, or if their parents are addicts. Other potential causes: Deprivation or overindulgence, shifts from too much to too little discipline or praise.

## HOW TO TALK WITH YOUR CHILD ABOUT SEX

Parents who want to give their children mastery of the facts about sexuality have to start early in the child's life. That's when to begin, too, to build the attitudes they will need to enjoy themselves as sexual beings and to respect the sexuality of others.

A child is born sexual, just as he or she is born with the capacities of walking and of talking. Parents delightedly help children to develop their ability to walk and talk but rarely treat sexual pleasure the same way. Once you understand and accept your children's sexuality as normal and beautiful— the same as their other human

endowments—you will be free to help them in their sexual socialization.

### Sexual Socialization

The process of socialization starts in infancy. We socialize our children in other natural functions such as eating. We praise them for using a spoon instead of plunging their hands into the cereal bowl and for other appropriate eating behavior.

A child also needs the guidance and support of parents in developing appropriate sexual behavior that fits in with the parents' own cultural norm and value system. The beginnings:

• Establish a sense of intimacy and trust with a newborn by touching and holding it. The cuddling, kissing and hugging should continue—do not stop when the child reaches three, when some parents feel awkward with physical demonstrations of affection, especially with boys.

• When you start the game of naming parts of the body, include the sex organs. Avoidance of the area between the waist and the knees causes confusion and lays the groundwork for problems in adult life.

• Don't interfere with a child's natural discovery and enjoyment of self-pleasuring. Genital play is normal. At six or eight months, a child learns to put its hand where it feels good. Don't slap on a diaper, pull the hand away or look upset or disapproving. Leave the child alone. As the child gets older, teach what you consider appropriate behavior. You don't want your child masturbating in the supermarket or living room even at 15–18 months, so you pick up the child and, smiling, carry it to its bedroom. Explain that the place to pleasure yourself is in your own room with the door closed—that sex is good but should be private.

• Parents need privacy, too. Tell children: "When our door is closed, you don't come in without knocking and being invited. When we see your door closed, we'll do the same for you. Everyone likes privacy during sex games." This is when you can introduce the idea tht sex games are something people who love and respect each other can play together.

• Sex play between children is usual. If parents banish the play, it will only drive the child underground. It's better to keep the lines of communication open and to reinforce socially appropriate sexual play. Inappropriate: Sex play with someone older. Child molestation is more commonly practiced by someone in the family or known to a child than by a stranger. The message: "You don't have to let anyone touch your body if you don't want them to. You are in charge, and you can say *No*. Tell me if anyone gives you a hard time."

### Communication

Few parents are aware of how much sex education is transmitted before nursery school by attitudes and body language—how parents react to scenes on TV, the tone of voice or facial expression in sexual conversations or situations, significant silences.

Children delight in affection openly expressed between their parents. Withholding such demonstrations can indicate sexual hang-ups.

Don't avoid opportunities to discuss sex or to answer questions. Always speak only the truth. You may wish to withhold some of the details until later. Explain appropriate behavior outside the home. "In our family, we are open with each other about sex. But most other families don't talk about it the way we do. So, we keep what we do private. It's a good thing to respect what other people believe."

A child who doesn't ask questions by the age of four or five has gotten the idea that the parent is uncomfortable about sex, that sex is not an open topic, or he was not given straight answers. But parents should be the ones to give children sexual information. Initiate a discussion. One idea: Tell your child about your own questions when you were the same age. If there is no response, try again another day to prove you're available.

Choose a time when you (or both parents) are alone with the child and have plenty of time. Be encouraging about behavior that is appropriate or shows maturation. Give recognition to a good line of thought.

Respond positively, even if you are criticized.

### Common Mistakes

The most damaging mistake is to associate sexual parts of the body with dirt, ugliness or sin. Guilt and shame transmitted about such a wonderful part of our human birthright will never be erased.

Parents should never lie. They may have to tailor the truth to the level of the child, however. Example: To a three-year-old who asks, "Do you have to be married to have a baby?" the correct answer is, "No, you don't, but. . . ." Then you go into your own value system about why marriage is important—on a level that a three-year-old can understand.

Talking with children about sex should be a shared responsibility. A harmonious front is important. Both parents should be clear on attitudes towards standards and rules and on what they agree and disagree on. If there are differences of opinion, call them that. Undermining the other parent shakes the confidence of the child in the one who's doing the undermining. Children trust parents who are for each other.

### After Six

If you have laid groundwork between birth and six or seven, then you can take advantage of the major learning years until 12. Before puberty is when to pour in reliable information about sexually transmittable diseases, reproduction, etc. Keep the lines of communication open. Give opinions when they're asked for. Avoid judgments—they tend to close off discussions. Express your own values frankly and give sound reasons. Young people will respect them, even if they don't share them.

**Source:** Interview with Mary Steichen Calderone, M.D., former medical director of the Planned Parenthood Federation of America and co-founder and president of SIECUS (Sex Information and Education Council of the US), New York.

# WHEN *NOT* KNOWING CAN BE HARMFUL

Ignorance about sex doesn't make people less promiscuous. Rather, it makes them feel guiltier—and more likely to have impulsive, unprotected sex. Lack of knowledge leads to irresponsible sexual behavior. Research finding: Sex education classes do little to change students' overall values.

**Source:** Robert Pollack, professor of psychology, University of Georgia, in *Self*, New York.

## TEENAGE CONFIDENTIAL

Virgins can become pregnant as the result of heavy petting with a boyfriend. If the male ejaculates outside the vagina, sperm could reach the vulvar mucosa, causing inadvertent insemination. It is important for youngsters to know this, since they often engage in this kind of sexual activity without realizing the risks.

**Source:** Dorothy DeMoya, R.N., and Armando DeMoya, M.D., writing in *RN*, Chicago, IL.

## FATHER/DAUGHTER TALKS ABOUT MEN, DATING AND SEX

When a daughter comes of age, it is often only the mother who has heart-to-heart talks with her concerning "life." But there is a role here for the father, too, since he can supply the male point of view on these vital topics.

These father-daughter discussions not only help the young woman in her understanding of life but initiate a healthy exchange of ideas and opinions that benefits both parties for the rest of their lives.

*Important prerequisites:*

• The tenor of a talk between a father and a 12- to 14-year-old daughter depends on their existing relationship. It is usually difficult for the father to take a young woman into his study and blithely talk about sex any better than he might with a son unless there is a feeling of trust and mutual understanding.

• The father must know what the mother has been telling the daughter about the facts of life.

Once these requirements are established,

the father begins the conversation along these lines: "You're getting to an age now where your mother and I notice your growing interest in boys and the facts of life and sexuality. Your mother has spoken to you about these things from the woman's point of view. I wonder if there are any questions you have about men, life, sex or anything else that you would like me to answer from the male view."

From here, the discussion could include a range of subjects. Example: If the father worries about the type of people his daughter is socializing with, this is the time to air those misgivings. Reiterate the family attitudes toward sexuality. Background: Talk with other parents to explore their rules and regulations concerning dating and sex. This will help provide backup facts in case the daughter says, "Mary's parents let her go out any night she wants."

Although the attitudes of other parents help in setting guidelines, the father still makes clear his views as to what is proper and healthy.

Point: Always level with your daughter, and don't hide behind excuses. If she has been going out with older boys who drive cars, explain why this is a worry to you—the fear that she will be drawn into premature sexual relationships, drinking and dangerous driving. Make clear that she need not feel pressured to go along with the crowd. Remind her that regardless of what other parents might allow, your family has its own set of standards.

These talks go more smoothly if you practice these ways to defuse conflicts:

Always welcome your daughter's male friends into your house. At times, you may have to swallow hard before being polite. But if you turn them away, most likely she will see them outside your house—and you'll lose contact with your daughter.

Guard against putting down her boyfriends. The jealousy of a father is often revealed in the disparaging remarks he makes about his daughter's male friends. Another sign of this jealousy: Overprotectiveness.

A father must realize that it is not uncommon today for girls around the age of 16 to engage in sexual activity. Make sure that your daughter knows the truth about sex. Certain myths still persist. Example: In one survey made not too long ago, 30% of the youngsters aged 14–16 believed that if you have sex standing up, the girl won't get pregnant.

Fathers can explain that men, when sexually excited, have an imperative desire for an orgasm. Contrast: Young girls are usually satisfied with holding, kissing and some petting. Two important considerations:

• The girl has a right to say that she is not ready for sex. The male will always want to go further because of his crushing need for orgasm. (Although this biological male urge may be helpful in repopulating the human race, it can be very destructive to human relationships.)

• Be sure your daughter knows it is all right to enjoy sexual feeling. The pleasures of her limited sexual experiences are nothing to feel guilty about. If sex takes on a blind negativity, the daughter will not be able to enjoy the riches of conjugal love after she is married.

A father can be surprisingly helpful to a daughter when she is breaking up with a steady boyfriend, especially if she feels she is hurting a decent person with whom she has shared a lot. The father can point out that since his daughter is a warm and giving person, her friend should be honored that he had the privilege of her exclusive company. Through this relationship the daughter has learned more about love, men and sex. Message: The love that lasts for a few months or a year or two years is the love with which the daughter tests herself. It's part of learning about life. When she finally decides to get married, she will probably make a better choice because of this experience.

Trap: A formidable obstacle in a father-daughter relationship is the daughter's sexuality. As the girl reaches puberty, a father may become frightened by his own response. The daughter he once kissed in greeting he now shies away from. Antidote: Be aware of this sexuality and don't be alarmed by it. If you kissed your daughter when you greeted her as a little girl, continue to do so when she becomes a young woman.

Key: The father is the first intimate male model the daughter has for the adult world. This is important in developing her sense of the opposite sex. Note: Although the father is a model, he must not fear showing his human frailty. At all costs, avoid hypocrisy. Be honest, even if it hurts—or makes you look like less than a god.

Best approach: Communication in which the father and daughter discuss things openly and freely. The most important of these talks occurs when a girl becomes a young woman. But they should remain part of a continuous, ongoing dialectic process. In the long run, the father learns as much as he teaches. He becomes more aware of the female side of the world—and that is something males cannot know enough about.

**Source:** Interview with Clifford J. Sager, M.D., clinical professor of psychiatry, New York Hosptial—Cornell Medical Center.

# HOW TO FIND OUT IF YOUR CHILD'S BEEN SEXUALLY ABUSED

Among the ugliest of crimes are the ones we don't talk about much—especially sexual crimes against children. But the problem of sexual exploitation of children, particularly incest, has started to surface. One out of every three girls under 18 and one out of every eight boys under 18 have reported incidents of sexual abuse. Although parents may warn their children about dangerous strangers, the fact is that 80% of the reported cases of sexual abuse involve relatives, friends of the family or neighbors.

Communication between parents and children about child sexual abuse is vital. If there are open channels of communication, children won't think that what has happened to them is a dark, shameful secret. They will feel free to talk to their parents about it. Most of all, every violated child needs to know he or she isn't alone.

### What Is Child Sexual Abuse?

We may think we know what constitutes sexual abuse of a child, but the borders aren't always clear, especially to children themselves. In order to protect our children, we have to be able to explain to them what is abusive and what isn't.

Sexual abuse occurs when a child is forced or tricked into sexual contact with an older person. What constitutes sexual contact: Touching of the child's genitals. Requests that the child touch or look at the genitals of an older person. . .participate in oral/genital contact with an adult. . .undress and/or be photographed in sexual positions with other children or adults. . . witness the sexual activities of adults. Sexual abuse may or may not include actual penetration.

Sexual abuse often develops gradually, occurring not as the result of violent attack but through subtle coercion over time. It may occur repeatedly before being detected. The older person uses coercive statements that may seem unconvincing to adults but can have enormous influence on children. Examples: "It's OK, everybody does it. It's just a game. I used to play this when I was your age. If you tell anyone I won't like you any more, or I'll have to go away. If you tell your parents, it will hurt them. If you like me, you'll do it for me. This is how you learn about sex. You're getting older, and I just want to check you out. Oh, you'll enjoy it, everybody does." Also: Bribery may be used, with promises of presents or special privileges.

### The Value of Communication

Parents have an important responsibility to educate their children about sexual abuse as part of their general sex education. This responsibility cannot be left to the schools or the child's peers. If the parents have developed communication and trust with a child, that child will feel free to come to them when something frightening has happened, sure that the parents will respond with concern and protectiveness.

What parents should communicate:

• There are "good" touch and "bad" touches. If the child feels uncomfortable about any kind of touching by anyone, including family members, he or she has the right to say, "No. I don't want to." The child should be told that not all adults care about children's feelings.

• If the child feels that something that just doesn't seem right is going on with an older person, whether it's a friend, family member or stranger, he or she should feel free to discuss it with you. No matter what kind of threats or promises have been made, you won't get angry or blame the child

• Make it very clear that if, by chance, the child doesn't feel free to tell you about a disturbing situation, he or she should talk to some other trusted adult. You might suggest a teacher, clergyman, friend or parent of a friend.

### Reading Your Child's Signals

Children, especially less verbal preschoolers, may give off nonverbal signals. Their silence, rather than their words, may indicate a problem. Danger signs: Change in appetite, nightmares, acting out or hyperactivity. The child may avoid or react fearfully or abnormally to a person he or she has usually felt comfortable with.

If you suspect sexual abuse, you will have to approach the child very carefully to get an honest answer. Questions such as "Is something wrong?" are likely to elicit simple denials. Better: "I know you're involved in something that's hurting, something you want to discuss, but maybe you're afraid I won't understand." Be positive in your questioning. Show empathy, compassion and understanding. If you come on like gangbusters, aggressively asking who, when, what and where, you'll frighten the child and get no answers.

### If Your Child Has Been Sexually Abused

• React calmly. If you get hysterical or visibly angry, you'll frighten the child.

• Talk about specific details, but don't push the child to reveal more than he or she feels comfortable with at any one time.

• Reassure the child that he or she is not to blame, that you don't doubt his/her word and that you will protect him/her against any repercussions from the accused person.

• Report any case of child sexual abuse to your local social services or law enforcement agency. If the abuser is a family member, contact the local chapter of Parents Anonymous or Parents United.

**Source:** Interview with Vincent J. Fontana, M.D., a pediatrician. He is medical director of the New York Foundling Hospital and chairman of the Mayor's Task Force on Child Abuse and Neglect.

## MISPLACED GUILT

Victims of child abuse are more likely to feel guilty than their abusers. In one study, half the victims of sexual abuse said they felt guilty "for disrupting the family or revealing the act." (Only 5% voluntarily reported the abuse.) But less than half of actual abusers either expressed any guilt or felt responsibility for the act.

**Source:** *Sex Care Digest,* Piscataway, NJ.

## HOW A CHILD CAN PROTECT HIMSELF

Child molesters are often deterred if the child simply yells or screams. Yelling helps the child translate fear into anger and overcomes the initial panic response. Good phrases: "Stop it!" or "Get away!"

**Source:** *Your Child Should Know* by Tamar Hosansky, Berkley Books, New York.

## WHY SOME ADULTS PREFER BAD KIDS

Many people who consider themselves sentimental child lovers actually have fond feelings only for docile, respectful children. They cannot embrace independent, free-thinking, quirky or opinionated children who are critical of adults. Problems: The defiant child magnifies adult impotence. The vulnerable child reminds us of our own frailty. The self-sufficient child proves we're not indispensable. Result: Some adults find it easier to believe that children are intrinsically bad. This frees them from responsibility, allowing them to be cruel and punitive.

**Source:** Letty Cottin Pogrebin, author of *Family Politics,* McGraw-Hill, New York.

## ANOTHER KIND OF CHILD ABUSE

Emotional abuse can stunt children's social growth, undermine their self-esteem, and lead to later mental disorders. Worst: When negative interactions between parents and children become repetitious. Common forms of abuse: Criticism that tells children that they're "bad" or worthless, rather than singling out a specific behavior. Constant teasing with the child as the butt of the joke. A failure to praise good behavior.

**Source:** *Parents,* New York.

## VIOLENCE THAT LEADS TO MORE VIOLENCE

Children who see physical violence between their parents are six times more likely to abuse their own spouses after they marry. If those children were also hit by their parents as teenagers, they are 12 times more likely to abuse their spouses.

**Source:** National survey of family violence, cited in *Medical Aspects of Human Sexuality,* New York.

## PITFALLS OF TOO MUCH TV

Children who watch violence on television are more likely to commit violent crimes as adults. This is the conclusion of a 22-year study. Also: Girls who often view violent television become mothers who use more physical punishment on their own children.

**Source:** Study at the University of Illinois, cited in *The Salk Letter,* New York.

• Heavy TV viewing lowers school achievement in all children. Bright kids are hurt the most. One explanation. . . Good students generally come from homes with books, magazines and stimulating games and have parents who encourage their use. The more time spent on TV, the less is left for these mind-sharpening activities.

**Source:** *Gifted Children Newsletter,* Bergenfield, NJ.

## TO BREAK THE TV HABIT

If your kids watch too much TV, you could restrict their viewing to one hour per day (makes children more discriminating viewers). Watch along with them; then discuss (or disagree with) the program's "message" (makes them more critical viewers). Or, substitute family games, reading or athletic activities.

## MAJOR PARENTAL FAILING

Poor discipline is perceived as the major failing of today's parents. In a recent poll, 37% said that parents were "too lenient" and that children "have it too easy." Second worst failing: Child neglect.

**Source:** Poll by The Gallup Organization, Inc.

## WHEN NOT TO SHOUT AT YOUR KID

Shouting at children under age five—even in dangerous situations—only confuses them and eggs them on. Very young children, according to recent research, react to the context in which words are given. A shouted command like "Don't chase that ball into the street!" has a lot of energy in it. To a toddler, that energy is interpreted as encouragement. (A shouted instruction to an older child—if the technique is not overused—will get his attention and, quite likely, his obedience.) Most effective with under-fives: Give commands in a soft or moderate tone of voice.

**Source:** Lee Salk, clinical professor of psychology in psychiatry and pediatrics, The New York Hospital-Cornell Medical Center, writing in *The Salk Letter,* New York.

## THE RIGHT AND THE WRONG WAY TO PUNISH

Hitting a small child as punishment only sets up a destructive pattern of escalation. Each occasion requires harder blows, and the relationship between parent and child deteriorates. Better: Withdraw a privilege or cancel a planned excursion.

**Source:** Lilian G. Katz, professor of early childhood education, University of Illinois at Urbana-Champaign, writing in *Parents,* New York.

• Don't withhold the allowance to punish a child. Reason: Doing so imbues money with moral and emotional values, which could distort financial decision-making later on. Better punishment: Temporarily withhold a non-monetary privilege such as television.

**Source:** *Better Homes and Gardens,* New York.

## DANGER OF MATERIAL REWARDS

Material rewards actually discourage children from learning or achieving for its own sake. When you pay your child for an accomplishment, you literally steal the personal satisfaction that came from doing it. Better: Offer children strong approval to enhance their self-esteem.

**Source:** *The Salk Letter,* New York.

## WHEN BOTH PARENTS WORK

When both parents work, children need help in coping with extra stress and pressure. Suggestions: (1) Don't yell at the kids. Be sure to tell them what they do right. (2) Be on time. Children may feel neglected or become scared when parents aren't home at the set hour. (3) Think smaller. Instead of ordering children to clean up their room, tell them to put away the toys. (4) Communicate with the kids. Leave a cheerful note or taped message for them to find.

**Source:** *Execu-Time Letter,* Lake Forest, IL.

## HELP FOR "LATCH-KEY" KIDS

Children left alone after school because both parents work often feel lonely or frightened. But two new services are helping the nation's estimated four million "latch-key" kids cope with the stress. One is a self-help program of the Campfire, Inc., youth organization. It consists of eight one-hour sessions that teach children how to act in normal and emergency situations when they're home alone. The other is Phone Friend, a Pennsylvania volunteer service that counsels children over the phone.

**Source:** *A Letter from Dr. Lee Salk.*

## WORKING VS. FULL-TIME MOTHERS

Full-time mothers average less than 10 minutes per day of play or reading with their preschool children—the same amount of time as mothers who work outside the home. Chief activities of the stay-at-home mothers: Household chores, followed by television watching.

**Source:** *Mother Care/Other Care* by Sandra Scarr, Basic Books, New York.

## HOW TO CHOOSE A SAFE DAY-CARE CENTER

A decent day-care facility offers clean quarters, good food, reasonable safety precautions and regular naps. Beyond that, parents should look for:

• A stable staff, with relatively little turnover... specialized training in child development or psychology... staff members assigned to specific children.

• A staff-to-child ratio of no less than one to three for infants, one to four for two-year-olds, and one to eight for children age three to six.

• Ambitious activities (trips to a zoo, a tour of the firehouse), but no heavy academic instruction.

• A welcoming attitude toward parental involvement, including unannounced visits.

**Source:** *Newsweek, NY.*

## TRAITS TO LOOK FOR IN A BABYSITTER

The ideal babysitter is warm, patient, outgoing, well-adjusted and interested in your child. Caution: Very domineering people will undermine your relationship with your child. People who are depressed or have other emotional problems will be more concerned with themselves and will not see to the emotional needs of your child.

## DIVORCE AND THE KIDS

Younger children (under the age of six) suffer less emotional damage in the long run, a new study suggests—even though they show the most distress at the time their parents break up. Theory: Younger children forget about life before the divorce more quickly than older ones.

**Source:** Study at Ohio State University in *Psychology Today, New York.*

• Divorce hurts preteen sons more than daughters, especially as they approach puberty. Reason: Boys of this age have an increased need for their same-sex parent. But 90% live with their mothers after a divorce.

**Source:** Study by John Guidubaldi, chairman of the Early Childhood Department, Kent State University.

• Single-parent children are more than twice as likely to get a divorce in adulthood as children from traditional homes. They also generally leave school earlier and earn less money.

**Source:** Study by sociologist Daniel P. Mueller of the Amherst H. Wilder Foundation, in *USA Today.*

## WHEN TO PUT OFF A DIVORCE

Father hunger commonly strikes young boys when families are split by divorce and the mother retains custody. Symptoms include insomnia, nightmares about the missing parent, and uncontrollable rages or crying jags. Most at risk: Boys between 18 months and 32 months. They need a man around for gender identification. Treatment: Frequent visits with the father, including a tour of his new living quarters. Even better, couples should consider postponing divorce to a less crucial stage of a boy's development.

**Source:** Alfred A. Messer, M.D., an Atlanta-based family psychiatrist, in *The Wall Street Journal*.

## LIVING BETTER WITH ADULT CHILDREN

We have entered the era of the nesters: Adult offspring (past age 18) who are living in the parental home. Twenty million young adults are proving Thomas Wolfe* wrong. They *can* go home again, and they're at least 25% more likely to do so than they would have been 15 years ago.

Nesting is a temporary phenomenon. Your children want to be self-sufficient. At least 90% come home for financial reasons. Education and housing cost more these days, and an entry-level job's paycheck buys less.

The great majority of nesters are "re-roosters." They've tried independent life, if only at a college dorm. Maybe they've lost a job or gone through a failed romance or a divorce. They're coming home to lick their wounds before venturing out again.

Six of our eight kids are grown, and all six have moved in and out at least a couple of times. (Our record-holder has completed six round trips.) At first it was a shock. I'd figured I owed them only 20 years apiece.

Over the years, however, it's become a very positive experience for us. Nesting offers parents a chance to develop close, adult relationships with their children. At last they can enjoy their kids as individuals, apart from the burdens of childrearing or the stresses of adolescence. It's time to reap the results of all that labor.

But, if mishandled, nesting can be hazardous to the family—even destructive. It can strain the parents' marriage and hurt the nester's growth. Key: You can't dictate to nesters nor smother them with indulgence. You must seek the middle ground. Your nesters need to make their own decisions to ease their transition to independence. Guidelines:

• Release your parental authority. When children reach adulthood, they should be treated accordingly. It's time to reshape your old roles. This adjustment can be toughest for fathers, who (like my husband) often deal with their children as authoritarians.

• Don't be too generous with advice or financial aid. For many parents, excessive giving may be an unconscious attempt to control the nester. Our motto: Don't offer, but don't refuse. Try to find a solution that preserves the nester's responsibility. Example: Your nester approaches you for an emergency loan. Rather than simply forking over the money, you agree to co-sign a bank note.

• Communicate. Sulking may be tolerated in a 10-year-old, but there's no excuse for it in adults. The issue may be trivial— breakfast dishes that don't get cleared, ice-cube trays that are never refilled. But if resentment is allowed to build, the entire family will suffer. Speak up about what's bothering you.

• Don't perform a nester's personal business. As adults, they are responsible for walking their dog, getting up in time for work and paying their taxes. They might as well learn now...there will come a day when you won't be around to bail them out.

• Share household chores equitably. Make a written list. A 23-year-old bachelor's standard of cleanliness may not mesh with your own.

• Ask that they contribute something toward room and board. My survey found that nesters with full-time jobs pay an average of $75 a month. (One-third pay nothing at all.) Fair formula: Propose that your nester pay 15% of take-home pay. Don't feel guilty about this. You're teaching a key survival skill: How to handle money and live within one's means. (If you really don't need the money, you can put it aside as a nest egg for when your nester leaves. But keep this a secret, or you'll defeat your purpose.)

• Remember that it's your roof and mortgage. If your adult children want to live in your home, they must abide by your rules and value system. In part, this is just basic consideration, such as limiting telephone or bathroom time. But it also applies to drugs or premarital sex. If you feel uncomfortable with certain behaviors, it's your right to forbid them. (Flexibility helps. Much as you might despise cigarettes, for example, you might let a nester smoke in his or her bedroom.)

• Keep in mind that house rules stop at the front door. What nesters do outside is their own choice, unless they bring their problems home (no drunk driving or drug dealing condoned). Our study found that curfews are unrealistic. Like it or not, much of a young adult's social life happens after midnight.

• Reject the notion (quite popular in this culture) that nesters are failures. Ignore any friend who suggests the same. You know better.

• Set a target departure date before the nester moves back in. This could be three months after college graduation or six months after a divorce. The date can be modified later on. But by affirming that your nester's stay is temporary, you'll relieve much anxiety on both sides.

**Source:** Interview with Monica Lauen O'Kane, author of *Living with Adult Children*, Diction Books, St. Paul, MN.

*Author of *You Can't Go Home Again*.

# 12. For Men Only/For Women Only

## WHY MEN MAY BE THE WEAKER SEX

Men are less hardy than women (more males are miscarried or stillborn or die in infancy). They wilt faster in the heat. Their blood clots more rapidly, making them more susceptible to blockages in the cardiovascular system. Their suicide rate is higher. And they are more aggressive. Because they take more risks, men are three times as more likely to die from accidents. Women mature faster than men. Their high ratio of body fat supplies a store of energy for such endurance activities as long-distance swimming. They have a lower metabolic rate, making it harder to lose weight. Women have sharper hearing in the higher ranges, better night vision and a stronger immune system. Their hormones give them a natural resistance to heart disease during their childbearing years. Bottom line: Women outlive men by an average of almost eight years.

## PATERNITY WITH CERTAINTY

The first foolproof paternity test—can even be performed before the baby is born. Today's tests rely primarily on biochemical analyses of blood cell proteins. And if proteins show up in the cells of a child, the test is considered positive.

In reality, though, there's a 10%–15% chance that such a conclusion is wrong. Reason: Different men can pass nearly identical cellular proteins on to their offspring. And current tests can be performed only after a child has been born—a discouraging prospect for a woman who has been raped.

New world: The new tests, which can be combined with amniocentesis, focus directly on the genetic material (DNA). And except for identical twins, no two people have the same DNA. . . . So if a man's DNA shares certain key similarities with the child's, paternity is conclusive. Bonus: DNA testing is easily automated . . . and it's expected to cost much less than the current $400/test.

**Source:** Roche Biomedical Laboratories (division of Hoffmann-La Roche), Burlington, NC.

## MEN AND ABORTION

Abortions are traumatic to men, as well as to women. A recent study also found that 91% of the fathers wanted to be in the recovery room. . . 69% wanted to be with their partner during the abortion. . .17% were so upset that they weren't sure they wanted to ever be faced with another pregnancy.

**Source:** Study by Arthur B. Shostak, sociology professor, Drexel University, Philadelphia.

## WHAT A REALLY GOOD PHYSICAL INCLUDES

A man's thorough physical includes these procedures: Blood pressure test (most important). Eye and eye pressure exam. Check of lymph nodes and thyroid for swelling. Stethoscopic exam of heart and lungs. Stress test (particularly for vigorous exercisers). Examination of the aorta. Testicle examination. Reading of pulse in legs. Proctoscopic exam of rectum and lower large intestine. Prostate examination. Stool sample for blood. Superficial neurological exam (reflexes and muscle strength). Laboratory tests: Blood sugar, cholesterol, uric acid, complete blood screening (every three years), triglyceride, kidney function and calcium. Cost: $100–$500.

**Source:** *M* magazine, New York.

# ALL ABOUT THE PROSTATE

At some point in their lives, most men will have prostate trouble. The major function of the prostate is the secretion of semen. Ninety-five percent of the ejaculate is fluid from the prostate; the remaining 5% is sperm.

The prostate is a doughnut-shaped organ about one and one-half inches in diameter and one and one-half inches deep. It encircles the urethra at its junction with the bladder. (The urethra is the tube that carries urine from the bladder to the end of the penis.) When the prostate is enlarged, it narrows the urethra, blocking the passing of urine.

There is no prevention tactic, but luckily most prostate ailments are minor and easily treatable. For those who develop prostate cancer, however, new treatments are now available that don't have the severe side effects of previous therapies.

In order to be healthy and active as long as possible, men should understand how the prostate works, what disorders it's subject to and what treatments are available. Most important: Every man over 50 must have an annual rectal exam. The earlier prostate cancer is detected, the better the chances of cure.

## Prostatitis

Prostatitis in an inflammation of the prostate which is most common among men in their twenties and thirties, although older men can also be affected.

• Causes: Infectious agents (bacteria) and noninfectious agents of unknown origin.

• Symptoms: Frequent urination, burning on urination, increased urgency to urinate.

• Diagnosis: Cultures of prostatic fluid to determine if an organism is causing the problem.

• Treatment: Antibiotics, sitz baths, abstention from sex during the acute period. Prostatitis isn't a serious ailment, but it can cause serious discomfort and should be treated by a doctor.

## Prostate Enlargement

Benign prostatic hypertrophy or prostate enlargement occurs in about 80% of middle-aged men. Although it's a benign condition, there are dangers. An enlarged prostate can obstruct the urethra, creating back pressure on bladder and kidneys. If left untreated, bladder infections, bladder stones and damage to the kidneys may result. The urinary infections of most middle-aged men are related to an enlarged prostate and consequent incomplete bladder emptying. The residual urine is a good culture medium for bacteria.

• Cause: We don't know a whole lot about the causes of prostate problems. Prostate enlargement probably relates to the changing balance of testosterone to estrogen hormone levels in middle age.

• Symptoms: Decrease in the force of the urinary stream, difficulty in initiating urination, increased frequency of urination and nighttime urination.

• Diagnosis: By physical examination. During a rectal exam, an enlarged prostate can be felt. Also: It frequently shows up on a kidney X-ray.

• Treatment: Varies according to the individual case. Only about half the men with enlarged prostates need treatment at all. The other half either have minimal enlargement or don't have any symptoms or signs of kidney problems. The half who require treatment must have an operation. There's no medication yet available to shrink an enlarged prostate, though researchers have been looking for one for years. An open or closed prostatectomy may be performed, depending on the amount of enlargement. An open prostatectomy is a formal surgical operation. An incision is made and prostatic tissue is removed. The alternative is a closed prostatectomy or TURP (transurethral resection of the prostate). For a TURP, a special "telescope" is inserted through the penis with an instrument that electrically removes the tissue. Recommended: A surgeon with extensive TURP experience. The more experienced surgeon will do a TURP even when the prostate is severely enlarged, saving the patient the trauma of major surgery. Side effects: None, aside from postoperative recuperation.

A prostatectomy will not cause impotence. Also: It does not remove the risk of prostate cancer. The operation involves removing 95% of the tissue inside the prostate capsule. The capsule itself remains. The 5% of remaining tissue can regrow and be a source of cancer. Removal of 100% requires a radical operation and does result in impotence.

### Prostate Cancer

Prostate cancer occurs in men 55 to 60 and over. It is the second most common cancer after lung cancer. It can turn up in men as young as 40. Of men diagnosed with prostate cancer, 40% will be in stage D, a metastatic disease that's spread to the bones. Another 40% will have stage C, a large tumor of the prostate extending outside the prostatic capsule but confined locally. Another 10% are in stage B, a solitary nodule on the prostate, and the final 10% are in stage A, which is discovered incidentally when an enlarged prostate is operated on and cancer cells are found. There's also substage A-1, a very small focus of minimally abnormal tumor cells.

• Cause: Unknown.

• Symptoms: Similar to an enlarged prostate. . .decrease in force of urine, hesitancy, increased frequency of urination. Also: Bone pain or backache. Problem: There may be no symptoms.

• Treatment: I recommend no treatment for stage A-1. For stages A or B, there's a choice of radical prostatectomy, where the prostate is completely removed. . .external beam radiation, where the entire area is irradiated. . .or interstitial radiotherapy, where radioactive particles are placed in the prostate and emit radioactive waves. The lymph glands in the pelvis are also removed in this procedure. For stage C, external beam radiation is used because the cancer is already outside the prostatic capsule and therefore beyond surgical curability. For stage D, there's no curative treatment, though symptoms can be managed and life prolonged with removal of the testicles or medication with female hormones.

• Side effects: Radical prostatectomy is a major operation. It always causes impotence and sometimes urine leakage. External beam radiation causes impotence in about one–third of patients, and may also cause urethral strictures from scarring, a shrunken bladder and blood in the urine. Interstitial radiotherapy, which we advocate at Sloan-Kettering, avoids these side effects by eliminating damage to tissues outside the prostate itself. Removal and biopsy of the lymph nodes also aids in a more accurate diagnosis.

• What you should know: Which treatment to use is the most controversial area in urologic cancer today. Some doctors feel that the prostate should be removed entirely so it won't provide a source for further cancer spread. Both radical prostatectomy and external beam radiation have a good long-term track record. Interstitial radiation is a relatively new procedure, and the long-term, large-scale follow-up isn't in yet. But so far, our five- to 10-year survival rates with several hundred patients are as good as for the other two treatments.

**Source:** Interview with Neil H. Bander, M.D., urology specialist and Cornell University Medical College and research associate at Memorial Sloan-Kettering Institute, both in New York City.

# MEN HAVE PLUMBING, TOO

As with women, the plumbing systems of men need maintenance. Fortunately, most of the problems respond to treatment easily of the early warning signs are not ignored. Some conditions to watch for:

### Enlargement of the Prostate

The prostate is a gland the size of a chestnut located below the neck of the bladder and encircling the urethra, the canal that carries away the urine. It is essential to fertility, although its exact functioning is not well understood. Enlargement of this gland is quite common, especially for men past the age of 60.

*Symptoms:* A change in urination patterns. It becomes harder to start and takes more time to finish. Since the bladder does not empty completely, the urge to urinate returns in about 10 minutes. Typical problem: A person is unable to start urinating despite a full bladder. This may occur after an evening that involves alcohol and a need to hold off urinating (a banquet with long after-dinner speeches, for example). Danger: Fluid backing up in the system may damage muscles at the opening of the bladder or kidneys.

*Treatment:* Some men live quite well for an extended period with a slight enlargement of the prostate and its mild symptoms. But for many, surgery is required to trim the gland. With the patient under general anesthesia, the surgeon reaches the prostate by entering through the penis with a slender instrument (transurethral resectoscope) suitable for the trimming process. Immediately after the procedure, a catheter is inserted for urination. It remains in place for about three days. After about five days, the patient goes home. He can usually resume sex and strenuous activity in a month to six weeks. Note: This partial resection of the prostate does not cause impotence.

Enlargement of the prostate is a natural result of the production of male hormone over the course of a man's lifetime. The only preventative measure would be the removal of the testicles in males over 40 years old. Doctors find this is not a popular idea. Although alcohol or spicy foods may irritate an enlarged prostate, abstention from these things does not prevent the ailment. Upshot: There are no practical preventative steps.

### Cancer of the Prostate

Although this is one of the most common causes of cancer death in men, cancer of the prostate is successfully treated if caught early.

*Symptoms:* Difficulty in urinating, as with the enlargement of the prostate. Major difference: How the gland feels during rectal examination. (Men should have this exam once a year after the age of 50.)

*Treatment:* Radiation is one option. It is done through the implantation of radioactive seeds in the gland or by external radiation. Preferred: Seeding. It takes less time, does not affect the patient's ability to hold

urine and should not lead to impotence.

The most reliable therapy is complete removal of the prostate. However, up to 10% of these patients will subsequently have difficulty holding urine. Although this surgery causes impotence, the impotence can be corrected by surgery.

*Prognosis:* If the cancer has not spread and the pelvic lymph nodes are unaffected, survival rates are very good with treatment . . . only five recurrences of cancer out of every 75 men treated. If the nymph nodes are involved, the outlook is much poorer—recurrence within two years in nearly half the cases treated.

### Bladder Cancer

This is much more common in men than in women. Warning sign: Blood in the urine. Therapy: Removal of the growth by simple surgery.

### Stones in the Urinary Tract

Bladder stones used to be fairly frequent among older men as a complication of prostate problems. Better detection and early treatment of prostate disease, however, have substantially reduced their occurrence.

Kidney stones crop up more often and are found in men of all ages. Symptoms: Sharp back pain just below the rib cage and blood in the urine.

Treatment: First wait. Often the stone is passed in the urine. If not, there are techniques (under anesthesia) for pulling the stone out through the bladder or sometimes through the kidney. The last resort is an open operation to remove the stone.

If there is a strong family history of stones, or if they have formed previously, have an X ray, followed by blood and urine tests. These tests determine if a structural abnormality makes formation of the stones more likely.

Drinking lots of fluid is recommended for everyone. Stones form when calcium in the urine fails to stay dissolved. This usually happens when there is not enough liquid.

**Source:** Interview with Ralph Devere White, M.D., a urologist at the Presbyterian Hospital, Columbia Presbyterian Medical Center, New York.

## WHAT'S YOUR CHANCE OF BEING RAPED?

One woman in 10 is raped during her lifetime. The typical victim appears vulnerable and helpless. To help prevent attack, women should stay fit, which in turns builds physical confidence. Especially helpful: Self-defense training.

**Source:** *Vogue.*

## PREMENSTRUAL-SYNDROME UPDATE

Premenstrual distress may be soothed by evening-primrose oil. Most women treated with the oil (sold as capsules in health-food stores) report less irritability, depression, fluid retention, headache, anxiety, anger and breast discomfort. Theory: An active ingredient in the substance modulates the influence of prolactin, a pituitary hormone linked with premenstrual syndrome. Warning: Don't exceed two grams a day of the oil.

**Source:** David Horrobin, M.D., Efamol Research Institute, Kentville, Nova Scotia.

## WOMEN AND EXERCISE

Menstrual irregularities are common among female athletes and dancers: 25%–40% of serious female athletes have fewer than three menses per year. Hypothesis: Low body weights and reduced fat supplies interfere with the body's ability to store female hormones. Problem: Low levels of hormones such as estrogen are associated with demineralization of bones. Nonmenstruating women athletes have been found to have decreased mineral content in their vertebrae. Such thinning of the bones (osteoporosis), which ordinarily does not begin before menopause, presents a real health hazard.

**Source:** *New England Journal of Medicine.*

## FOODS TO WATCH OUT FOR

Eating too many carrots may interfere with menstruation. Women with menstrual dysfunction were instructed to eat less carrots, broccoli, spinach, pumpkin and squash— vegetables with high levels of the yellow pigment carotene. The patients also added more protein to their diet. Result: They began to menstruate within four months. Others in the group whose high carotene levels were not restricted found that their problem persisted.

**Source:** *RN.*

## EXERCISES THAT RELIEVE MENSTRUAL CRAMPS

Relief from menstrual cramps: Bicycling, which increases blood flow and breaks up pelvic congestion. For premenstrual pain: On your hands and knees, bend your elbows and place your forearms on the floor at right angles to your body, fingertips overlapping. Rest your head on the floor in front of your arms. Keeping your buttocks high, try to touch the floor with your chest. Hold this position until the discomfort ceases. Repeat as needed.

**Source:** *Total Sexual Fitness for Women* by Kathryn Lance and Maria Agardy, Rawson Associates, New York.

## LAST-DITCH HELP FOR CRAMPS

Menstrual cramps can be relieved by a heart drug if other treatments fail. In one study, 25 of 35 women with severe cramps were helped dramatically by nifedipine, taken in capsule form. Pain relief lasted up to five hours. Side effects: An increase in heart rate, a slight decrease in blood pressure and a brief facial flush. But none of these was considered serious when the drug was taken under a doctor's supervision.

**Source:** Study by Ulf Ulmsten, M.D. at the University of Lund, Sweden.

## GOOD AND BAD NEWS ABOUT DIURETICS

Diuretics are effective in relieving menstrual bloat, but they're dangerous if taken every day to lose weight. Reason: The loss of so much salt and water can cause an acute potassium shortage. Potential problems with abuse: Erratic heart rhythms, metabolic disturbances and deteriorated kidney function. Diuretic withdrawal can be difficult, and users often require hospitalization for as long as 10–14 days.

**Source:** Emmanuel Bravo, M.D. the Cleveland Clinic, in *McCall's*, New York.

## TOXIC-SHOCK SCREEN

A simple blood test can identify the 5% of the adult population who are susceptible to this frightening disease. Everyone carries the staphylococcal germs that can be triggered to produce the toxins causing toxic shock syndrome. But not all adults have the antibodies in their blood that fight the toxin. These people should take extra precautions against the disease. Such women, for example, should be very careful in their use of tampons. Individuals without the antibodies should be alert to the symptoms of toxic shock: High fever, vomiting, diarrhea, rash.

**Source:** Dr. Merlin S. Bergdoll, researcher at the University of Wisconsin who developed the blood test, quoted in *Medical World News*.

## ABOUT BREAST LUMPS

• Fibrocystic disease of the breasts probably is not a disease at all. About 50% of women have nodules in their breasts. At autopsy, 90% of women have cystic structures. It is now felt that painful irregular breasts are not diseased, but are showing an increased hormonal response. This is not a significant risk factor for cancer.

**Source:** Susan Love, M.D., Sidney Farber Cancer Institute, Boston, writing in *American Family Physician*.

• Breast lumps are not cancerous in eight out of 10 cases. A woman in her childbearing years most likely has a benign cystic or fibrocystic condition from plugged ducts (due to hormonal changes), bruises or injuries.

**Source:** American College of Obstetricians and Gynecologists, Washington, DC.

## TREATING BREAST LUMPS

Wear a supportive bra that isn't too tight. Drink less fluid to control swelling before menstruation. Cut down on caffeine. Get checked for thyroid disease. In severe cases, ask your doctor about treatment with Danazol, a male hormone derivative that permanently cures breast problems for 60% of women treated. Drawbacks of Danazol: Weight gain, hot flashes, irregular periods. The good news: There is no persuasive evidence that women with a history of breast lumps are more likely to get cancer.

**Source:** *Working Woman*.

## CAUSES OF BREAST DISCHARGES

A milky discharge from the breasts of women (outside of motherhood) is generally harmless and no reason for getting alarmed. Most common causes: Breast stimulation, sexual intercourse, stress, use of blood-pressure medication or the Pill. If excessive discharge becomes embarrassing, it can be controlled with a drug called bromocriptine. Other types of discharges should be checked by a doctor.

**Source:** *The Lancet*.

## WHERE VAGINAL YEAST INFECTIONS COME FROM

Vaginal yeast infections are most commonly linked with overuse of antibiotics (either oral or vaginal). Reason: The drugs upset the natural balance of microorganisms, disrupting natural defenses. Other factors: Pantyhose, tight jeans, exercise clothing or wet bathing suits. Medicated or scented douches, bubble baths or bath oils. Concentrated sexual activity. Poorly controlled diabetes. Estrogen or progesterone treatment. Pregnancy.

**Source:** Jack D. Sobel, M.D., infectious-disease specialist at the Medical College of Pennsylvania, Philadelphia.

## Rx FOR URINARY TRACT INFECTIONS

Extended sex play can help a woman avoid urinary-tract infections. Reason: Vaginal lubrication prevents irritation during intercourse that can promote infection.

**Source:** *RN.*

## NEW HELP FOR BLADDER PROBLEMS

Involuntary urination when laughing or coughing is common among women who have had several pregnancies. Traditional treatment involves major surgery. New alternative: A small incision is made in the vagina. Needles are inserted from above the pubic bone to the bladder neck, giving added support to the bladder. Most patients leave the hospital the second day after surgery. Success rate: 95%, with virtually no complications.

**Source:** *Internal Medicine News.*

## FACIAL-HAIR CONFIDENTIAL

Women with excessive hair on their faces have been helped by a drug originally developed to lower blood pressure. Spironolactone has been found to regress the growth of body hair within two months in 95% of test patients at the University of California (La Jolla). By inhibiting the production of male hormones, the drug reduces both the amount of body hair and its rate of growth. Endocrinologists—specialists in hormones—can evaluate the safety and advisability of a woman's using spironolactone.

## TRUTH ABOUT DOUCHING

Frequent douching has no medical value—and it can even be harmful. Reasons: It dries out the vagina by removing natural lubricants. Some commercial douches may cause allergic reactions. A strong spray can even spread an infection from the vagina into the uterus.

## HYSTERECTOMY FACTS AND FICTIONS

Hysterectomy (removal of the uterus) rarely results in a decline in sexual activity or enjoyment, contrary to belief. At least 80% of women have sexual relations within eight weeks of surgery. Virtually all resume sex at some point. About half find intercourse more enjoyable after the operation. Another half find their enjoyment unchanged. Only about 5% report less pleasure. In some cases this minority can be helped by taking testosterone.

**Source:** *Sex Over Forty.*

## ALL ABOUT KISSING

Whether it's a peck on Aunt Sadie's cheek or a deep, romantic clinch with your spouse, kissing is a universal communication that says many things. Added benefit: In a study by a West German life insurance company, men who kissed their wives every morning before going to work were found to live longer, healthier lives than the average. Examples of style:

• The French kiss. This originated with an ancient Chinese belief that a woman has a "jade spring" of vitality under her tongue that a man can tap by kissing her. It is still the most popular form of kissing between lovers.

• Warm, open kiss. Leaves room to get passionate or to stay friendly (your partner can decide).

• Kiss on the cheek. A cordial and warm greeting.

• Soft, brief kiss. Shows affection but not necessarily passion.

**Source:** Interview with Danny Biederman, author of *The Book of Kisses,* Dembner Enterprises Corp., New York.

## RETURN TO PETTING

The pleasures of petting were missed by

many modern couples when the sexual revolution relaxed the restrictions on pre-marital intercourse. Happy revival: Leaders of sex seminars report a renewed interest in the techniques of foreplay—the kind of necking activity previous generations spent years perfecting before marriage. The joys of hand holding, hugging, stroking and French kissing are making a comeback.

**Source:** Sharon Goldsmith, RN, a Los Angeles sex educator and host of *Human Sexualtiy* on the Cable Health Network.

## SEXY BLUSH

The blush that humans experience when embarrassed or frightened is believed to be descended from the sexual flush that occurs just before or after orgasm. Like other sexual messages, this flushing may have evolved as a signal of appeasement. Today, the blush remains tinged with erotic feelings, perhaps a sign of an inner passion that the rules of society force people to deny.

**Source:** Harvard psychiatrist J. Stephen Heisel as quoted in *American Health.*

## LACTATION AND LIBIDO

Does breast-feeding heighten sexual desire, as Masters and Johnson once suggested? No, according to new research. Of nursing mothers queried, 62% reported less desire or none while lactating and not menstruating; 26% said they had the same desire. Only 11% reported a heightening of sexual desire.

**Source:** *Journal of Family Practice.*

## DELAYED DESIRE

A minority of women feel their greatest sexual drive right before menstruation, rather that midcycle. Doctors suggest both physical and psychological reasons. Physically, estrogen/progesterone stimulation may excite them. Psychologically, relief from worrying about conception and an emotional need for affection may make them more open to sex.

**Source:** Dr. Ewa Radawanska, University of Arkansas College of Medicine, Little Rock, writing in *Medical Aspects of Human Sexuality.*

## 5 "T"s FOR GOOD SEX

Trust, touch, time, tease and talk. Key ingredient: The "talk" must be in bed and about sex. Ritual silence during lovemaking can only impede change, variety and maximum enjoyment.

**Source:** Domeena Renshaw, M.D., director, Loyola University Sex Clinic, Maywood, IL, in *Medical Aspects of Human Sexuality.*

## EROGENOUS ZONE UPDATE

A woman's breasts may not be erogenous, and she should not feel sexually inadequate if her partner's fondling of them is not exciting or satisfying to her. Alfred C. Kinsey found in his early sex studies that nearly half the women he interviewed were not sexually stimulated by having their breasts stroked. More recent studies have confirmed that women vary widely in the parts of their bodies that give them the greatest sexual satisfaction.

**Source:** Michael Carrera, M.D., Hunter College School of Health Sciences and chairman of the Sex Information Council of the United States.

## SHARING SEXUAL FANTASIES

Sexual fantasies don't have to be of the whips-and-chains variety. By liberating the imagination, even simple fantasies such as pretending to be in an exotic place or role-playing a character you would like to be can add playfulness to a relationship. Fantasies can allow partners to communicate real needs in a nonthreatening way. A good start for the shy: Write down a fantasy in detail and read it aloud to your partner.

**Source:** *How to Make Love to Each Other* by Alexandra Penney, G.P. Putnam's Sons, New York.

## MEN'S SEXUAL FANTASIES

• Men's sexual fantasies are being affected by the women's liberation movement. College-aged men today are more titillated by sexual stories in which the male and female partners are equally assertive then they are by descriptions of dominant-passive situations.

**Source:** Study by Mark Sirkin of the University of Connecticut at Storrs, presented at the annual meeting of the Society for the Scientific Study of Sex.

• Most common sexual fantasies (for heterosexual men): replacement of the established partner; forced sexual encounters with women; observing others' sexual activity; sexual encounters with men; group sex. Among homosexual men, sexual encounters with women represented the third most common fantasy.

**Source:** Study by Drs. Mark Schwartz and William Masters in *American Journal of Psychiatry*.

## WHY MEN FAKE ORGASMS

Orgasms are faked by men, as well as by women. Reasons: Fatigue and the desire to sleep; concern that they can't achieve a second orgasm in the same session; protection of their partners' feelings or their own egos.

**Source:** Research by sex therapists Linda Levine and Lonnie Barbach, cited in *Mademoiselle*.

## WOMEN AND SEX

Only about 30% of women reach orgasm during intercourse. Another 30% have orgasms only with masturbation (by themselves or with their lovers). Another 30% have virtually no orgasms at all. And 5% have emotional problems that make orgasm impossible. Key: A woman must feel free to teach a man what gives her pleasure.

**Source:** Ruth Westheimer, Ph.D., sex therapist and adjunct associate professor at New York Hospital-Cornell University, in *Playboy, Chicago*.

## ORGASM AND SLEEP

It's commonly believed that satisfactory sex with orgasm leads to better sleep for both partners. But a recent experiment did not prove it. The sleep of volunteers who deprived themselves of sex with their wives for one week was compared with the sleep for those same volunteers following sexual satiation. Result: No difference in the quality of sleep, nor in how rested each person felt on awakening. Upshot: There are widespread individual differences in response to orgasm. Some people even feel more energetic after sex.

**Source:** Charles Fisher, M.D., director of the sleep laboratory, Mount Sinai School of Medicine, New York, writing in *Medical Aspects of Human Sexuality*.

## TRUTH ABOUT MASTURBATION

Until recent years, the medical profession believed masturbation had harmful effects. This was less a scientific view than an adoption of the prevailing Judeo-Christian injunctions against it. Since the Kinsey Report came out, however, the thinking has gradually changed.

### "Normal" Masturbation

Update: The medical profession now sees masturbation as a rehearsal stage for normal adult sexual activity. Not only is it not harmful, but if you inhibit it in a child or make him/her feel guilty, the inhibition or guilt may carry over into the child's adult sexual expression. If you were to take the sexual history of a person who had prohibitions against masturbation in childhood, you would be more likely to find sexual problems later in life than with a person who masturbated normally as a child.

Pathological effects: Masturbation, however, can be used to avoid regular outlets for sex by those who have problems relating normally to the opposite sex. Some who are afraid to have sex in a normal manner masturbate compulsively and then are not able or are not moved to function sexually with a partner.

### Guilt

Onanism is still considered a sin by the Orthodox Jewish and Catholic religions, but is not considered sinful by the majority of other religious groups. Today, people tend to feel less guilty about the act itself than about the fantasies that accompany it. Each person has his/her own script. If it isn't completely straight and normal (male-female in a conventional sex act), guilt may result.

To relieve anxiety: I point out to my patients that atypical sexual fantasies are normal. The fantasy is simply a way of allowing oneself to have pleasure, not a sinful or harmful act. Also reassuring: Most people don't enjoy acting on their fantasies. If they could do what they think about, they would hate it, and they know it.

### Common Practices

• Sex therapy: Masturbation can be a help for people with a history of tense inhibition.

• Women: Masturbation is especially effective in treating those who do not know how to have orgasms. The therapist first teaches the patient how to have an orgasm alone. Acquaintance with her own body gives a woman the rehearsal experience she missed as a child, the necessary transitional phase to having normal sex with another person.

• Men: In sex therapy, masturbation may be recommended for men who experience retarded ejaculation. As with women who have difficulty experiencing orgasm, it is helpful to men as a transitional stage to normal sex.

• People without sexual partners: The decision about whether to remain sexually active is an individual preference. For tense, upset people who have no sexual outlet, masturbation is a reasonable alternative if it is part of their value system and they can accept it. Other people are not frustrated or unhappy without a sexual outlet. Abstinence is not a health problem if the choice is made consciously and not on a neurotic basis.

• Older people: Masturbation may be useful, particularly for men over 50 when they are not active for a time and then resume sexual activity. After a period of abstinence, a man may fear he is not able to perform. But if he continues some form of sexual activity, even self-induced, it is proof that his genitals are still functioning.

### AIDS and Herpes

Acquired immune deficiency syndrome (AIDS) is a fatal disease. It destroys the body's immune defenses against disease, leaving victims vulnerable to many terminal illnesses. There is no known cause or cure for AIDS. Medical experts believe it is transmitted through sexual contact and blood transfusions. Masturbation has become a social aid for male homosexuals, who make up the majority of the AIDS victims. Rather than run the risk of genital contact, they have increasingly turned to masturbation as an alternative.

Likewise, partners of herpes sufferers may choose masturbation during periods of eruption. Herpes is more a "media hype" problem than a serious medical problem. Not to minimize the suffering of those few people who have a low resistance to the virus, most victims become resistant in short order. After the first few attacks, genital herpes is often no worse that the fever blister on your lip.

**Source:** Interview with Helen Singer Kaplan, M.D., Ph.D., a New York City specialist in the treatment of sexual disorders.

# SEXUAL PROBLEMS MAY BE PHYSICAL NOT PSYCHOLOGICAL

• At least 20% of sexual problems have physical causes. In a recent British study, many women with orgasm problems were found to have a minor nerve defect that weakened a clitoral reflex.

**Source:** Dr. Alan Wabrek, Hartford Hospital, Hartford, CT.

• Impotence isn't always psychological in origin. In fact, endocrinologists who evaluated 42 men with erectile dysfunction detected underlying physical problems in 90% of the cases. Most often involved were nerve and blood vessel disorders. Also discovered by these physicians: An apparent link between impotence and vasectomy. Further study is planned at UCLA to validate this association.

**Source:** *Medical World News.*

## WHAT'S CHANGED IN THE SEX-THERAPY FIELD

What's changed recently in the sexual problems you are seeing and the way these problems are treated? Are there any new developments?

Yes, there have been changes. Fifteen years ago, when Masters & Johnson published their pioneering study, *Human Sexual Inadequacy*, most patients came with very specific sexual problems: Premature ejaculation or erectile difficulties in men; orgasm problems, painful intercourse and vaginismus in women.

Today, we are seeing specific problems of premature ejaculation and lack of orgasmic response less frequently. The explosion of sexual information in the media and the acceptance of a freer life style have lessened inhibitions and taught both sexes to deal with some problems on their own, without professional help. Popular works such as *The Hite Report* have enhanced couples' sexual experience by reassuring them that many women do not experience orgasm during intercourse, and that there are many other ways to achieve satisfaction.

The problems of impotence and the fear of not "performing" adequately are still with us, as they have been for centuries, but today, as a result of new research and scientific methods of treatment, help is available. There is no statistical evidence that impotency is increasing. However, it may be that, in the context of women's becoming more sexually interested and being more accessible, men with problems are more likely to feel free to seek help.

A major change in the area of erectile difficulties is that it is now recognized that 50% of impotence is due to organic causes, whereas we had previously estimated that 95% was due to psychological causes. Of course, psychological and physical causes are often interwoven. As a result of the recognition of the many physical and medical causes that may contribute to the problem of impotence, new treatment methods have been developed, and the prognosis for a more favorable outcome has improved.

Another development since the early days is that we now treat single people, as well as partners, because of the large group of singles who wish to improve their sexual functioning.

What kinds of problems are you seeing in your practice now, as opposed to 15 years ago?

What we're seeing now is much less clear-cut. The sexual problems are interwoven with the other problems in the relationship, or there are problems within the individual that affect his or her sex life. A problem has emerged that we didn't recognize then—lack of desire. That's the major change. Usually one person in the couple reports a lack of interest, saying something like: "I love my partner, I'm really attracted to him or her, but I don't feel like making love. I'd rather read a book or watch the late show."

What's at the bottom of that?

We can only speculate. We don't know specifically, since there's no single cause. A thorough evaluation is indicated. Lack of desire may be caused by a low level of depression that's strong enough to reduce the libido. Some people just can't risk the close connection that sex represents. Or one partner may be angry at the other and able to express it only by withholding sex. It can even be chemistry: Sometimes a person wants to feel attracted, but that spark just isn't there. Ironically, sex therapists may have contributed to this problem: With the sexual revolution and all the how-to information we've spread throughout the media, there is now a lot of pressure to be sexual. It's become another area in which people feel they must excel.

Do outside pressures play a part?

Absolutely. One big cause of lack of desire today is stress. People invest so much in their jobs that they feel drained at the end of the day and just want to be left alone. I see more and more of that in the population I treat—ambitious young professionals. I'm astounded at how these "yuppies" routinely work 10 or 12 hours a day. Their lifestyle and priorities put sex near the bottom of the list. I used to see only older couples (age 40–60) experiencing lack of desire as a problem. Now my patients in their early thirties are complaining of it.

Is lack of desire treatable?

If it's due to inhibitions because of background or conditioning, it will respond easily to therapy. But you don't see that much anymore, because society itself has become therapeutic in overcoming inhibitions.

Generally, treating lack of desire doesn't rank high on the list of successful sex therapies. But it can be treated, depending on the particular issues. If it's caused by anger or resentment in the relationship, the couple needs to work on that. If the root is fear of intimacy, the focus shifts to individual therapy, which emphasizes developing the ability to become vulnerable and trusting, as one must be in a relationship. If the problem is stress, and the relationship is basically a good one, the couple must start reordering their priorities. An interesting sidelight: People who complain about lack of desire usually enjoy the sexual experience once they're in it.

What did you think of the Ann Landers column that polled women on whether they'd rather have sex or just cuddle?

I discussed that on the Phil Donahue Show and a lot of other programs. I'm fascinated by it. You can't just dismiss the responses of the 72,000 women who preferred cuddling out of the 90,000 polled. Even though the question was loaded because it didn't offer any in-between position as an answer, it does show that for many people making love has become "the act." Part of the reason is the great emphasis on sex as intercourse or oral-genital contact without a similar emphasis on the emotional aspect. I never hear people talking about love. I fall into that trap myself. Often when I'm giving a lecture, someone asks, "What above love?" Sex is more than just who does what to whom. It's a wide panorama of experience that most people enjoy when it's within a close, loving relationship.

What about the difference between the sexes on this issue?

Feminist awareness has been creating a gradual change, but you can't overturn something so ingrained in a few years. Men are still fearful of showing their feelings and being vulnerable. Actually I think we're reinforcing machismo again. The model of the successful man is at a high premium today, not only financially but also in status and recognition. I think, however, that there's a biological basis to the sexual differences between men and women. Women simply need more time to get aroused—they need more touching. That's one of the few differences in the sexual responses of men and women. A man can watch football or TV all day and then move to the bedroom very quickly. But his wife becomes very insulted, complaining that he didn't talk to her all day but now he wants to have sex. Women need a transitional period...and more auditory arousal (that's plain old talk).

**Source:** Interview with Dr. Shirley Zussman, director of the Association for Male Sexual Dysfunction in New York City.

## CURE FOR SEXUAL BOREDOM

Sexual boredom often afflicts men with the most active sex and fantasy lives. Sex becomes a merry-go-round leading nowhere, eventually leaving them dissatisifed or impotent. Causes: Promiscuous, superficial sex...a preoccupation with pornography...performance anxiety...a fear of commitment. Treatment: Open communication (outside of sex) with a partner the man truly cares about.

**Source:** Lorna and Philip Sarrel, co-directors of the Yale Human Sexuality Program, in *Gentlemen's Quarterly*.

## HEADACHE CONFIDENTIAL

Post-orgasm headaches often reflect a troubled relationship. Reason: Repressed emotional stress and anxiety often surface as physical ailments. Tension headaches may result if a person senses a lack of warmth or sharing with a spouse—a condition most acute and obvious just after lovemaking. Common victims: People who are competitive, perfectionist or inarticulate about feelings. Women are affected more often because they are less likely to vent their anger verbally or to make sexual requests. Treatment: psychotherapy and/or marital counseling, heat and massage, muscle-relaxing tranquilizers.

**Source:** *Harper's Bazaar, New York.*

## FACTS ABOUT DESIRE

Low sexual desire may be a problem for as much as 20% of the adult American population. Sex counselors have termed the disorder Inhibited Sexual Desire (ISD). Not a reaction to the sexual revolution, ISD has simply become better known. A study of couples with an ISD problem at New York's Mt. Sinai Hospital suggests that the problem is less physical than psychological. The study so far also suggests that ISD is not necessarily debilitating—the subjects are happy, loving people who are successful at their jobs but feel a lack of fulfillment in their sex lives.

## APHRODISIAC BREAKTHROUGH

Scientists seem to be closing in on a safe and effective treatment for human sexual (libido) dysfunction in men and women. Research focus: Yohimbine hydrochloride, a compound derived from the sap of certain evergreen trees. Human tests with the drug are just beginning, but recent studies in laboratory rats yielded remarkable results. Animals injected with the drug displayed intense sexual arousal and performance. They sought to mate twice as frequently as untreated animals. Although researchers aren't sure how the drug produces its miraculous effects, recent findings seem to indicate that it stimulates the production of norepinephrine (a naturally occurring brain chemical that mediates the body's response to pleasure).

**Source:** John T. Clark, PhD., department of physiology, Stanford University, Stanford, CA.

## IMPOTENCE CURE

A device that corrects psychogenic (psychologically-based) impotence is now in clinical trials. The goal: To free men from lengthy psychoanalysis or the surgery required for implanting a prosthesis. How it works: A small plastic unit (about $7/8'' \times 3''$) is inserted into the rectum, where it is positioned near the nerve center responsible for initiating erections. Next, a tiny transmitter hidden in a piece of jewelry signals the battery-powered insert to generate an electrical field. This prompts a "natural" erection. The device is completely portable, requires no surgery and can be inserted and removed at will by the user.

**Source:** Biosonics, Inc.

## IMPOTENCE AND DIABETICS

Impotence resulting from diabetes may be psychological rather than organic in many cases. Finding: About one-third of men previously diagnosed as permanently unable to have an erection due to physical causes actually had erections while asleep. About 20% regained enough erectile ability to have intercourse after behavior modification therapy.

**Source:** American Diabetes Association.

## IMPOTENTS ANONYMOUS

Impotents Anonymous, a self-help group modeled after Alcoholics Anonymous, provides information and emotional support to the 10 million chronically impotent men in the US, most of whom are very reluctant to talk about the problem. IA was founded by a Washington businessman who finally sought (and found) help after 10 years of silence. I-Anon is a companion organization for wives.

**Information:** IA, 5119 Bradley Blvd., Chevy Chase, MD 20815. Anonymity is guaranteed.

## PRESCRIPTION-DRUG ALERT

Prescription drugs were the villains for

25% of men with impotence problems, a recent study concluded. Possible sex spoilers: Topical antibiotics, antihistamines, blood pressure medications, antianxiety drugs (such as Valium) and antidepressants. If drugs and lessened desire coincide: Ask your doctor about alternative medications.

**Source:** *Self.*

# SEXUAL SIDE EFFECTS OF WIDELY USED MEDICINES

Many illnesses can themselves cause lack of libido and impotence, but, in other cases, is the medication that brings on changes in sexual desire and capability. Research in this area is scanty, and the sexual side effects of many drugs are not universal. Discuss your own situation with your doctor. However, the following drugs are known to have affected the sex lives of many who take them regularly:

### High Blood Pressure Medicines

• Esimil and Ismelin (guanethidine) may cause impaired ejaculation and lack of potency in men.

• Aldomet, Aldoclor and Aldoril (methyldopa can decrease sexual desire and make holding an erection difficult for men. In rare cases, they cause a man's breasts to develop.

• Diupres, Exna-R, Rau-Sed, Regroton, Salutensin, Ser-Ap-Es and Serpasil (reserpine) can cause reduced libido and potency, delayed ejaculation and enlarged breasts.

• Catapres (clonidine) may produce impotence in men and failure to achieve orgasm in women.

• Eutonyl and Eutron (pargyline) may bring on impotence, delayed ejaculation or delayed orgasm.

• Inderal and Inderide (propranolol) rarely cause side effects, although difficulty with erections have been reported.

### Digestive-Tract Drugs

Many of the older, commonly prescribed ulcer drugs such as Banthine, Bentyl, Donnagel, Donnatel, Pamine, Pathibamate and Pro-Banthine have been associated with ual problems. The more recent medication Tagamet (cimetidine) has been reported to reduce male potency and enlarge breasts when given in very high doses.

### Tranquilizers

Librium and Valium have quite opposite effects on different individuals. For some, these drugs reduce inhibitions and increase sexual desire. In other cases, they decrease libido.

### Birth Control Pills

Regardless of brand, the sexual effects vary among women. Many report increased libido, which may simply be a release from the fear of pregnancy. Some women claim decreased sexual desire on the Pill, which may be caused by the drug's effect on hormonal regulation.

### Anti-depressant Drugs

Depression itself often causes a lack of interest in sex. Antidepressant drugs sometimes increase libido and sometimes decrease it. Other sexual side effects vary widely and are not well recorded. Possible problems include impotence, testicular swelling, breast enlargement and milk secretion, impaired ejaculation in men and delayed orgasm in women.

### Anti-psychotic Drugs

Many medications used to treat mental illness have adverse sexual side effects that have not been fully documented. Among the symptoms are impotence, difficulty in ejaculation, irregular menstruation, abnormal lactation, increased and decreased sexual desire and even false positive pregnancy tests.

**Source:** Interview with Joe Graedon, a pharmacologist and author of *The People's Pharmacy* and *The People's Pharmacy-2*, Avon Books, New York.

# COLD-REMEDY ALERT

Temporary impotence can be a side effect of using medications for the common cold. Although it isn't generally mentioned in the packaging, antihistamines and decongestants (components in virtually all over-the-counter cold remedies) have properties that interfere with the ability to have an erection. Don't worry about a temporary inability to have sexual intercourse. Side effects usually wear off about 12 hours after medication is discontinued.

**Source:** *Sex Over Forty.*

## ZINC ALERT

Male impotence can be caused by a zinc deficiency, according to a recent study of dialysis patients. After 50 milligrams of zinc acetate daily for six months, the men's sperm counts and serum testosterone were up significantly. The men also had improved sex drive and more frequent intercourse.

**Source:** *Vegetarian Times.*

## SMOKING MAY BE BAD FOR YOUR SEX LIFE

Cigarette smoking can be a prime factor in male impotence. Reason: Smoking leads to constriction of the blood vessels, which can in turn impede erections. In a recent study, 35% of men with proved impotence eliminated their problem simply by swearing off cigarettes for six weeks.

**Source:** *Sex Over Forty.*

## BEST POSITION FOR PREMATURE EJACULATORS

Premature ejaculators may do better in the female-astride position. Reason: When a man lies on his back, his muscles are more relaxed. He's better able to reflect on and edit his biological response, rather than simply react. Added advantage: This position may help the woman achieve more rapid orgasm.

**Source:** *Bedside Manners* by Dr. Theresa Larsen Crenshaw, Pinnacle Books, New York.

## 2 VIRILITY MYTHS

• Male-virility myths notwithstanding, women are more likely to complain that a penis is too large than it is too small. Reason: Intercourse can become uncomfortable for a woman when penetration is too deep.

**Source:** Dr. Theresa L. Crenshaw, director, The Crenshaw Clinic, San Diego, in *Medical Aspects of Human Sexuality.*

• Overlong intercourse can be more painful than exciting for women. Comfortable limit for many women: 10–15 minutes of continuous thrusting. More than that, even with adequate lubrication, might cause soreness and discomfort.

**Source:** *Bedside Manners* by Theresa L. Crenshaw, Pinnacle Books, New York.

## SOLUTION TO VAGINAL DRYNESS

Vaginal lubrication in sexually stimulated women decreases sharply after menopause, with 40% of post-menopausal women describing their lubrication as "inadequate" for sexual intercourse. Two simple solutions: More foreplay. . .use of a commercially prepared sexual lubricant.

**Source:** *Love, Sex and Aging* by Edward M. Brecher, Consumer Reports Books, Mount Vernon, NY.

## OFTEN MISDIAGNOSED PROBLEM

Vaginismus is an involuntary spasm of muscles near the vaginal opening. Commonly misdiagnosed, it makes intercourse painful or even impossible. Treatment: a combination of limited psychotherapy and supervised dilation usually works within two to three months.

**Source:** *Bedside Manners* by Dr. Theresa Larsen Crenshaw, Pinnacle Books, New York.

## BEST TIME FOR OLDER MEN TO HAVE SEX

Older men who have trouble attaining erections at night can do better with morning sex. Testosterone levels are higher earlier in the day.

Source: *Medical Aspects of Human Sexuality.*

## SEXUAL DYSFUNCTION IN MEN OVER 50

The most common causes, according to a study of men over 50, are the use of anti-hypertension medication (reported by 18% of those surveyed)...prostate surgery (13%)...heart attack (10%)...diabetes (6%). Leading causes in women: Hysterectomy (34%)...ovariectomy (removal of both ovaries) (18%)...antihypertension medication (18%)...mastectomy (5%)... diabetes (4%)...heart attack (4%).

Source: *Love, Sex and Aging* by the editors of Consumer Reports Books, Consumers Union, Mount Vernon, NY.

## ALL ABOUT MATURE SEX

Middle age can be an opportunity to make sex better and more satisfying than ever before. Basic reasons: People of mature years have had more experience in lovemaking. (Research shows that many women don't experience a climax until they are in their thirties, though this is beginning to change as men learn more about orgasm.) The pressures of career building are less frantic, leaving couples with more time to share. The children have grown up and left home, giving adults more privacy and fewer demands on their time. And, as men age, they lose the pressure to get right to intercourse and a quick climax. They can concentrate on a fuller sensual and sexual experience in lovemaking.

Most common mistakes about age and sex:

• Believing that your sex life is essentially over by the time you're in your fifties. Society tends to reinforce this notion with its emphasis on youth. The tendency is particularly evident in the absence of advertisements showing older people as objects of sexual interest. People behave according to the expectations that the culture sets for them and begin to give up on their sexual lives at middle age. This is, in many ways, the equivalent of giving up on life itself.

• Failing to understand that the physiological changes affecting sexual function are normal and can be adapted to without the loss of sex life. Middle-aged men suppose that these changes are signals that sex is (and is supposed to be) over for them. They become fearful that they can't function any longer. Once this fear sets in, sexual function really is affected seriously. Example: Many men age 55–60 or over worry when they don't get a spontaneous erection at seeing their partner undress as they did when they were 20 or 30. But this does *not* mean sexual function is over for them. It means only that they now require more direct stimulation. Many men put off having intercourse until they get a spontaneous erection for fear their wives will think they have some sexual problem. Sex in these circumstances becomes less and less frequent, and this is what causes wives to be fearful that their husbands are no longer interested in them.

• Believing that sex requires a climax every time. As men get older, they need longer and longer periods between ejaculations. A man in his sixties may require a full day or even several days between ejaculations. This does not mean that he cannot enjoy intercourse and lovemaking in between. Sex partners get into serious trouble when they think climaxes are essential and that the male, particularly, must have one. (The man feels he must because his partner expects it. The woman feels that if he doesn't, he no longer cares for her.) You can enjoy all the sensations of sexual arousal without climax. Remember how pleasurable it was just to neck in the back of a car in your younger days, when sex was less permissive?

Lack of lubrication, the problem for aging women: Estrogen, cycled with doses of progesterone, will alleviate this condition. The fear that estrogen might cause cancer of the uterus has prevented many women who needed it from receiving this treatment. Recent studies have shown that estrogen, when given with progesterone in cycles, is not only safe, but probably offers some protection against cancer of the uterus. Another benefit: Women taking such medication show a much decreased incidence of osteoporosis (the condition that causes bones to break easily). Several times as many aging women die of fractured hips every year as die of cancer of the uterus. There is also early evidence that estrogen may decrease the incidence of heart disease. And there is no clear evidence showing a negative relationship between estrogen therapy and incidence of breast cancer in women.

The problem of impotence: Many factors can cause impotence. Contrary to the opinion that has prevailed since Masters and Johnson did their research, not all impotence is caused by psychological problems. More and more recent research shows that a variety of physical problems can cause impotence and that these are treatable. (Included are hormonal problems and vascular and neurological conditions.)

Impotence may be being caused by medical or organic factors (rather than psychological ones) if:

• Medications are being taken to lower blood pressure. . .or antidepressants, tranquilizers, antihistamines or decongestants are being used.

• Alcohol is being overused. That has very strong negative effects on sexual function, including possible long-term problems such as reduced production of the male hormone, decreased sperm production and reduced sex drive.

• A major illness, especially diabetes, thyroid disease or arteriosclerosis, is experienced. Illness doesn't dictate erection problems but should be considered as a possible cause.

• The man has lost his sexual desire (as well as capacity).

Impotence is likely being caused by psychological factors if:

• There are firm erections under some circumstances (waking at night or in the morning, during masturbation, etc.). This indicates that the physical mechanism is in good working order and that emotional factors are the more likely cause of impotence.

• Firm erections are lost just before or after entry. The odds here greatly favor an emotional cause.

• The problem started suddenly, over the period of a month or less. More likely this is an emotionally caused impotence, since physical problems affect sexual function more gradually. Caution: There are exceptions. Emotional causes are not always sudden in their effect. And medical causes can be sudden in their effect, especially if a drug is prescribed.

• The problem started after a very stressful emotional experience (the death of a spouse, the loss of a job, a divorce, rejection by a partner).

**Source:** Interview with Saul H. Rosenthal, M.D., editor of *Sex Over Forty.*

# THE PILL AND VITAMINS

Using birth control pills on a long-term basis can reduce the levels of vitamin C, some B vitamins and zinc in the bloodstream. A deficiency in vitamin B6 may be the cause of the depression and sluggishness some birth control pill users complain of.

**Source:** *Psychosomatic Medicine.*

# WHY YOU MAY NOT NEED A CONTRACEPTIVE

Fertility problems (or outright sterility) affect 1.4 million American men. Recommended: Husbands should have a sperm count before their wives needlessly take birth control pills or else should have surgical sterilization.

**Source:** Cappy Rothman, M.D., a Los Angeles fertility expert, in *Nursing Life.*

# RATING THE CONTRACEPTIVES

The latest data on the newest. . .and oldest contraceptive techniques:

• Sterilization (male or female). It's the most popular form of birth control in the US. Drawback: Depending on the procedure used, reversal ranges from difficult to impossible. Cost: $1,180 for tubal ligation, $241 for vasectomy. Pregnancy rate:* Less than one.

• Oral contraceptives. The newest birth control pill releases different levels of hormones to accommodate different stages in a woman's reproductive cycle. It seems to reduce the frequency of ovarian, breast and uterine tumors and pelvic inflammatory disease. It can lead to depression, weight gain and cardiovascular problems in women who smoke, but this occurs rarely. Average cost per year: $172, including the cost of a visit to the doctor. Pregnancy rate: 2–4.

• Condoms. They're not foolproof because they can tear, leak or slip off during intercourse. Buy they are the best current protection against sexually transmitted disease. Average cost per year: $30. Pregnancy rate: 10.

• Intrauterine devices (IUD). An effective form of birth control, but can cause cramping and infection. Not recommended for women who have never been pregnant or who have many sex partners. Average cost per year: $131, including the visit to physician for insertion. Pregnancy rate: 5.

• Diaphragm. Helps combat sexually transmitted diseases, and must be used with a spermicide to be effective. Average cost per year: $70. Pregnancy rate: 15–9.

• Spermicide. Protects but does not safeguard against venereal disease. For maximum protection against pregnancy, follow instructions precisely. Average cost per year: $50. Pregnancy rate: 18.

• Contraceptive sponge. As good as spermicides at preventing VD. Average cost per year: $150. Pregnancy rate: 9-15.

• Withdrawal. Popular but highly unpredictable. Average cost per year: $0. Pregnancy rate: 23.

• Natural family planning. Various systems are used to determine a woman's fertile period. The couple abstains from sex during that time. Average cost per year: $0. Pregnancy rate: 24.

• Cervical cap. Never achieved wide acceptance due to difficulty of insertion and removal. Not yet approved for general use in the US. Drawback: Level of effectiveness has not been documented yet. Presently available in only a few sizes, which don't fit all women. Average cost per year: $100.

**On the Horizon**

• An agar gel diaphragm that protects against conception and then liquifies within several hours.

• Hormone-releasing vaginal rings that protect against conception.

• Hormone injections that prevent ovulation for three to six months.

• A penile cap made from contraceptive film. These caps cover the head of the penis only, and are made of a very thin film that is washed off after use. It's in the early stages of development.

• An under-the-skin implant for women that works like an oral contraceptive. Bonus: A single implant prevents pregnancy for five years. One type is already being used in several countries, and a second version is being tested for use in the US.

One dark cloud: Research on a male oral contraceptive has been disappointing. Injecting a man with a synthetic version of the hormone that controls sperm production seems to reduce but not stop it, and has caused temporary impotence.

*Number of pregnancies per 100 couples in one year.

**Source:** Interview with M.D., Jane O. Galasso, a gynecologist/obstetrician in private practice in New York.

## COMMONEST FORM OF BIRTH CONTROL

• Sterilization is the most common form of birth control in the US, primarily because of the increasing number of men undergoing vasectomies. Another factor: Decline in popularity of birth-control pills among women. Among couples who don't intend to have more children, sterilization is by far the most popular method. However, women who use the Pill still outnumber women who have undergone sterilization.

**Source:** Study by the National Center for Health Statistics, Hyattsville, MD.

• Three out of four people aged 35–44 prefer male or female sterilization to other methods, a recent survey found. Also: Women dislike condoms and diaphragms more than men do.

**Source:** Survey at the University of Florida, Gainesville.

## TWO STUDIES—TWO VIEWS OF VASECTOMY

• Vasectomy does not lead to later impotence, according to a six-year study of 10,590 vasectomized men. The results, which contradicted an earlier, smaller study at UCLA, found that 162 of the men developed impotence or sexual dysfunction five to 14 years after the operation. That compared well with 155 men in an equal-sized control group.

**Source:** Report by Dr. Frank J. Massey, professor of biostatistics at the UCLA School of Public Health, in *Medical World News*.

• Vasectomy and impotence have been linked in a recent study of men over the age of 50. One-third of the impotent men had had vasectomies. Many underwent the operation up to 20 years ago, when it was less common. The vasectomies may have been a contributing cause to organic troubles that hamper the ability to have an erection. Thus for the first time a shadow of suspicion has been cast on the consequences of the operation.

**Source:** A survey of 42 non–diabetic men over 50 years old at the Sepulveda VA Medical Center, Los Angeles, as reported in *Medical World News, Houston*.

## 4-MINUTE VASECTOMY

Vasectomies in the US will soon be done with an ultrafine cauterizing needle (no incision). The relatively painless procedure, used now in England, takes less than four minutes.

**Source:** *New Scientist*.

## GOOD REASON TO USE BARRIER CONTRACEPTIVES

Barrier contraceptives (condoms, diaphragms and spermicides) may protect women from more than just pregnancy.

First episodes of pelvic inflammatory disease (PID) are significantly lower for women who use barrier contraceptives than for those who use the Pill or IUDs, according to government studies. Theory: Since initial PID problems are associated with sexually transmitted vaginal infections, the barrier contraceptives prevent penetration by bacteria as well as by sperm.

**Source:** *Journal of the American Medical Association*.

## HOW MANY HOURS IS IT SAFE TO WEAR A DIAPHRAGM?

Women who use a diaphragm as a contraceptive device risk toxic shock syndrome if they leave it in place for 24 hours or more. Bacteria growing in the vagina and cervix are blocked from exit. Best: Remove the device within 12–18 hours after intercourse. Diaphragms that are too big can cause recurring urinary tract infections. Too large a device presses on the bladder neck, preventing the bladder from emptying completely. The lingering urine spawns bacteria.

**Source:** *Ladies' Home Journal*.

## GOOD NEWS ON THE PILL

A definitive national study has confirmed that women who use oral contraceptives incur no added risk of breast cancer. This includes women with benign breast disease or a family history of breast cancer. The research also confirmed that the Pill tends to protect women against cancer of the ovary and endometrium.

**Source:** National Institute of Child Health and Human Development and the Centers for Disease Control, reported in the *Journal of the American Medical Association*.

## MORE GOOD NEWS

The Pill is now considered more a health aid than a health hazard. The new-generation Pill (with lower doses of estrogen and progestin) helps to prevent ovarian or endometrial cancer, pelvic inflammatory disease and ectopic pregnancy. It also protects against iron-deficiency anemia, ovarian cysts and benign breast disease. Bottom line: The Pill is an appropriate contraceptive for 85% of women between 13 and 35. (It is best if you discuss this with your doctor.)

**Source:** Studies by the Centers for Disease Control, cited in *Discover*.

## MOST HAZARDOUS BIRTH-CONTROL PILLS

Some birth-control pills apparently are more hazardous than others. A study of 314 women found that those taking pills high in progestogen content were far more likely to develop breast cancer and cervical cancer than other women. Implicated: Ovulen, Demulen, Ovral, Enovid 10, Norinyl 10, Ortho-Novum 10, LoOvral, Enovid 5 and Norlestrin.

**Source:** Study by Seattle researchers reported in *The New York Times*.

## ANTIBIOTICS THAT DEFEAT BIRTH-CONTROL PILLS

Women who use oral contraceptives should be aware that their effectiveness is neutralized by some antibiotics. Contraceptive failure has been linked with tetracycline (Achromycin, Panmycin, Sumycin), ampicillin (Amcill, Omnipen, Pensyn), chloramphenicol (Chloromycetin), sulfamethoxypyridazine (Midicel) and rifampin (Rifamate, Rifadin and Rimactane). Particularly susceptible: Low-dose estrogen contraceptives like Brevicon, Demulen 1/35 and Modicon.

**Source:** *RN*.

## CONDOM ALERT

Why condoms fail: They deteriorate with age or improper storage. Petroleum jelly is used as a lubricant (it can break down rubber). They aren't used until just before ejaculation (after some semen has already leaked).

**Source:** *Medical Aspects of Human Sexuality*.

• Condoms often fail because they pull off prematurely, particulary in the women-on-top position. For more security: Use contoured condoms instead of the straight-sided variety. Or, simply hold the condom at its base during intercourse. (This method adds to the stimulation of the woman, too.)

## WHAT TO DO IF YOU'RE ALLERGIC TO A CONDOM

Condom allergies can lead to itching and skin eruptions (similar to eczema) on the penis. Obvious solution: Switch from rubber condoms to natural "skins" made of processed sheep's intestine.

**Source:** M.D., Alexander Fisher, clinical professor, department of dermatology, New York University Post-graduate Medical School, New York, in *Medical Aspects of Human Sexuality*.

## SPERMICIDE SAFETY

There is no link between the use of spermicide contraceptives and birth defects in infants, according to a recent series of tests by researchers at the National Institute of Child Health and Human Development. Even the use of spermicides after the onset of pregnancy does not appear to affect the health of the child.

## WRONG TIME TO USE A FOAM

Contraceptive foam does little to prevent pregnancy if used after sexual intercourse. Reason: Sperm reach the fallopian tubes too fast to be affected by the foam, which stays in the vagina. Best postcoital contraceptive: Large doses of estrogen administered by a physician.

**Source:** *Medical Aspects of Human Sexuality*.

## CONTRACEPTIVE GELS AND THE LAW

Contraceptive gels are still considered safe by most experts, despite a court ruling linking them with birth defects. Fact: Although thousands of women become pregnant each year when spermicides fail, the rate of birth defects is normal.

**Source:** Solomon Sobel, M.D., Food and Drug Administration, in *USA Today*.

## CONTRACEPTIVE SPONGES

Four cases of toxic shock syndrome (TSS) have been reported from the use of sponges, but the actual risk is very low—about equal to the risk from tampons now. Users should be aware of the possible link between the sponge and TSS. But, they should also realize that there are risks in alternative contraceptive methods, all of which must be weighed against the risk of pregnancy.

**Source:** Steve Cochi, M.D., cited in *Contraceptive Technology Update*.

## THE "PILL" FOR MEN

The search for a safe, effective oral contraceptive for men could be coming to an end. Researchers have found a natural substance (derived from the Ecballium elaterium—or squirting cucumber—plant) that renders men temporarily infertile for up to eight hours. Result: Contraception better than that provided by virtually every other method short of total abstinence... better than foams, jellies, condoms—even diaphragms and intrauterine devices.

How it works: Taken 30 minutes before intercourse, the pill immobilizes sperm by acidizing ejaculate. (Sperm need a slightly alkaline medium to function.) And sperm cannot fertilize an egg if they can't reach it. Bonus: Because the substance is free of steroids, hormones and other potentially harmful chemicals, the male pill is apparently free of adverse side effects. (Test subjects indicate that taking the pill actually increases libido.) Projected cost: About 50¢ per capsule.

**Source:** Rational Alternative Corp., Mission Viejo, CA.

## CONTRACEPTIVE SALVE FOR MEN

A contraceptive salve may turn out to be the male version of the Pill. Now under testing, the salve combines testosterone with estradiol, an estrogen found in small quantities in men. The salve is rubbed on the stomach at regular intervals. When it is absorbed into the bloodstream, it signals the hypothalamus to shut down sperm production. Side effects: Fewer than those with oral contraceptives, according to preliminary animal experiments.

**Source:** Research by Larry Ewing, Ph.D., a reproductive biologist at the Johns Hopkins School of Public Health.

## PERSONAL RHYTHM CLOCK

Birth control will soon be possible by microcomputer. University of Florida researchers are testing a battery-powered bedside clock-thermometer-computer that takes daily temperature readings, interprets temperature fluctuations and lets the woman know when she's fertile. The "personal rhythm clock" is manufactured (and already on the market) in England.

**Source:** *Medical World News*.

## WHEN CONDOMS PREVENT DISEASE AND WHEN THEY DON'T

Condoms offer protection against some venereal diseases (gonorrhea, nongonococcal urethritis and yeast infections). They are less effective against herpes, venereal warts and chlamydia, which are small enough to pass through the pores of the condom. If either partner has an active urethral infection or genital lesion, the only safe course is sexual abstinence.

**Source:** Dr. Michael Carrera, professor of health sciences, Hunter College School of Health Sciences, City University of New York.

## VENEREAL-DISEASE PREVENTION

Urinating within a few minutes after sex significantly reduces the chance of contracting a venereal disease. Also good: Washing with soap and water. Dubious: Douching for women. It may force organisms into the cervix or mask disease symptoms.

**Source:** *American Health.*

## RESTROOM REASSURANCE

Although the risk cannot be entirely ruled out, researchers say there is no evidence that diseases such as herpes, hepatitis and gonorrhea can be contracted from public toilet seats or faucets. For extra security: Don't touch the toilet seat (use a seat cover or make your own from toilet paper). Avoid using the first few sheets of toilet paper. Flush with your foot. Most important: Wash your hands.

**Source:** *Self.*

## GONORRHEA UPDATE

Men who are exposed just once to a woman with gonorrhea have a 22%–40% chance of catching the disease. But some men won't catch it even after repeated exposures. Why: They have antigonococci organisms in their urethras or residual immunity from previous infections. To decrease risk: A condom.

## BAD NEWS FOR TEENAGERS

The greatest risk for gonorrhea occurs during adolescence, particularly among those who are less sexually experienced. Extrapolated statistic: The annual incidence of reported gonorrhea approximates 3,000 per 100,000 sexually active women who are 15 to 19 years old. Contrast: 20- to 24-year-old women have a ratio of 1,600 cases per 100,000. More bad news for adolescents: Risk of pelvic inflammatory disease, caused by gonorrhea, is higher among infected teenagers than among infected women over 20 years old.

**Source:** H. Hunter Handsfield, M.D. director, STD Control Program, Seattle, writing in *Medical Aspects of Human Sexuality.*

## NEW DRUG COMBATS GONORRHEA

Penicillin-resistant gonorrhea may soon be treated with a new drug called *norfloxacin.* This promising drug has so far been 100% effective in curing gonorrhea in cases where penicillin therapy had not worked.

**Source:** Steven Crider M.D., Naval Hospital, San Diego, CA, in *New England Journal of Medicine.*

## HERPES UPDATE

Just because herpes has faded a bit in the public eye doesn't mean it's gone away. It's still around, and just as contagious as ever. The good news: A new drug for herpes has just been approved by the FDA.

### The New Drug

Oral acyclovir, known in its ointment form as *Zovirax,* made by Burroughs-Wellcome, is available through prescription. Zovirax, the only drug available so far, is most effective for the first outbreak. After that it won't get rid of lesions, although it somewhat lessens their intensity and duration.

The newly approved acyclovir in *oral* form totally prevents lesions in 91% of patients. The drug has a few mild side effects in 3% of patients, but it doesn't cause cancer or birth defects. When given in the last trimester to a pregnant woman with a history of herpes, it prevents an outbreak during delivery. Although herpes in adults is a very minor illness, it can cause blindness and other severe deformities in newborns, who lack sufficient immunity.

For adults with herpes, acyclovir has been declared safe to take permanently on a regular basis to prevent outbreaks. However, if the drug is discontinued, outbreaks will recur. The first outbreak after discontinuance is sometimes more virulent than usual. The decision whether or not to take acyclovir regularly will be up to each individual and his doctor.

### Refresher Course

Herpes is a virus that causes a highly infectious and transmittable sore, usually on the lips or genitals. Type one herpes, the more benign variety, commonly known as a cold sore, almost always used to occur above the waist. Type two always occurred below. But now, oral sex has changed that pattern.

The herpes sore appears two to seven days after exposure to the virus. After the first episode, 60%–70% of patients have a recurrence. The virus resides in its dormant form at the spinal root, occasionally traveling down a nerve to the outbreak site on the penis or vagina. No one can say how far apart the recurrences will be or what causes each new outbreak. Sometimes menses can bring it on. Stress does too.

Normally, the recurrences are slightly longer and more severe early in the history of the disease. Then they get farther and farther apart and more and more benign. The disease eventually burns itself out. I occasionally see herpes in people in their forties, but rarely after age 50. Nobody knows why that is.

### Myths and Realities

• Myth: Herpes is a devastating disease that can ruin your life. Reality: People tend to panic when they get herpes, both because it's so dangerous to the newborn and because of guilt and shame at having contracted a sexually transmitted disease. Actually, genital herpes is a very minor affliction, no more dangerous than a cold sore. The only long-term danger to adults is a somewhat higher cervical cancer rate in women with herpes. However, cervical cancer is almost 100% curable if caught in its early stages. A woman with herpes who has a Pap test every six months doesn't have to worry.

• Myth: If you wear a condom, you won't get herpes. Reality: This is not 100% certain. Herpes is a virus, which, unlike bacteria, may be small enough to pass through the pores of a condom. However, condoms are very good venereal disease preventives in general, and we'd see a lot less venereal disease if more men used them.

• Myth: If both sexual partners already have herpes, they don't have to worry about giving it to each other. Reality: They do. One partner may pick up a new strain and give it to the other partner. For instance, a woman who has an outbreak on one spot in her vagina may be infected by her partner with herpes at another spot. The new infection will travel up the nerve and can then break out at a new site. Recommended: Don't have sex during an outbreak, even if both partners have herpes.

• Myth: Children with herpes on the lip should be kept out of school. Reality: This is ridiculous. Herpes is dangerous only to the newborn. By the time children can toddle they have antibodies to protect them.

• Myth: There are no warning signs before a herpes episode. Reality: Frequently people who get herpes and cold sores experience a prodome phenomenon. A prodome phenomenon, which is a tingling on the lip, penis or vagina, is an accurate outbreak predictor. The blisters usually break out within a day. If you're going to have tests to determine whether or not you have herpes, it's best to come in the day after the prodome, when the blisters are fresh. Don't have sex during the prodome—it's part of the contagious period.

• Myth: Herpes can be transmitted even when dormant. Reality: It's perfectly safe to have intercourse as long as you don't have the prodome phenomenon or lesions. You should wait until all the lesions have crusted over and the crusts have fallen off, exposing new pink skin underneath. Then, and only then, is intercourse safe. You must also keep in mind that during the first outbreak, a lesion may be deep inside the vagina for a woman—and consequently undetectable. A watery discharge may be the only signal. During subsequent outbreaks, however, lesions will almost always occur on the outer lips of the vagina, where they are easy to detect.

**Source:** Interview with Mary Ellen Brademas, M.D., assistant professor of dermatology and attending physician at the Skin and Cancer Clinic, New York University Hospital, New York City.

## WHAT YOU MUST KNOW ABOUT SAUNAS AND HOT TUBS

Sitting on plastic seats in whirlpool baths, saunas or hot tubs can be risky. The *herpes simplex* virus can live for up to four hours on these seats because of the hot, humid environment. (Note: Seats of nonplastic material weren't tested.) The virus lives on the seats. It doesn't live in the water—but some other bacteria can live in the water. Recommended: Bathe both before and after using whirlpools, hot tubs or saunas.

**Source:** Study by John L. Sever, M.D., Ph.D., in *Journal of the American Medical Association.*

## VACCINATION MYTH

Smallpox vaccinations for herpes don't help, and they can be dangerous. Basic rule: Have a smallpox vaccination only for smallpox.

**Source:** *Harvard Medical School Health Letter.*

## HERPES DATING SERVICES

Though herpes dating services may help ease rejection and loneliness, they can also make participants sicker. Reason: There are several different strains of herpes. A person who has one variety can still be infected with another.

**Source:** Benjamin Raab, M.D., University of Chicago School of Medicine.

## FROM FATHER TO BABY

Herpes simplex (an often fatal disease for infants) can be transmitted to babies by fathers as well as by mothers. In two recent cases, fathers with cold sores were traced as the source of infection. Precaution: Infected family members should refrain from kissing newborns and should wash their hands carefully and often.

**Source:** *RN.*

## HELP IS ON THE WAY

Herpes help is on the way for the millions of Americans who may be exposed to the disease. At least four vaccines are being tested. One, developed by British virologists at the University of Birmingham, seems particularly promising: Of 300 subjects frequently exposed to herpes who received the vaccine, only two developed infections. The promising vaccine won't be thoroughly tested for another two years.

**Source:** *Time.*

## HERPES AND THE LAW

Pending in court are cases in which people who contracted herpes are suing those who gave it to them. Prerequisite: The victims asked the infected partner if he/she had herpes before sexual contact was made. Precedents: Successful cases against carriers of other venereal diseases and tuberculosis.

**Source:** Arthur Miller, professor, Harvard Law School, Cambridge, MA.

# 13. What You Should Know about Technology and Drugs

# What You Should Know about Technology and Drugs

## HOME MEDICAL TESTING REVOLUTION

Home medical testing is on the rise, with Americans already spending about $350 million each year for diagnostic tests and devices. In the privacy of your own home, you can test urine for sugar, blood, nitrites, infection and pregnancy hormone. Blood can be tested for anemia and diabetes . . . teeth for plaque. . . and feces for hidden blood. There are tests for measuring lung capacity, breath alcohol and breath carbon monoxide.

Many doctors favor home testing when such tests are used as screening devices in high-risk patients or for monitoring the progress of those under treatment (for example, those with high blood pressure who are taking medication). Physicians stress, however, that self-diagnosis is dangerous and that a negative test result should never discourage the patient with symptoms from seeking professional help.

### Accuracy

Home pregnancy tests claim accuracy levels in the 90% range.

However, there are many factors that can influence the results of tests for other conditions. Physical exertion, for example, may cause some glucose or protein to appear in the urine of certain individuals.

Many medications affect test results. For example, cortisone-like drugs and water pills can cause false positive results in urine glucose tests.

Diet, too, can influence test results. For example, some kits designed to detect traces of blood in the stool give false positive results if you've eaten red meat within a few days before taking the test.

Other critical factors determine how accurate the results will be. Instructions must be followed carefully. For instance, some urine specimens are to be collected immediately upon awakening, while other tests are to be performed on the second specimen of the morning. Also, tests must be performed at the prescribed time of day or month. At $10 per pregnancy kit, it is unwise to use the kit before levels of HCG (the pregnancy hormone the test measures) are high enough to be detected— about 10 days after a missed period.

### Additional Considerations

Check the expiration dates on supplies you're using. Be certain they're sealed properly. Some chemicals lose their potency when exposed to air or moisture.

Be certain your equipment is in good working condition. Check the accuracy of your blood-pressure machine with your doctor so that he can determine whether the cuff size is correct for you. (If it's not, you may get inaccurate pressure measurements.)

Your physician and pharmacist are good sources to contact if you have any questions about a home test. In addition, some test manufacturers have a toll-free number you can call if you need further information about their products. Surgical supply store representatives can also give guidance.

Most home tests can be obtained through pharmacies and surgical supply stores. Other devices must be ordered from their manufacturers or through mail-order catalogs.

**Source:** Rachelle Kess, a registered nurse and specialist in medical writing.

## DO-IT-YOURSELF URINE TEST

Worried about kidney dysfunction or the possibility of diabetes? Urine can now be tested at home. Urinalysis kits are available in drugstores. Cost: $14.95 (includes cost of analysis and report). The urine sample is mailed to the laboratory in a specially designed container in a postage-paid mailer. Confidential results are returned within days, along with a copy of the report for the patient's physician, if desired.

**Source:** Bruce Yaffe, M.D., gastroenterologist in New York.

## 160 MEDICAL TESTS YOU CAN DO WITHOUT A DOCTOR

Check your health without a doctor. A new book details 160 tests you can do yourself, some with no more equipment than an ordinary match. Especially useful: A sphygmomanometer (blood pressure machine), $70–$200. A reading at home may be more accurate than one taken during a stressful doctor visit.

**Source:** *Do-It-Yourself Medical Testing,* Facts on File Publications, New York.

## MEDICAL SOFTWARE OF THE FUTURE

Medical software that runs on home computers is coming soon. Programs will compile medical records, make diagnoses and even suggest treatment. Data obtained with self-care equipment (such as blood pressure gauges) will be entered either through sensors or manually on the keyboard. Health-oriented software will then advise the user on matters such as diet, nutrition and biofeedback.

**Source:** *Medical Economics,* Oradell, NJ.

## 2 DUBIOUS TREATMENTS

Medical quackery is booming in the US, and the federal machinery for keeping it in check is too cumbersome to be effective. Consumers must be wary of dubious cures and treatments lacking FDA approval. Current FDA concern: Body wrap salons and passive exercise centers that employ electronic muscle stimulators. No body wrap treatment has received an FDA blessing, and electronic muscle stimulators have been approved for use only under a doctor's prescription for specific health problems. Reducing, body shaping and wrinkle removing are not among them.

**Source:** Arthur Hull Hayes, Jr., commissioner, Food and Drug Administration, quoted in *Changing Times,* Washington, D.C.

## MEDICAL RIPOFFS

Surgical procedures that are often performed unnecessarily: Knee surgery, prostate removal, hysterectomy, repair of deviated septum of the nose and podiatric surgery. Finding: When the state of New York required about one million people on state insurance policies to get second opinions on these procedures, the number of actual operations dropped significantly.

**Source:** Nelson Carpenter, associate director, Governor's Office of Employee Relations, New York State, quoted in *Business Insurance,* Chicago, Il.

## A MEDICAL PROCEDURE THAT CAN CAUSE HARM

Cut down X ray exposure by asking if fewer pictures can be taken. Make sure that only the area of concern is exposed to radiation. Avoid repeats by sitting still and holding your breath while films are taken. Insist on lead shields to protect your reproductive organs.

**Source:** *The Complete Book of Medical Tests* by Mark A. Moskowitz, M.D., W. W. Norton and Co., New York.

## BIOPSIES: BETTER, CHEAPER, FASTER, SAFER

Totally nonsurgical biopsies: Ultrasound imaging system's next generation could be the first step—lets physicians examine internal tissues about as closely electronically as is done currently with "knife and microscope." Bonus: Eliminates harmful X rays and radioactive tracers. Background: Ultrasound, which creates images of muscle, fat, organs, etc. within the body via harmless high-frequency sound waves, has been around for years. But, until now, it had been of limited use because the images generally were fuzzy and difficult to interpret. Breakthrough: New ultrasound device incorporates a computer to produce images two to four times clearer than those produced by conventional noncomputerized systems. For the first time ever, physicians can focus the waves precisely to determine, for example, not only whether there is a tumor, but also whether it is benign or malignant. (Fetal abnormalities and heart disease can also be detected more easily with this superior scanning capability.) Impact: Examinations are quicker, more precise and more detailed than was previously possible.

**Source:** Acuson, Mountain View, CA.

# NEW BLOOD SUBSTITUTE

An emergency blood substitute has been developed in Japan. Fluosol (trade name) has the oxygen-carrying properties of hemoglobin. A petroleum-based chemical made from compounds called perfluorocarbons, the product has been used successfully in the US during surgery on patients who refuse to have blood transfusions for religious reasons. Unlike blood, the synthetic has no clotting ability. It leaves the body within 72 hours as natural blood supplies rebuild. Advantage: No worries about its carrying hepatitis or AIDS. Possible uses: Treating carbon monoxide poisoning, sickle cell anemia and the acute stages of heart attacks.

**Source:** *New England Journal of Medicine*, Boston, MA.

# BLOOD TRANSFUSIONS AND HEPATITIS

Six percent of patients who have transfusions contract a strain of hepatitis that isn't detected in blood screening. (Hepatitis types A and B are picked up in blood tests.) Blood banks do not accept donors with any history of hepatitis infection or exposure or with a low-grade liver inflammation, but these precautions are not foolproof. To protect yourself: Before elective surgery, donate enough of your own blood over the preceding weeks to cover your needs at the time of the operation.

**Source:** Dr. Bruce H. Yaffe, a gastroenterologist in private practice in New York.

# PRIVATE BLOOD BANK

Surgery patients at some hospitals can now store their own blood before the operation to ensure safer transfusions. Eligibility: Anyone who is free of anemia or blood impurities. The patient donates a pint a week to a blood bank, which freezes it until needed.

# WHY SOME ACNE SUFFERERS SHOULDN'T GIVE BLOOD

Acne sufferers who are taking the drug Accutane should not donate blood. If the blood is transfused into a pregnant woman—or even into a woman who becomes pregnant shortly afterwards—the drug could endanger the fetus.

**Source:** Federal Drug Administration, Washington, D.C.

# ROBOTIC SURGEON

Robotic neurosurgery may soon replace human neurosurgery in delicate and hard-to-reach areas of the brain. CAT scans or NMR scans accurately map out a tumor in the brain, translating it into computer images that control a robotic arm with a laser scalpel that surgically obliterates the abnormal tissue. Advantages: The size of the surgical opening in the skull is considerably smaller.

Patients leave the hospital generally within two days instead of a typical two weeks. And . . . the chances of human fallibility are removed.

**Source:** Yik San Kwoh, M.D., Memorial Medical Center, Long Beach, CA.

## SKIN ZIPPER FOR NO-SCAR SURGERY

Plastic strips that close surgical wounds with a zipper-like action will probably change the way most people think about surgery. Why? Because scarring is so dramatically reduced with the new technique that you'd have to look carefully to find it. Background: Millions of operations are performed each year, and all of them require some form of wound closure. Fine stitches are ideal for cosmetic work, but they're ineffective and far too time-consuming for most general surgery. Surgical staples were invented several years ago. They permit surgeons to close large wounds very quickly. But they still have one big problem: They leave very obvious, unsightly scars.

To the rescue: Dermizip. It's fast, cost-effective and leaves only minimal scars (just a series of pin-sized dots—which eventually disappear). When the wound is healed, the pins and tracks are removed. Outlook: Expect zippers to become the big method of surgical closure—perhaps displacing staples altogether.

**Source:** Biomet, Inc., Warsaw, IN.

## BLADDER-CONTROL OPERATION

Artificial sphincters can help people with urinary incontinence resulting from spinal or pelvic injuries, surgery, etc. The surgically implanted bladder control is operated manually by the patient. Success rate: 85%.

**Source:** Urologists Zafar Khan, M.D., and E. Douglas Whitehead, M.D., Beth Israel Medical Center, New York, quoted in *Vogue*, New York.

## NEW HELP FOR LEG FRACTURES

Resistant leg fractures no longer automatically lead to amputation. A new surgical procedure uses a "spare part" of the other leg's fibula to replace the damaged or diseased part of the thicker tibia. Result: Within 12 months, the reconstructed leg can bear the body's full weight.

**Source:** Harold M. Dick, M.D., director of orthopedic surgery, Columbia University Medical Center, New York.

## DRUG TO AID TRANSPLANT PATIENTS

A new transplant drug could double the number of successful transplants, increasing the kidney survival rate from 50% to 80%. Cyclosporine A (marketed by Sandoz under the name Sandimmune) apparently lowers the body's tendency to reject a foreign substance but doesn't interfere with the body's ability to fight infection. Additional benefits: Doctors are optimistic that the drug will also help heart and lung transplant patients.

## MEDICAL DREAM COME TRUE

A natural body substance could be the key to new methods of speeding the healing of wounds and surgical incisions. . . treating symptoms of arthritis and diabetes. . . repairing damaged heart tissue without the cost or risk of bypass surgery. . . and treating and diagnosing stubborn cancers.

Miracle: *Angiogenin,* a protein that stimulates production of blood vessels. Scientists predicted the existence of such a substance years ago, but they were unable to identify it because it is found in the body in very small concentrations. The protein's chemical composition has at last been determined, and scientists have cloned the gene needed to produce large quantities of the protein.

Inside story: Every cell in the body, healthy or diseased, depends on networks of blood vessels to deliver nutrients and remove waste products. When vessels become clogged (as in coronary heart disease or stroke), or when they are severed (as in cuts, wounds or incisions), surrounding tissue quickly dies. Now: Angiogenin promotes growth of blood vessels to replace or supplement damaged vessels. Clogged arteries could be "bypassed" without bypass surgery. . .and wounds could be made to heal twice as fast as usual.

Exciting opportunity: A tumor cannot usually grow in the body without the growth of additional blood vessels to allow for the tumor's rapid metabolism. Angiogenin-*inhibiting* agents could control tumor growth without dangerous radiation or toxic drugs. More: Special probes are being developed to spot high levels of angiogenin in a patient—a likely sign of tumor growth somewhere in the body.

Future: Angiogenin-related treatments for diabetic retinopathy (damage to blood vessels in the eye that often leads to blindness), rheumatoid arthritis, and other vascular disorders. Angiogenin is even being investigated as a *baldness* remedy. (Some researchers believe baldness may be caused by atrophy of blood vessels in the scalp.)

Status: Research is still in early stages, but two patent applications have already been filed. Funding the research: Monsanto, St. Louis, MO. (Monsanto will have first dibs on developing commercial products.) Investigators: Bert L.Vallee, M.D., and colleagues at Harvard Medical School. (Harvard University will retain patent rights.)

## WHY DRUG-USE MAY BE DOWN

Prescription drug use has fallen 7% since 1975, despite the new drugs added to the market. The biggest declines are in Valium prescriptions (from 62 million to 31 million) and sleeping pills (from 40 million to 21 million). Reason: Americans, more conscious of the negative effects of drugs, are trying to find alternatives.

**Source:** Study from the National Institute of Mental Health, Rockville, MD.

## WHAT A GOOD PHARMACIST WILL DO FOR YOU

Choose a pharmacist who keeps a "drug profile"—a log for each patient listing the medications used and the prescribing doctors. Advantage: If a new medication is incompatible with an old one the patient is still taking, the pharmacist will spot the problem before filling the new prescription.

**Source:** *Harvard Medical School Health Letter,* Cambridge, MA.

## MEDICINE CABINET ALERT

In 1978, the FDA required drug companies to put expiration dates on *all* over-the-counter medications (the ones you can buy without a prescription) unless:

• The medication carries no dosage limit, and

• The medication will remain stable for at least three years.

What to do: Check the medicine cabinet for OTC drugs with no date. . .meaning they were packaged prior to 1978. Discard them and buy replacements.

The FDA also requires expiration dates on all prescription medication containers. Trap: Consumers rarely see the container because pharmacists transfer the drugs from big bottles into the familiar brown plastic ones.

Solution: Ask the pharmacist to type the expiration date on the container given to you. If you receive the drug within a month or two of its expiration date, request that your prescription be filled from a more current batch.

**Source:** Frank Coran, Consumer Safety Officer and assistant to the director, US FDA, Washington, DC.

## EXPIRED DRUGS

If a product has been stored as recommended, prescriptions should maintain 90% of labeled potency through the last day of the month indicated on the package. Beyond that, it's best to get a pharmacist's advice. The active ingredients may have lost their effectiveness or, in rare instances, deteriorated into toxic compounds.

**Source:** *US Pharmacist.*

## PEOPLE LEAST LIKELY TO FOLLOW DIRECTIONS

Forty percent of all Americans don't follow directions in taking prescription drugs. Least compliant patients: Men, people between the ages of 18 and 24 and college graduates.

**Source:** *Drug Topics,* New York.

## EASY WAY TO KEEP TRACK OF YOUR MEDICATION

Pill dispenser helps you to remember which medications to take and when. The Mediplanner has 28 plastic compartments to organize a week with up to four doses a day.

**Source:** Apex Medical, Bloomington, MI.

## EASIEST WAY TO SWALLOW A CAPSULE

Avoid the natural inclination to bend your head back when swallowing a capsule. It's better to tilt your head or upper body forward. Then the lighter-than-water capsule can float toward the throat.

**Source:** *Modern Maturity.*

## TO MAKE A PILL GO DOWN

To swallow a pill, stand up and sip a liquid to lubricate the esophagus. Then swallow the pill with an entire glassful of the liquid. Remain standing for at least 90 seconds.

Bedtime pills: Take them 30 minutes before retiring, since salivation and swallowing taper off with sleep.

**Source:** *Self,* New York.

## SELF-ADMINISTERED INTRAVENOUS ANTIBIOTICS

Infectious problems often require lengthy treatments with intravenous antibiotics in a hospital. Now, however, physicians are training patients to self-administer the medication intravenously at home. When patients are trained correctly, there's little risk of complications. Benefits: Less expensive. Avoids the possibility of picking up infections commonly found in hospitals. Saves time.

**Source:** *Medical Tribune.*

## BEWARE OF INACTIVE INGREDIENTS

Medication side effects may be caused by inactive ingredients not listed on the label. Prime offenders: Coatings, binders, fillers, colorings and flavorings. Recommended: Ask your doctor or pharmacist if your reaction might be caused by an inactive ingredient. A similar, equally effective drug with different ingredients may be available.

**Source:** *New England Journal of Medicine.*

## ASPIRIN: FACTS YOU SHOULD KNOW

Aspirin overuse can lead to kidney damage, a recent study found. About 20% of patients on kidney dialysis may be there because of too much aspirin or some other analgesic. How much is too much? Two kilograms in six years—just three regular tablets a day—can seriously impair the kidney's cleansing function.

**Source:** Dr. William Bennett, Oregon Health Science University, Portland.

## COMMON REMEDIES THAT CONTAIN MORE ALCOHOL THAN A CAN OF BEER

Cold remedies and dental products may contain more alcohol (in one daily dosage) than a can of beer. This could be dangerous for anyone who shouldn't touch it. Most at risk: Recovered alcoholics, young children, pregnant women, people using sedatives or sleep aids, and peptic ulcer patients. Highest: Terpin Hydrate and Codeine Elixir (40% alcohol). Listerine mouthwash (26.9%). Nyquil Cough Syrup (25%). Phenobarbitol Elixir (25%). Scope mouthwash (18.5%). Vicks' Formula 44 Cough Mixture (10%). Contac Jr. Liquid (10%).

**Source:** *RN* magazine, Chicago, IL.

## COUGH MEDICINES THAT DON'T DO WHAT THEY ADVERTISE

The Federal Drug Administration is beginning to agree with an increasing number of independent doctors who say commercial cough remedies are of little benefit. Basic drawback: Virtually all commercial medications interfere with the body's natural way of clearing the respiratory tract, which is coughing. Doctors are especially concerned with:

• Antihistamines, which they say work by thickening, not thinning, lung secretions. Good only for allergies.

• Decongestants, which might be good for extreme stuffiness but are otherwise of doubtful effectiveness.

• Expectorants, which drug companies say loosen mucus and phlegm, although the evidence is scanty.

• Suppressants, which suppress the brain's cough reflex. They are especially hazardous for people with asthma or bronchitis who rely on coughing to breathe when their lungs are not clear.

Skeptics of cough medications say home remedies may be more effective and less risky. Chicken soup and fruit juices may work as well as an expectorant. Vaporizers and humidifiers offer relief, as does a drop of honey on the back of the tongue.

**Source:** Dr. Sidney Wolfe, M.D., and others, quoted in *Executive Fitness*, New York.

## TWO DRUGS THAT DON'T GO TOGETHER

A potentially dangerous drug combination: Cimetidine (Tagamet), the biggest-selling ulcer drug in the US, and theophylline, a drug commonly used for asthma. They have often been prescribed together for patients with asthma and ulcers. But recent studies show that the drugs interact, causing the body's theophylline levels to build up. This can lead to potential toxicity, irregular heart beats and irritability. Safer: Renitidine (Zantac). It has the same results as Tagamet, but doesn't cause the theophylline buildup.

**Source:** *The Archives of Internal Medicine*, New York.

## PRESCRIPTION DRUGS AND DRIVING

Prescription drugs are a leading factor in automobile accidents. Worst hazard: Psychoactive medications, including tranquilizers, sedatives, stimulants and antidepressants. These can both alter drivers' judgment and make them sleepy. Also dangerous: Painkillers (especially codeine and other narcotics), muscle relaxants, ulcer drugs, heart medications, eye drops and over-the-counter antihistamines. Worst combination: Drugs and alcohol, which can intensify each other's effects. Ask your doctor about potential side effects of every drug you take. Take the first dose of a new one at home.

**Source:** *Drugs and Driving*, a study by the National Institute on Drug Abuse, Rockville, MD.

## DRUG BREAKTHROUGHS

• Taking heart. *Milronone*, a new compound, can aid the heart's contractions without the side effects linked with digitalis. Future hope: Milronone may prove most effective when used in conjunction with digitalis.

• New anti-ulcer drugs, the prostaglandins, both heal the disorder and prevent the quick recurrence that is a common problem with current drugs such as Tagamet and Zantac. One prostaglandin, Enprostil, has already proved effective in tests.

• A new tranquilizer, *Buspar,* calms anxiety without affecting mental alertness. Unlike Librium or Valium, it allows users to drive or work without impairment. Bonus: Buspar has no significant interaction with alcohol.

• Good as gold. *Ridaura,* a new oral gold preparation, appears to control rheumatoid arthritis without the significant side effects of injectable gold or other potentially toxic drugs.

• New blood-pressure drugs won't leave patients depressed, fatigued or impotent (common with current medications). Angiotensin-converting-enzyme (ACE) inhibitors are designed to make a patient feel better as well as get better. The pioneer is Capoten, by Squibb. Unfortunately, it's been associated with several serious side effects. Other ACE inhibitors are now in the medical pipeline.

• Cure for the common cold? Sniffing interferon sharply reduces the number of viruses in the nose—the battleground of the cold. Result: Symptoms are eased significantly. Possibility: Interferon may also help prevent colds if used after exposure to another person who has the virus.

• High blood pressure will soon be treated with a seven-day skin patch, a major advance over the daily medications now in use. Advantages: Patients will be much less likely to forget to take their medication. And because a patch allows a drug to ease gradually into the bloodstream, there will be fewer side effects.

• Insulin by a nose. Diabetics of the future may be able to take insulin by nasal spray rather than by cumbersome, painful shots. The spray lasts up to five hours.

**Source:** Bruce H. Yaffe, M.D., is a gastroenterologist in private practice in New York.

## WHEN ANTIBIOTICS DON'T WORK

A new drug may soon wipe out bacteria that previously resisted antibiotics. Augmentin, from Beecham Laboratories, contains penicillin and another chemical that blocks the bacteria's protective enzymes. Prime targets: Children's ear infections, respiratory- and urinary-tract infections.

**Source:** Mile Hilton, manager of public relations, Beecham Laboratories, Bristol, TN.

## NEW APPROACH TO NARCOTIC DRUGS

Narcotic drugs have a legitimate role in medicine—to relieve periods of acute pain. Problem: These drugs are addictive. Understandably, doctors have carefully meted out a minimum of the drugs in an effort to cut down on that risk. New approach: Prescribing narcotics every four hours. With pain relief so readily available, patients tend to refuse many doses and to take less overall. Added benefit: If a drug is not perceived as a desperate need, it is less likely to become an addiction.

**Source:** Bruce Yaffe, M.D., a gastroenterologist in private practice in New York.

## TAMPER-PROOF CAPSULES

New pharmaceutical manufacturing process produces capsules that are tamper-proof, leak-proof, and gas-tight (contents will not degrade on contact with oxygen). Bonus: The new capsules, made of hard gelatin, are thinner and cheaper than the soft-gelatin capsules and have always been used with liquid and oil fillings. Key: Hermetic sealing of capsule halves. Makes it possible to reduce the gripping surface on the lower half of the capsule. . . so tampering cannot take place without damaging the original capsule. Final heat-sealing step locks capsule halves in place but does not alter the contents in any way. The inventors find the new capsules suitable for encasing powders, pastes, liquids, oils, pellets, microspheres—or any combination of these. Outlook: About a dozen large pharmaceutical firms have already expressed interest in the technology.

**Source:** Capsugel AG (Division of Warner-Lambert), Basel, Switzerland.

# 14. The Mind: Problems and Solutions

# The Mind: Problems and Solutions

## MOST COMMON KINDS OF MENTAL ILLNESS

Mental illness affects one adult in five. Most common: Anxiety disorders or phobias (13.1 million people). Alcohol or drug abuse (10 billion). Depression (9.4 million).

**Source:** Study by the National Institute of Mental Health.

## ADDICTIONS, OBSESSIONS AND COMPULSIONS

Americans are always striving for the biggest and the best. As a result, we are extremely vulnerable to excessive behavior. This can lead to a variety of illnesses, including obsessive-compulsive neurosis and various addictions. Although the terms are often used interchangeably, their meanings are actually quite different. Since the addictive process is the major one in America—and the most dangerous—it's useful to know the difference between addictions, obsessions and compulsions. The chances are that you or someone you know is suffering from one of them.

### Obsessive-Compulsive Neurosis

Obsessions and compulsions are linked, but they don't always go together. *Obsessions* are repetitive thoughts. The most common ones are thoughts of violence, contamination and doubt. *Compulsions* are repetitive actions. The most common are handwashing, counting, checking and touching.

Obsessive thoughts, such as fear of contamination, are linked to compulsive actions (such as constant handwashing). We're all familiar with common (and mostly harmless) compulsions—constantly checking to see if you're on time or repeatedly touching your pocket to make sure your keys are there. Many of us are assailed by obsessive thoughts, such as worrying about having said the right thing or whether you shut off the light in the kitchen when you left the house.

The distinctive quality of obsessions and compulsions is that, unlike addictions, they give no pleasure and are not actively sought out. They're essentially repetitive, meaningless, trivial and ritualistic thoughts or actions that reduce anxiety. Also, unlike addictions, they don't involve tolerance withdrawal, abstinence or destruction to bodily functions.

Neurotic obsessions produce loss of energy, ambivalence and doubt that may destroy mental functioning. Example: A person who becomes obsessed with hatred of his boss for not giving him a raise may be unable to work productively.

With neurotic compulsions, the behavior is experienced as being against one's will. Example: Someone who can't start work until all his pencils are sharpened to the same length may know his behavior is bizarre, but he feels compelled to perform the ritual anyway.

In both obsessions and compulsions, there is always awareness of the pain and dysfunction, and sometimes a conscious need to hide the thoughts and actions because of embarrassment. Although obsessive-compulsive neuroses are not as destructive to the self or others as addictions are, they can be painful and sometimes crippling. The individual often seeks help because he is usually conscious of how unpleasant and non-functional his obsessions and compulsions are. The addict, on the other hand, tends to deny that there is anything wrong him.

## Addiction

Addiction is a process. It is not limited to drugs, alcohol or other substances—you can be addicted to anything. Food, cigarettes, gambling, television, work, sex, spending money and even jogging are other common addictions.

Characteristics common at every stage of the addictive process:

• There is an overpowering desire or need for a substance, object, action, interaction, fantasy or milieu that produces a "high."

• This reaction is sought repetitively, impulsively and compulsively.

• In the early stages of addiction, it is felt as a pleasurable way of coping with an intolerably painful psychic conflict or stress. However, the initial sense of relief diminishes as the process continues.

• Relationships with friends and family deteriorate, and the addict can no longer deny the pain. Symptoms appear when "hangover phenomena" (tension, depression, rage, guilt and physical distress) start to predominate.

The addictive process may not be continuous. It can be occasional or cyclic, but it always involves tolerance, abstinence and withdrawal. The addict builds up increased tolerance, needing more and more of whatever he is addicted to—while he gets less and less satisfaction from it. When he tries to abstain from his addiction voluntarily, he undergoes unpleasant or painful withdrawal symptoms. Sometimes, a person shifts from one form of addiction to another, but the process remains the same. Example: Cigarette addicts often become addicted to food when they give up smoking.

In true addiction there is almost always excessive use of pleasurable activities to cope with unmanageable conflict or stress. The very fact that pleasure is being used to cope makes it difficult for both a diagnostician and an addict to recognize and treat the addiction. The addict cannot identify his pain or admit that his addictive behavior is excessive.

## Causes of Addiction

Vulnerability to addiction seems to run in families. Although constitutional and genetic factors may be involved, upbringing is very important. Every addicted adult I've treated has told of excessive inconsistency, deprivation or overindulgence in early life. Common: Shifts from too much to too little love, protection or discipline. A chaotic family situation with frequent separation, divorce or experimental living arrangements. A parent who smokes, drinks, eats or works too much or who is drugged or overeroticized. Parents who have little ability to delay gratification and a low frustration tolerance.

Addicts suffer from low self-esteem. They have excessive expectations of themselves, but little ability or willingness to be self-disciplined. Society also contributes by swinging from prohibition to permissiveness. Example: Commercials for fattening foods are often followed by exhortations to diet.

## How to Change

Before doing anything about either an obsessive-compulsive neurosis or an addiction, it should be diagnosed. Since obsessive-compulsives are consciously aware of their pain, they're more likely to seek help voluntarily. Since addicts tend to deny their problems, it's wise to seek help if your friends or family have been complaining about your behavior. If someone close to you, whom you generally respect, thinks you're an addict, you probably are.

Self-help groups can be very effective for addicts. They provide supportive mentors in former addicts who have conquered their addiction. There are self-help groups for drugs, alcohol, food, gambling and smoking. Unfortunately, self-help groups do not yet exist for addictions to work, sex, overspending, TV or multiple addictions. In some cases, even a family member, friend, co-worker or former addict can be an effective helper. But if the problem is severe, the addict should seek professional help.

**Source:** Interview with Lawrence J. Hatterer, M.D., a psychiatrist and psychoanalyst and associate professor of psychiatry at Cornell University Medical School.

# HOW TO RECOGNIZE MENTAL ILLNESS

A change...a difference in behavior... that is the chief clue that somebody close to you is experiencing painful mental problems and needs help.

Once you begin to sense a difference that makes you uncomfortable and worried, put your powers of observation into high gear. To confirm your feelings about a change for the worse, one that calls out for professional help, there should be a pattern of differences in behavior—changes occurring in more than one area.

### Sight and Smell

Be alert to a marked difference in the way a person dresses. A shift to comply with fashion is, of course, insignificant. But, a mild-mannered, conforming woman suddenly begins to wear excessive makeup and to push people around. A neat dresser starts to look unkempt. Or, a casual dresser becomes overly fastidious. Uncombed hair and dirty or torn clothes also signal trouble.

By the time a person begins to smell bad, indicating a lack of concern about personal cleanliness, you can assume that the trouble is pretty far advanced. Individuals usually have to be in severe distress to ignore well-established standards of personal hygiene. (Even in a mental hospital, professionals can detect a difference in smell between the patients who are recovering and those who are still acutely ill.)

### Sudden Mood Shifts

A common sign is rapid shifts in mood and emotion—from anger to playfulness, from sadness to giggles.

You might also find that you get little or no emotional feedback from the person. It's common for a person in trouble to develop what is called a low-information face—a blank look that leaves you confused as to how the person is reacting to what you say.

A sudden change to expansive gestures that are beyond a person's means—for example, impulsive invitations to take everybody out for lunch, or major buying sprees—are also a warning sign. Possibilities: Manic behavior...or drug use.

A descent into sadness and melancholy is another common warning sign. (If this tendency appears regularly and then disappears, and the individual is a woman, the problem could be premenstrual syndrome.)

More clues:

• A previously polite and caring person suddenly becomes insensitive.

• A person begins to behave inappropriately with those in authority.

• A person who is usually energetic and creative acts tired and indifferent.

• A decisive person begins to vacillate, postpones decisions, upsets schedules, and seems foggy in his or her thinking.

• A persons talks from subject to subject without connection. He or she seems pressured to continue speaking, is repetitive and rambling, and rarely pauses to let the other person enter into a dialogue.

### False Family Loyalty

Many of these symptoms are ignored within families because of false loyalties. Parents, especially, often blind themselves to evidence of severe problems with their children because they view the children as extensions of themselves and defend them right or wrong.

Most important clue: A child who is consistently a loner, and is clearly living a fantasy life needs professional help. If you find yourself excusing this pattern of behavior by suggesting that your child is too bright to play with others, beware! Chances are that it is too painful for you to face the prospect of your child's trouble—but ignoring it hurts the child.

In most cases, when children or young adults finally commit acts of violence that are evidence of severe mental problems, a close examination will show that the clues have simply been ignored.

Examples: A series of pets have mysteriously disappeared...A teacher suggested to the parent years ago that the child be taken to a psychologist.

### Let's Go Together

When the pattern of difference in a person's behavior is very clear to you, tell the person—but in a very caring, non-threatening way. Don't say: You're acting strange. Better: I can't put my finger on it, but something seems different about you. I care for you and think you should talk to somebody skilled about it. I know a person I've talked to myself. Maybe we can go together. I'll introduce you.

In a family, the clear message should be: I'm with you all the way in this. Even in a business situation, this approach can work if a supervisor plans carefully with a professional.

Example: A high-level executive suddenly began to act violently toward people around him. After consultation with a local psychiatrist, the president of the company suggested to the executive that he talk to someone the president had talked to himself. He offered to walk with him to the psychiatrist's nearby office—continuing the sense of caring and friendship. The walk itself was part of the plan to diffuse the executive's rage.

**Source:** Interview with Milton M. Berger, M.D., co-director, American Short-Term Therapy Center.

## SCHIZOPHRENIA UPDATE

Schizophrenics' brains may literally be scrambled. Nerve cells from 10 victims were wildly askew, according to a recent study of autopsy specimens. Cause: Still unknown. Area of worst disorder: The hippocampus, which helps us express emotion and process sensory data.

**Source:** Arnold Scheibel, M.D., University of California, in *Discover, New York.*

## WHEN SHORT-TERM THERAPY WORKS AND WHEN IT DOESN'T

Short-term therapy often resolves a patient's problem with a fraction of the time and expense of traditional psychoanalysis. Duration: From one to about 20 sessions. Brief therapy works best when a patient can target a single problem, such as a troubled marriage. It's also effective in crisis intervention, as in the death of a loved one or loss of a job. Added benefit: Short-term treatment makes a patient less dependent on the therapist. (Note: It's not good for drug addicts, alcoholics or people with psychiatric illnesses.)

**Source:** Joseph H. Weissberg, Ph.D., a psychoanalyst and director of the Association for Short-Term Psychotherapy, a New York research group.

## ALL ABOUT FANTASIES

An active fantasy life is as crucial to the mental health of adults as it is to children. We tend to think that as we grow up we must leave our fantasies behind along with other childish things. The reverse is true. Without fantasy, we'd never dare to push or grow psychologically. We'd become bland and constricted half-people. To understand why fantasy is so important, you should know the role it plays in keeping us aware, awake and alive.

### Fantasy and Children

For children, fantasy is so important that a child who doesn't fantasize may be seriously mentally ill. Play and fantasy are intricately associated. For a slightly older child, fantasy helps to master anxiety, aggression and guilt.

Example: Every child has imaginary monsters. The monsters are a projection of anger toward parents and self-punishment for feeling that anger. Small children often can't get angry with their parents directly because their need for love is too great and the fear of abandonment too strong.

Little by little, children are shamed out of their fantasies. The first six years are the magic years. The start of school means fantasy will be reined in by teachers and parents, but the child who can maintain the ability to fantasize freely will probably become a creative adult.

### Fantasy and Creativity

Fantasy, when connected to reality and given free expression, makes for creativity. The creative person shares his fantasies with us—something we're often afraid to do because it makes us feel so vulnerable. Although fantasy sharing can be very liberating, the vulnerability can become too frightening for some people and cause them to curtail their fantasy lives.

Creative writers and artists are commissioned by society to be our fantasizers. They're given free rein to keep the child within them alive, and we pay them to do so. When we're very moved by a painting, film, book or other work of art, it is probably that an unexpressed fantasy in ourselves has been touched by the artist.

### Fantasy and Everyday Life

Adolescents move to adulthood by fantasizing the roles of people they admire and would like to be. To make any moves in life, we must fantasize what we want.

Examples: Anyone who contemplates a job or career change first fantasizes what it would be like to do other kinds of work. People who make a lot of money often start by fantasizing about ways to get rich.

Business, although not traditionally thought of as particularly creative, in fact does involve creativity arising from fantasy. From envisioning a new product to imagining its uses and potential customers, the businessperson allies fantasy and thinking. You can try something out in your mind without actually having to do it. Fantasy is a way of testing concepts and ideas.

### Other Functions

• Fantasy helps us master negative emotions and events. If we're very depressed over a loss or other unhappy event, we can allow ourselves to feel better by imagining something that makes us feel good. Fantasy can relieve boredom or an unpleasant experience. We've all fantasized through a traffic jam.

• Fantasizing can mean the difference between life and death in truly traumatic situations—war, solitary confinement, etc. Diaries of concentration camp survivors attest to this.

• In sex, fantasy has been touted as an enhancer of pleasure. How much of this is helpful is disputable. Fantasy during sex can be one way of tuning out and avoiding intimacy with the other person. Better: Sharing sexual fantasies to enhance intimacy.

• Fantasy has a reparative function. Many people who have had unhappy childhoods go through life blaming their parents, which is nonfunctional. Fantasy can help us—not to re-create the past, but to make more sense of it and restructure the way we see it.

Example: We forget things our parents did that were nice. In order to see the past as having been good, as well as bad, we might imagine something good they did, even if it is a fantasy, because it's probably built in part on something that actually happened.

• Love relationships are predicated on fantasy. We project onto the loved one our fantasy of the ideal lover. This is an obstruction in one way, because it keeps us from seeing the real person, but if we didn't do it, we wouldn't fall in love at all. That's why fantasy always has to be checked by reality. Without fantasy, we'd never get involved, but to stay involved, we have to switch to reality.

• Fantasy displaces fear. We displace frightening things through fantasy as adults, just as we did as children. Paranoid persons do it by fantasizing people who are out to destroy them, while it's really their own aggression displaced onto other people. Ordinary people, on the other hand, imagine that harmful things will happen elsewhere—that someone else and not them will have a car accident, for instance.

### The Danger of Fantasy

Fantasy must always be tempered by reality in order to remain a positive force. A child who fantasizes that he's Superman must realize he isn't Superman or he might wind up jumping off a ledge.

When children's real lives are extremely traumatic, they may withdraw into a fantasy world and stay there, becoming psychotic. Adults also become psychotic when their fantasy lives take over to the exclusion of reality.

When we retreat into a fantasy world untempered by reality, there is the real danger of becoming nonfunctional—not getting out of bed in the morning or not taking care of the routine matters that ensure our daily existence.

Example: We may fantasize that a deceased loved person is still alive. Up to a point this can be normal, at least during acute mourning, but if it continues, professional help is needed. When the deceased is hallucinated as actually present, there is the risk of irretrievably crossing the frontier between reality and nonreality, "normality" and psychosis.

Grandiose fantasies are also a problem. If we have a vision of ourselves as something we can't be, we might become seriously depressed.

It's crucial to maintain the fantasy/reality balance in our lives.

**Source:** Interview with Simone F. Sternberg, Ph.D., a psychotherapist and psychoanalyst in private practice with both children and adults in New York.

## DAYDREAMING'S NOT A WASTE OF TIME

Daydreaming isn't a form of laziness or irresponsibility. It's more than just a pleasure you allow yourself occasionally. Daydreams are necessary for your health, happiness and creativity. Not only do they provide opportunities to lower stress, but you can use them to rehearse the emotions of a scene. . .flash back to relive your first romance. . .flash forward to punch the boss in the nose without facing the consequences of either scene.

**Source:** *Whole-Brain Thinking* by Jacquelyn Wonder, William Morrow & Co., New York.

• Daydreams help to reduce restlessness, tension and depression. Bizarre fantasies can provide a harmless outlet for anger. And daydreams about activities—whether work or a softball game—can actually help you perform those activities better. An obsessive daydream may mean you have an important problem that needs to be resolved.

**Source:** *The New York Times Guide to Personal Health* by Jane Brody, Avon Books, New York.

## SHOULD YOU BE DEPENDENT ON YOUR SPOUSE?

Strong men who are towers of strength in business may cave in if something goes wrong in their personal lives. Since they don't feel free to be dependent on anyone at work, they must establish relationships elsewhere to satisfy their dependency needs. A wife is an obvious choice. But being too dependent on one's wife can be psychological dynamite in the event of separation, divorce or death. What this type of man actually needs: A wide range of dependencies—friends, colleagues and family.

**Source:** *Levinson Letter.*

## MACHISMO TRAP

The strong silent type pays for his machismo with a shorter life span. Reasons: This "typical" male often ignores his health, takes more risks (in driving or sports), bottles up his emotions, and reacts to stress by drinking , smoking or overeating. By denying his vulnerability, he's pretending he's immortal. His body, of course, has no such illusions.

**Source:** Dr. Marc B. Lipton, psychologist, Johns Hopkins University.

## HOW TO BE EMOTIONALLY INTIMATE

Physical intimacy—touching, hugging, caressing—is not the highest level of communication. While physical communication is more intimate than intellectual communication, the highest level of all is emotional intimacy. Most people, unfortunately, haven't been taught to be emotionally intimate. Emotional intimacy is more than sharing a daily life with another person. It involves sharing on an inner level, valuing human relationships above all and being mutually available without criticism.

There can't be a really intimate relationship between a superior and an inferior.

**Source:** *Successful Saleswoman.*

## HOW THE SEXES VIEW EMOTIONAL SUPPORT

Emotional attachment is not always viewed in the same way by men as by women. Insight: The apparent independence of men is based on their feeling that they will be cared for by a woman. The certainty that another person will supply emotional support permits this independence. Contrast: Young girls learn early that they must rely on themselves. They sense that no one else will take care of them emotionally. Result: Women in counseling often equate the expectation of emotional care from another person with weakness and childishness.

**Source:** *What Do Women Want? Exploding the Myth of Dependency* by S. Orbach and L. Eichenbaum, Putnam, New York.

## DEPRESSION MYTHS AND REALITIES

Common as it is, depression is shrouded in popular misconceptions. Whether short-term and mild or more serious and longer-lasting, those feelings of low self-esteem, aimlessness and conviction that nothing much is worth doing afflict many people periodically. Depression needs to be understood for what it is.

### Major Fallacious Notions
• If you're feeling depressed, the cause must be psychological. Fact: Not necessarily. Many psychiatrists consider much emotional distress to be caused by genetically inherited body chemistry. Also, a variety of physical illnesses, such as viral infections, can cause low psychological moods for a period.

• People who lack ego strength and character are more likely to get depressed than those with strong personalities. Fact: If anything, it's the strongest characters who are most subject to feelings of depression and low periods. Reason: Loss of self-esteem is one of the main causes of depression. People who might be described as weak personalities are generally more content with what they are. Strong personalities have very high standards of success and morality. They take themselves seriously and have high competitive and ego needs, all of which make them more vulnerable to feelings of depression.

• Men and women are equally susceptible to depression. Fact: Women are more likely, by a ratio of two to one, to develop feelings of depression. On the other hand, men tend to have more serious depressions and a higher rate of suicide. Possible reason: Men are much less likely than women to seek professional help.

• Depression will affect you psychologically but not physically. Fact: Prolonged and serious periods of depression can result in weight loss, sleeplessness and other stress that can make the sufferer vulnerable to serious physical problems. There is a high correlation between emotional distress and heart attacks, multiple sclerosis and other illnesses. People who have begun to get help for their emotional problems often notice, quite soon, that they don't get as many colds as before, for example.

• Falling in love will lift you out of depression. Fact: People who are feeling low and emotionally distressed are too internally preoccupied to be either very interested or successful in handling relationships. When you're at an emotional low point, you see others in a much darker, more pessimistic way. Usual distortion of this mood: "Anyone I like, anyone worthwhile, wouldn't be interested in me." Feelings of depression also cause a decrease in the sexual impulse.

• Help for depression can come only from long-term psychotherapy. Fact: There are ways of combating depression effectively that don't require long-term therapy. Anti-depressant drug therapy may lift a depression in several weeks. People who are having a mild, short-term depression may profit from seeing a therapist or a counselor for a period, in order to help themselves to understand the dynamics of their feelings and the causes. Such periods usually will end of themselves. However, serious and disabling depression that continues for months does call for professional treatment.

• Tranquilizers will help you combat feelings of depression. Fact: People who take Valium or alcohol to overcome feelings of depression are only magnifying the problem. These are both depressants themselves, as are all tranquilizers. The only medications that work are the antidepressant drugs, which must be carefully prescribed.

• The cause of your depression is usually obvious. Fact: The cause that seems most obvious is most often not the real one. Reason: Depression has to do with unconscious conflict. For example, one of the frequent causes of depression is repressed hostility. When that hostility is acknowledged, the depression usually lifts. (The person has ceased attacking himself as a substitute for expressing his real hostility to his employer, wife, etc.).

• You always know when you are depressed. Fact: There are common forms of depression in which people do not know how they feel. Such people express their depression in other ways. Example: Obese people often may not feel depressed, but their obesity is the equivalent. The same holds true of alcoholics. People who feel their depression have a greater advantage because they at least have a chance to do something about it.

• There are usually some after-effects from depression. Fact: It's possible, after a period of feeling depressed, to jump right back to where you were with no residuals. Depression does not change the psyche.

**To Cope with Depression**

• Avoid isolation. Talk with someone who can provide counsel. If a period of depression lasts for more than a few weeks, or if your ability to function is impaired, more professional help is needed.

• Recognize that your outlook during a low period is going to be pessimistic and distorted. In such a period, your judgments of yourself, of your situation and of other people are not based on reality.

• Difficult as it may be, try to be active, do things and see people. People who are most successful at coping with feelings of depression are those who fight them.

**Source:** Interview with Michael Levy, M.D., a psychiatrist in private practice in New York.

# DRUGS THAT FIGHT DEPRESSION

An estimated 12 million Americans suffer from serious, life-disrupting depression. The good news: Most cases of this devastating mental disease are treatable. A major breakthrough has been the discovery that much depressive illness is biologically determined and responds to antidepressant medications. In fact, if someone has suffered from a continuous depression for a month or more, chances are a biological factor is at work, and an antidepressant will help. An effective antidepressant begins to work within six weeks.

### Major Types of Depression and Antidepressants

*Bipolar* depression, with its wild swings from manic stages to deep depression, is relatively rare. Treatment with lithium allows many manic-depressives to lead normal lives with only periodic visits to a doctor to have their blood levels checked.

*Unipolar* depression involves no contrasting highs. Much more common, it takes a number of forms, including the depression that follows the death of someone close or serious emotional stress. This reactive depression seldom requires medication. Unipolar depressions that do respond to antidepressant drugs:

• *Chronic endogenous* depression is a biologically involved illness characterized by loss of interest and pleasure in life, food and sex and an inability to sleep or to concentrate. Left alone, it can become very serious. Treatment with one of the tricyclic antidepressants (Elavil or Tofranil) is very effective.

• *Phasic endogenous* depression, another biologically involved illness, staggers clearly defined episodes of depression with periods of normalcy. The tricyclic antidepressants are helpful in treatment.

• *Atypical* depression is similar to other types of depression in some ways—patients show little interest in life or sex—but very different in other ways. Patients sleep and eat too much and are extremely lethargic. Most successful treatment: The monoamine oxidase inhibitors (MAOI) such as Nardil and Parnate.

**Source:** Interview with Fred Quitkin, M.D., director of the Depression Evaluation Service, New York State Psychiatric Institute, Columbia Presbyterian Hospital, New York.

## THE IMPORTANCE OF HOPE

Hope sustains life. Hopelessness is a prelude to death. That startling premise is the conviction of a practicing physician/psychiatrist. People can change a negative passivity into an assertive way of life. Awakened hope is possible if you work for it.

There are two kinds of hope, one positive, one negative. Active hope: An inner force that moves the will to action. Those with active hope make dreams come true. Passive hope: Nonaction or inhibited action. It is the attitude of those who dream their lives away. It may signal an unconscious preoccupation with death. Passive hopers never spread their wings. When dreams give out, they may sink into a depression.

Depression is a morbid sadness. It is different from grief, which is realistic. Main causes of depression:

• Failure in sexual functioning.

• Criticism from others and the risk of rejection.

• Lack of success, as judged by one's self or measured by professional standards.

• Success itself, when the person feels unworthy of praise or prosperity.

• Failure to act when action is necessary.

Steps to a happier existence:

• Try to understand the deep causes of your fears.

• When your brain is clear, write down a program of action for times of confusion.

• If necessary, seek professional help.

**Source:** *Hope: The Dynamics of Self-Fulfillment* by Arnold A. Hutschnecker, M.D., G.P. Putnam's Sons, New York.

## Rx FOR DEPRESSION

Head off depression by isolating and then discarding your "favorite" bad feeling, the one you fall back on in most unpleasant situations—anger, envy, etc. Write a list of all the ways you can make yourself feel that emotion. Then write a second list of the ways you can deal with that emotion and get back to feeling happy. Use the second list whenever needed.

**Source:** Gisele Richardson, Richardson Management Associates, Montreal.

## THE DEPRESSION/PAIN CONNECTION

Many patients with chronic pain have associated depression, often secondary to the pain. The depression in turn makes the feelings of pain worse. By treating the depression, one can often decrease the need for narcotics and other pain medications.

## WHAT KINDS OF EXERCISE FIGHT DEPRESSION?

• Vigorous exercise is a good antidote for occasional depression. When depressed women pedaled a stationary bike four times a week, their mood improved with their fitness. Essential: Aerobic intensity. Light exercise that doesn't raise the pulse has little effect on mood.

**Source:** Study by Elizabeth Doyne, M.D., University of Rochester, Rochester, NY.

• Jogging can be an effective treatment for depression. Doctors discovered that jogging often leads to a natural high which can be effective as a treatment for the low of depression. Forty-five minutes of moderate to heavy exercise or an hour of brisk walking four to six times a week is adequate to produce this high. In addition, many drug-addicted individuals have used the exercise program with great success.

**Source:** Dennis Coffee, M.D., Del Amo Hospital, Torrance, CA.

## DEPRESSED PEOPLE MAY BE SUFFERING A CHEMICAL IMBALANCE

A chemical deficiency in the brain may be the key both to depression and suicide. In a study of brain samples from 11 suicide victims, researchers found almost 44% more serotonin receptors than in a control group. This was an apparent compensation by the brain to absorb what little of the chemical there was.

**Source:** *The Lancet,* London.

## DO-IT-YOURSELF-DEPRESSION TEST

If you're depressed for no good reason, it might be a hormone deficiency. How to check: Place an oral thermometer on your bedside table. As soon as you awaken, tuck the thermometer into your armpit for 10 minutes. A temperature below 97.8 may point to low thyroid or adrenal activity. Possible treatment: Prescribed medication.

**Source:** Dr.Stephen Langer, Berkeley, CA, quoted in *Family Circle.*

## WHY SUNLIGHT IS NECESSARY FOR YOUR MENTAL HEALTH

Natural-light deprivation causes depression. The less you are exposed to natural unfiltered light, the more depressed you are likely to feel. Sunlight appears to stimulate the production of melatonin, a hormone that influences mood, sleep and fertility. Normal artificial light does not provide the spectrum of light needed. Solution: Try to spend at least 15 minutes a day outside, or install a full-spectrum light bulb that provides light similar to the sun's.

**Source:** Duro-Lite Lamps, Inc., North Bergen, NJ.

## WHO CHOOSES SUICIDE?

• About four times as many men as women commit suicide. But almost three times as many women attempt suicide. Most suicides occur in the spring, but there is usually a rash of them around Christmas. Favorite methods: Women prefer toxic substances. Men go for violent means, such as guns or leaps. Lowest suicide rate: Married people. Note: Each rise of a single percentage point in the national employment rate brings an additional 318 suicides.

**Source:** *Dealing with the Crisis of Suicide* by Calvin J. Frederick, Public Affairs Pamphlets, New York.

• Suicide among young people age 15–24 has risen 300% in recent years. Suspected factors: Death of a parent in childhood or adolescence, scattering of the family, passivity and social detachment. The highest suicide rate is still held by older whites. Suicidal patients of all ages are not only depressed…they're also evasive, angry, manipulative, provocative, withdrawn and help-rejecting. Sad: Suicide-prevention centers have not lowered the suicide rates.

**Source:** *Suicide in America* by Herbert Hendin, W.W. Norton, New York.

• Psychiatric patients with a family history of suicide are at very high risk for suicide attempts. In one study, 49% of these patients had attempted suicide. Early parental loss (before age 11) is also associated with attempted suicide. Aggressive treatment is warranted when an individual with a family history of suicide or early parent death exhibits suicidal preoccupation.

**Source:** *Archives of General Psychiatry,* New York.

# THE BRAIN/IMMUNE SYSTEM CONNECTION

Exciting new research into the immune system has proved a definite link between the brain and the body's ability to fight disease. Does this mean that as individuals we now have the power to avoid or cure ourselves of cancer or other dreaded diseases? We're not at that stage yet, but all the indicators are good that medicine will soon find a way to use the human mind to heal the body.

To find out more about how the mind and body interact, we interviewed psychologist Dr. Robert Ader and immunologist Dr. Nicholas Cohen of the University of Rochester, who pioneered much of the most convincing research in this area.

How did you make your basic discovery about the brain/immune system connection?

Actually, it was by accident. We conditioned an aversion to saccharin in rats by injecting them with a substance that gave them a stomach ache after they drank saccharin. During the course of the experiment, some of the rats died for no obvious reason. We found that the animals had not only learned to avoid the saccharin solution but had learned to impair their immune systems' competence as well. This was due to a second property of the drug that suppressed the immune system. The rats had apparently learned to associate the suppression of their immune systems' competence with saccharin also. So at the same time that we were conditioning an aversion to saccharin in the rats, we were also inadvertently conditioning the suppression of their immune systems. If immunity were suppressed, the animals might have been more vulnerable to any disease-causing agents in the environment. The data we gathered opened up a whole new area of research with respect to the relationship between the brain and the immune system.

Hadn't this connection ever been investigated before?

No. It challenged a cherished assumption that has always existed in immunology—that the immune system is an independent agency of defense against disease; that it is self-regulating and not influenced by any other systems. Now we come along and say, wait a second, that assumption may not be true. We proved that the immune system, like any other system of the body, is integrated and interacts with all other systems, and thus is regulated by the brain. The reason we know so little is that nobody ever asked these questions before. What we've done simply indicates that, just as it's possible to condition behavioral and physiological responses, it's also possible to condition changes in immune response. It means that the immune system may be one of the means by which psychological factors influence disease susceptibility. There is already solid evidence for the influence of psychosocial factors on the hormone and central nervous systems as they relate to disease. But up until now, the immune system was—well, immune.

Have studies been done on people?

The human studies that have been done usually relate specifically to stress, rather than being an attempt to understand how the brain influences the immune system. For obvious reasons, people can only be studied after the fact. There is new evidence from Australia and the work of Dr. Marvin Stein at Mt. Sinai Hospital in New York City that stress is associated with changes in immune function. The Mt. Sinai study is the primary example. They picked a group of subjects under severe stress—men whose wives had died of cancer—and found that their immune response was markedly lowered during the first two months after the wife's death. Normal response returned about four months later. A long-term study will show whether that depression in immune response alters susceptibility to disease.

There has been a lot of controversy about the mind/body connection in regard to cancer, especially when it comes to alternative treatments. Cancer victims tell of being cured by methods such as change in diet and lowered stress. What do you think of such treatments?

It's one thing to describe case histories and another to provide unequivocal data of a causal chain of events. But to deny the existence of such phenomena is to hide your head in the sand. There's no question that such cures sometimes work. We simply don't understand *how.* I don't think certain alternative cancer therapies can do any harm, and I see no reason why it shouldn't be employed as an adjunct to—but not instead of—more traditional cancer therapy.

Is there a relationship between the immune system and heart disease?

Maybe. Some data suggest an immunological involvement in a lot of diseases that previously we didn't think were related to the immune system. Examples are atherosclerosis and some forms of diabetes. Getting the most attention at the moment are AIDS (acquired immune deficiency syndrome) and herpes, both of which have an immunological component.

Are any personality traits associated with lowered immunity?

That's the jump people are making. They take one from column A and two from column B and put it all together before any data exist. There are no good data yet on the relationship of personality characteristics to immune function.

Will people eventually learn to regulate their own immune systems?

It's theoretically possible, but it would be far more difficult than regulating responses such as blood pressure or heart rate. A primary reason is that the ability to feed back changes within the immune system, or even in the hormone system, is not technically feasible at the moment. With the nervous system, for example, rapid feedback can be given in the form of electrical impulses. If you could translate hormonal or immunological changes into a rapid feedback system, self-regulation might be possible. But there's not likely to be such a system for several years.

Do you think the Far East, whose yogis can control functions such as breathing and heart rate, has something to teach us in this area?

There's no question that mind and body are inseparable. Unfortunately, we've become very chauvinistic about things Western, which does not, by definition, make them better. We are missing out on

a great deal of human potential by not studying such phenomena. The ability to regulate internal states behaviorally is an established fact—and it's an ability that can be learned.

**Source:** Interview with Robert Ader, M.D., department of psychiatry, and Nicholas Cohen, M.D., department of immunology, University of Rochester Medical Center, Rochester, NY.

## WHY UNEMPLOYMENT MAY BE BAD FOR YOUR HEALTH

Unemployment greatly increases the risk of hospitalization. Workers who are unemployed more than 50% of the time are seven times more likely to enter a psychiatric clinic than those who are regularly employed. And the chance of admission to medical and surgical wards is almost twice as high among the chronically unemployed.

**Source:** A survey of bricklayers in Risskov, Denmark, as reported in the *Journal of the American Medical Association,* Chicago, IL.

## WHAT DOCTORS DON'T ALWAYS TELL YOU

Why is the mind/body connection playing a more prominent role in medicine today?

Antibiotics and modern medical technology have wiped out the infectious diseases that were major killers in the past. The treatment of disease today can no longer be a matter of finding the "magic bullet." People don't die quickly any more. They tend to live for a long time with chronic illnesses. Examples: Diabetes, arthritis, heart disease, multiple sclerosis, respiratory disease, ulcers and even cancer, which may go into and out of remission. Treating a chronically ill patient is a matter of dealing with that person's whole life: Body, mind and spirit. Not only drugs but also adjustments in lifestyle, family patterns, exercise, diet, stress management and coping techniques must be used against such diseases.

Why have doctors been so resistant to this approach?

The new techniques haven't been around long enough or been sufficiently tested to make doctors feel comfortable with them. Although people who have undergone these treatments are often very enthusiastic, their experiences are anecdotal. Systematic independent evaluation is necessary to separate the wheat from the chaff. That's one reason our institute was founded—to filter out what works from what doesn't and to legitimize the effective techniques so the mainstream medical establishment will start taking them seriously.

How is this going to happen?

It's very important to build bridges. It's not an adversarial process, with the doctors on one side and the "flakes" on the other, even though some of the spokespeople from both are rigid and adversarial. In the past five years, the walls between the two camps have eroded, and there's been a lot of crossover. One reason: The medical consumer is becoming more aware and wants to understand what's happening. Patients have become less likely to accept whatever their doctor tells them blindly.

What are you looking into now?

We're looking at a whole range of treatments, most of which are psychological or behavioral. We're examining biofeedback, relaxation exercises, meditation, imagery and visualization exercises, and various techniques grouped under stress management. We're also interested in the effects of exercise and diet on the healing process.

Which branch of medicine is most responsive to your point of view?

Family practitioners. It's very interesting that recently there's been a resurgence of family practice. Harvard Medical School, among others, is seeing growth in that specialty, although it had virtually disappeared. The young students in family practice are criticizing medicine's over-reliance on technology, and they're pushing for a more humanistic approach. Also, doctors who treat chronic diseases are increasingly discovering that their treatments are more successful if they take the broader perspective into consideration. Even the most technical specialties, such as surgery and anesthesiology, are being affected. Recent research has found that patients who are under anesthesia at some level "hear" what is being said in the operating room. So, if the surgeon remarks, "Looks like this guy isn't going to make it," that comment becomes a serious matter.

Can you mention some other interesting discoveries that have been made in this field?

There is some evidence that immune system levels are positively affected by imagery and visualization exercises. In these, the patient concentrates on a mental image of his body healing itself. A good number of studies have showed that diabetes, heart disease, postsurgical recovery and even arthritis can be markedly improved with relaxation exercises. Some kind of relaxation regimen seems to help most people. A number of studies have been seeking to pinpoint the particular characteristic that makes some people more responsive than others to stress-management techniques. What seems to be important is the individual's sense of control. This is why the partnership between the doctor and patient is so important. The patient who participates in the healing process is the one who gets better.

How about the placebo effect?

Placebo is being taken seriously as a phenomenon. Positive suggestion definitely helps people get better. If you use a drug plus a placebo, you get a better response than by using either singly. On the other hand, a negative suggestion can cancel out the effect of a drug. The context in which treatment is given is very important. The placebo effect brings up ethical issues, however. Do you give everyone a sugar pill and say, "This is going to make you better"?

Then there's the miracle-cure phenomenon. The patient doesn't know what's wrong. His treatment hasn't worked so far. Then his doctor walks in, flanked by two important-looking specialists, and they tell him he's had a new treatment that has cured everyone. How can the guy not get better? He'd be letting down the medical establishment. It is a known phenomenon that a drug works better when it's first discovered. The excitement of something new is a powerful positive suggestion.

How can people help themselves?

Always get a second opinion. This can't be emphasized enough. Not only may your doctor be wrong, but it gives you a feeling of participating in the decision. And with so many options today, there's tremendous room for disagreement. Medical history is rife with interventions that have gone out of fashion. (Just a few examples are lobotomies, hysterectomies, radical mastectomies, cesarean sections and coronary-bypass surgery.) In his book *The Healing Heart,* Norman Cousins speaks about his own heart attack. He was told he would be dead in a year without bypass surgery. Three years later he's still around.

It's also important to find a doctor with whom you can enter into a partnership—someone who makes you feel comfortable and informed. Doctors are increasingly urged to get into this kind of relationship with patients.

Finally, you must start seeing health as an ongoing part of your lifestyle. If you attend to your diet, exercise, work and family patterns, it can have a lot to do with getting sick less often.

**Source:** Inteview with M. Barry Flint, executive director, The Institute for the Advancement of Health, New York.

# SOME REASONS TO CONSIDER ACUPUNCTURE

Many health problems can be helped by acupuncture. The sex and age of patients are not important factors, but their attitude is. They must not fight the treatment mentally. They should be believers.

The sensation of the needles varies among patients. Some feel only the slightest prick and others find it painful. The more pain a patient feels, the more resistance and stress there are in the related part of the body. As in deep massage, where the patient must "work through" the pain to get real relief, we help him get through the painful part of acupuncture until he gets some positive effect. Actually, acupuncture goes even deeper than massage because it stimulates the nervous system.

**Problems That Respond to Acupuncture**

• Back pain. First, we ease the discomfort by working on the circulation in the spinal area. Then we try to analyze the cause of the problem. It could be posture, weight, or a poor mattress. Or the patient may need a better diet and more exercise. The object is to keep the pain from recurring. Success rate: 95%.

• Insomnia. We try to relax the natural functions of the body through the nerve system to get the patient into a natural rhythm of feeling energetic when he wakes up and sleepy at night. Success rate: 90%.

• Addictions: Whether the substance is cocaine or nicotine, the user must want to shake the habit. Acupuncture helps people get into a healthier, more energetic cycle. When cocaine users feel good naturally, they won't need the high from the drug. With smokers, we try to counteract nicotine withdrawal symptoms by reprogramming nerves to the lungs and the adrenal gland. Success rate with patients who really want to quit: 80%.

• Excess weight. Businesspeople do a lot of nervous eating. Acupuncture relaxes them and strengthens their sense of well-being. They can then better burn off fat and control eating. Success rate: 80%.

• Depression. Many people don't know how to cope in our kinetic society. They tire and get nervous too easily. We give them more energy with acupuncture and a combination of herbs and vitamins. Success rate: 80%.

• Hearing loss. We can help if the problem is the result of some (but not all) kinds of nerve damage. Success rate for hearing improvement: 80%.

• Impotence: Sometimes people lose sensitivity and desire because they are tired. Acupuncture can contribute to general well-being and appetite and can specifically stimulate the nerves of the sex areas. Success rate: 70%.

• Hair loss. Acupuncture can increase circulation to the scalp and may be helpful to men under 50. I take this treatment myself as a preventive measure.

### General Therapy

Acupuncture should be your first therapy rather than a last resort. We recommend monthly treatments for general good health. These "tune-up" sessions rejuvenate the thyroid, lymph and digestive glands to head off other problems before they surface. For a specific problem, such as back pain, patients usually need 10 visits for sustained relief. Expect to pay around $50 for a visit of 45-60 minutes.

Look for a good acupuncturist who is certified by your state's licensing board. If you find a practitioner by word of mouth, be sure he has the proper credentials.

**Source:** Interview with Zion Yu, a 20th-generation acupuncturist in Beverly Hills, CA.

# WHAT ISAAC ASIMOV BELIEVES

Do you believe in the power of witch doctors to cure people or strike them dead?

Of course. That sort of thinking works not only in New Guinea or Africa but even in our own culture. If the doctor tells you you're going to be all right—the operation worked, this medicine will surely help you—your chances of surviving increase. If you are told, "I'm terribly sorry, but you'd better make out your will," your chances decrease. I suppose it's quite clear that the mind does have an effect on the body, that the will to live is important, and that a cheerful disposition will help you more than an apprehensive one.

And if you are told that you will die next April 17 and thoroughly believe it, I wouldn't be surprised if you did. That's the well-known phenomenon of death by suggestion.

What about witches?

My feeling is that witches are practitioners of a religion that is not the religion of the person labeling them witches. Witches pretend—or are believed—to control the universe, in a way. They have spells and enchantments that will cause the gods or demons to do their will. And, of course, if they don't use the precise magic that you use, you'll feel that they're serving the devil, and they're evil. You yourself have different spells, different magic. You call your people "priests" and you say that they are serving God. But one man's witch is another man's priest.

During World War II, weren't the English witches enlisted to brew up storms so the Germans couldn't send their invasion army?

In various countries and houses of worship, people get together to perform spells and say prayers. When they work, you remember them. You try to influence the course of the war by praying against the enemy. Prayer is legally permissible witchcraft, and, conversely, witchcraft is prohibited religious practice. Prayer doesn't work any better than any other kind of witchcraft, either.

Do you believe in firewalking?

James Randi, author of *Flim-Flam: Psychics, ESP, Unicorns and Other Delusions** and famed debunker of Uri Geller, watched people walk on hot coals without injury, and he admitted that he couldn't understand it. I don't know that I can explain it either. I presume there are people who can do it. There are all sorts of theories that the perspiration on the feet protects them, but I don't know whether anyone really understands how firewalking works.

Can you expound on other ways the mind influences and heals the body?

The mind is part of the body; the body is part of the mind. There's no question that mental attitudes can affect the body.

Do you agree with Norman Cousins that watching Marx Brothers films can help cure an illness?

I suppose that pleasure produces a bodily state that is more conducive to curing. Maybe it affects your immune mechanisms favorably. It surely can't hurt! Personally, I am perfectly convinced that I'm never going to catch the flu. The last time I had the flu was in 1937. While I can't believe completely that it's a matter of mind over body, nevertheless, the fact that I'm always confident about not catching the flu helps me.

How much can the mind cure the body?

I suspect that its influence is important. A healthy mind helps one have a healthy body. I agree with Norman Cousins that cheerful, happy people have fewer health problems than miserable people. Of course, there are also people who enjoy being sick, but that's another subject.

And the laying on of hands?

The laying on of hands is another facet of the influence of the mind over the body. If you really believe that a person has some sort of conduit to powers beyond, and that if he puts his hands on you somehow goodness will flow from the infinite into you, it increases your security and your certainty of getting better. It will help, perhaps.

I think much the same thing happens when a doctor gives you a placebo—when he feels that there's nothing very seriously wrong with you but you believe there is. You won't feel comfortable unless the doctor does something obvious, like giving you an injection or an antibiotic. Even just a sugar solution will make you feel a lot better. The laying on of hands comes under the same category.

\* Prometheus Books, Buffalo, NY.

**Source:** Interview with Isaac Asimov, biochemist, teacher and prolific writer of both science fiction and science for the layperson.

## SURVIVAL TECHNIQUE

Denying the seriousness of an illness often helps a patient survive. This denial is a coping mechanism that enables some people to put aside their fears. Result: Less stress, which encourages healing. Those with the ability to deny are usually born so.

**Source:** Thomas P. Hackett, M.D., professor of psychiatry at Harvard Medical School and chief of psychiatry at Massachusetts General Hospital, Boston.

## THE HEALING POWER OF HOPE

Hope helps heal the sick and may even keep you from getting ill in the first place. Heart disease and sudden death are more likely to strike a person who is troubled by bereavement, divorce, business failure or retirement. Cancer victims with high "hope scores" did significantly better in fighting their disease.

**Source:** Studies by the American Psychiatric Association, cited in *Medical World News,* Houston, TX.

## BETTER HEALTH THROUGH RELAXATION RESPONSE

Most of us have experienced the power our minds can exert over our bodies. You dream that you are being chased—and awaken perspiring, your heart pounding in your chest. A mosquito buzzes in your ear—and soon you are scratching all over. You feel insects crawling on your skin, even when nothing is there!

Audiences at *Lawrence of Arabia* flocked to buy drinks. These moviegoers were not really suffering from a lack of liquids, but their identification with scenes of hot deserts provoked in them overwhelming thirst.

Conditions our minds perceive to be real become real for our bodies through the messages transmitted by our brains.

### The Faith Factor

Physicians have long been aware of the importance of their patients' beliefs in effecting cures—from the life-preserving will to live to the less dramatic but much more common placebo effect, in which a patient believes a treatment will help him, and therefore it does.

It has been estimated, in fact, that 75% of all patients who visit their doctors have conditions that will eventually get better by themselves. Only 25% are illnesses or injuries that require specific medication or surgery.

For many, the simple act of seeing a trusted physician is enough to bring relief. The doctor's reassuring manner interacts with the patient's faith in modern medicine and in his doctor's ability, producing measurable physiological changes in the patient.

Even without direct medical intervention, the patient's condition improves. Any treatment is likely to have greater success if the patient has a profound faith in his physician's efficacy or a belief that a higher spiritual force is at work in his body.

### The Relaxation Response

Deep relaxation or meditation also produces physiological changes in the body. . . lowered heart rate and blood pressure, slowed breathing and brain waves, and a generally reduced rate of metabolism. Physicians call this set of physiological changes the *relaxation response.*

The process reverses the self-perpetuating cycle of anxiety, in which worries trigger the central nervous system to react (heart rate and blood pressure increase, intensifying anxiety, which again triggers the central nervous system . . . aggravating the symptoms of stress-related ills).

Regular practice of the relaxation-response technique has proven benefits: Relief from headaches, backaches, hypertension, hyperventilation, panic attacks and insomnia; reduction of high blood pressure, angina pectoris pain and cholesterol levels; enhancement of cancer therapy and other specific treatments; increased inner peace and emotional balance.

The procedure is simple:

(1) Assume a comfortable position in a quiet environment.

(2) Close your eyes and consciously relax your muscles.

(3) Breathe slowly and naturally.

(4) On the exhale, repeat a focus word or phrase of your own choosing.

(5) Maintain a passive attitude, gently dismissing intrusive thoughts and returning to your focus word.

(6) Continue for 10–20 minutes, once or twice a day.

### Combining the Relaxation Response with the Faith Factor

The human mind exerts its power over the body better when it is provided with a positive focus for belief—faith in a healer or a pill, for example. Likewise, patients show improved response to the relaxation-response technique when they choose a positive focus word or phrase that has deep personal meaning. (Avoid words such as health or calm, which might draw your attention to your medical problems.)

Example: A Greek Orthodox patient was told to practice his relaxation-response technique. His doctor suggested that he focus on the number *one.* A few days later his condition had worsened. The doctor learned that the patient had negative associations with the word one, and together they arrived at *Kyrie eleison.** The patient then improved rapidly.

Choosing a focus word or phrase with personal meaning can activate and reinforce your belief system, providing a more calming effect on your mind than a neutral—or negative—focus word. But more importantly, it will increase the likelihood of your regular practice of the technique.

### Suggestions

The technique works best on an empty stomach, so plan your sessions accordingly.

Try to suspend your expectations, and do not worry about how well you are doing. Noticeable results may take four to six weeks—or longer—so allow your practice to become as routine as brushing your teeth.

It is normal for your mind to wander. When thoughts intrude, quietly return to your silent repetition.

Place a clock or a watch where you can peek at it. (Don't set a jarring alarm.)

Allow yourself a few minutes when your session is over to just sit quietly with your eyes closed. Jumping immediately to your feet may produce a slight dizziness.

The ultimate benefit of the relaxation-response technique is to reinforce your belief in your body's capacity to heal itself— and thereby its ability to do so.

*Lord, have mercy.

**Source:** Interview with Herbert Benson, M.D., associate professor of medicine at the Harvard Medical School and director of the division of behavioral medicine and hypertension at Boston's Beth Israel Hospital.

## KISS OF DEATH

Strong, supportive families have always been assumed to sustain the chronically ill. Surprise: In a recent study of dialysis patients, those who enjoy close family ties suffered more complications and died sooner. Probable reason: When family members interact well, a chronic illness is a more profound stress on the entire unit. In such a case, death may represent a collaboration—the patient dies so the family can survive.

**Source:** Research by David Reiss, M.D., of the Family Research Center, George Washington University, in *Medical World News*, New York.

## GRIEF KILLS

Husbands whose wives died still had suppressed immune systems two months after the deaths. Their systems were still acting somewhat subnormally a year later, making the men vulnerable to illness and earlier death. Suspected cause: Dysfunction of the hypothalamus, which is also linked with depression and anxiety.

**Source:** Study at Mount Sinai Hospital in New York.

## TRUTH ABOUT MEDITATION

Meditation isn't inherently mystical or religious, though often used for those purposes. Nor is it a problem-solving technique. Actually, the content of your thoughts while meditating isn't important. Meditation is simply an attempt to clear your head of discursive, ruminating thoughts. It can be a very good relaxation technique once you learn to turn off your verbal, symbolic thinking temporarily.

**Source:** Herbert Benson and Miriam Klipper: *The Relaxation Response*, Avon, New York; and Alan Watts, *The Way of Liberation*, Weatherhill, New York.

## BREATHING FOR RELAXATION

One benefit of Zen meditation is the breathing exercise. It helps you clear your mind and relieve stress. Try this exercise when you are tense or need to think more objectively:

First get into a comfortable position, either standing or reclining. Then take a deep breath, slowly, through your nose. Hold the breath for a second and try to push the air down to your stomach. (Your exhalation should be slower than your inhalation.) Important: Concentrate on the flow of your breath going in and out.

**Source:** Interview with Shihan Tadashi Nakamura, founder and chairman of the World Seido Karate Organization in New York.

## HOW HYPNOSIS WORKS

The sharp voice of your boss/teacher/spouse startles you. "You haven't heard a word I've said!" "I'm sorry," you explain. "My mind was on something else."

Sound familiar? If you have been so absorbed in a train of thought that you were barely aware of the activity around you, chances are you were in a state similar, if not identical, to a hypnotic trance.

Trance is a state that occurs naturally in the vast majority of people, a state of aroused intense concentration—the opposite of sleep—that can occur spontaneously whether one intends it or not. And hypnosis is, quite simply, the formal use of this natural capacity for attentive, receptive concentration.

Our everyday consciousness is balanced between whatever our attention is focused on and our awareness of peripheral activity. The hypnotized person is able to focus his attention entirely on a single issue while increasing his peripheral awareness.

Health-care professionals regularly use hypnosis to treat problems ranging from chronic pain to fear of flying. The use of hypnosis is an active part of a wider trend to enlist the strengths and resources of the individual patient in his or her own healing.

Hypnosis is not something that is done *to* you. You are not in someone's power. You do not "go under" or "pass out." Rather, hypnosis seems to be a matter of shifting attention to the right hemisphere of the brain (the side that is more emotional, visual, creative and analogical) while the left brain (verbal, analytical and rational) "idles." Hypnosis is something that people can be taught, quickly and easily, to do for themselves—a technique that can give them greater control over their lives than they have ever had before.

### Who Can Be Hypnotized?

About 30% of people are not hypnotizable. This group includes persons who are mentally ill, who have suffered brain damage, who are of very low intelligence, or whose ability to concentrate has been otherwise impaired. The remaining 70% of the population have a measurable amount of "trance talent." Ten percent of people have the ability to achieve a light trance. They are known as "ones" on a scale of zero to five. About 50% have medium ability. They are the twos and threes. Finally, there are the remaining 10%, the highly hypnotizable fours and the ultra-talented fives.

An individual's capacity for achieving the trance state seems to be a given and does not change appreciably over time.

One indicator of trance capacity is the eye roll. The subject, seated comfortably, is asked to roll his eyes toward the top of his head and at the same time to close his eyelids slowly. The amount of white showing just before the eyes close indicates the degree of trance capacity. "High rollers" (the easily hypnotizable) have no iris showing. "Low rollers" (poor candidates for hypnosis) are barely able to roll their eyes.

Personality traits also indicate trance talent. People with a strong preference for the left-brain mode (practical, analytical) fall on the low side of the scale—the zeros and ones. People who are distinctly right-brained (creative, intuitive) are the fours and fives.

### How Does Treatment Work?

Just because a person has little trance talent does not mean that hypnosis can't help him. Motivation is equally important. For example, a person who is highly motivated to quit smoking through hypnosis has a high probability of success, even if he has only modest trance talent. And motivation can be increased.

Hypnosis increases our responsiveness to suggestion, whether the messages are directed by a hypnotist or later reinforced through self-hypnosis. A general rule for success seems to be to accentuate the positive. Example: Certain therapists use "aversion therapy" to help their hypnotized patients quit smoking by suggesting that cigarettes taste and smell like manure. Although this technique may work briefly, it is rarely effective in the long run because the patient knows the premise to be untrue. A far more successful strategy is to suggest to the smoker that cigarettes are poisonous to the body. . .that we need our bodies to live. . .and that we are responsible for our bodies as for a beloved child or pet.

### Ways Hypnosis Is Helpful

Although hypnosis cannot do anything that psychotherapy can't, it does greatly accelerate the process. Hypnosis has been particularly successful in the following areas:

• Overcoming phobias. The success rate for one-time treatment of fear of flying is higher than for any other clinical syndromes, and many other phobias are overcome with hypnosis.

• Eliminating undesirable habits. Symptoms such as hair-pulling, teeth-grinding and nail-biting are overcome.

• Conquering addictions, such as those to nicotine, food or caffeine. Hypnosis has proved least successful with alcohol and drug problems, possibly because these substances interfere with a person's ability to concentrate.

• Controlling pain. Subjects are taught techniques to "filter the hurt out of the pain" with impressive success. Migraine headaches, childbearing, dental work and, in some cases, even major surgery can be rendered painless, while the subject remains relaxed and awake.

• Mastering insomnia and anxiety. The sensation of "floating," often mentioned to describe the feeling of trance, is particularly useful in problems relating to anxiety. In the "screen technique" a subject is instructed to make his mind a blank screen and to place his anxieties on one half of it while conjuring up a restful scene on the other half. He can then focus entirely on the second screen until he is calm.

• Enhancing concentration, memory and creativity. When the constraints of left-brain thinking are temporarily relaxed, "creative leaps" are facilitated.

As a person gains control over one problem through hypnosis, his self-respect is increased, and he may gain control in other areas.

There do not seem to be any negative effects associated with hypnosis. The Svengali-like hypnotist creating a zombie-killer is pure myth.

Hypnosis by itself is not the same thing as treatment. You don't visit a hypnotist to have a tooth extracted, and you shouldn't expect medical treatment from anyone who is untrained in medicine. Referrals to accredited practitioners of hypnosis can be obtained from your physician or from a professional association.*

Hypnosis is not useful for everyone. But for the 70% of us who are gifted with trance capacity, it is a quick, simple, inexpensive and pleasurable way for us truly to use our minds.

*American Society of Clinical Hypnosis, 2400 E. Devon Ave., Des Plaines, IL 60016. Society for Clinical and Experimental Hypnosis, 129-A Kings Park Dr., Liverpool, NY 13088. International Society of Hypnosis, 111 N. 49 St., Philadelphia 19139.

**Source:** Interview with Herbert Spiegel, M.D., clinical professor at Columbia University's College of Physicians and Surgeons and in private practice in New York.

## SELF-HYPNOSIS SECRETS

The word *hypnosis* is actually a misnomer. The Greek word for sleep, it is actually the opposite of sleep. While hypnotized, you're tuned in to what the hypnotist is saying. It's basically an altered state of consciousness in which there is heightened attention. It is useful for giving yourself certain suggestions that will "take you someplace you want to be."

Hypnosis can be used to help you stop smoking, overeating, using drugs or drinking excessively or to control any other compulsive behavior. It can help you overcome anxiety, give you relief from pain or help you get to sleep. In these stressful times, hypnosis is an invaluable relaxation technique. It uses neither magic nor hocus-pocus, but our untapped human potential to cure some of what ails us.

### Hypnosis at Its Best

As a therapeutic tool, hypnosis is most effective as an adjunct to treatment rather than as a treatment itself. Exception: Pain control or other non-psychological problems that can be helped by hypnosis alone. Many problems that seem simple are actually multi-faceted, and no one-shot treatment can provide a lasting cure.

For any self-hypnosis technique to be meaningful, it must be tailored to you as an individual, to reflect your particular problem. Example:

A man goes to a hypnotist to lose weight because he has a family history of diabetes and is terrified of getting the disease. His self-hypnosis technique will include visualization of an insulin needle, being hooked up to a kidney machine, etc. If you want to lose weight but don't have this particular fear, your technique will be quite different. Each person has to find the one that works best for him or her.

Hypnosis also works as a diagnostic tool to uncover the secret fear that is keeping a person from reaching a goal. I ask my patients while hypnotized to visualize themselves without the problem they've come to me to cure. During the visualization, I ask them, "What's wrong with the picture?" Example:

A happily married overweight woman, when asked what was wrong with the picture while she was visualizing herself at her ideal weight, said, "I'm cheating on my husband because I'm getting more attention from men and feeling sexier." In order for self-hypnosis to work for this woman, she had to confront her fear and deal with what she perceived as a threat to her marriage.

Hypnosis will work only for the highly motivated person who isn't lookng for an instant magic cure but is willing to make some sacrifices to reach the goal.

### Using Images

The visualization of images during self-hypnosis, both negative and positive, is at the heart of the technique. The hypnotist aims to find out what your hot button is. Then you work on coming up with an image that will have a strong impact. You close your eyes and imagine yourself as a character in a movie. Examples:

• You want to stop smoking. Visualize yourself 10 years from now in a chest specialist's waiting room. The receptionist calls you into the doctor's office, telling you your X rays have just been developed. The doctor points to a dark mass on the X ray and tells you it's inoperable. Nothing can be done. You have only six weeks to live, and you'd better start making arrangements for your family.

• You want to lose weight. Visualize yourself at your favorite restaurant with your usual dinner companion. Dinner is over, and the waiter asks if you want dessert. Your partner orders chocolate cake, but you ask just for coffee. See yourself watching that person eating the cake without feeling deprived or competitive.

Important: The scene you visualize should be as detailed as possible. The type of image used will depend on the problem. Negative images can be very useful with something that you can avoid completely, like cigarettes, alcohol or drugs. For such substances, negative imagery also serves as an aversion technique. If you hypnotize yourself and imagine that the first drink will taste like urine, a strong aversion to alcohol can be created.

Negative imagery doesn't work in weight control, however. You can't give up food completely, and no matter how often you imagine a chocolate-chip cookie tasting like sawdust, eventually you'll try one and it will taste good. The point of self-hypnosis for weight control is to take a rational approach to food, so that it becomes just food—not comfort or friendship.

### Hypnotizing Yourself

I teach people self-hypnosis in two or three sessions. During the first session I take a detailed history of the problem in order to tailor the hypnotic routine individually. Then I hypnotize the person, later explaining how it can be done at home, repeating the process until the person feels comfortable doing it alone. How it works:

• Sit down near as little distraction as possible, preferably at night, in a comfortable chair you don't usually sit in. Roll your eyes up, keep them there, take a deep breath and hold it. Close your eyes slowly, exhale very deeply and normally, and concentrate on a floating sensation. Feel the sensation spread from the top of your head to the tips of your toes. Deepen the sensation by visualizing a staircase of ten steps. As you walk down the staircase, the floating sensation doubles with every step. When you get to the bottom, use your visualization exercise.

• Imagine yourself in control. The whole essence of hypnosis is gaining control, and self-hypnosis puts you in perfect control. You're not distracted as at other times, but are totally tuned in to yourself. So use that moment to see yourself in control, able to resist temptation.

### Finding a Reputable Hypnotist

Hypnosis is a field riddled with quacks. There are no officially recognized licensing or accrediting procedures. Anyone can hang out a shingle, claiming to be a graduate of this or that school of hypnosis. It might have been just a mail-order course. Since anyone can learn to hypnotize another person in five minutes, quacks are attracted.

But to be effective, self-hypnosis must be individually structured. That requires education and training. To find a reputable professional, contact the American Psychological Association or the American Psychiatric Association. They will refer you to a psychologist or psychiatrist who is qualified and experienced in hypnosis. Although a variety of professionals (chiropractors, podiatrists, etc.) and non-professionals hold themselves out to the public as hypnotists, you are generally best off going to a qualified mental health professional.

**Source:** Interview with Ronald Jay Cohen, Ph.D., a clinical psychologist in private practice in New York.

# A NEW LOOK AT BIOFEEDBACK

When biofeedback was first introduced in the 1960s, it was touted as a cure-all. When later results from better studies showed that it wasn't as effective as the initial research indicated, it was largely deserted.

Now, with some time and distance from the first enthusiasm, we can see that biofeedback is neither the 20th century's panacea nor a total waste of time. The truth, as always, lies somewhere in between. Biofeedback can have amazing to mediocre results, depending on the disorder being treated and the skill of the person treating it. And practitioners are constantly coming up with new ways to use biofeedback, not only to treat disease but to enhance human potential.

### When to Try Biofeedback

Biofeedback has been shown to be helpful in the following conditions:

• Tension headache. Biofeedback has shown spectacular success in treating this problem and is now one of the treatments of choice. Electrodes on a forehead band are connected to an electromyograph (EMG), which monitors and feeds back muscle-tension levels that are ordinarily too small for the person to notice. Thus he "learns" how to control his tension level.

• Migraine headache. Biofeedback will work in some cases if the migraine sufferer can be trained properly. Migraine, in some cases, is caused by blood rushing through vessels that were previously constricted due to tension. Temperature biofeedback teaches the migraine victim to increase the temperature in his extremities (the tips of

the fingers or feet) when he senses a migraine coming on. This pushes blood away from the head, forestalling the migraine. It doesn't always work. There's still a lot to learn about migraines.

• High blood pressure (essential hypertension). This is a very exciting area in biofeedback because hypertension is such a killer, and many of the drugs used to control it have harmful side effects. The use of the EMG to lower general muscle tension has produced promising results. There has generally been a reduction of 10–25 points in the blood pressure readings. This approach is especially helpful in patients with borderline essential hypertension, but it may also be helpful in cases. Often, this approach can lead to a decrease in required medication.

• Other conditions. Biofeedback has shown some success with functional diarrhea, bruxism (teeth grinding), insomnia, premenstrual tension, intestinal disorders resulting from stress, including spastic colon, certain types of substance abuse, anxiety and depression, and painful muscle spasms. Recommended: It's worth trying biofeedback in any disorder with no organic cause that may be stress-related, especially if the alternative treatment is a drug with undesirable side effects.

### New Techniques

One problem with the initial biofeedback craze was that inexperienced people were using biofeedback without knowing how it fit into behavior and personality. The lack of success that resulted was not the fault of biofeedback itself, but of practitioners who were not familiar with a variety of techniques that could be effectively used with biofeedback training.

We're now using techniques borrowed from transcendental meditation (TM) and behavior modification, together with more traditional forms of psychotherapy, to show patients how to relax. The patient uses these techniques while hooked up to the biofeedback machine so he can see what works and what doesn't. Example: A phobic patient was afraid to speak in front of a group. Using behavior-modification imaging techniques, he was instructed to imagine progressively more threatening situations, staying with each one until the machine indicated he felt relaxed with it. Also helpful: Relaxation exercises where you ask a person, as he breathes out, to feel the tension leave his body. The machine gives the patient a sense of the distinctions in levels of tension.

### New Horizons

One of the most difficult but also potentially most exciting and innovative biofeedback areas is brain-wave biofeedback. Brain waves are measured by an electroencephalograph (EEG), and this information is fed back to the person. Problem: Impulses sent out by the brain are far less intense than the impulses sent out by muscles in the forehead. To pick them up, the machine must be very sophisticated, and there isn't much of the high-level machinery around. The original studies of EEG biofeedback found that many of the results were faulty because eye movements, fluorescent lights or radio waves influenced readings.

What the EEG measures: People put out different levels of brain waves. If you're attentive or anxious, you might put out anywhere from 13 to 14 cycles per second or more. Below that is the alpha state, 8–12 cycles per second. Theta is 5–8 cycles and delta is 1–4, deep sleep.

My personal favorite area of work is theta, which I've found can on occasion provide significant relaxation effects and increase creativity. Theta can be compared to that stage when you go from wakefulness into sleep. If you have a problem, sometimes when you're in a theta state, the answer will just pop into your head. For some people, biofeedback may be able to train the brain to go into theta at will when there is a need to solve a particular problem.

### Finding a Good Practitioner

Some people doing biofeedback are inexperienced and inadequately trained in relevant disciplines such as behavior, physiology, etc. There is still no completely trustworthy accreditation in this field. Recommended: Go to someone licensed in the area of your concern—a physician, psychologist or physical therapist who uses biofeedback as part of his or her practice.

**Source:** Interview with John Hudesman, Ph.D., a psychoanalyst specializing in stress management in New York.

# GOOD POSTURE TIP

Stand straight to think straight, says Dr. Raymond Harris, chief of cardiology at St. Peter's Hospital, Albany, NY. Reason: Good posture promotes greater lung expansion. Since more air is inhaled, more oxygen reaches the brain, increasing alertness and decreasing fatigue.

# YOU CAN BEAT FATIGUE WITHOUT FIGHTING IT

Fighting fatigue is a concept of success-oriented people that actually makes them fatigue-prone. You can't do battle with fatigue. Rather you must recognize it and be sensitive to its message. Fatigue is your mind creating a symptom to get your attention—to tell you there's something wrong with the way you live. To beat fatigue, you have to get your life back in balance. If you ignore or "fight" fatigue, it will probably get worse.

### Out of Balance

When you were a child, you never got tired. You got up early, went to school, ran around during recess, went home, ran around again until dinner, did your homework, went to bed under protest, and woke up the next morning raring to go.

Most of us haven't felt that kind of energy since childhood. We stop going through the day with that innate rhythm. Part of it has to do with losing the natural balance of physical exercise to mental exercise. We overemphasize head work at the expense of body work. Most of us also live in cities and work in offices, where the environment is stacked against us.

### What Is Fatigue?

The tiredness we feel after jogging, for instance, is not what we think of as fatigue. Fatigue is an absence of energy, *joie de vivre*, interest. . . . It's a blunting of sensation, a shutting out of stimuli. Behavioral clues: Difficulty in getting going or persevering. . . not having the energy to do things you know you enjoy. . . having trouble waking up or getting to sleep. . . taking too many naps.

The main cause of fatigue is a monolithic lifestyle, in which the rational sense is used to the exclusion of the other senses such as touch and smell, movement (in the kinesthetic sense) and the emotions.

### Who Is Most Vulnerable?

• People who do virtually the same thing all day, every day. Example: The executive who spends his work hours hunched over a desk, grabs a sandwich at lunch, takes a break only to talk to co-workers about business, and goes home to a set routine with his family each evening. Monotony is at the root of fatigue. A person who does a lot of different things during the day will be less fatigued.

• People whose lifestyles are contrary to their natural inclinations. Each of us has a rhythm of activity with which we are most comfortable. Example: If a natural doer is forced to lie on a beach in the Bahamas for two weeks, he'll come back exhausted. Important: To discover the proportion of activity versus repose and socializing versus alone-time that makes you feel best.

### To Eliminate Fatigue

• Analyze your lifestyle. Write down what you do every day. Be sure to include the amount of physical exercise you get and the kinds of demands (emotional and otherwise) that are made on you. Include your time with people and your time working alone. Also: How is your evening different from your day? Document the times when you feel fatigued. Is it at work or at home? Is it better or worse around other people? Correlate your fatigue diary with your activity record, and look for patterns.

• Try some small changes in your work style. If your job puts you under constant pres-

sure, take minibreaks to do some gentle stretches. If you spend a lot of time with other people, make some private time for yourself. If you do paperwork alone, schedule some social breaks.

• Pay attention to diet and eat regularly. A breakfast of complex carbohydrates such as whole-grained toast and protein will keep you going until lunch. People who skip meals or have an erratic eating pattern are more fatigue-prone.

• Stick to a regular, moderate exercise regime—not weekend overexertion. Best: Walking. Besides being healthful and safe, it also gives you time alone to notice the outside world and reflect on your inner life. Aerobic exercise stimulates the brain to produce endorphins, the body's natural painkillers and anti-depressants.

• Look within yourself. Do you like your job, friends, home life? Could you admit it to yourself if you didn't? If, for the next two weeks, you could do anything you wanted, what would it be? Is there a way of incorporating that fantasy into real life? What's the biggest price you have to pay for your current lifestyle? Once you identify problems, see what you can do about them. Example: If you like your job but hate the long commute, maybe you can stagger your hours to work fewer days a week—or move closer to the office.

• Get a physical checkup. Although there is no physical basis for fatigue in 99% of the people who visit doctors complaining of it, occasionally a health problem is a factor. Most common medical cause of fatigue: Mild low thyroid, which occurs more commonly in women.

**Source:** Interview with Mary E. Wheat, M.D., an internist at Mt. Zion Hospital and Medical Center, San Francisco.

# HOW TO INCREASE YOUR RESISTANCE TO STRESS

In today's fast-moving, success-oriented world, it seems as though one must be able to withstand a very high stress level in order to get ahead and stay ahead. Many ambitious people put themselves under a crushing stress burden for years, eventually paying the price in heart disease, ulcers, and so on.

But there are busy, high-achieving people who are seemingly immune to stress. They deal with demanding workloads and high pressure year after year and show every evidence of thriving on their lifestyle. Such people have certain personality traits that insulate them against the ill effects of stress. They have something to teach us on how to increase our own stress-resistance.

### Who Is Stress-Resistant?

Studies have determined that people who display three main qualities are the most stress-resistant:

• Seek out and enjoy change. They see it as a challenge. This is extremely important. How we view a stressful event determines how our bodies and minds react. If an event is seen as a threat and we feel victimized, the actual physiology of the body changes to meet the threat. If we see change as a challenge, with potential for growth and excitement, the body's response is entirely different. Crucial: How we view our past performance. Although some people do as well as others at a particular task, they always feel they haven't done well enough. These are the perfectionists—a very stress-vulnerable group. Perfectionists are always condemning themselves for not having coped well enough in the past. When a new challenge comes along, they view it as just another threat to their self-esteem.

• Feel at one with what they're doing. It's almost as though they've selected or adjusted to what they do so it's an extension of their personalities, rather than something foreign. This quality is important because we don't see stress as dangerous or threatening if we feel that it's something we've chosen—not something that's been laid on us. Identifying with our work enables us to deal with stress.

• Have a sense of control over what goes on in their lives. If you participate in the planning and problem-setting, are then involved with handling your part, and also get a sense of completion at the end of a particular task, there's a clear sense of control. This is why top managers are under less stress than middle managers.

### The Vicious Cycle of Stress

When a situation is viewed as a threat, the body's fight-or-flight syndrome is activated. More energy goes to the muscles and brain, to the exclusion of other organs. Blood pressure, heart rate and blood sugar all go up. The gut tightens and the hormones alter. The body literally tears away at its inner structure to deal with threat.

This alarm system was programmed into our genes to deal with the actual physical dangers faced by early man. For animals, the fight-or-flight syndrome disappears in a few hours. They rest and regain internal balance. With humans, however, the alarm system is called into play when there's a psychological threat...and then persists. Rebalancing does not occur because we continue to ruminate about the problem. Even when we rest or sleep, we're still thinking or dreaming about it. We wake up still tight and tense, and therefore less able to deal with the problems of the next day. A perpetual cycle of chronic distress builds up, eventually resulting in body-system breakdowns. Many overstressed people are so accustomed to living with this syndrome that they don't even realize they're under stress until they get physically sick. About 80% of the people who visit physicians are actually suffering from chronic stress.

### Building Your Stress-Resistance

• Change your expectations. The difference between expectations and perception of reality is the measure of how much stress you will experience. Example: If you begin the day with an attitude of "the world is changing, finances are fluctuating, nothing stays the same," and you perceive that to be so, you'll experience very little stress. If, instead, you assume that tomorrow will be the same as today and that things will go as you planned, you'll experience a lot of stress if your expectations aren't met. Either the environment or your own performance will displease you. Remedy: Diminish your expectations and pay attention to your perceptions of reality.

• Ask for feedback. You won't be able to deal with stress if you feel that your past performances have been inadequate. You'll assume that you'll just fail again. Remedy: Find out the average or expected performance for any given job and gear yourself to that. You may find out you've been failing for very different reasons than you thought. People under stress tend to feel extremely anxious and afraid. These feelings often come across to others as anger rather than fear. If people see you as hostile (even though it is not really so), it may adversely affect any evaluation of your performance.

• Seek a socially cohesive work situation. In England during World War II, there was less illness and higher performance among Londoners who weathered the bombings than before, or after, the war. Great social cohesiveness was provided by an external enemy. That same kind of cohesiveness occurs in any organization geared toward a strong goal.

### Learn to Relax

• Do relaxation exercises.* The purpose of these is to get the focus on a nonlogical part of the body. It's the constant logical planning and rumination that keep stress going. Best: Approaches that focus on breathing. Proper breathing triggers other parts of the body to relax. The body is born with the innate ability to produce the opposite of the stress response. These exercises allow you to get in touch with that feeling, and, eventually, you'll be able to call upon it at will.

• Make time to do something relaxing. Take some time away from your desk to window-shop or do something "silly." Eat lunch out of the office. Plan something pleasurable each week, and then follow through. Caution: If you eat while under stress, you'll have a 50% higher cholesterol level after the meal than if you were relaxed.

• Physical exercise helps only if you do it right. For instance, if jogging is just another chore that you don't enjoy, but you squeeze it into a heavy schedule because you feel you should, it only puts an extra load on your heart. Exercise while under stress can be dangerous. But if you see the trees and smell the air and feel high and good after running, you're doing it right. Exercise that makes you feel good is as helpful as any relaxation technique.

*Recommended: Herbert Benson's *Relaxation Response;* Stroebel and Hartford's *Quieting Response;* Patricia Carrington's *Freedom in Meditation.*

**Source:** Interview with Kenneth Greenspan, M.D., phychiatrist and director of the Center for Stress and Pain-Related Disorders, Columbia Presbyterian Medical Center, New York City.

## HOW TO PROTECT YOUR IMMUNE SYSTEM

Stress depletes your immune system. The extent depends on your individual personality.

The production of immunoglobulin-A (a virus fighter found in the saliva) was monitored by researchers at Harvard. They checked students during the first year of an accelerated program. Students in the test were divided into two personality types: (1) Those motivated by a need to be best and (2) Those motivated by a desire for close personal relationships. Every student's level of immunoglobulin-A dropped during the year, reaching a low during a particularly difficult exam period. The students driven to succeed had consistently lower levels of immunoglobulin-A throughout the study. Their opposites, who seemed to be more content with their work and more relaxed about the demands of the program, maintained higher levels.

Conclusion: The key to raising your immunity to disease may be learning to relax under pressure.

**Source:** *Science 84,* Washington, DC.

## THE CHOLESTEROL/STRESS CONNECTION

High cholesterol levels may reflect stress more than diet. When a group of accountants felt under heaviest pressure at their jobs, their serum cholesterol rose an average of 20% even though their diets remained the same. Other cholesterol links: Depression, anger, fear, aggression and hostility.

**Source:** Lorenz van Doornen and K. F. Orlebeke, Dutch psychophysiologists, writing in *Journal of Human Stress,* Shelburne Falls, MA.

## BOREDOM CAN BE DANGEROUS

Boredom can cause as much personal stress as pressure does, and the effects may be even worse. Drug addiction, for example, can often be traced back to boredom. The best way to avoid general boredom is always to be learning something new. . .and planning something to look forward to. Helpful: Sear off mental opiates such as soap operas and pulp fiction.

**Source:** David Reuben, Ph.D., quoted in *Thrive on Stress* by Richard Sharpe, Warner Books, New York.

## WHY IT PAYS TO PANIC

Executives who are least prone to panic may be most susceptible to stress. The most competent decision makers are those who approach problems from a variety of perspectives, combining all plausible ideas into one effective action plan. Studies show these multi-dimensional managers have fewer psychiatric problems than others but a higher incidence of intestinal upsets and cardiac irregularities.

**Source:** Siegfried Streufert, professor of behavioral science, Pennsylvania State University's College of Medicine, cited in *Management Focus*, New York.

## KILLER JOBS

People whose work takes the worst physical toll are laborers, secretaries, inspectors, clinical laboratory technicians, office managers, foremen, managers and administrators. Their jobs are the high-stress occupations. Criteria: Rates of death, heart and artery disease, hypertension, ulcers, nervous disorders and mental health admissions.

**Source:** Study by the National Institute for Occupational Safety and Health in *Workrights* by Robert Ellis Smith, E. P. Dutton, Inc., New York.

• The job stress that puts workers most at risk for heart disease is a combination of high psychological demand and low control over how the job is done, according to recent studies in both the US and Sweden. Example: Machine-paced assembly line workers were found to be 70%–200% more likely to develop heart disease than low-level managerial personnel. Other occupations with dangerously low decision control and high psychological demand: Fireman, waiter/waitress, salesclerk, telephone operator, cashier, cook, freight handler, garment stitcher and mail worker. Jobs traditionally thought to be most stressful—manufacturing or sales manager, real estate agent, physician, policeman, high school teacher—were found to be less damaging to physical health. Individuals in these jobs are in a position to make their own decision about what needs to be done and how to go about doing it.

**Source:** Robert A. Karasek, Ph.D., director of the studies and assistant professor of industrial engineering, Columbia University, quoted in *The New York Times.*

## BEST DAYS OF THE WEEK

Blue Mondays are a myth. In tests to learn about stress in married men, a tangential discovery was made—that Mondays are no more difficult (for those interviewed) than any other day of the week. Upbeat days: Saturday and Sunday. Maybe Mondays only seem blue by comparison.

**Source:** Findings of psychologists Arthur A. Stone and John Neale at the Long Island Research Institute and the State University of New York at Stony Brook.

## HOW DO YOU HANDLE ANXIETY?

• Yogi Berra, The New York Yankee baseball great: "I spend lots of time on the golf course, often with my son, who is also a ball player. And I like to work out at my racquetball club in Fairfield, New Jersey, too."

• Jane Brody, *New York Times* science writer

and author of the best-selling *Jane Brody's Nutrition Book* and the new *New York Times Guide to Personal Health:* "I find the best way to avoid anxiety is to exercise. I drop everything and do something physical—jog, swim, whatever. I clear the slate and calm down. When I come back, things don't seem so bad. Another thing—I keep a continuing calendar and try not to let too many things pile up at once. And I have also learned the fine art of saying 'No.'"

• Joyce Brothers, TV personality: "Whenever I get anxious, I swim. (Studies indicate that 15 minutes of strenuous exercise have amore tranquilizing effect than strong drugs.) Another good way to fight stress and anxiety is to take a long, brisk walk, which I really enjoy, on our farm."

• Dr. Frank Field, NBC science editor: "The key word, for me, is *awareness*. Once I am aware of my anxiety, I stand back and look at it. If someone tells me that I am shouting, I try to do something about it—not just deny it. I get swept up with so many things that often I am unaware that I am becoming anxious. So then I take control of myself.

• Eileen Ford, Ford Model Agency: "I do yoga deep breathing and changing breaths. The tension just flows from my body."

• Roger Horchow, founder of The Horchow Collection: "I don't have much anxiety in my life. When I do, I guess it is when I eat too much. But mostly I try to work harder to eliminate what is bothering me. . .try to accomplish more and deal with the source."

• Reggie Jackson, baseball player: "My best cure for anxiety is working on my collection of old cars. I also enjoy building cars, and I find that doing physical work can relieve stress for me. Reading the Bible also puts my mind at ease and gives me spiritual comfort."

• Ann Landers, syndicated columnist: "I first try to avoid anxiety, and I do a fairly good job. My life is not stressful in that I can make my own schedule without anyone looking over my shoulder. My work is not anxiety-producing, but occasionally, if there is a hitch, I get into a hot bath, take the phone off the hook and count my blessings. I have a great deal to be thankful for, and I know it."

• Marvin Traub, chairman, Bloomingdale's: "I have no problem with anxiety, so I really don't have to deal with it. I enjoy my job very much, and I don't feel any stress."

• Dr. Ruth Westheimer, prominent sexologist: "When I get anxious, I say 'Ruth Westheimer, get hold of yourself!' The important thing is to recognize your anxiety. Sometime this makes it go away. If it were a really serious anxiety, I would go for professional help."

## GUIDELINES FOR THE OVERWORKED

Busy people incur more than their share of dangerous stress. If you have more work than you can handle: Get better organized. Establish priorities, and then concentrate on doing one job at a time. Recognize your limitations. Don't dwell on failure. Remember past successes. Ask for and use help when you need it. Bottom line: The American Medical Association reports that 80% of our diseases are either caused by or aggravated by stress.

• Job involvement can be overdone. Obsessive people create elaborate (but impractical) systems, work by formula, can't take criticism and often immerse themselves in details to avoid big decisions. They lie awake worrying about their jobs, too. But the only result is lost sleep and decreased mental alertness.

**Source:** *Insight*, Waterford, CT.

## TO REDUCE STRESS AT YOUR DESK

• Make certain that your chair is comfortable.

• Quiet your telephone's ring.

• Alter the lighting to reduce glare. . .or increase brightness.

• Personalize your work space with photos,

posters, etc.

• Adopt at least a partial closed-door policy for your office. (If you have no way to be alone in your office, find a place elsewhere in the building where you can take breathers.)

• Avoid tight shirt collars. . .they can cut blood flow to the brain and result in light-headedness and panic attacks. Tightly cinched belts are troublesome, too.

• Establish a regular time for meals, especially lunch.

**Source:** *The Termination Trap* by Stephen Cohen, Williamson Publishing, Charlotte, VT.

## GOOD WAY TO FIGHT STRESS

Mentally conjure up something that promotes an inner smile or glow—the face of an adored person or your dog bounding out to greet you when you get home. Such "melt moments" provide perspective. They induce calmness, reduce heart rate, relax muscle tension and give a sense of well-being—all incompatible with stress.

**Source:** Theodore S. Kurtz, Ph.D., writing in *Registered Representative*, Newport Beach, CA.

## EASY STRESS REDUCER

1. Sit relaxed with arms in lap. Clench fists and hold tightly for a count of five, then relax. Repeat five times.

2. Press right fingertips against left ones (as if on a mirror). Relax, and repeat 10 times.

3. Use each thumb to massage the opposite palm. Work hardest on muscles at the base of the opposite thumb and on the web between thumb and forefinger. Continue until you feel a warm sensation.

4. Drop hands to sides and shake them well. Then briefly rub them together.

**Source:** James McClernan, psychologist, John C. Lincoln Hospital, Phoenix, AZ quoted in *The National Enquirer*, New York.

## BREATHING TIP

Chest breathing can induce anxiety and panic attacks. Reason: Chest breathers take in too little oxygen and blow out too much carbon dioxide. To make sure you're breathing from your diaphragm: Slouch down in your chair until you can see your stomach, and work on making it move up with each inhalation and down with each exhalation. Bonus: This is a good relaxation exercise when done for five minutes three times a day.

**Source:** *The Termination Trap* by Stephen Cohen, Williamson Publishing, Charlotte, VT.

## WANT TO RELAX? GET A FISH TANK

The aquarium in your dentist's office is not just decoration. Watching fish swim lazily about can have a positively tranquilizing effect. In fact, recent tests showed that fish-watching is as calming as hypnosis or meditation before a tooth extraction.

**Source:** Study by Aaron Katcher, M.D., associate professor of psychiatry, University of Pennsylvania.

• Although tropical fish won't fetch your slippers, they can relieve stress. Watching fish lowers blood pressure for most people.

**Source:** *Medical Self-Care*, Inverness, CA.

## THE SIGNS OF ANXIETY

Highly nervous people believe that physical signs of their anxiety are visible to others, but this is not the case. Reassuring: Anxious people rated their sweaty palms and twitches as being much more apparent than did others who observed them.

**Source:** Kimberly McErvan, psychologist, University of Calgary, Alberta, Canada, quoted in *Psychology Today*, New York.

## AN END TO ANXIETY

It's about time: An anti-anxiety drug without the troublesome side effects and addictive potential of Valium (diazepam). Our pharmaceutical industry insiders predict that Buspar (buspirone) will become the drug of choice in the treatment of anxiety. . .and that's big, big news in the $600 million/year oral anti-anxiety drug market. Valium now has a 40% share of that market.)

Buspar is as effective as Valium in reducing anxiety and its related disorders (heart palpitations, insomnia, nausea, etc.). . .but Buspar doesn't cause drowsiness or affect motor coordination, so it's completely safe to take while driving or using machinery. An "anxio-selective" drug, Buspar zeroes in on anxiety receptors and leaves the rest of the body's nervous system unaffected. Even better: Buspar is completely nonaddictive. In contrast, studies show that patients taking Valium for as little as six weeks can suffer withdrawal symptoms when the drug is discontinued. (The withdrawal symptoms are commonly mistaken for anxiety. Consequently, patients continue on the drug not because they are anxious, but because they are physically dependent on it.)

Other advantages: Buspar doesn't interact with alcohol or barbiturates. . .and it causes fewer adverse effects than Valium in patients taking other medications. (Note: Buspar is not as effective as Valium in treating muscular symptoms of anxiety—tension headache, backache, etc.)

**Source:** Mead Johnson Pharmaceuticals (a subsidiary of Bristol-Myers), Evansville, IN.

## ANXIETY ANGST

A study comparing *alprozolam* (Xanax) to *diazepam* (Valium) concludes that alprozolam has the same anti-anxiety effectiveness with decreased sedative effect.

**Source:** Bruce Yaffe, M.D., a gastroenterologist in private practice in New York.

## CHOCOLATE VS. VALIUM

That Tootsie Roll can help relieve stress—and with minimal side effects. Reason: Chocolate is loaded with pyrazines, which are structually similar to life-essential amino acids. Pyrazines stimulate the pleasure center of the brain, which interrupts stress signals and helps cheer you up. And the sugar in chocolate raises the level of brain serotonin, a natural chemical that soothes frazzled nerves.

**Source:** Susan Schiffman, a psychology professor at Duke University Medical Center, quoted in *Self*, New York.

# 15. What You Should Know about Doctors and Hospitals

# What You Should Know about Doctors and Hospitals

## HOW TO GET THE BEST FROM YOUR DOCTOR

With medical care getting more complicated, and with the growing number of specialties and even subspecialties, the field of doctoring is becoming more of an impersonal industry. To the person with no medical problems, that's usually an academic point. But for the ill and elderly, the new situation is causing additional heavy burdens.

What used to be a simple doctor-patient relationship is now very complicated. For example, how do you . . .

• Maintain reasonable continuity of your medical records when you move from one specialist to another?

• Identify the right doctor to diagnose and treat various illnesses?

• Evaluate the medical advice you're given—and find the many alternative treatments that may be better for you than the conventional ones?

### Active Role

Increasingly, patients are discovering they can no longer be passive in the doctor-patient relationship. They have to take an active interest to be sure they get not only the best care, but, in some instances, just adequate care—as the soaring number of medical malpractice suits seems to indicate.

Here is a valuable checklist of potential problems and advice for dealing with today's doctors. . .

• Checkups: The usual procedure is for a doctor to perform a physical checkup and do lab work-ups during the examination. Then, a few days later, the doctor's nurse calls and relates an oversimplified assessment of the lab results.

Instead: Arrange for a preliminary visit so that lab work can be done before the physical exam. That way, the doctor can go over the results of the tests in detail, answering any questions during the regular exam. If there is need for further lab work, it can be done later.

• Medical records: In most cases, your medical records are kept by the doctor. So if you move, decide to change doctors or subsequently see a specialist, you have to go through a long procedure to get your records.

Instead: Ask for copies of all records and keep them in your own permanent file. Especially useful: Electrocardiograms, blood tests and X rays. The doctor might charge you a nominal fee to make copies.

• Selecting professionals: It's generally very hard to find out whether a doctor treats your particular problem or uses the procedure you need until you visit the office—a waste of your time and money, since you'll probably have to wait for the appointment and pay for the visit.

Instead: Try to get the information on the telephone. Obstacle: Most office staffs tend to overprotect doctors from such calls—even, on occasion, contrary to the doctor's inclination. Trick: Refer to yourself on the phone as "doctor." It's amazing how that can open doors with medical professionals. Not all people feel comfortable with such deception, but given the payoff, it should be considered.

• Doctor-patient relations: Doctors usually prefer to be called "Doctor." Yet they frequently call patients by their first names. That small difference helps to perpetuate the role of doctor as parent and patient as child—where the patient isn't expected to question the doctor's orders. This leaves the patient in a position of not sharing responsibility for his own health.

Instead: As a symbolic gesture, settle whether the two of you are on a first- or last-name basis.

### More Ways to Win

• If the doctor always keeps you waiting, call before you leave for your appointment. Even better: Ask someone else to call and explain that your professional duties make your schedule very tight.

• If the doctor diagnoses an illness and prescribes drugs, take notes on the name of the condition and the drugs being prescribed.

• If you're overcome by the news of the illness (which isn't unusual), call the doctor after you've had some time to calm down and frame any questions about the prognosis and the method of treatment. Also, arrange to bring a relative or friend with you to emotionally charged doctor visits. That'll give you the emotional space to "collapse" or to go temporarily "deaf" to bad news, while your companion is able to listen, ask questions and interpret what the doctor says. The period right after serious illness is disclosed is hard to handle, so make arrangements to compensate for it.

### Drugs

Since even the "safest" drugs usually have some side effects, it's prudent to insist that you be included in any decisions about prescriptions.

Frequently, the decision isn't only which drug to take, but whether one should be taken at all. In some cases, there are alternatives to drugs...changes in diet, life-style or exercise. Many doctors believe, perhaps correctly, that most patients don't feel that on office visit for an illness is complete unless a pill is prescribed. Make it clear that you don't feel that way.

• Insist that the druggist include the manufacturer's fact sheet with any prescription you're given. Read it. It's technical, but with the aid of a medical dictionary you may discover things about the drug you'll want to discuss with the doctor. It's hard, if not impossible, for doctors to know current information on all drugs. You may discover that the dose is excessive or that the drug is no longer considered effective for your condition.

• If you do take a drug that has side effects (dizziness, stomach distress, etc.), start taking it during a weekend or when you're home, so you'll be in a safer and more comfortable place when they hit.

• If you or the doctor feel that the drug you're taking may not be fully effective—but is the best currently available—consider doing some of your own research.

Sources: Check medical journals that specialize in the condition you have. Also, some brokerage firms run stock analyses of leading drug companies and include comprehensive reports on new drugs. One of the best: Kidder, Peabody & Co., 10 Hanover Sq., New York 10005. The problem then, is to find a doctor running clinical studies with the new drug. Only that doctor can legally use it if it doesn't have FDA approval. Be aware, too, that you're a risk in using the drug. However, some new drugs have already been given full approval in other countries.

**Source:** Interview with Susan G. Cole, editor of *The Practical Guide to Cancer Care*, Health Improvement Research Corp., New York.

# MEDICAL CARE AND SEX DON'T MIX

Sexual contact between women and their medical doctors is as emotionally damaging as affairs with their psychotherapists. Especially harmful: Liaisons in which the woman has a history of sexual victimization.

**Source:** Study at the University of Washington at Seattle, reported in *The Journal of Consulting and Clinical Psychology*.

# HOW TO PROTECT YOURSELF FROM YOUR DOCTOR

The best doctors are sometimes the ones with the poorest personalities. Bedside manner is not necessarily a relevant criterion. The prime do's and don'ts:

• Do ask questions. Many patients are intimidated by the doctor's professional status. Don't be. Ask your prospective doctor about his medical philosophy. Pose specific questions—for example, does he believe in taking heroic measures in terminal cases? Look for a doctor who is attuned to the patient/doctor relationship. Be wary of a doctor who puts you off, who takes a question as a personal affront, or who says things like, "Don't worry, I'll take care of it.".

• Don't be impressed by the diplomas on the wall. Many are probably from organizations that the doctor joined for a fee. What you should know: Is the doctor *board certified* in his specialty?

• Do find out about the doctor's hospital affiliation. Is he on the medical staff of a hospital? Is it a local hospital of good reputation?

• Don't go straight to a specialist when you're having a problem. Specialists can be blind to any ailment that doesn't fall into their specialty. Have a generalist or internist assess your problem and send you to the appropriate specialist.

### What Else to Consider

A doctor should be willing to re-evaluate and reassess. Too many doctors are ready to write off a patient as neurotic. I've had any number of cases in which people judged neurotic had something physically wrong with them

A patient has an absolute right to a second opinion. The mere fact that the doctor doesn't suggest it is no reason to assume you don't need one. Many doctors become unpleasant when a patient mentions getting a second opinion. Ignore that and get one anyway if you have any questions as to a doctor's evaluation or if surgery is recommended.

You have a right to your medical records. You'll need them for the second opinion. Most states have statutes that make it mandatory to give patients a copy (not the original) of their records.

### Obstetric Malpractice

Since obstetrics is the most common area of malpractice today, there are certain points that pregnant women should be aware of:

• The doctor, not the nurse, should give the care. Nurses can take a blood pressure or pulse reading, but the doctor should do the internal examinations.

• Any woman in a high-risk group should get special attention. Women over 35 with their first baby need that special attention. So do women with a history of toxemia in the family and women with a cardiac, renal or diabetic condition

• Make sure your obstetrician does all the basics—asks a lot of questions, does regular urine tests, and pays attention to your weight and changes in uterine height. Special attention should be given to swelling, headaches and post-term pregnancy.

### Hospital Malpractice

In a hospital you can't interview everyone who will be giving you care. But there are some things you can do:

• Voice your complaints. . .and I don't mean about the tasteless food. Complain about things like an IV bottle that's been empty for an hour, or a catheter left in, or a doctor who says he'll be back in 10 minutes and instead returns the next day. Make friends with the nurses. Be polite but firm about what you need.

• Make sure the doctors and nurses know what you're allergic to. Be sure the allergies are adequately documented in the health records.

• Find out, especially in a teaching hospital, who is giving you care. Not everyone in a white coat is automatically qualified. You have a right to know how much training the doctor administering your treatment has received.

• Make sure you have given informed consent to any invasive procedure. The biggest issue in my office is patients who routinely sign anything that's put in front of them. Find out the risks and alternatives to any invasive procedure. Request an oral explanation in layman's terms. Make sure you totally understand anything you sign.

• Learn the names of the drugs you're getting. Find out what they're for and what their side effects are. Then, if someone hands you a drug you don't recognize, question it. If you're taking drugs from more than one doctor, be sure each knows what the other has prescribed, including over-the-counter medications.

• Ask the reason for each test you're given.

• Tell the doctor or nurse your full health history. Should malpractice occur, you won't have a leg to stand on in court if you've withheld vital information.

• Before you're discharged from the hospital, get full instructions about what you should do after you leave. Write down your questions about diet, bed rest, exercise, medication or anything else that concerns you.

• If you believe that you have been injured by the hospital or the doctor, consult a lawyer who specializes in malpractice. Don't wait too long. There are different statutes of limitatiion in various jurisdictions.

**Source:** Interview with Leonard C. Arnold, M.D., J.D., Chicago.

## WHY YOU MAY BE INTERVIEWED BY A COMPUTER

Patients generally reveal more about themselves to a computer than to a physician during a diagnostic interview. They are less inhibited because they're not receiving any judgmental or negative feedback via facial expression, body language and/or vocal intonation.

## HOW TO KEEP YOUR MEDICAL RECORDS PRIVATE

Confidential medical information, often revealed without a patient's consent or knowledge, can seriously damage a career, boost insurance premiums and cause embarrassment. Sometimes you can protect yourself.

### Risk Factors

• Socially stigmatized medical conditions.

Venereal disease, alcoholism, sexual dysfunction, nervous conditions and the like can endanger your reputation and your job.

• Company plans. Any condition for which you file a claim may come to the attention of your employer. Commom problems such as diabetes, heart disease, cancer or even insomnia may affect your future with the company.

• Seeing a specialist. You may have a verbal agreement with your family doctor not to release any but the most specific or innocuous information to other sources, such as employers or insurance companies. Although doctors are usually good about protecting information, they routinely disclose medical histories to other physicians without the patient's consent. Since you do not have a personal relationship with the specialist, knowledge of your record may proliferate from there.

• Computerized records. Purchasers of health insurance should be aware of the Medical Information Bureau, a computerized service that keeps extensive medical records on over 11,000,000 Americans for their insurance company subscribers. The computer stores medical information and may also contain personal items, such as participation in dangerous sports, drunk-driving citations, criminal associations and large life insurance purchases.

### How to Protect Yourself

Use the doctor/patient relationship. The basis of confidentiality is largely contractual and is not covered by laws. Review this issue with your doctor and with every new doctor or specialist you go to. You might devise a written form for each physician requiring your permission for the release of any information about yourself.

Never sign a blanket medical release form. The only medical release forms you sign should specifically identify the following: Information to be released, who is releasing the information and who is to receive it. Releases are not self-limiting as to time. A form you signed 10 years ago can still be used to obtain information. A period of one year is suggested.

Do not use your company insurance plan.

378 / DOCTORS AND HOSPITALS

in sensitive areas. If you need treatment for an emotional problem, venereal disease, etc., pay for it yourself if at all possible.

### Legitimate Inquiries

Insurance companies, potential employers and current employers all have the right to know a fair amount about your health. However, if you protect yourself as outlined, you can minimize the information revealed in a legitimate inquiry. Physical examinations required by a current employer have been upheld in the courts and so must be complied with. The American Occupational Medical Association, to which company doctors belong, has a code of ethics provision precluding occupational physicians from turning over a patient's full record.

### Getting Access to Your Records

• You have a right to see your medical records in about half the states. In states that don't have specific statutes, your legal right to see your records would probably be recognized by the courts.

• You do have a right to rebut what your medical record says. In states with right-of-access, you can often force removal of damaging information from your record, or at least have your rebuttal included in the record. In states without right-of-access, you can challenge by filing a lawsuit.

Bottom line: Take preventive action before confidential medical information about you has reached the wrong parties.

**Source:** Interview with Robert R. Belair, former counsel to the National Commission on Confidentiality of Health Records. He is co-author, with Dr. Alan Westin, of *Medical Confidentiality: A Guide for Practioners, Administrators and Other Users of Personal Health Data,* Aspen Systems Corp., Rockville, MD.

## HOSPITAL TIMING

Put off non-emergency surgery and medical tests until late fall if you can. Reason: In the cycles of medical education, new residents—the least experienced doctors on a hospital staff—take up their duties on July 1. Senior staff physicians often take summer vacations. Bottom line: The hospital is more likely to run smoothly after the new residents have worked into the routine

and the senior staff is back from vacation.

**Source:** Jo Ann Friedman, president, Health Marketing Systems, New York.

## HOSPITAL-STAY SURPRISE

Hospital stays vary more with where one lives than with the ailment. In general, doctors in the East keep their patients hospitalized longer. Longest average stay: 13.1 days, in New Jersey. Shortest average: Six days, in California. Conundrum: Length of stay seems to have little effect on a patient's recovery.

**Source:** Study by the Congressional Office of Technology Assessment.

## HOW TO GET VIP TREATMENT IN A HOSPITAL

The first thing an admitting clerk does when you're brought into a hospital is slip a plastic tag with an identity number onto your wrist. From that point on, like it or not, you are a number to most of the hospital staff.

Being a number instead of a name can be an awful shock. It means that you may be treated as if you have no identity—except for your symptoms, vital signs and medical treatment.

Fortunately, there are steps you can take to improve that treatment. And those steps, if successful, not only will make you feel more comfortable and human during your hospital visit, they could dramatically affect your state of health by the time you're ready to be discharged. In fact, it may be the issue that determines whether you leave alive or dead.

### What You Can Do

Think of a hospital as a sort of huge, complex hotel—however, one that dispenses more than food, entertainment and lodging.

As you obviously know, a hospital dispenses both life-saving and life-threatening services. A moment's inattention at a hospital can lead to tragedy.

So how do you get the hospital to treat you like a person instead of a number?

In general, you've got to use the same techniques you use in other aspects of your personal and business life. The key word is assertiveness. That's not to say you should complain and be demanding—although, as you'll see, that may be necessary under certain circumstances.

### Finding the Right Doctor

The first step in getting VIP treatment in a hospital should be taken long before you're admitted—and that's finding a doctor who can provide the leverage you'll need. You want someone with more than an M.D. after his name.

Every community has a clique of doctors who have "political" clout. Usually, these are physicians who serve on the local hospital's board of directors. Be aware, however, that a doctor with clout doesn't necessarily have the skills or any other attributes that make a physician a superior healer. Do you want such a person as your personal physician? Generally speaking, the answer is no, but there are exceptions. If you're satisfied that such a doctor can serve double-duty, so to speak, then you need go no farther.

The drawbacks: Aside from the possibility that such a doctor may be more expert in a boardroom than an operating room there are other potential problems.

The most serious: He may be more interested in keeping his professional calendar and the institution's beds filled than in your welfare. Of course, there are ways to get around that. If he wants to admit you to the hospital for treatment and there is any doubt in your mind about this decision, ask for a consultation.

Generally speaking, it's always wise to get a consultation for any complex medical procedure—and the likelihood is that the procedure he's recommending is relatively complex if he wants to hospitalize you. So by asking for a consultation, you're not showing lack of faith in your doctor.

Caveat: However, we've heard of many instances where doctors are annoyed when a patient announces that he would like a consultation or second opinion. If you ever face a less-than-cooperative response to such a request, it would be prudent to seek out another doctor immediately. It's well within your rights to consult with as many physicians as you wish.

### The Personal Touch

To guarantee better attention once you know that you're going to spend time in hospital, make a date with the hospital administrator. He may or may not be a doctor—but in any case, he is a businessman, so you can be sure he speaks the same language as you. Introduce yourself. Tell him that you're a little concerned about your hospital stay and that you'd appreciate it if he'd take a personal interest in your case.

He'll get the message, and in all likelihood, he'll take steps to be sure that you're well cared for. Now that you've made your presence known, he will probably, out of courtesy, call the head of nursing and the admitting office and tell them you are coming to the hospital and that they should be expecting you. It's just such words, without pressure, that may make all the difference in the way you're subsequently treated.

### Once You're in the Hospital

Even if you've failed or haven't had the time to take the above steps, there are still things you can do to ensure good treatment, if not VIP treatment.

If you're not physically up to it, your spouse or a friend or relative may have to help you, but if you're feeling well enough, you can take the following steps yourself.

• During the admission procedure, ask what rooms are available. You may prefer a private room, or for the sake of company, you may want to share a room with someone else. If you do want to share, ask about your potential partner's medical status to be sure that you can deal with his illness.

• After settling into your room, ask to see the dietitian. Explain that you understand that the hospital is not a hotel, but within reasonable bounds, and limited by doctor's orders, there are foods that you do and do not like. Itemize them. If you present your request with tact, the dietitian will probably try to meet your reasonable requests.

• Go out of your way to be polite to the nursing staff. They are your lifeline—literally. If the nurses take a dislike to you, the recuperation period will not be smooth.

• It's not tacky to provide small favors, such as a box of candy, and even flowers, on each of the three nursing shifts: the 8 A.M. to 4 P.M., the 4 P.M. to midnight, and midnight to 8 A.M. Don't offer a gratuity until you're ready to be discharged. Nurses are professionals, and most would resent the offer. But if you received extra special care from a nurse during your stay, a tasteful gift isn't inappropriate.

• Make it clear that you'd like to know what medication or treatment is being given to you *beforehand*. That will require a discussion with your doctor. Most doctors work on the premise that patients don't want to know too much, and so only provide information as it's necessary or if the patient specifically requests it.

### Why You Should Want This Information

Unfortunately, mistakes are made now and then, but if you ask the nurse "What are these pills?" or "What exactly will you be doing to me?", and she has orders from your doctor to provide that information on request, then it gives the staff the opportunity to double-check what they are doing and it gives you a chance to say "Wait a minute!" if an obvious error is being committed.

### How to Complain

If you're not happy with your care, explain your complaint firmly and politely to the nurse. If that gets you no place, ask to speak to the head nurse. And if that fails, you may have to speak to either your doctor or the hospital administrator. Usually, when you reach that level, and you're not being unreasonable, steps will be taken to satisfy your complaint and resolve your problem.

## WRONG PILLS IN HOSPITALS

Since 1962, when a study of hospital medication practices uncovered an error in every six doses given to patients by nurses, the handling of drugs in U.S. hospitals has changed appreciably. A majority now have central pharmacies that make up unit doses to be dispensed by nurses and/or technicians in most of their departments. Where unit dose systems are in place, errors average only three per 100. However, that 3% can be fatal, and the number of errors in departments and hospitals not served by the central pharmacy is still very high (8%–20%). The problem: Overworked nurses, confusing and similar drug names and packaging, and illegibly written prescriptions. How to protect yourself: Be sure you know exactly which drugs and what dosages your doctor has ordered for you. Never accept medication without knowing what it is and what it is for.

## BEST HOSPITALS FOR MAJOR SURGERY

• Doctors who operate frequently have better safety records because they maintain their skills. Guideline: A minimum of 40–50 operations a year, even more for heart surgery. Aim for a hospital that does many similar operations. Best bets: Teaching and specialty hospitals. A good one substantially improves the chances of avoiding serious complications or death.

## WHAT TO ASK A SURGEON

To protect against unnecessary surgery, ask the physician hard questions beforehand.

• What are the risks?

• What is the mortality rate for this operation?

• How long will it take to recover?

• What is the likelihood of complications?

• Are there ways to treat this condition medically?

• How many people have you seen with similar symptoms who have chosen not to have surgery?

• How many of these operations have you done in the past year?

Always get a second opinion.

## HOW TO CHOOSE AN ANESTHESIOLOGIST

It is common knowledge that patients should consult more than one doctor before proceeding with any kind of surgery. But when it comes to the selection of an anesthesiologist, we tend to be much more passive. However, the quality of the care we receive from our anesthesiologist is as important—or more so—as the quality of surgical care. Anesthesiologists' work involves not only the administration of potentially lethal drugs but also the monitoring of the patient's vital signs during the surgery.

### For Aggressive Health-Care Consumers

Typically, the first contact with the anesthesiologist is in the hospital, the night before the operation. Better: Ask your surgeon for the name of the anesthesiologist he plans to use when the operation itself is discussed . Meet the proposed anesthesiologist well before the operation.

Ask your surgeon how often he has worked with this anesthesiologist. Ask your family doctor if he knows him and what he thinks of him. Ask anyone you know who works at the hospital—nurses, volunteers, etc.—for the hospital grapevine's assessment of the anesthesiologist.

Unless someone volunteers the information, you won't be able to find out whether anyone has ever sued this anesthesiologist for malpractice. However, you can call the licensing board of your state and ask if any complaints have been made against him and how they were resolved.

The fact that one complaint has been made does not necessarily mean the doctor is guilty of any misconduct. But if the doctor has inspired a number of complaints, this should tell you something. Make sure the doctor is board certified. Look up his credentials (in any medical-specialist book at any public library) to find out where he trained and how long he has been practicing.

The hospital may want to assign a nurse anesthetist. An individual nurse anesthetist may be well qualified to administer anesthesia.

Interview the proposed anesthesiologist. Ask him to explain the options available to you and to tell you why he recommends a particular course. There is greater risk in general anesthesia than in local anesthesia. Can the operation you are having be done with local anesthesia? Feel free to discuss anything that bothers you.

If you are at all dissatisfied with the proposed anesthesiologist's qualifications or competence, request another one...and check him out. If that can't be arranged, seriously consider changing to another surgeon and/or hospital. The choice is always the patient's.

**Source:** Interview with Leonard Glanz, associate professor of health law, Boston University School of Public Health.

## PATIENTS' RIGHTS

People who are asked to sign medical consent forms are often in the worst possible psychological shape to make a decision about anything. Serious illness is a terrible shock. It brings out the part of human nature that wants to abdicate responsibility and put fate in the hands of an omnipotent being—in this case, the doctor. It's important to understand before you get sick what your rights as a patient are and what medical consent actually means.

### Informed Consent

The law in this country guarantees the patient an informed consent. That means the patient must be thoroughly informed in advance about all significant aspects of the proposed treatment. Consent is necessary in all non-emergency situations in which there are invasive* procedures or treatments involving risks unknown to most lay people. This includes not only surgery but also more minor procedures such as invasive diagnostic tests or injections of any substance with negative side effects.

The essence of informed consent is what takes place between the patient and the doctor. A consent form signed by the patient does not in itself constitute informed consent. The form is simply evidence collected by doctors and hospitals as protection in case of an eventual lawsuit. In all states the patient has the right to an explanation and must understand the procedure. And in some states the informed consent must be obtained by the procedure. Example: The risks of anesthesia must be explained by the anesthesiologist. The explanation must be in simple language the patient can understand. If the patient speaks only Urdu, it's the hospital's responsibility to make a good-faith effort to find an Urdu translator. Basics:

• Consent for a medical procedure on a child or unconscious adult can be given over the telephone, but hospitals and doctors will want it confirmed in writing.

• Consent can be revoked at any time prior to the procedure. Medical consents are not legally binding prior to the procedure, and you don't give up any rights when you sign a form and then change your mind.

• Consent must be to a specific procedure. A general consent form is not evidence of consent for those specific procedures which require that specific information be imparted to the patient to make him "informed." Recommended: Sign general consent forms for basic hospital care. After you're admitted, it's still the hospital's and doctor's responsibility to explain any specific procedures in order to obtain consent that's informed.

• Consent is not necesssary for an emergency procedure where the patient is incompetent or unconscious and no one authorized can be located to consent. Emergency: Any procedure that is medically necessary to treat a condition dangerous to life or health.

## What the Patient Must Be Told

• Purpose: For what reason the procedure is being done.

• Procedure: What exactly will be done and how. What the procedure entails.

• Benefits: What the doctor hopes to achieve by performing this procedure.

• Alternatives: What else could be done besides what the doctor is recommending.

• Risks: This is the stickiest area. It gives rise to the most malpractice suits. The doctor is supposed to inform the patient about

what the law calls material risks. These are risks that are high in frequency or severity or that might have an impact on decision-making. Example: Anesthesia sometimes results in brain damage. This is a high-severity, low-frequency risk, but you're entitled to know anyway. Determination of material risk varies with each procedure and the condition of each patient.

## Who Can Consent

• Any conscious, competent adult (over 18 in most states) can give an informed consent. A mental patient may be considered competent to consent even though he may be hallucinating, as long as he can understand objective medical data and make reasoned decisions concerning his medical treatment.

• An emancipated minor or a minor who is married or a parent can give consent.

• Consent for a medical procedure on an unconscious adult can be given by: Spouses, adult siblings, parents, adult offspring, court-appointed guardians. If a hospital cannot find an authorized relative, it can go to court for guardianship.

• A parent can consent for a medical procedure on a child. A competent adult can refuse medical treatment for himself. But a parent cannot refuse treatment for a child. This issue comes up in cases of religious-sect members who don't believe in blood transfusions and parents of defective children who don't want them treated with extraordinary measures.

## When You Can Sue

You can sue for malpractice on the basis of lack of informed consent without other malpractice claims, irrespective of whether you were injured. The jury award may be limited, however, if you sustained no physical or psychological injury.

Occasionally an informed consent can legitimately not be taken. These are what doctors and hospitals usually use as legal defenses:

• When the risks are well-known. Example: An appendectomy will cause a scar.

• The patient was informed about risks, but

he couldn't make up his mind and told the doctor to decide for him.

• The patient refused to be informed, telling the doctor to go ahead and do whatever he thought best.

• It wasn't possible to find someone competent who was authorized to consent, and it was an emergency procedure.

• The doctor claims that knowing about the risks would adversely affect the patient's medical condition. In such a case, he is obliged to inform the family, if not the patient.

**Source:** Interview with attorney Natalie J. Kaplan, a former hospital legal consultant, now in private practice in New York.

*Invasive: any object entering the body through the skin or orifices.

## HOW TO HANDLE INFORMED CONSENT

The process of giving medical consent is often so psychologically charged that many patients don't remember giving an informed consent. In six-month follow-ups, patients have been shown videotapes of their consent and still not remembered. If they do remember anything, it's having alternatives explained to them (more than any other aspect of the consent procedure).

Since making a decision about treatment of a serious illness is so traumatic, there are things you should do to be sure your decision is the right one:

• Some hospitals provide patient representatives. Ask for one to sit in on the informed-consent procedure.

• Write down all your questions in advance.

• Take notes or use a tape recorder for the answers.

• Ask the doctor for recommended reading about your illness and its treatment.

• Get second (or third) opinions.

• Take a friend or relative with you. Someone uninvolved will be cool-headed enough to get more information.

• Don't agree to anything just to get it over with. Listen closely to the alternatives and risks.

• There is usually a time gap between the time you consent and the actual operation. Use this period to do research about the procedure. Go to your hospital's medical library. If you're too ill to do your own research, ask a friend to do it.

• If you feel that the advice of your physician is more than conservative than you wish, look for alternative medical sources in your area. Example: When statistics indicated that lumpectomies might be just as effective as radical mastectomies, some physicians were more quickly convinced than others to try the new procedure.

**Source:** Interview with attorney Natalie J. Kaplan, a former legal consultant now in private practice in New York.

## UNDERSTANDING HOSPITAL TALK

A hospital patient may have considerable difficulty understanding some of the jargon used by nurses and other hospital personnel. Here is what some commonly used terms mean:

NPO—Sign placed by the bed of a patient who is not to get anything to eat or drink.

Emesis basin—Basin brought to patients who are sick to their stomach.

Ambulate—Take the patient for a walk.

Force fluids—Encourage intake of lots of liquid.

Void—Urinate.

IV—Intravenous.

OOB—Out of bed.

IPPB—Intermittent Positive Pressure Breathing machine to aid the breathing.

HS—Medication before sleep.

BP—Blood pressure.

HR—Heart rate.

Medication Schedule:

QID—4 times a day.

TID—3 times a day.

BID—2 times a day.

OD or QD—Once a day.

OOD—Every other day.

## INFECTION ALERT

Hospital-acquired infections may be caused by rings worn by hospital staff. At the hospital that was tested, two out of every five nurses had disease-causing bacteria on the skin under their rings

**Source:** Study at a London hospital, in *Prevention*, St. Emmaus, PA.

# HOSPITAL-BILL WARNINGS

Check hospital bills carefully. Errors are fairly common. According to one insurer, Equitable Life Assurance Society of America, every dollar it spends on audits of hospital charges recovers $3–$4 for the company in billing mistakes.

• Hospital bills almost always contain mistakes. An auditor's study found errors on 98.1% with unsubstantiated charges. Erroneously entered items are common, as is failure to make adjustments when tests or medications are canceled or reduced by the doctors.

**Source:** Study by Equifax Services, Atlanta, cited in *Innovation & Performance Report*.

# HOW TO PROTECT YOURSELF FROM HOSPITAL BILLING ERRORS

When the mechanic hands you a bill for $500, it's unlikely that you'd pay it without a glance at the charges. But when given a hospital bill for $5,000, most people tend to do just that.

As it turns out, hospitals and doctors are far from infallible when it comes to billing. According to the New York Life Insurance Company, which has been auditing hospital bills for the past three years, the averaage hospital bill contains $600 worth of erroneous charges. This money comes not only out of the insurance company's pocket, but also out of yours. You can save money by knowing how the system works and how to spot billing errors.

### Why Bother?

With the rising costs of health care, the current trend in the insurance industry is to have the insured employee share in the cost of health care. Under major medical plans, employees are usually responsible for a fixed dollar amount, termed out-of-pocket expenses, which includes deductibles and co-insurance. In addition, many employees pay a portion of their health-care premium, so it is to their advantage to keep health-care costs down to avoid unnecessary increases in premiums.

How it works: Let's say the out-of-pocket limit is $1,000. The insurance company usually pays 80% (and the patient 20%) of all non-room-and-board charges until the $1,000 out-of-pocket expense limit is reached. After that, insurance takes over 100%.However, most patients don't reach the out-of-pocket limit, since they'd have to run up at least $5,000 worth of non-room-and-board hospital expenses or other health-care costs to do so. Therefore, while your contribution to out-of-pocket is still adding up, it clearly pays to keep costs down.

### Why and How

There are many billing errors for the simple reason that many hospitals have inefficient billing systems. Major problem: Hospitals are geared to making sure that patients are billed for services provided, and not toward verifying charges.

Typical mistake: Because of a clerical error, a $50 electrocardiogram is entered onto your bill at a $500 charge. Since you may not know the typical cost of an EKG, the error goes undetected.

Another example: A lab technician comes in to draw blood and finds that the patient is no longer there. However, he's still charged. Reason: Billing starts from the day the charges are entered in the book, and his charges are never canceled.

Similar mistakes occur with drug prescriptions. Example: The doctor might order 10 days of penicillin and then switch to tetracycline after seven days. If the unused three days' worth of penicillin is not returned, the patient is billed for it.

### The Four Major Mistake Areas

• Respiratory therapy. Equipment such as oxygen tanks and breathing masks isn't credited when it's discontinued. Sometimes it's not even removed promptly from the room.

• Pharmacy charges. Credit isn't given for drugs that were returned, or unused drugs are not returned.

• Lab tests. Cancellations of tests aren't noted.

• Central supply items. Hospital staff or nurses may run out of something and borrow it from another patient. They intend to give credit or return the item, but often they don't get around to it.

### What You Can Do

• Keep track of the most basic things, such as how many times your blood was drawn. Suggestion: If you're able, jot down what happens daily. Note: If the patient is too sick to keep track of services rendered, a family member should try to keep track of the charges. Although it may be difficult to know how many routine things such as blood counts or X rays were done, someone who visits regularly is likely to know about nonroutine services, such as barium enemas or cardiac catheterizations.

• Ask questions. Ask the doctor to be specific about tests. If he orders X rays, ask him what type of X rays. If he doesn't answer the question to your satisfaction, ask the nurse. Always ask. It's the most important thing a health-care consumer can do. Reassuring change: The newer generation of doctors is more willing to involve the patient in his own care.

• Insist on an itemized bill, not just a summary of charges.

• Check room and board charges. Count the days you were in the hospital and in what kind of room. Are you being charged for a private room, even though you were in a semi-private? Some hospitals have different semi-private rates for two-bed and four-bed rooms. Check your rate.

• Review the charges for TV rental and phone.

• Be equally careful with doctor bills. Often these bills are made out by the doctor's assistant, who may not be sure of what was done. Most common errors: Charges for services in the doctor's office, such as a chest X ray or an injection, that weren't actually performed. Charges for routine hospital physician visits on days that the doctor was not in attendance.

**Source:** Interview with Janice Spillane, manager of cost containment in the group insurance department of New York Life Insurance Co., New York.

# HOME VS. HOSPITAL CARE

Many hospital procedures can be managed at home effectively and efficiently to spare the patient's pocketbook. A home chemotherapy program run by M. D. Anderson Hospital in Houston saved an average of $1,500 per patient. Home recipients of intravenous feedings through a Cleveland Clinic project cut an estimated $100 a day from their bills. In Nashua, NH, patients who took intravenous antibiotic therapy at home instead of in the hospital saved $286 a day. Bottom Line: Check with your doctor about local home-care programs the next time a family member is hospitalized.

**Source:** A study conducted by *Voluntary Effort Quarterly*, reported in *Physician's Management*.

# THE WORLD OF LESS EXPENSIVE HEALTH CARE

As recently as five years ago, people had few options when it came to health care. If you woke up with a high fever or needed to have a wart removed, you saw your family doctor. If your child fell off his bicycle and broke his arm, you went to the hospital.

Today there is an alternative: Ambulatory, free-standing clinics. You walk in, receive care at your convenience (and considerably less expense), and walk out again—all in the same day.

It's an idea whose time has come. There are now 2,000 free-standing "emergicenters" nationwide. They deal with a wide range of health crises: Respiratory illnesses, gastrointestinal problems, fractures, sprains and lacerations. Although these clinics lack the blood banks or equipment to handle major emergencies (such as a stroke or cardiac arrest), they can stabilize such patients until they reach a hospital.

In addition, there are 200 "surgicenters" (up from 10 in 1974) for minor elective operations. As surgery becomes more sophisticated and less invasive, many procedures that once required a hospital stay can now be done on an ambulatory basis, with local anesthesia. You may not be able to play golf later that afternoon, but you can go home.

These procedures range from plastic surgery to foot and skin surgery and hernia repair. In any given clinic the areas covered depend, of course, on the specialties of the participating doctors

The most obvious advantage of the free-standing clinic (particularly to employers, who wind up paying most of the bills) lies in its economy. Comparable care typically runs at least one-third less than it would in a hospital. Examples: Treatment of a fractured arm costs on average $157 in a hospital emergency room but only $71 at a free-standing clinic. Influenza with fever: $159 at a hospital, $30 at a clinic. Arm laceration and suturing: $133 at a hospital, $75 in a clinic.

The clinics can charge less because of lower overhead. They aren't supporting expensive labs, high-tech machinery or large numbers of peripheral staff. They are usually very efficient. Although ambulatory clinics may make more extensive use of nurse-practitioners and physician assistants, they don't stint on the level of care. In fact, patients are often treated by the same doctors who work at the hospital down the block or across town—only in a different setting.

If anything, clinic patients may get more quality time and attention from the doctors. They're not competing for priority with a triple bypass on the next corridor as they might be at a hospital. Result: Operations are virtually never delayed or "bumped" for rescheduling.

The free-standing clinics also score heavily for convenience. Many are open from 7 A.M. until 11 P.M. Some stay open 24 hours a day, seven days a week. Suppose you need to have a bunion removed but don't want to lose a day of work. You could leave your office around 4 P.M., enter the surgicenter, get picked up at 10 that night, and go to work the next morning. Or you could arrange for a procedure on Friday evening and convalesce over the weekend.

The case could be made that ambulatory clinics are better for your general health than hospitals. By skipping an overnight stay, you're avoiding long hours in a germ-ridden environment. Nurses aren't interrupting your sleep. And studies have shown that patients recuperate more quickly in the comfortable familiarity of their own homes. It comes down to the first question asked by most hospital patients after surgery—not "How did it go?" but "When can I go home?"

Free-standing clinics have gained their widest acceptance in the Sun Belt, where licensing requirements are generally less stringent. But they've also become common in Illinois and Ohio, and they will probably begin to penetrate the Northeast within a few years.

**Source:** Interview with Robert Williams, executive director, the Freestanding Ambulatory Surgical Association, Phoenix, and Phil Wolfe, staff member, National Association of Freestanding Emergency Centers, Dallas.

# ALL ABOUT THE RIGHT TO DIE

Life-prolonging medical equipment is proliferating to such a degree that very few Americans have escaped the traumatizing experience of watching a terminally ill loved one suffer terribly through the hookup to life-support machines. And in different ways the family and friends often suffer more than the patient. Efforts to have the equipment removed are frequently stymied by the doctor or the hospital.

American courts and legislatures are still in the process of confronting the legal issues of the right to die, but guidelines are emerging.

### Why Is There a Problem?
Doctors are ambivalent about terminally ill patients. The Hippocratic oath tells them to preserve life, but it also directs them to relieve suffering. These two goals too often conflict.

### Your Rights Now
Twenty-three states have what's called living-will legislation. It recognizes the right of an individual to have honored a written

statement that he doesn't wish his life to be artificially prolonged if there is no expectation of recovery. Living wills have been tested and upheld in three courts. Informed consent provides the legal basis for living-will legislation. No doctor in the US should now be able to perform a procedure without the patient's or a family member's express permission. Problem: Such laws are written in varying ways, providing different degrees of protection.

Examples: California law makes a living will a binding document two weeks after the person has been diagnosed as having a terminal condition, which does nothing for the stroke or accident victim. Most of the laws have no provision for a severely brain-damaged, comatose person. Some states allow a witnessed oral statement instead. In Florida there's a whole list of family members who can be consulted if there's no written document.

The one thing legislation does: It protects health-care providers from liability should life-sustaining treatment be withheld or withdrawn from a dying patient. Irony: Doctors and hospitals don't really need this legal shelter. No doctor or hospital has ever faced criminal or civil charges for stopping treatment of a terminally ill patient, as opposed to a handicapped infant such as Baby Jane Doe.

**What You Can Do**

As with all social problems, legislation often follows what has become common practice. Many hospitals and doctors honor a living will whether or not the state has living-will legislation. And many honor the wishes of the family, quietly allowing a patient to die the way he and his family request.

Problems arise when the doctor and/or the hospital refuse to go along with the patient's or the family's wishes. The family can always petition the court for an order to turn off the equipment. But no one in such an emotionally traumatic situation wants to hire lawyers and face judges. There are a number of alternatives available before going to court—whether or not there is a living will:

• If there is a living will, make sure it's been shown to the doctor and is on the patient's medical chart.

• Ask the doctor if there is any chance the relative will ever return to his or her former condition. If not, ask why the hospital is maintaining the patient. The dictor has to answer this question.

• Try for interim measures. Try to get a "do not resuscitate order" put on the chart. If you're trying to get a dying person off tubes, the last thing you want is the cardio-vascular rescue team running in to start the patient's heart when it fails.

• If the doctor refuses to do what you want, find out why. Then talk to the hospital's patient representative or ombudsman, if there is one. This person often is the interface between patients and staff and can can be helpful.

• If the doctor is uncooperative, try to get a more cooperative doctor assigned to the case. Failing that, try to get the person transferred to another hospital.

• Finally, you can ask to see the hospital attorney and say, "This is assault and battery. My relative did not give consent for this procedure." If that's the case, you can sue the hospital if its staff doesn't take the patient off the equipment.

• As a last resort, you can take the person home to die. It's been done. A hospital can't hold a patient against his or her will.

• No matter how desperate you feel, don't pull the plugs yourself. That's murder. Although mercy killers are generally found not guilty in this country, such a trial is a terrible ordeal.

• Call Concern for Dying for advice.

**Source:** Interview with executives at Concern for Dying, an educational council, 250 W. 57 St., New York 10107.

# 16. Getting a Good Night's Sleep

# Getting a Good Night's Sleep

## WHY WE SLEEP

All about sleep. No one really knows why humans sleep, but two theories have been proposed. The prevailing view: We sleep so that cells and chemicals depleted from the body during the day can be restored. Flaw in that view: Not a single such chemical has been identified. New idea on sleep: Early man adapted to nighttime sleep because he was vulnerable to predators and accidents during the hours when he couldn't see. Mammals bigger than man sleep less than we do. Elephants, for example, sleep only two hours a night. They have no predators, but possibly they need the other 22 hours to find enough food for their huge bodies. Grazing animals, always at the mercy of predators, sleep only intermittently in groups where some members are always awake.

**Source:** Dr. Wilse Webb, quoted in *Psychology Today.*

## UNDERSTANDING SLEEP

Although most people sleep seven or eight hours a night, others may log from 4 to 11 hours without ill effects. There is a natural spread of sleep needs.

Sleep deprivation does not actually cause any mental or physical derangement. Main effect of sleep loss: Decreased alertness.

The quality of sleep changes with age. Young adolescents sleep so soundly that very little disturbs them. Contrast: The normal sleep of the elderly is light and fitful.

Does sleep physically help the body and mind to mend and rejuvenate? Scientists are not exactly sure. One certainty: After strenuous exercise, such as a marathon run, people have longer nondreaming stages of sleep. During these stages a growth hormone that repairs tissue damage is secreted.

## NAP NEWS

There are two kinds of naps: Recreational snoozes and sleep-replacement dozes. Recreational naps are brief, self-terminating and refreshing. Rest-replacement naps—the result of too little sleep the night before—are deep-sleep periods that leave you feeling groggy and terrible. Bottom line: A brief, light nap during the day is fine, but if you need more nighttime sleep, go to bed earlier.

**Source:** Study by Dr. Wilse Webb, University of Florida, Gainesville.

## RIGHT WAY TO TAKE A NAP

Napping won't bother your nighttime sleeping if it is done correctly. Keep your naps short, about 10–20 minutes. This clears your head without making you drowsy. Try to nap at the same time every day, so your body can accommodate the nap into its rhythms.

**Source:** Dr. Charles Polak, director, Sleep-Wake Disorders Center, New York Hospital-Cornell Medical Center.

## HOW TO BUY A MATTRESS

The quality of sleep makes the quantity less important. To enable you to relax, your mattress must provide proper support for your body, yet be resilient enough for comfort.

The old-fashioned double bed gives each sleeper only 26 inches of space, about the same width as a baby's crib. The current most popular size—queen—is seven inches wider and five inches longer than the old double bed. King size is an additional 16 inches wider.

Mattress prices depend on the materials, quality of construction, size number of layers of upholstery and the store's markup. (Prices may be lower in small, neighborhood stores with low overhead.)

Standard mattresses have two different kinds of construction, inner-spring or foam rubber. Top-quality-innerspring mattresses have covered metal coils, cushioning material and an insulator between the coils to prevent them from protruding.

Foam mattresses are made of a solid block of urethane, high-resiliency foam or laminated layers of varying density sandwiched together. A good foam mattress is at least five to six inches high and feels heavy when lifted. A high-density foam mattress costs about $300 in queen size and should last 10–15 years. Foam mattresses can be used on a wooden platform for extra firmness or with a conventional boxspring.

How to shop for a mattress:

• Sit on the edge of the bed. The mattress should support you without feeling flimsy, and it should spring back into shape when you get up. A reinforced border increases durability.

• Lie down. (If the bed is to be used by a couple, both partners should test it lying down.) Check several different firmnesses to choose the one you're most comfortable with. Next, roll from side to side and then to the center. The mattress should not sway, jiggle or sag in the middle. If you hear creaking springs, don't buy it.

• Examine the covering. Best: Sturdy ticking with a pattern woven in, not printed on.

• Check for handles on the sides for easy turning, small metal vents to disperse heat and allow air to circulate inside, and plastic corner guards.

Up to 80% of the sleeper's weight is borne by the boxspring. The finest mattress won't be effective unless it's accompanied by a boxspring of equal quality. When a new mattress is needed, both the mattress and spring should be repaced to ensure that the support system is specifically designed for the mattress.

Queen-size innerspring sets should be used in a sturdy bed frame with a footboard or in a six-leg heavy steel support. Twin and double size can use a four-leg metal frame.

A good innerspring sleep set should last 15–20 years.

There is no proven medical advantage to sleeping on a hard surface, so consider comfort the key factor. According to Dr. Hamilton Hall, an orthopedic surgeon who specializes in techniques to relieve pain, there is no single perfect mattress. "What's perfect for one person may be uncomfortable for another."

Best advice: Only buy a sleep set made by a manufacturer with a good reputation and sold by a reputable dealer. Be very wary of advertised bargains.

# GETTING TO SLEEP...AND SLEEPING THROUGH THE NIGHT

Sleep disturbances are usually the temporary symptoms of life changes...bereavement or joy...getting a new home or job...passing a milestone (turning 40).

Weight loss can also be a cause of poor sleep. Those with slightly higher than normal weight sleep better. Although uninterrupted sleep becomes less and less common after the age of 50, fewer total hours of sleep are required.

Long-term sleep disturbances can arise from poor daily habits. Worst offenders: Smoking, and drinking alcohol or caffeine within four hours of bedtime. Daytime naps make falling asleep difficult for some people. Sleeping pills are not recommended.

### To Combat Sleeplessness

A regular daily schedule is the best guarantee of natural, comfortable sleep. This means rising at the same time every day. To catch up on lost sleep: Go to bed early the next night, instead of sleeping late.

Keep the bedroom cool. Ideal sleeping temperature: 64–66 degrees. Use the bedroom only for sleep and sex. All of the room's associations should be pleasurable ones, unconnected with work or any other such activity.

Wait until you are sleepy to go to bed. If sleep does not come within 15 or 20 minutes, get out of bed. If hunger pains keep you awake, eat a light, easily disgested snack. Best: Cereal and milk. The ami-

392 / GETTING A GOOD NIGHT'S SLEEP

no acid trypotophan, found in milk and tuna fish, helps some people sleep.

If falling asleep remains a problem, the three-step "easy sleep" technique may help:

• Lying in bed, relax the muscles, starting from the head down—scalp, eyes, facial muscles, the mouth area, the tongue, down the arms to the fingertips, down from the chest through the legs, all the way to the tips of your toes.

• Imagine yourself having a good night's sleep. Think what this would be like.

• Imagine yourself at the center of a relaxing, pleasant scene. Examples: Sitting at the beach watching the waves. Relaxing on a porch swing. Dozing in a rocking chair before a fire.

**Source:** *Get a Good Night's Sleep* by Elliott Phillips, M.D., Prentice Hall, Englewood Cliffs, NJ. *Get a Better Night's Sleep* by Ian Oswald, M.D., and Kirstine Adams, Ph.D., Arco Publishing, New York. *Easy Sleep* by John J. Gnap, M.D., with Nancy Flaster, Stein & Day, Scarborough House, Briarcliff Manor, NY.

# HELP IS ON THE WAY

Sleep problems—from real insomnia to occasional restless slumber—can be cured.

The first step in the cure is to become aware that you're not alone—and that something can be done.

Occasional insomniacs usually contribute to their problem by worrying that theirs is a serious problem—and a symptom of even more sleep problems in the future. Occasional means anything from one sleepless night a week to one a year. In most cases, sufferers should dismiss those symptoms. They are usually caused by some specific and temporary stress or anxiety.

How do you know when your occasional insomnia has become a chronic disorder?

To be a chronic problem, the loss of sleep must have a real effect on your daytime functioning. A good question to ask yourself is, "What would I be doing differently during the day if I were getting eight hours sleep at night?" In other words, what benefit would being able to sleep bring you?

Sometimes, a person is simply not sleeping as much as he thinks he should, but his daytime functioning is not adversely affected. In those cases, the individual probably is trying to sleep more hours than he needs to.

Prescription for the occasional insomniac: Condition your sleep environment. Learn to associate your bed and your bedroom with sleep.

How to do it:

• Pay attention to bedroom conditions, such as light, heat, noise. Shut off telephones if necessary. Keep temperature cool (around 68°). Make sure your mattress and your sleep clothing are comfortable.

• If you don't fall asleep right away, get up, leave the bedroom, and go do something else. Don't lie awake thinking about it. Staying in bed for hours trying to get to sleep accentuates the problem. You begin to associate your bed and bedroom with trying to sleep instead of with sleeping.

• Stick to a regular bedtime schedule. Go to bed at the same time every night— weekdays and weekends. Some insomniacs have the idea they'll catch up on missed sleep on the weekends. You can't do it. Trying to do it simply disrupts your biological rhythms.

Other popular sleep inducers or aids:

• Sleeping pills. Doctor-prescribed sedatives are very useful in temporary situations where a particular emotional or physical upset is the cause of the insomnia. Problem: Tendency to become dependent on them, and a worsening of the quality of sleep as more pills are used.

How to handle pills: Use for no more than a week or two. Expect that sleep will be very disturbed on the first night or two after stopping the pills. That's perfectly normal. Expect it and accept it.

• Nonprescription, over-the-counter sleeping pills are absolutely useless. Studies have shown "sugar pills" to be just as effective.

• Exercise. Early in the day is okay. Late in the evening is too stimulating.

Exception to the rule: Sexual activity, within a comfortable relationship where no tension or anxiety exists, is helpful.

• Caffeine. Coffee, tea, soft drinks act as stimulants. Avoid completely.

• Alcohol. May help you get to sleep but interferes with quality of sleep. Wears off after several hours.

• Widely advertised insomnia cures like vibrating beds, prerecorded cassette tapes, sleep masks are fine if they relax you.

**Source:** Dr. Frank Zorick, former clinical director of the sleep disorder center at Cincinnati Veterans Administration Hospital and the University of Cincinnati.

## HOW TO FALL *BACK* TO SLEEP

Agony: Awakening in the middle of the night and not being able to fall back to sleep. Prime cause: Advancing age. People over 50 have middle insomnia. Those under 50 often have difficulty falling to sleep.

How to cope: Do not become angry when you find yourself awake at 3 A.M. Anger only excites you, preventing sleep. Instead, fix your mind on a single relaxing image. Example: Visualize a flickering candle. If you are still awake after 30 minutes, go to another room. Watch an old movie on TV, or read a book or magazine. When you feel sleepy, return to bed. If sleep still eludes you, go back to the other room and read some more. Frustrating and useless: Tossing and turning in bed, waiting for sleep to arrive.

Preventive steps:

• Eliminate daytime naps if they have been a habit.

• Do not go to bed too early. This only increases the chances of middle insomnia.

• Set your wake-up alarm an hour earlier than usual. This makes you more tired for the following night. Advance the alarm by 15-minute increments until you are sleeping through the night. Then slowly extend your sleep period until you are back on a normal schedule.

**Source:** *A Good Night's Sleep* by Jerrold S. Maxmen, M.D., Contemporary Books.

## PROFILE OF AN INSOMNIAC

Chronic insomniacs are less active physically and mentally during the day and are also less involved in their work and with other people than good sleepers. Insomniacs are also more preoccupied with self, quieter . . . and, oddly, less worried. They spend more time watching TV during the day, shopping and relaxing. Good sleepers pass their time studying, working and doing active things around the house. Unknown: Whether the habits of insomniacs are the result of poor sleep or its cause.

**Source:** Study conducted by psychologists at the University of California, San Francisco, and the Pacific Graduate School of Psychology, Palo Alto, CA.

• Insomnia-prone people are generally unable to discharge anger and stress outwardly. Insomniacs are characteristically inhibited, anxious and depressed. Their internalized emotions lead to physiologic activation, preventing sleep at night.

## RELAXATION MAY BE THE KEY

Insomnia is often stress-related and is frequently treated by relaxation therapy. Sleeping pills can cause morning drowsiness and poor-quality sleep. Some techniques: Hypnosis, progressive relaxation (tensing and relaxing muscle groups), biofeedback (including relaxation and breathing exercises), meditation (focusing the mind on a single point), and yoga. It's important to reduce outside stimuli—no reading, eating, or TV-watching in bed. Avoid: Worrying, especially about getting to sleep.

## SLEEPING-PILL ALERT

Avoid sleep medications until the source of insomnia is traced. Reason: The drugs can be harmful, even deadly, to people with sleep apnea (a disorder in which breathing ceases momentarily.)

## INSOMNIA REMEDY

Chronic insomnia remedy: Two grams of L-Tryptophan, an amino acid available in health food stores. Take it 30 minutes before bedtime on three successive days, followed by four days without medication and repeat as long as necessary. The usual treatment duration is four months. In one study L-Tryptophan was completely effective for at least half of the severe insomniacs tested. For the other insomniacs, intermittent treatment was all that was needed to correct sleep abnormalities.

**Source:** *Internal Medicine News.*

# HOW TO STOP SNORING

• Put a brick or two under both of your bed's pillow-end legs. Elevating your head will keep the airway open. Counterproductive: Using extra pillows. They'll only kink the airway.

• Avoid all depressants a few hours before bed. Take no alcohol, tranquilizers, sleeping pills or antihistamines late in the day.

• Lose weight. Three of four snorers are at least 20% over their ideal weight.

• Wear a cervical collar. It keeps the chin up and the windpipe open.

• Wear a "snore ball." Cut a small, solid-rubber ball in half. Using two patches of Velcro, attach the flat side of the half-sphere to the back of your pajama top. If done right, it should keep you off your back—the position for virtually all snoring.

**Source:** *Prevention.*

# HOW TO GET OUT ON THE RIGHT SIDE OF THE BED

• Stretch each leg and flex each foot.

• Rotate your feet (inward and outward circles).

• Roll your head slowly from side to side.

• Open your eyes wide. Move them from side to side while keeping your head still.

• Open your mouth wide. Yawn four times.

• Stretch your arms up to the ceiling, inhaling deeply.

• Lying on your back, clasp your hands behind your head. Slowly lift your head until your chin touches your chest.

• Use both hand to pull one knee to your chest.

• Massage your face with the knuckles of both hands.

• Gently wipe the corners of each eye with your middle fingers.

• Do a sit-up with bent knees.

• Take a deep breath. Relax and think of something pleasant.

**Source:** SmokEnder's founder Jacquelyn Rogers, in *American Health.*

# CLOCK FOR THE SIGHTED AND THE BLIND

Braille clock with raised numbers and hands is a boon to the sighted who are bothered at night by the electronic glow of digital clocks. It is, of course, also useful to the blind. Made by Seiko.

# 17. What You Should Know about Drugs and Smoking

# What You Should Know about Drugs and Smoking

## THEORIES OF ADDICTION

What leads a person to become an alcohol abuser, drug addict or compulsive gambler? According to a study by the National Academy of Sciences, these traits are typical: Impulsive behavior, with a pull toward immediate gratification. More esteem for nonconformity than for conventional goals and achievements. A sense of social alienation. A sense of heightened stress.

• There may be a distinct connection between personality and choice of drugs. People who cope with stress or feelings of low self-esteem by avid TV-watching or food binges tend to use depressants. Workaholics and high-risk takers opt for stimulants. People involved in obsessive artistic or spiritual pursuits are likely to pick hallucinogens.

**Source:** Study at Bellevue Hospital Center, New York, reported in *Psychology Today*, New York.

## CHANGING DRINKING HABITS

Americans are drinking less than at any time since 1969. Only 65% drink beer, wine or hard liquor even occasionally—down from 71% in 1977. And 29% say they have cut back on alcohol over the last five years (although 11% are drinking more). Exception: In the 18–29 age group, 21% have increased consumption.

**Source:** *Reader's Digest/* Gallup survey.

## IT'S WHAT YOU *THINK* YOU'RE DRINKING THAT COUNTS

What you think you're drinking may be at least as important as what it really is. Men became more aggressive and sexually aroused when they drank only tonic water but *thought* it was mixed with vodka. They were less aggressive when they drank vodka and tonic but believed it was straight tonic.

**Source:** Study at the University of Washington, Seattle.

## DRUGS AND DRIVING

In the most recent study of fatal automobile accidents, 81% of male drivers between the ages of 15 and 34 had alcohol and at least one other drug in their bloodstreams at the time of the accident.

**Source:** Insurance Institute for Highway Safety, Washington, DC.

• Even after eight hours of sleep following a night of heavy drinking, you should not drive a car. Driving ability is impaired as much as 20% the morning after a bender—whether you feel rotten or not. Your reactions are slowed down after a bout of drinking alcohol even if your head and stomach have escaped the classic hangover symptoms. Stay away from the wheel until afternoon at least.

**Source:** Study by the Swedish National Road and Traffic Institute, reported in *Journal of the American Medical Association*, Chicago.

• Alcohol is involved in 55% of fatal car accidents, 80% of boating deaths, and 10% of fatal private-plane crashes.

**Source:** Study by the National Transportation Safety Board, Washington, D.C.

## WALKING AND ALCOHOL DON'T MIX

Intoxicated pedestrians are more than

three times more likely to be injured in a traffic accident than sober walkers. Those who are not drunk but still have alcohol in their blood run an accident risk that is 1.5 times higher than that of abstainers. Contrary to popular thinking, drinkers suffer more serious injuries in such accidents than victims who are sober.

Source: A study of pedestrians made in Belfast, Northern Ireland, as reported in the *British Medical Journal, London.*

## HEART DISEASE AND CHRONIC DRINKERS

A single drink of hard liquor can lead to cardiac rhythm disturbances in chronic drinkers with a history of heart disease. Even healthy hearts can fall prey to "holiday heart syndrome"—arrhythmias that commonly result from weekend imbibing. Bottom line: Modest "social" drinking may not be as universally harmless as once thought.

Source: *RN* magazine, Oradell, N.J.

## GOOD AND BAD NEWS ABOUT ALCOHOL AND SEX

Alcohol delays orgasm in men and women up to 12 minutes past the normal time. Bright side: Alcohol taken in moderation does increase sexual arousal without a significant loss in performance.

Source: *The Playboy Advisor on Love and Sex* by James R. Peterson, Perigee Books, New York.

• Excessive alcohol and sex don't mix for either gender. It's well known that an intoxicated man may have trouble attaining an erection. But recent clinical observation suggests that a woman often fails to lubricate after six or more drinks. And, although women may be more compliant when intoxicated, there's no evidence of increased sexual response or satisfaction.

Source: Wallace Mandell, director of the Johns Hopkins Hospital clinical alcoholism program, Baltimore, in *Medical Aspects of Human Sexuality*, New York.

## THINKING AND DRINKING DON'T MIX

Heavy drinkers tend to lose their ability for high-level, abstract thinking—even when sober. Slightly tipsy (one drink beyond the usual daily quota) imbibers' thinking scores drop dramatically. Drinking may take a greater toll on the mind than aging does.

Source: Research psychologist Elizabeth S. Parker, quoted in *American Health* magazine, New York.

## BLOOD PRESSURE ALERT

Alcohol contributes to high blood pressure in hypertensive men. Those who regularly drink as much as 2.8 ounces of alcohol a day (about three drinks) can significantly lower their blood pressure by going on the wagon. And, according to research, a return to drink will bring levels back up again.

Source: Study at Dudley Road Hospital, Birmingham, England, reported in *The Lancet*, London.

## DANGER OF BINGE DRINKING

Binge drinkers face an increased risk of stroke and brain hemorrhage, according to Finnish researchers. It's unclear, however, whether this applies only to regular heavy drinkers, to occasional heavy drinkers, or to both groups.

Source: Study reported in *The Lancet.*

## THE DANGERS OF MODERATE DRINKING

Moderate drinkers—people who have even two drinks or less a day—live longer on average, are more relaxed and have less risk of heart attack than either heavy drinkers or teetotalers.

However, these benefits are reversed whenever the moderate drinker exceeds his two-drink limit. Recent tests show that even light social drinking affects mental performance for longer than expected.

398 / DRUGS AND SMOKING

Everyone knows that drinking during the day reduces efficiency. Now it appears that cognitive abilities continue to be adversely affected after the alcohol has left the bloodstream. Reason: Once irritated, the central nervous system remains disturbed even after the cause has been removed.

The dulling effects of alcohol are usually noticeable on the day following a night of three drinks or more. But the effects of two drinks are often too subtle to be noticed by moderate drinkers. Bottom line: If you must think fast, you give something away by drinking the night before.

### Controlling Alcohol Intake

The dangers of excessive alcohol for moderate drinkers come less from lack of control than from careless measuring. Two drinks means two 1½-ounce servings of 80-proof liquor (the contents of two shot glasses)....or two four- or five-ounce glassses of wine...or two 12-ounce bottles of beer. Most drinks served at parties and bars these days contain considerably more than an ounce and a half. In fine restaurants, it's not unusual to be served three ounces of liquor in a single drink. So, one drink can put you beyond your safe limits.

Moderate-drinking rules:

• Take no more than two drinks on any single occasion.

• Reduce the limit to one drink the night before an important meeting or other occasion when you want to have your wits about you.

• Drink no more than once a day.

• When drinking liquor, use a mixer. Reason: Diluted drinks reduce the irritant effects of alcohol on the system.

• Measure how many ounces your wineglasses hold, and learn to estimate the four to five ounces that constitute a drink.

**Source:** *How Much Is Too Much? The Effects of Social Drinking* by Leonard Gross, Random House, New York.

## MODERATE DRINKING PLUS

Moderate drinking apparently does more

than soothe jittery nerves. According to recent research, it also lowers chances of developing cardiovascular disease and gallstones.

**Source:** Study at the University Department of Medicine, Bristol Royal infirmary, Bristol, England, reported in *The Lancet*, London.

## NEW HELP FOR ALCOHOLICS

Lithium carbonate may help some alcoholics abstain from drinking. In a recent study, some alcoholics were given the lithium compound, others a placebo. Result: 75% of those given lithium stayed off alcohol for 18 months, as compared with 50% of those given the placebo. Lithium's surprising effect suggests alcoholism may be associated with a genetically transmitted biochemical marker.

**Source:** Study by Jan A. Fawcett, M.D., Rush-Presbyterian-St. Luke's Medical Center, reported in *Medical World News*, N.Y.

## HANGOVER HELP

There is no cure for inebriation nor any magic formula to prevent the headache and general malaise that follow an evening of drinking too much alcohol too quickly. However, some measures can keep a night on the town from being a total disaster.

• Eat fatty or oily food before you have the first drink. That lines your stomach and slows the body's absorption of alcohol. (Cheese and nuts are good choices.)

• Eat starches while you drink to soak up the alcohol. (Bread or crackers work.)

• Avoid spirits with high levels of congeners (additives that can cause toxic effects). Brandy, red wine, dark rum and sherry are the worst. Vodka and white wine are the least adulterated.

If you wake up with a hangover, you can only try to treat the symptoms and help bring back to normal all the bodily functions disrupted by alcohol. Some suggestions:

• A dry mouth is a sign of dehydration.

Drink plenty of water to replace the lost fluid.

• Alcohol depletes the system of many nutrients, particularly vitamins A, B, $B_6$ and C and minerals such as niacin, calcium, magnesium and potassium. Take a multivitamin that includes minerals.

• Take charcoal tablets to speed up the removal of the congeners (four tablets if you are small and up to six for larger people). Cabbage and vitamin C are reputed to help in this area as well.

• To work the alcohol out of your system (actually to metabolize it), a little exercise is useful. It increases your intake of oxygen, and oxygen speeds up this process. So does the fructose found in honey and fruit juices.

• For pain or nausea, over-the-counter analgesics or antacids are the antidote.

• "A little hair of the dog that bit you" is an old cure that has some basis in reality. The brain cells affected by alcohol can return to normal quite suddenly. This explains the supersensitivity to noise and smells associated with hangover. A small amount of alcohol (one to one-and-a-half ounces) can ease your brain back into awareness. Recommended: If you try this panacea, mix the spirits with something nutritious like cream. Other possibilities: A can of beer. A Fernet Branca, a packaged alcoholic mixture that includes herbs, and folk-medicine standbys like camomile and aloe.

**Source:** *The Hangover Handbook* by David Outerbridge, Harmony Books, New York.

## ALCOHOL WITHOUT HANGOVERS

Some hangover discomfort is caused by congeners (toxic chemicals formed during fermentation). Vodka has the lowest congener content, gin next. Blended scotch has four times the congener content of gin. Brandy, rum, and pure malt scotch have six times that amount; bourbon, eight times.

Retard the absorption of alcohol by eating before and during drinking (especially foods, such as cheeses, containing fatty proteins).

Use water as a mixer. Carbonation speeds the absorption of alcohol.

If you get a hangover anyway, the only known cures are rest, aspirin, and time. Endless rosters of other remedies—ranging from cucumber juice and salt to a Bloody Mary— have more to do with drinking mythology than with medical fact, although according to psychologists who have studied hangovers, if you believe in a cure, it may help.

## HIGH-SCHOOL SENIORS' DRUG CHOICES

Marijuana remains the most popular illicit drug among American youth. In a 1982 survey of 17,700 high school seniors, 59% said they had used marijuana at least once (up from 47% in 1975). Also used: Stimulants, 36% (up from 22% in 1975). Cocaine, 16% (up from 9%). Sedatives, 15% (down from 18%). Tranquilizers, 14% (down from 17%). Hallucinogens, 13% (down from 16%). How many had tried heroin? Only 1%.

**Source:** *Statistical Bulletin*, Metropolitan Life Insurance Co., New York.

## PLAIN TRUTHS ABOUT COCAINE

The pleasures of cocaine stem from the short-lived but intense euphoria it imparts. Sexually, cocaine may increase sensual awareness. However, it does not improve performance, and, in fact, it is often associated with impotence. Users often justify cocaine by citing its lack of physiological dependence. Problem: Many users are consumed by an overwhelming desire to continue cocaine ingestion to perpetuate the euphoria. Result: This psychological compulsion breeds its own strong dependence.

**Source:** Robert H. McDonald, M.D., University of Pittsburgh School of Medicine, writing in *Medical Aspects of Human Sexuality*, New York.

## WHY PRETEENS SHOULDN'T SMOKE MARIJUANA

Preteens who smoke marijuana are risking

their health more than older cigarette smokers. Reason: Marijuana contains more of some carcinogenic substances than tobacco does, and young lungs are especially vulnerable to the damaging effects of the smoke.

**Source:** American Lung Association, New York.

## NARCOTICS MAY BE BAD FOR YOUR SEX LIFE

Narcotics and sex are often an incompatible mixture. Complaints of heroin addicts and those on methadone maintenance: Reduced sexual drive, impotence or delayed ejaculation in men and inability in women to reach orgasm. Withdrawal from the drugs usually reawakens sexual interest. But for men, this is frequently accompanied by nocturnal emissions and premature ejaculation. Only after detoxification are the effects of the opiates on orgasm reversed.

**Source:** Roger D. Weiss, M.D., Harvard Medical School, Boston, writing in *Medical Aspects of Human Sexuality* journal, New York.

## AGE WHEN CIGARETTE SMOKING BEGINS

Virtually all serious cigarette smokers picked up the habit between the ages of 12 and 18.

**Source:** *Harvard Medical School Health Letter*, Cambridge, MA.

## ANOTHER REASON WOMEN MAY OUTLIVE MEN

Men live as long as women if they don't smoke. On the average, women live to be 77.9 years old, 7.6 years longer than men. But a study shows that men who never smoked (or were not killed by violence) lived as long as women. Lesson: The heavy smoking of men is the overwhelming cause of women's relatively greater longevity. Bad news: Teenage girls now surpass their male counterparts in percentage of smokers, which could shorten the life span of women.

**Source:** A study of the case histories of 4,394 people who died in Erie County, PA, by, Gus H. Miller, M.D., of Edinboro, PA, and Dean R. Gerstein, M.D., of Washington, DC.

## THE COST OF SMOKING

Another reason not to smoke: There's strong evidence now that cigarette smoking causes a host of digestive dysfunctions—including heartburn, peptic ulcers (smoking also delays ulcer healing) and esophageal cancer. Also, some drugs (for example, propranolol for heart patients and Tagamet for ulcer patients) aren't properly metabolized by the liver in smokers. Middle-aged men who are heavy smokers will spend an average of $59,000 in extra medical bills and lost earnings over a lifetime.

**Source:** *Vegetarian Times*, New York.

## SMOKING AND MENOPAUSE

Heavy smoking tends to bring on earlier menopause. According to recent research, women aged 48 to 51 who smoked more than 14 cigarettes a day were far more likely to have passed menopause than nonsmokers in the same age group.

**Source:** *Prevention* magazine, Emmaus, PA.

## SMOKING, COMPUTER GAMES AND YOUR HEALTH

Smokers under stress run the highest risk of chronic heart disease, according to recent research. Stress test subjects: Young men who played a video game (a mildly stressful event) immediately after having a cigarette. Their blood pressure and heart rate rose at least twice as much as those of smokers who had either played without smoking or smoked without playing.

Postscript: Many smokers claim cigarettes "calm their nerves" and aid their concentration. But the study found that the performance of game-players—even habitual smokers—declined after their first cigarette.

**Source:** A study at the Stress and Cardiovascular Research Center, Eckard College, St. Petersburg, FL, reported in *The Journal of Human Stress.*

## INSURANCE BREAKS FOR NONSMOKERS

Nonsmokers will soon pay less for health insurance.(Smokers cost 54% more than nonsmokers in their use of health services.) The National Association of Insurance Commissioners is also urging incentives for people who maintain proper weight and blood pressure.

Nonsmoking men will pay significantly lower life insurance premiums, beyond the discounts they are currently offered. A recent study of 8,300 people in Erie County, PA, found that men who had smoked fewer than 20 packs of cigarettes in their lifetime lived virtually as long as women.

**Source:** Robert W. MacDonald, president of ITT Life Insurance Corp., Minneapolis, MN.

Nonsmokers are getting bigger breaks on car insurance premiums. . .and they're being offered by more companies: Range: 12%–25% off for liability, collision, and no-fault medical-payment coverage.

**Source:** *Working Woman* magazine, N.Y.

## TRUTH ABOUT CIGARETTE FILTERS

Filters on cigarettes reduce smoke particles by 20%–96%. But, as the cigarette shortens, the particle count increases. If one closes off the ventilating holes on the sides of the filters with one's fingers while inhaling, the filter becomes even less effective. For example, with the vent holes blocked, Barclay exceeded unfiltered Marlboro in the number of particles inhaled.

**Source:** *Archives of Environmental Health*, Washington, D.C.

## LOW-TAR CONFIDENTIAL

Low-tar cigarettes will not save smokers'

health. Because low-tar brands also have less nicotine, smokers often compensate by drawing more deeply or frequently or by closing off ventilation holes in the filter with lips or fingers. Concerning one brand (Barclay), the Federal Trade Commission has challenged the manufacturer's claim of "1 mg. tar." The FTC found that normal pressure from the smoker's lips would block air channels in Barclay's special filter. Result: More smoke inhaled and 3–7 mg. of tar per cigarette.

**Source:** *Consumer Reports*, Mount Vernon, N.Y.

## LOW NICOTINE RIPOFF

Low-nicotine cigarettes do not cut down on the amount of nicotine in the system, according to recent studies. By testing the blood of smokers, researchers discovered that concentrations of nicotine in the human system were inversely correlated with the measurements of nicotine produced by smoking machines. (The tobacco industry uses machines to measure nicotine and tar content.) What did make a difference: The number of cigarettes smoked per day.

**Source:** *New England Journal of Medicine*, Boston.

## PASSIVE SMOKING IS BAD FOR YOUR HEALTH

How truthful are tobacco industry ads claiming that inhaling smoke is not harmful to nonsmokers?

In my opinion, "passive smoking" is very harmful.

Lung cancer does not occur for two or three decades after the exposure to smoking, and, of course, the amounts of smoke inhaled from a room are not as easily measured as the number of cigarettes smoked daily. So, for smokers, the correlation between smoking and lung cancer is more clearly seen and understood.

However, two major studies have shown that there is a positive correlation between "involuntary" smoking and lung cancer. These studies involved measuring the incidence of cancer in the nonsmoking wives of smokers. These wives were found to have a higher chance of getting lung cancer than the wives of nonsmokers. More heart disease and chronic lung obstruction have also been found in such "involuntary" or passive smokers as these.

Though the effects of smoke on nonsmokers are harder to measure, it is perfectly reasonable to conclude that the carcinogens in cigarette smoke are harmful even when diluted by secondhand inhalation.

**Source:** Interview with Joseph Cullen, M.D., deputy director, Division of Cancer Prevention and Control, National Cancer Institute, Bethesda, MD.

## YOUR SPOUSE MAY GIVE YOU CANCER

Nonsmokers married to smokers are 54% more likely to develop lung cancer than those whose spouses don't smoke.

**Source:** Study at the Department of Environmental and Preventive Medicine, St. Bartholomew's Hospital Medical College, London.

## WHY QUITTING SMOKING IS SO DIFFICULT

Cigarette smoking is a form of drug dependence that leads to compulsive use. Because it is an addiction, it is difficult to stop. Relapse is common, even years after quitting. Of the millions who try to quit, only 20% succeed.

How this addiction works: The first cigarette of the day sends a burst of nicotine to the brain, producing an immediate euphoria and satisfaction. The smoker tries to hang on to this glowing feeling for the rest of the day by smoking a series of cigarettes.

Oddity: The nicotine in cigarettes affects the body in different ways. Under stressful conditions, it works like a tranquilizer. In serene situations, it serves as a stimulant, like an amphetamine.

The first few days of withdrawal after quitting bring decreases in heart rate, blood pressure and the production of hormones that act on the nervous system, along with

occasional headaches and gastrointestinal discomfort. And mood changes plague many of those who abstain.

Frequent mysterious side effect: Weight gain, even among those who don't compensate by eating more.

The most important single influence on whether or not a person smokes: The behavior and attitude of family and friends.

Support and understanding are critical when the smoker tries to kick the cigarette addiction.

**Source:** William Pollin, M.D., director of the National Institute on Drug Abuse, testifying before the US Senate.

## ANTI-SMOKING GUM

The latest weapon against smoking is nicotine chewing gum. It was approved by the Federal Drug Administration for prescription use only. Aim: To help smokers kick their habit without new problems in nicotine withdrawal. Withdrawing from the gum is then relatively easy. Early returns: An English study found that more than 45% of patients tested were helped to quit. Caution: The gum should not be used by pregnant women or patients with heart conditions.

## HYPNOSIS: ONE WAY TO STOP SMOKING

I had smoked heavily for 35 years, at least two packs a day, and I had to give it up. But I lacked the conscious willpower. I had read that it is dangerous to play around with hypnosis, so I went to a professional. He hypnotized me and told me I could do it myself—and I did.

Whenever I thought of smoking (many times a day), I'd say, " I do not like to smoke cigarettes. The taste is repugnant." I'd repeat it again in bed before going to sleep, to carry it with me all night.

It took me about three months really to succeed. One morning, I got up and instinctively reached for a cigarette. I lit it and, as I drew on it, I said, "Yuck! This is terrible!" I put it out. That was nearly eight years ago.

You can't hypnotize a person who is unwilling to be hypnotized. You have to want to do it yourself. I really wanted to stop smoking. Since then, I've felt no desire at all. My closest friend smokes like a chimney. I sit and watch her, but it does nothing to move me back to cigarettes. I feel like a million dollars! I'm alert! I feel good!

**Source:** Interview with Hope Bryson, head of Selmore Advertising Agency, Los Angeles.

• In a followup study of 100 smokers who had averaged 1.2 pack a day, 78% were still off cigarettes one year after hypnosis therapy.

**Source:** Harold B. Crasilneck, Ph.D., Dallas, in *Journal of the American Medical Association*, Chicago, IL.

## HELP TO BREAK THE HABIT

SmokeBreak is a smokeless cigarette that uses tobacco- or menthol-flavored wicks to simulate the smell of real cigarettes. It's part of a behavior modification system that satisfies the smoker's desire to put something into his mouth. It also satisfies the taste craving.

**Source:** Apex Medical, Bloomington, MN.

## SECOND-BEST TREATMENT FOR SMOKERS

Two drinks per day may cut a smoker's risk of emphysema by more than 50%, a new study suggests. Whereas 26% of nondrinking smokers had emphysema, only 10% of the smokers who had two drinks daily developed the condition. Obviously, the best preventive treatment is to discontinue smoking, but the second-best treatment for smokers may be to have two drinks (and no more) per day.

**Source:** Philip Pratt, M.D., Durham VA Center, Durham, NC.

## CLOVE-CIGARETTE ALERT

Clove cigarettes, a teenage fad imported from Indonesia, can be dangerous and even fatal. One youth recently died of pneumonia after smoking a clove cigarette (*kretek*) while recovering from the flu. Hundreds of other smokers have complained of getting asthma, nosebleeds and lung infections and of coughing up blood. The suspected hazard: Eugenol, a natural anesthetic that is found in cloves.

**Source:** Frederick Schecter, M.D., a thoracic surgeon at Humana Hospital, West Anaheim, CA.

## WHAT SMOKELESS TOBACCO MANUFACTURERS DON'T TELL YOU

Smokeless tobaccos, such as snuff and chewing tobacco, have not proven to be harmless alternatives to cigarettes. Among heavy users of three years or more, 60% develop mouth lesions. . .and an oral cancer link is strongly suspected. Potential time bomb: It's estimated that 25% of high school and college males are regular users.

**Source:** *Oncology Today* magazine, New York.

## DON'T SMOKE BEFORE YOU HAVE AN OPERATION

Quit smoking at least 12 hours before surgery to reduce the risk of organ damage and complications. Reason: The carbon monoxide produced by smoking combines with the blood's hemoglobin, reducing its capacity to carry oxygen to body tissues. After 12 hours of abstinence, capacity returns to normal.

**Source:** Bruce Yaffe, M.D., a gastroenterologist in private practice in New York.